Dermatological Emergencies

Dermatological Emergencies

Edited by

Biju Vasudevan, MD (Dermatology)

Department of Dermatology, Base Hospital
Lucknow, Uttar Pradesh, India

Rajesh Verma, MD (Dermatology)

Department of Dermatology, Army College of Medical Sciences
New Delhi, India

CRC Press
Taylor & Francis Group
Boca Raton London New York

CRC Press is an imprint of the
Taylor & Francis Group, an **informa** business

CRC Press
Taylor & Francis Group
6000 Broken Sound Parkway NW, Suite 300
Boca Raton, FL 33487-2742

First issued in paperback 2020

© 2019 by Taylor & Francis Group, LLC
CRC Press is an imprint of Taylor & Francis Group, an Informa business

No claim to original U.S. Government works

ISBN-13: 978-0-8153-7807-5 (hbk)
ISBN-13: 978-0-367-77860-6 (pbk)

Contents

Foreword

If dermatology is alluded to as a panoramic canvas with myriad presentations, dermatological emergencies are its epicenter. In the preceding decades, dermatology as a speciality has grown exponentially to transcend heretofore unforeseen frontiers. These advancements are most evident in the spectrum of dermatological emergencies, with the enhanced comprehension of underlying etiopathogenesis and novel investigational modalities, including a well-researched and focused therapeutic armamentarium to address these challenging disease conditions

A dermatology ICU, which was a distant dream in India in the past, was initially established at Armed Forces Medical College and Command Hospital (Southern Command), Pune, and is now an emerging reality in the country. Many acute conditions necessitating advanced care, such as toxic epidermal necrolysis, DRESS, pemphigus, connective tissue disorders, vasculitis, angioedema, staphylococcal scalded skin syndrome, etc., are being managed primarily by the dermatology fraternity in synergy with allied specialists, who provide augmented support. It is widely accepted that dermatologists cogently understand the pathophysiology and clinical status of these conditions, as well as therapeutic approaches. This evolving paradigm implores us to have the requisite preparedness for efficient management of these complex challenges. This book is an earnest endeavor

to facilitate the improved acumen for effective management of dermatology-related emergencies. It also encompasses the various acute conditions in leprosy, sexually transmitted diseases, and dermatosurgery, thus providing a holistic perspective.

Customized treatment and individualized management as per the needs of patients including diseases and comorbidities are a few of the important imperatives. As Sir William Osler remarked, "The good physician treats the disease. The great physician treats the patient who has the disease." Scientific protocols, SOPs, supportive care, counselling, prerequisites of the dermatology ICU, and the training and preparedness of caregivers are equally significant in mitigating these severe conditions.

I am confident that this book, with its unique and informative contents, contextual relevance, cogent articulation, and lucid presentation, will be a quantum value addition to the knowledge, skills, and perspective of postgraduates, practitioners, faculty, and academicians in dermatology, as well as allied specialists and general physicians.

Rajan S. Grewal
MD (Dermatology)
Prof ACMS , New Delhi, and Ex Prof (Armed Forces Medical College and Command Hospital), Pune, India

Preface

Dermatological emergencies are less written about in the medical literature. Dermatology, which is one of the most rapidly growing branches of medical science, is faced with many challenges clinically, diagnostically, and therapeutically when it comes to dermatological emergencies. With this text we attempt to make these emergency conditions more comprehensible for dermatology residents, practitioners, and academicians, as well as for other specialities. This is especially important to those in countries where dermatological emergencies are most prevalent.

This project is meant to help all concerned in diagnosing various dermatological emergencies correctly and early, investigating them appropriately, and treating them to the best of the abilities and facilities available. It also will help postgraduate students to understand the disorders better, aiding in both practical and theoretical preparation for their exams.

Every topic has been chosen keeping in mind the relevance of dermatological emergencies in today's world.

Emergencies in clinical dermatology, venereology, and leprology are included, and cutaneous manifestations of systemic emergencies are also incorporated. Relevant images are provided to highlight the textual matter.

Authors with special expertise in these topics have been handpicked for the various chapters. The section editors have reviewed the chapters and made their contributions to both the text and images.

The text aims to be a benchmark for approaches to dermatological emergencies. The logical flow of the chapters with relevant images and coverage of diagnostic and therapeutic approaches lends a unique format that will help all involved in managing these conditions. We acknowledge and appreciate the efforts of all those who have contributed to this text and hope this text proves to be a valuable resource for all those interested in dermatological emergencies.

Biju Vasudevan
Rajesh Verma

Editors

Biju Vasudevan received his MD (Dermatology, Venereology, and Leprology) degree from Armed Forces Medical College, Pune and FRGUHS (Dermatosurgery) from Bangalore Medical College, India. Presently he is a Professor at Base Hospital Lucknow and is a recognized postgraduate examiner at Maharashtra University of Health Sciences, King George's Medical University, and West Bengal University. He has published 88 indexed publications (14 international) and 30 chapters in various books and is the the chief Editor of the *IADVL Colour Atlas of Dermatology*, *Clinical Correlations in Dermatology*, and *Procedural Dermatosurgery* textbooks. He has been a part of various research projects, has conducted 24 international/national/state level quizzes, is on the editorial board of four journals, and is presently the deputy editor of the *Indian Journal of Dermatology, Venereology, and Leprology*. He has delivered 76 guest lectures and conducted eight workshops at various conferences. He has been the organizing/scientific secretary of seven conferences, served as the past joint secretary of the IADVL, and was awarded the Young Dermatosurgeon Award by the Association of Cutaneous Surgeons (I) in 2018 and LN Sinha Memorial Award in 2019. His interests in dermatology include vasculitis, connective tissue disorders, skin in systemic medicine, and dermatosurgery.

Rajesh Verma received his MD (Dermatology, Venereology, and Leprosy) degree from Armed Forces Medical College, Pune, India, and completed Diplomate National Board (Dermatology and Venereology) and Membership of the National Academy of Medical Sciences qualifications. He is presently serving as a Professor of Dermatology at the Army College of Medical Sciences, previously having served as Professor and Head of the Departments of Dermatology at Armed Forces Medical College, Pune, and Command Hospital, Lucknow. For standing first in MD Dermatology, he was awarded a gold medal by Pune University. He is passionate about teaching Dermatology to undergraduates and postgraduates and has been a guide and recognized postgraduate teacher and examiner at Maharashtra University of Health Science, Rajiv Gandhi University of Health Sciences, King George's Medical University, Lucknow, and various other universities. His awards include Gaurav Sammaan by Uttar Bhartiya Sangh, Pune, for contribution in the field of education in 2013, and Teacher par Excellence by the Indian Association of Dermatology, Venereology, and Leprology (IADVL) in 2014. In 2008 he served as Vice President of the Indian Association for the Study of Sexually Transmitted Diseases and AIDS and in 2014 as Vice President of IADVL. He has contributed 20 chapters in various textbooks, published 70 papers, delivered more than 50 invited lectures, and has been principal worker and coworker in various completed research projects. He has organized national-level CME programs and conferences in dermatology. His interests in dermatology include dermatological emergencies, cutaneous drug reactions, vasculitis, and pregnancy dermatoses.

Contributors

Saniya Akhtar MD (Dermatology)
Registrar
Department of Dermatology
Government Medical College and Associated Hospitals
Srinagar, Jammu and Kashmir, India

K. P. Aneesh MD (Dermatology)
Consultant Dermatologist
Department of Dermatology
Koya's Hospital
Kozhikode, Kerala, India

K. B. Anuradha DNB (Dermatology)
Consultant Dermatologist
Aster Medcity
Kochi, Kerala, India

Sandeep Arora MD (Dermatology)
Professor and HOD
Department of Dermatology
Command Hospital Bangalore
Karnataka, India

Pradeesh Arumugam MBBS Resident (Dermatology)
Department of Dermatology
Base Hospital
Lucknow, Uttar Pradesh, India

Afreen Ayub MBBS Resident (Dermatology)
Department of Dermatology
Base Hospital
Lucknow, Uttar Pradesh, India

Ambresh Badad MD (Dermatology)
Assistant Professor
Department of Dermatology
Mahadevappa Rampure Medical College
Kalaburgi, Karnataka

Anupama Bains MD (Dermatology)
Senior Resident
Department of Dermatology
All India Institutes of Medical Sciences (AIIMS)
Jodhpur, Rajasthan, India

Santanu Banerjee MD (Dermatology)
Associate Professor
Department of Dermatology
Military Hospital
Secunderabad, Andhra Pradesh, India

Safiya Bashir MD
Senior Resident
Department of Dermatology
Venereology and Leprology
Government Medical College
Srinagar, Jammu and Kashmir, India

Sukriti Baveja MD (Dermatology)
Professor and HOD
Department of Dermatology
Command Hospital
Pune, Maharashtra, India

N. S. Beniwal MD (Dermatology)
Department of Dermatology
MH Kirkee
Pune, Maharashtra, India

Neetu Bhari MD (Dermatology)
Assistant Professor
Department of Dermatology and
Venereology
All India Institute of Medical Sciences
New Delhi, India

Ramesh Bhat MD (Dermatology)
Professor
Department of Dermatology
Father Muller Medical College Hospital
Kankanady, Mangalore, India

Yasmeen Jabeen Bhat MD (Dermatology)
Assistant Professor
Department of Dermatology
Government Medical College
Srinagar, Jammu and Kashmir, India

Riti Bhatia MD (Dermatology)
Assistant Professor
Dermatology and Venereology
AIIMS Rishikesh
Uttar Pradesh, India

Ruby Bhatia MD (Gynae and Obs)
Associate Professor
Department of Obstetrics and Gynecology
Government Medical College
Patiala, Punjab, India

Anuj Bhatnagar MD (Dermatology)
Assistant Professor
Military Hospital
Dehradun, Uttar Pradesh, India

O. Biby Chacko DM (Cardiology)
Consultant Cardiologist
Muthoot Medical Centre
Pathanamthitta, Kerala, India

Manas Chatterjee MD (Dermatology)
Professor and HOD
Department of Dermatology
INHS Asvini
Mumbai, India

Rajesh Chilaka MBBS Resident (Gen Medicine)
Army Hospital Research And Referral
Delhi Cantonment, New Delhi, India

Ajay Chopra MD (Dermatology)
Professor and HOD
Department of Dermatology
Base Hospital
Delhi Cantonment, New Delhi, India

Rajeshwari Dabas MD (Dermatology)
Associate Professor
Department of Dermatology
Command Hospital
Bangalore, Karnataka, India

Anupam Das MD (Dermatology)
Assistant Professor
Department of Dermatology
KPC Medical College and Hospital
Kolkata, West Bengal, India

Mahashweta Das MBBS Resident (Dermatology)
Department of Dermatology
Base Hospital
Lucknow, Uttar Pradesh, India

Pankaj Das MD (Dermatology)
Department of Dermatology
Armed Forces Medical College (AFMC)
Pune, Maharashtra, India

Dipankar De MD (Dermatology)
Additional Professor
Department of Dermatology
Post Graduate Institute of Medical Education and
Research (PGIMER)
Chandigarh, India

Rasya Dixit MD (Dermatology)
Consultant Dermatologist
Dr Dixit Cosmetic Dermatology Clinic
Bengaluru, Karnataka, India

A. P. Dubey DNB (Medical Oncology)
Consultant Oncologist
Department of Oncology
New Delhi, India

Renu George MD (Dermatology)
Professor
Department of Dermatology
Christian Medical College and Hospital
Vellore, Tamil Nadu, India

Vinay Gera MD (Dermatology)
Assistant Professor
Department of Dermatology
Base Hospital
Lucknow, Uttar Pradesh, India

Kunal Ghosh MCh (GI Surgery)
Consultant GI Surgeon
Base Hospital
Delhi Cantonment, New Delhi, India

Rajan Singh Grewal MD (Dermatology)
Professor
Army College of Medical Sciences
Delhi Cantonment, New Delhi, India

Ankan Gupta MD (Dermatology)
Assistant Professor
Department of Dermatology
Christian Medical College and Hospital
Vellore, Tamil Nadu, India

Vishal Gupta MD (Dermatology)
Assistant Professor
Department of Dermatology
All India Institute of Medical Sciences
New Delhi, India

Sanjeev Handa MD (Dermatology)
Professor
Department of Dermatology
Post Graduate Institute of Medical Education and
Research (PGIMER)
Chandigarh, India

Sushila Hansda MD (Dermatology)
Senior Resident
Indira Gandhi Institute of Medical Sciences
Patna, Bihar, India

Neirita Hazarika MD (Dermatology)
Assistant Professor
Dermatology and Venereology
AIIMS Rishikesh
Uttar Pradesh, India

Arun Hegde MD (Medicine), DNB (Rheumatology)
Assistant Professor
Command Hospital
Pune, Maharashtra, India

Ruchi Hemdani MBBS Resident (Dermatology)
Department of Dermatology
INHS Asvini
Mumbai, India

Manjunath Hulmani MD (Dermatology)
Associate Professor
Department of Dermatology
SSIMS and RC
Davangere, Karnataka, India

Arun C. Inamadar MD (Dermatology)
Professor and Head
Department of Dermatology
Shri B.M. Patil Medical College
Hospital and Research Center
BLDE University
Bijapur, Karnataka, India

Soumya Jagadeeshan MD (Dermatology)
Assistant professor
Department of Dermatology
Amrita Institute of Medical Sciences
Kochi, Kerala, India

Sridhar Jandyala MD (Dermatology)
Department of Dermatology
INHS Asvini
Mumbai, India

Manasa Shettisara Janney MD Resident (Dermatology)
Department of Dermatology
Command Hospital
Bangalore, Karnataka, India

Nidhi Kaeley MD (Medicine)
Assistant Professor
Department of Emergency Medicine
All India Institute of Medical Sciences
Rishikesh, India

Divya Kamat MD (Dermatology)
Senior Resident
Department of Dermatology
PGIMER
Chandigarh, India

Rajan Kapoor DM (Clinical Hematology)
Hematologist and Hemato-Oncologist
Army Hospital (R and R)
New Delhi, India

Subuhi Kaul MD (Dermatology)
Senior Resident
Department of Dermatology
All India Institute of Medical Sciences
New Delhi, India

Sujay Khandpur MD (Dermatology)
Professor
Department of Dermatology
All India Institute of Medical Sciences
New Delhi, India

Vidya Kharkar MD (Dermatology)
Professor
Department of Dermatology
Seth GS Medical College and KEM Hospital
Mumbai, India

Piyush Kumar MD (Dermatology)
Associate Professor
Katihar Medical College
Bihar, India

Sheetanshu Kumar MD (Dermatology)
Senior Resident
Department of Dermatology
Post Graduate Institute of Medical Education and
Research (PGIMER)
Chandigarh, India

M. Kumaresan MD (Dermatology)
Professor
PSG Hospitals
Coimbatore, Tamil Nadu, India

M. R. Kusuma MD (Dermatology)
Consult Dermatologist and Dermatosurgeon
Cutis Academy
Bangalore, Karnataka, India

Radha Ramesh Lachhiramani MSc (Diploma in Clinical Dermatology, Cardiff University, United Kingdom)
Consulting Dermatologist
Imperial Healthcare Institute
Dubai

D. V. Lakshmi DVD (Dermatology)
Consultant Dermatologist
Bangalore, Karnataka, India

Niharika Ranjan Lal MD (Dermatology)
Assistant Professor
Department of Dermatology
ESI-PGIMSR and ESIC Medical College
Joka, Kolkatta, West Bengal, India

Sandeep Lal MD (Dermatology)
Resident
Department of Dermatology
Command Hospital
Bangalore, Karnataka, India

R. Madhu MD (Dermatology)
Senior Assistant Professor
Department of Dermatology (Mycology)
Madras Medical College
Chennai, Tamil Nadu, India

C. Madura MD (Dermatology)
Consultant Dermatologist
Dermatosurgeon Cutis Academy
Bangalore, Karnataka, India

S. Yogesh Marfatia MD (Dermatology)
Professor and Head
Department of Dermatology
Medical College Baroda
Gujarat, India

Madhulika Mhatre MD (Dermatology)
Assistant Professor
Lokmanya Tilak Municipal Medical College and Hospital
Sion, Mumbai, India

Debdeep Mitra MD (Dermatology)
Assistant Professor
Department of Dermatology
Base Hospital
Delhi Cantonment, New Delhi, India

Rashmi Modak DDVL (Dermatology)
Consultant Dermatologist
Ra'Derm Clinic
Mulund, Mumbai, India

Anuradha Monga BDS MBA (Healthcare Administration)
Health Care Consultant
New Delhi, India

Swetha Mukherjee MD (Pediatrics)
Assistant Professor
Department of Pediatrics
Command Hospital
Pune, Maharashtra, India

Aswin M. Nair MD (Dermatology)
Assistant Professor
Department of Dermatology
Christian Medical College and Hospital
Vellore, Tamil Nadu, India

Tarun Narang MD (Dermatology)
Assistant Professor
Department of Dermatology
Post Graduate Institute of Medical Education and Research (PGIMER)
Chandigarh, India

Shekhar Neema MD (Dermatology)
Associate Professor
Department of Dermatology
Armed Forces Medical College (AFMC)
Pune, Maharashtra, India

B. Nirmal BMD (Dermatology)
Associate Professor
Department of Dermatology
Velammal medical college and research institute
Madurai, Tamil Nadu, India

Tanmay Padhi MD (Dermatology)
Assistant Professor
Department of Dermatology
Medical College
Sambalpur, Odisha, India

Aparna Palit MD (Dermatology)
Professor and Head
Department of Dermatology
All India Institute of Medical Sciences (AIIMS)
Bhubaneswar, Odisha, India

V. Hari Pankaj PhD (Cutaneous Mycoses)
Associate Professor
Mycology Division
Department of Microbiology
Bhaskar Medical College and General Hospital
Hyderabad, Telangana, India

Vikas Pathania MD (Dermatology)
Assistant Professor
Department of Dermatology
Command Hospital
Pune, Maharashtra, India

Manoj Pawar MD (Dermatology)
Assistant Professor
Department of Dermatology
Dr Vasantrao Pawar Medical College
Nasik, Maharashtra, India

Indrashis Podder MD (Dermatology)
RMO cum Clinical Tutor
Department of Dermatology
Calcutta Medical School and District Hospital
Kolkata, West Bengal, India

B. R. Harish Prasad MD (Dermatology)
Consultant Dermatosurgeon
Vitals Klinic, Bangalore
Karnataka, India

K. Leksmi Priya MD (Dermatology)
Assistant Professor
Department of Dermatology
Base Hospital
Lucknow, Uttar Pradesh, India

Deep Kumar Raman MD (Pathology)
Professor and HOD
Department of Pathology
Command Hospital
Lucknow, Uttar Pradesh, India

Raghavendra Rao MD (Dermatology)
Additional Professor
Department of Dermatology
Kasturba Medical College
Manipal University
Manipal, Karnataka, India

Meryl Sonia Rebello MD (Dermatology)
Senior Resident
Father Muller Medical College
Mangalore, Karnataka, India

Tanumay Roychowdhury MD (Dermatology)
Consultant
Tata Medical Centre
Kolkatta, West Bengal, India

Sunmeet Sandhu MBBS Resident (Dermatology)
Department of Dermatology
Armed Forces Medical College (AFMC)
Pune, Maharashtra, India

Neerja Saraswat MD (Dermatology)
Assistant Professor
Department of Dermatology
Base Hospital
Delhi Cantonment, New Delhi, India

Nilendu Sarma MD (Dermatology)
Associate Professor and Head
Department of Dermatology
Dr B C Roy Post Graduate Institute of
Pediatric Science
Kolkata, West Bengal, India

Suneel Singh Senger MD (Dermatology)
Assistant Professor
Department of Dermatology
Index Medical College and Hospital Research Centre
Indore, Madhya Pradesh, India

Mitanjali Sethy MD (Dermatology)
Department of Dermatology
Kalinga Institute of Medical Sciences
Bhubhaneshwar, Odisha, India

Iffat Hassan Shah MD (Dermatology)
Professor and HOD
Department of Dermatology
Government Medical College and Associated Hospitals
Srinagar, Jammu and Kashmir, India

J. Ruchi Shah MBBS Resident (Dermatology)
Department of Dermatology
Medical College Baroda
Gujarat, India

Aseem Sharma MD (Dermatology)
Assistant Professor
Lokmanya Tilak Municipal Medical College and Hospital
Sion, Mumbai, India

G. K. Singh MD (Dermatology)
Assistant Professor
Department of Dermatology
MH Kirkee
Pune, Maharashtra, India

Jatinder Singh MD (Dermatology)
Department of Dermatology
Military Hospital
Ambala, Punjab, India

Sanjay Singh MD (Dermatology)
Department of Dermatology
All India Institutes of Medical Sciences (AIIMS)
New Delhi, India

Saurabh Singh MD (Dermatology)
Assistant Professor
Department of Dermatology
All India Institutes of Medical Sciences (AIIMS)
Jodhpur, Rajasthan, India

Anwita Sinha MBBS Resident (Dermatology)
Department of Dermatology
Armed Forces Medical College (AFMC)
Pune, Maharashtra, India

Asmita Sinha MBBS Resident (Dermatology)
Department of Dermatology
Base Hospital
Lucknow, Uttar Pradesh, India

Preema Sinha MD (Dermatology)
Associate Professor
Department of Dermatology
Armed Forces Medical College (AFMC)
Pune, Maharashtra, India

Vishal Sondhi MD (Paediatrics), DM (Pediatric Neurology)
Department of Pediatrics
Armed Forces Medical College (AFMC)
Pune, Maharashtra, India

Aradhana Sood MD (Dermatology)
Professor and HOD
Department of Dermatology
Base Hospital Lucknow
Lucknow, Uttar Pradesh, India

N. Srilakshmi MBBS Resident (Dermatology)
Department of Dermatology
SSIMS and RC
Davangere, Karnataka, India

Sahana M. Srinivas DNB, DVD (Dermatology)
Consultant Pediatric Dermatologist
Indira Gandhi Institute of Child Health Bangalore
Bangalore, Karnataka, India

Radhakrishnan Subramanian MD (Dermatology)
Department of Dermatology
Armed Forces Medical College (AFMC)
Pune, Maharashtra, India

M. R. L. Sujata MD (Dermatology)
Consultant Dermatologist
Mumbai, India

Anup Kumar Tiwary MD (Dermatology)
Consultant Dermatologist
New Delhi, India

S. S. Vaishampayan MD (Dermatology)
Professor and Head of Department
Department of Dermatology
Index Medical College and Hospital Research Centre
Indore, Madhya Pradesh, India

Resham Vasani MD (Dermatology)
Assistant Professor
K J Somaiya Medical College
Sion, Mumbai, India

Biju Vasudevan MD (Dermatology)
Professor Department of Dermatology
Base Hospital
Lucknow, Uttar Pradesh, India

Ruby Venugopal MD (Dermatology)
Department of Dermatology
Command Hospital
Pune, Maharashtra, India

Rajesh Verma MD (Dermatology)
Professor
Department of Dermatology
Army College of Medical Sciences
Delhi Cantonment, New Delhi, India

P. Vijendran MD (Dermatology)
Consultant Dermatologist
Apollo Hospitals and RT Skin Clinic
Bangalore, Karnataka, India

Vishalakshi Viswanath MD (Dermatology)
Professor and Head
Department of Dermatology
Rajiv Gandhi Medical College
Thane, Maharashtra, India

Vijay Zawar MD (Dermatology)
Professor
Department of Dermatology
Dr Vasantrao Pawar Medical College
Nasik, Maharashtra, India

PART 1

Introduction to Dermatological Emergencies

ANKAN GUPTA

Dermatological emergencies: What the term encompasses and key features in their diagnosis

INDRASHIS PODDER AND BIJU VASUDEVAN

BACKGROUND

Dermatology has traditionally been considered to be an outpatient-centered specialty, with very few emergencies and lethal conditions; so the term *dermatological emergencies* may seem like an oxymoron. However, there are several life-threatening dermatological conditions that may become lethal in about 8% of cases, unless adequate emergency care (prompt management and monitoring in the intensive care unit) is provided, contrary to popular belief [1]. Although dermatologists may encounter several such conditions in their career, proper awareness of them is still lacking in many parts of the world.

Recently, most of these conditions have been incorporated under the broad term *acute skin failure*, where there is extensive structural disruption and total functional impairment of the skin [2,3]. Acute skin failure is an acute emergency characterized by aberration of thermoregulation, fluid electrolyte imbalance, loss of proteins resulting in malnutrition, and failure of the mechanical barrier to prevent entry of infective organisms and other foreign materials. Thus, prompt diagnosis and emergency intervention are needed to revive the patient. Although this condition is as severe as other organ dysfunctions, viz. cardiac, renal, pulmonary, or hepatic failure, this condition is still not well known, and the need for intensive care in dermatology is often overlooked. This entity is discussed in detail in a separate chapter. The aim of the current chapter is to provide a brief introduction to these different dermatological emergencies.

ETIOLOGY

Several conditions may present as dermatological emergencies in both the pediatric (including neonates) and adult populations, which may pose diagnostic and therapeutic challenges. These conditions encompass both primary cutaneous disorders and dermatological manifestations of severe systemic disorders. Some of the important etiologies have been tabulated in Tables 1.1 and 1.2 [3–5].

ETIOLOGY BASED ON CLINICAL PRESENTATION

Although dermatological emergencies have been classified according to the underlying cutaneous/systemic disorder, often such a diagnosis becomes difficult in the emergency. So we have provided a set of conditions that may lead to dermatological emergencies, based on their clinical presentation. Skin rash is the most common presentation in the dermatology emergency, with or without fever. We have highlighted several causes based on the characteristic of skin rash (Table 1.3) [6,7].

APPROACH TO DIAGNOSIS

Whenever a patient presents to the dermatological emergency, prompt diagnosis and early management should be our aim to reduce morbidity and mortality. Like all other diseases, this process involves adequate history and physical examination to arrive at the correct diagnosis.

History

A detailed history regarding the nature of rash and other key aspects is of paramount importance to arrive at the accurate diagnosis. However, the first priority is to assess whether the patient is seriously ill and needs immediate management or is relatively stable to provide history. Some important points

Table 1.1 Causes of neonatal and pediatric dermatological emergencies

Disorders that can manifest as emergencies

A. Neonatal erythroderma
  - Ichthyosiform erythrodermas (bullous/nonbullous/lamellar/X-linked/harlequin)
  - Collodion baby
  - Netherton syndrome
  - Immunodeficiency disorders (Omenn syndrome, graft versus host disease, severe combined immunodeficiency disorder)
  - Papulosquamous disorders (congenital erythrodermic psoriasis)
  - Drug induced (vancomycin, ceftriaxone)
  - Others (diffuse cutaneous mastocytosis, Leiner disease)
B. Neonatal cutaneous infections
  - Bacterial (staphylococcal scalded skin syndrome, necrotizing fasciitis)
  - Viral (neonatal varicella, neonatal herpes infection)
  - Fungal (congenital/neonatal candidiasis)
C. Vesiculobullous disorders (epidermolysis bullosa, pemphigus)
D. Metabolic disorders (biotin deficiency, essential fatty acid deficiency)
E. Vascular complications (Kasabach-Merritt phenomenon)
F. Others
  Purpura fulminans
  Kawasaki disease
  Sclerema neonatorum

Table 1.2 Causes of dermatological emergencies in adults

1. Erythroderma (idiopathic, dermatitis [atopic/seborrheic], psoriasis, pityriasis rubra pilaris, drug induced, other keratinization disorders, Sézary syndrome)
2. Drug reactions (Stevens-Johnson syndrome, toxic epidermal necrolysis, drug hypersensitivity syndrome)
3. Acute generalized pustular psoriasis
4. Immunobullous disorders (pemphigus vulgaris and foliaceus)
5. Infections (staphylococcal scalded skin syndrome, febrile viral exanthemas)
6. Emergencies where systemic involvement is seen in association with dermatological manifestations
   i. Connective tissue disorders
   ii. Vasculitis
   iii. Malignancies
7. Emergencies related to dermatosurgery:
   i. Anaphylaxis (adverse reactions to intravenous antibiotics, local anesthetics, and other allergens like latex rubber)
   ii. Syncope—vasovagal
   iii. Lignocaine-related emergencies like syncope, anaphylaxis, bleeding, cardiac arrhythmias, etc.
   iv. Bleeding
   v. Acute stroke, status epilepticus, cardiac arrest in the operating room
   vi. Hypotension
   vii. Hypoxia
8. Emergencies related to Hansen's disease or leprosy
   i. Type 1 reaction that can be upgrading/downgrading type
   ii. Type 2 reaction—multisystem involvement along with skin lesions called erythema nodosum leprosum
   iii. Lucio phenomenon
9. Sexually transmitted diseases associated emergencies

Table 1.3 Nature of skin rash and possible dermatological emergency

Nature of skin rash	Possible dermatological emergency
• Erythrodermic (redness with scaling >90% body surface area)	Causes listed in Tables 1.1 and 1.2
• Maculopapular	Viral exanthem (may be associated with hemorrhagic features and shock as exemplified by dengue hemorrhagic fever and dengue shock syndrome, respectively, to form a dermatological emergency)
• Purpuric/petechial	Vasculitides, purpura fulminans/disseminated intravascular coagulation, Rocky Mountain spotted fever, meningococcemia, scarlet fever
• Pustular	Disseminated candidiasis, pustular psoriasis, acute generalized exanthematous pustulosis
• Vesiculobullous	Neonatal herpes simplex, pemphigus, bullous pemphigoid, herpes zoster
• Hemorrhagic/erythematous	Vasculitis, Kawasaki disease, erythema multiforme, Stevens-Johnson syndrome, toxic epidermal necrolysis

Table 1.4 Important elements of history for acute dermatological emergencies

- Mode of onset—acute onset or acute exacerbation of a chronic disorder
- Distribution/spread—localized (zoster, vasculitides)/ generalized (varicella, staphylococcal scalded skin syndrome, erythroderma)
- Site of onset
- Family/contact history—to rule out contagious diseases
- Travel history—to exclude endemic conditions, e.g., Rocky Mountain spotted fever
- Animal exposure
- Drug history—to rule out drug reactions, e.g., erythroderma
- Any history of allergy (drug/chemical)
- Occupational history
- Vaccination status
- Sexual history
- Any exacerbating/relieving factor, e.g., climate, chemicals, etc.
- Associated symptom—fever/itching or pain

need to be evaluated during this process as given in Table 1.4. Though a detailed history is necessary, some facets may be curtailed depending on the situation and dermatologist's experience.

Physical examination

Physical examination should follow history taking in order to narrow down the list of differentials, involving general, dermatological, and systemic evaluation. A few aspects of general and systemic examination should be undertaken in all cases:

- Pallor, cyanosis, jaundice, edema, clubbing, lymph nodes, and vitals should be checked thoroughly to rule out any systemic disease or life-threatening condition like sepsis or anaphylaxis.
- If any systemic disorder is suspected, specific attention should be paid to some conditions:
  - Any murmur, particularly new onset
  - Generalized lymphadenopathy
  - Hepatosplenomegaly
  - Arthritis
  - Oral, conjunctival, or genital lesions
  - Any sign of neurological dysfunction like meningeal irritation

Dermatological examination

A proper dermatological examination is mandatory to arrive at the correct clinical diagnosis and initiate appropriate management at the earliest opportunity. Some

important points need to be kept in mind during cutaneous examination:

- Dermatological examination involves checking the hair, skin, nails, and mucosae (oral, genital, ocular) apart from skin.
- Examination should be performed from head to toe after undressing the patient, in adequate illumination to appreciate any subtle color/textural change of the skin.
- Any cream/makeup should be removed, which may obscure the true nature of the lesion.
- Inspection and palpation are the components of cutaneous examination. A magnifying glass may be used if clarity is needed. An overall inspection of skin lesion/ rash is necessary, as many skin diseases can be diagnosed by their characteristic appearance or morphology of the lesions [8].
- The entire lesion should be palpated with a gloved finger to assess its texture and detect any blanching or bleeding under pressure.

A focused approach is needed regarding the dermatological examination, to save time and arrive at the correct diagnosis promptly. We look out for the types of skin lesions and their other aspects during cutaneous examination.

TYPE OF SKIN LESION

Skin lesions can be broadly categorized into two types: primary and secondary. Primary lesions are basic physical changes in the skin that are caused directly by the disease itself, while these lesions mature over time to give rise to secondary changes. Primary and secondary skin lesions are presented in Tables 1.5 and 1.6.

OTHER IMPORTANT ASPECTS OF SKIN LESIONS

After determining the nature of a skin lesion (primary/ secondary), we need to evaluate the other aspects of these lesions, such as morphology, color, arrangement, distribution, extent, and evolutionary changes, to obtain further clues regarding the disease.

Investigations

Investigations form an essential part of patient evaluation, as they help us to confirm the suspected diagnoses. They can be categorized under two heads:

- Bedside diagnostic procedures
- Laboratory investigations

BEDSIDE DIAGNOSTIC PROCEDURES

Some simple bedside diagnostic procedures may be performed to diagnose and differentiate different skin problems at the first instance [7]:

- *Diascopy*: Diascopy is a technique in which a glass slide is pressed firmly against the lesion to exert pressure on the lesion. It is primarily used to distinguish

Table 1.5 Primary skin lesions

Name of lesion	Characteristic feature
Macule	Circumscribed area of color change, flat lesion; <0.5 cm in diameter
Patch	Circumscribed area of color change, flat lesion; ≥0.5 cm in diameter
Papule	Solid, circumscribed raised skin lesion, diameter <0.5 cm; many additional features have been described like domed, flat-topped, umbilicated
Plaque	Solid, raised plateau-shaped skin lesion, ≥0.5 cm in diameter
Nodule	Raised solid lesion with deeper infiltration (height more than width)
Tumour	Skin swelling >2 cm in diameter
Vesicle	Well-circumscribed, clear fluid–filled lesion <0.5 cm in diameter
Bullae	Well-circumscribed, clear fluid–filled lesion ≥0.5 cm in diameter
Pustule	Circumscribed, elevated lesions containing pus; are commonly infected (as in folliculitis) but may be sterile (pustular psoriasis)
Wheal	Edema of skin, evanescent lesions

Table 1.6 Secondary skin lesions

Name of lesion	Characteristic feature
Erosion	Total or partial loss of epidermis; does not heal with scarring
Ulcer	Total loss of epidermis with or without dermal involvement, heals with scarring
Excoriation	Scratch marks, may result in erosions/ulcers
Fissures	Crevices in skin that may extend upto the dermis
Scale	Flakes of dead and dry skin
Crust	Dried-up purulent material, blood, or other exudate
Atrophy	Loss or thinning of epidermis, dermis, or subcutaneous tissues; skin appears white, papery, and translucent with loss of surface markings
Pigmentation	Hypo- or hyperpigmentation that may occur as part of disease process or after healing (post inflammatory)
Striae	Linear, atrophic lesions due to degeneration of connective tissue that may appear pink/red depending on stage; common site of topical corticosteroid abuse

hemorrhagic and inflammatory lesions. While inflammatory lesions blanch with pressure (e.g., erythema), hemorrhagic lesions remain nonblanchable (petechiae or purpura).

- *Nikolsky sign*: This sign refers to sloughing and erosion of skin when a shearing force is applied on normal skin in the perilesional area. This sign is positive in superficial blistering diseases like pemphigus, toxic epidermal necrolysis, and staphylococcal scalded skin syndrome (SSSS). It may be seen in severe cases of erythema multiforme, epidermolysis bullosa, pemphigoid, and variegate porphyria.
- *Bulla spread sign*: This is helpful in bullous disorders and confirms the location as epidermal like in pemphigus.
- *Grattage and Auspitz sign*: Taking out scales leads to positive grattage, while pinpoint bleeding after further scratching leads to the Auspitz sign, which is characteristic of psoriasis.
- *Dermatographism*: This sign refers to exaggeration of the physiologic triple response of Lewis (whealing tendency) on application of pressure. This is the hallmark of physical urticaria.
- *Wood lamp*: This is a useful clinical screening tool for several conditions like porphyria. It is an ultraviolet lamp with wavelength of 360–365 nm.
- *Dermoscopy*: Dermoscopy is a relatively new diagnostic maneuver often helping in the bedside diagnosis of several dermatological conditions, such as melanoma (atypical pigment network and vessels, blue-white veil, regression structures, irregular streaks, eccentric homogeneous pigmentation, and asymmetrical pigmented globules) and nonmelanoma skin cancers, such as squamous cell carcinoma (central yellow keratinous plugs with arborizing vessels centrally and hairpin vessels peripherally) and basal cell carcinoma (multiple blue-gray dots, globules and ovoid nests, leaf-like areas, arborizing vessels, erythema, erosions, and ulceration) [9]. These malignancies need a hasty diagnosis to avoid complications including metastasis and lethality.
- Swabs may be taken from discharge/ulceration for microbiological examination.
- Gram staining is a vital tool to detect and classify bacterial infections.
- Skin scrapings and microscopy may be done to confirm fungal infections (potassium hydroxide exam [KOH test]) or ectoparasite infestations such as scabies.
- Tzanck smear may be done if viral infection (herpes, varicella) or bullous disorder is suspected.

LABORATORY INVESTIGATIONS

Laboratory investigations include venereal disease research laboratory (VDRL), rapid plasma reagin (RPR), enzyme-linked immunosorbent assay (ELISA) for HIV, antinuclear antibody (ANA), and other such investigations to confirm the various clinical diagnoses.

Differential diagnoses

When a patient presents to the dermatological emergency with skin rash, a plethora of differential diagnoses need to be considered. It is often a challenge for the emergency physician to differentiate benign skin disorders from the more serious, fatal conditions that require immediate intervention.

The authors classified five major types of skin rash that may be encountered in the emergency: (1) maculopapular, (2) erythematous, (3) petechial/purpuric, (4) pustular, and (5) vesiculobullous.

All of these varieties of rash have been discussed briefly along with the major differentials and possible diagnostic workup based on clinical presentation. After a suspected diagnosis has been made, efforts should be made to confirm the same (tests discussed above) and then stabilize the patient.

MACULOPAPULAR RASH

Maculopapular rash is the most common type of skin rash, which can be differentiated based on its distribution and systemic features as given in Table 1.7 [7].

ERYTHEMATOUS RASH

An erythematous rash is characterized by diffuse redness of the skin due to capillary congestion. Some of the differentials are not immediately life-threatening, like SSSS, while others like toxic shock syndrome, anaphylaxis, and certain drug reactions are potentially lethal and demand immediate intervention. Such a rash may have the following differential diagnoses in the emergency setup:

- *With fever*: SSSS, toxic shock syndrome, scarlet fever
- *Without fever*: Anaphylaxis, alcohol flush

- *History of intake of certain drugs*: Stevens-Johnson syndrome, toxic epidermal necrolysis

PETECHIAL/PURPURIC RASH

Petechiae/purpura refer to extravasation of blood into the skin/mucosae; thus, lesions are non blanchable. Further, purpura may be classified into palpable/non palpable. The presence of concomitant fever/systemic toxicity suggests a sinister diagnosis and requires hasty intervention. A suggested approach to petechial/purpuric rash is as follows:

- *Palpable lesions*: With fever—meningococcemia, Henoch–Schönlein purpura. Without fever—cutaneous small vessel vasculitis.
- *Non palpable lesions*: With fever—purpura fulminans/disseminated intravascular coagulation. Without fever—thrombocytopenic conditions such as idiopathic thrombocytopenic purpura (flat, subcutaneous hemorrhages).

PUSTULAR RASH

Pustules are well-circumscribed pus-filled lesions on the skin surface. They can be either infective or noninfective in origin, characterized by the presence or absence of fever, respectively. The morphology is also important to arrive at the correct diagnosis as follows:

- Pustular lesions with fever, suspect infective origin such as impetigo, folliculitis
- Pustular lesions without fever (sterile pustules)
  - Coalescing pustules to form lakes of pus—pustular psoriasis
  - Noncoalescing discreet pustules—acute generalized exanthematous pustulosis (corroborative drug history may be obtained in almost 90% of cases)

VESICULOBULLOUS RASH

Vesiculobullous rash is characterized by the appearance of vesicles and bullae (Table 1.8). These rashes are a source of concern for both the patients and their physicians. However, a simplified diagnostic approach has been given based on its distribution and the presence or absence of fever.

Table 1.7 Differential diagnoses of maculopapular rash

Features of rash	Possible diagnosis
Centrally distributed rash with systemic toxicity	Viral exanthema Lyme disease Typhus fever
Centrally distributed rash without systemic toxicity	Cutaneous adverse drug reaction (history of drug intake positive)
Peripherally distributed rash with systemic toxicity	Secondary syphilis Meningococcemia Rocky Mountain spotted fever Erythema multiforme Stevens-Johnson syndrome (early)
Peripherally distributed rash without systemic toxicity	Scabies Eczema Psoriasis

Table 1.8 Differential diagnosis of vesiculobullous lesions

Generalized distribution	Localized distribution
• With fever—varicella/chickenpox, purpura fulminans/disseminated intravascular coagulation • Without fever—pemphigus vulgaris, bullous pemphigoid	• With fever—hand, foot, and mouth disease; necrotizing fasciitis • Without fever—contact dermatitis, herpes zoster, insect bite hypersensitivity

Management

The management of these conditions is discussed in subsequent chapters. A basic framework is provided that needs to be initiated at the earliest time [7]:

- Some conditions require the patient's immediate admission to the intensive care unit and emergency treatment, e.g., causes of acute skin failure (Table 1.2).
- Few conditions need observation in the emergency department for at least 24 hours before deciding the future course of treatment, such as anaphylaxis and acute urticaria.
- Patients with most of the other conditions can be provided emergency resuscitation and advised to seek treatment in the outpatient department on the following day.

Following are a few vital points that should never be missed while evaluating any dermatological patient in the emergency department:

- One should always examine the mucosae, including the genitalia and eyes, in these patients to rule out certain conditions like Stevens-Johnson syndrome and toxic epidermal necrolysis. Ophthalmologic opinion must be sought in these patients.
- Patients with extensive skin desquamation and blistering should be admitted to a burns unit/intensive care unit setup for proper management.
- Patients presenting with anaphylaxis should be resuscitated immediately (airway, breathing, circulation). Epinephrine is needed for hemodynamic support.
- The presence of systemic involvement (fever, renal dysfunction, neurological dysfunction, severe arthralgia/arthritis, respiratory distress, etc.) suggests a life-threatening condition and must be dealt with adequately.

CONCLUSION

Dermatological emergencies are being given their due only in recent times. Acute skin failure forms a major portion of these emergencies. Proper history taking, understanding the morphology of the presenting skin lesions, looking for associated systemic features, and investigating appropriately will pave the way for managing these conditions in the right manner.

KEY POINTS

- Dermatological emergencies are not uncommon
- Recognizing them early is the key to efficient management
- Identifying the type of rash, good history taking and examination is key to management
- Appropriate investigations are adjuvants to successful therapy

REFERENCES

1. Chowdhury S, Podder I, Saha A, Bandyopadhyay D. Inpatient mortality resulting from dermatological disorders at a tertiary care center in Eastern India: A record-based observational study. *Indian J Dermatol* 2017;62:626.
2. Inamadar AC, Palit A. Acute skin failure: Concept, causes, consequences and care. *Indian J Dermatol Venereol Leprol* 2005;71:379–85.
3. Samudrala S, Dandakeri S, Bhat RM. Clinical profile of dermatological emergencies and intensive care unit admissions in a tertiary care center—An Indian perspective. *Int J Dermatol* 2018;57:575–9.
4. Inamadar AC. Neonatal dermatological emergencies. *Indian J Dermatol Venereol Leprol* 2010;76:328–40.
5. Chakravarthy M. Management of dermatosurgical emergencies. In: Venkatraman M (Ed.). *ACSI Textbook of Cutaneous and Aesthetic Surgery*. 2nd ed. New Delhi: Jaypee Brothers Medical Publishers; 2017;236–42.
6. Chacon AH. Dermatologic emergencies. *Cutis* 2015;95:E28–31.
7. Senthilkumaran S. Dermatological emergencies. In: David SS (Ed.), *Clinical Pathways in Emergency Medicine*. Volume 1. India: Springer; 2016:437–56.
8. Gropper CA. An approach to clinical dermatologic diagnosis based on morphologic reactionpatterns. *Clin Cornerstone* 2001;4:1–4.
9. Bowling J. *Diagnostic Dermoscopy: The Illustrated Guide*. Oxford, UK: Wiley Blackwell; 2012:35–81.

2

Acute skin failure

S. S. VAISHAMPAYAN, SUNEEL SINGH SENGER, RADHA RAMESH LACHHIRAMANI,
AND ANKAN GUPTA

INTRODUCTION

Acute skin failure (ASF) is defined as disruption of the cutaneous integrity and loss of function of the skin that can lead to multiorgan failure and needs specialized care [1]. Loss of function includes barrier function, thermoregulatory function, and loss of proteins, water, and electrolytes. A large number of dermatological conditions and therapeutic interventions, especially drugs, can lead to this outcome. This concept is relatively new, and there is very little literature dealing with this subject. We discuss the management of ASF based on pathophysiology and practical knowledge gathered over the past 25–30 years of dermatological practice.

EVOLUTION OF THE CONCEPT

Sam Shuster from Newcastle, United Kingdom, in 1967 delivered the "Parkes Weber Lecture" at the Royal College of Physicians of London on "Systemic effect of skin disease." He became the first dermatologist to relate disturbed thermoregulation, anemia, hypoalbuminemia, and hemodynamic disturbances to the condition called erythroderma [2]. His pioneering work on systemic effects of skin diseases is the basis for the concept of skin failure. Rene Touraine from Lyon Sud University Hospital, France, first established an intensive care unit (ICU) in a skin department in 1974 [3]. Catriona Irvine in 1991 defined skin failure as a distinct entity that is comparable to any other major organ dysfunction [4]. Jean-Claude Roujeau of Paris mentioned the term *acute skin failure* in a paper to describe the systemic effects of toxic epidermal necrolysis (TEN). He pleaded for

the management of such cases in a specialized dermatology intensive care unit (DICU) rather than in burn units [5].

WHY IS ACUTE SKIN FAILURE AN EMERGENCY?

A prompt and effective treatment is paramount, as along with failure of skin, other vital organs like liver, kidneys, lungs, heart, and hematological system are also affected, which may lead to death or development of permanent sequelae [6].

ETIOPATHOGENESIS OF ACUTE SKIN FAILURE

The skin functions not only as a barrier to prevent entry of foreign materials and loss of fluid and electrolytes, it also helps in thermoregulation to maintain the core body temperature. Unlike burns, the pathogenesis in ASF continues until the disease process is controlled or there is clearance of the metabolite of the drug. The depth of tissue destruction, underlying vascular injury, and subcutaneous edema are more in burns than ASF.

The most common groups of disorders causing ASF are as follows:

1. Stevens-Johnson syndrome/toxic epidermal necrolysis complex (SJS/TEN complex)
2. Drug reaction with eosinophilia and systemic symptoms (DRESS)
3. Erythroderma due to any reason
4. Immunobullous disorders

5. Mechanobullous disorders/epidermolysis bullosa
6. Infections like staphylococcal scalded skin syndrome and varicella
7. Pustular psoriasis
8. Graft versus host disease
9. Acute lupus erythematosus

PHYSIOLOGY OF SKIN

To understand the pathology of ASF, one has to understand the physiology of the skin.

Main functions of normal skin are

- *Thermoregulation*: To maintain core body temperature by preventing heat loss and blocking the adverse effects of extreme changes in external environmental temperature on the body
- *Barrier function*: Preventing entry of any foreign materials (including infections, physical agents like rays and gases, chemicals) and protection against mechanical damage; also prevents loss of body fluids and protein
- *Immunological function*: Keratinocytes and Langerhans cells initiate immune response against many external agents [7]
- *Psychosexual function*: Helps in improving appearance
- *Wound healing*

ALTERED PHYSIOLOGY IN PATIENTS WITH ACUTE SKIN FAILURE

- *Fluid and electrolyte imbalance*: Due to increased transepidermal water loss (TEWL), an average daily fluid loss in adult TEN patients with 50% body surface area (BSA) involvement may be 3–4 L (400–1000 mL/day is normal) [8,9]. There is a reduction in the intravascular volume and a hyperosmolar state ensues that clinically manifests as dehydration, decreased urinary output, electrolyte imbalance ($\downarrow$Na+, $\uparrow$K+, and $\downarrow$PO4^{3-}), and raised serum levels of urea and creatinine. Patients with acute generalized pustular psoriasis may also have associated acute hypocalcemia secondary to severe hypoalbuminemia.
- *Altered thermoregulation*: Due to increased cutaneous blood flow, heat loss through radiation and convection increases, leading to a state of hypothermia. However, hyperthermia may be seen as a premonitory sign of sepsis or a part of illness due to excessive interleukin-1, produced by damaged keratinocytes [5,10–12]. A condition akin to poikilothermia develops.
- *Changes in hemodynamics*: Peripheral vasodilatation, anemia, and increased cutaneous blood flow lead to increased cardiac output (two to three times above normal), which can lead to high-output cardiac failure and decreased perfusion of vital organs [13]. An increase in vascular endothelial growth factor (VEGF) and vascular permeability factor (VPF) causes capillary leakage, expansion of extracellular space, and resultant edema, adding to the existing cardiac problem [14].

- *Metabolic abnormalities*: Basal metabolic rate (BMR) increases as a compensatory mechanism for hypothermia. Increased BMR leads to negative nitrogen balance, increased urinary nitrogen, and hypoalbuminemia. Hypercatabolic state due to destruction of cells results in hypoproteinemia, hyperglycemia, glycosuria, decreased insulin secretion, relative insulin resistance, and pancreatitis. Shivering, which is a compensatory mechanism for hypothermia, also increases energy consumption [8,13]. Hypoproteinemia (mainly hypoalbuminemia) results due to loss of protein in oozing. Combined protein loss may amount to approximately 150–200 g/day in TEN [5,15]. Diffuse scaling in exfoliative dermatitis and psoriasis leads to protein loss of approximately 50–100 g/day [16]. Hypoproteinemia also leads to delayed healing.
- *Loss of nutrients*: There is impaired absorption of iron, vitamin B12, and folic acid with increased excretion of these elements during exfoliation and in the exudates leading to anemia [15].
- *Changes in immune function and infection*: ASF leads to failure of keratinocytes and dendritic cells to initiate immune response. It also results in lymphopenia, neutropenia, impaired chemotaxis and phagocytosis by granulocytes, leading to immune dysfunction [11]. All of the above factors may allow endogenous and exogenous organisms to grow, causing systemic infection, septicemia, and death [8]. The presence of exudates also supports growth of organisms.
- *Pulmonary complications*: Severe pulmonary edema (secondary to capillary leak syndrome), adult respiratory distress syndrome (ARDS), and aspiration pneumonitis are common complications, especially in erythroderma [17]. Overzealous correction of hypovolemia can give rise to overt pulmonary edema [5].

The summary of pathophysiological alterations in ASF is provided in Figure 2.1.

PROGNOSTIC CRITERIA

1. *Body surface area (BSA)*: More the BSA involvement more is the morbidity and mortality. "Rule of nine" helps in BSA calculation (Figure 2.2) [2].
2. *Severity of illness score for toxic epidermal necrolysis (SCORTEN)*: It is a TEN-specific score, computed within 24 hours of admission and is used to predict the chances of mortality. Tuberculosis and diabetes can have been suggested as new prognostic markers in TEN [18].

INVESTIGATIONS

After the assessment, baseline investigations for patients with ASF include the following:

- Skin biopsy for histopathological examination and immunofluorescence studies (to confirm the diagnosis)
- Complete blood count

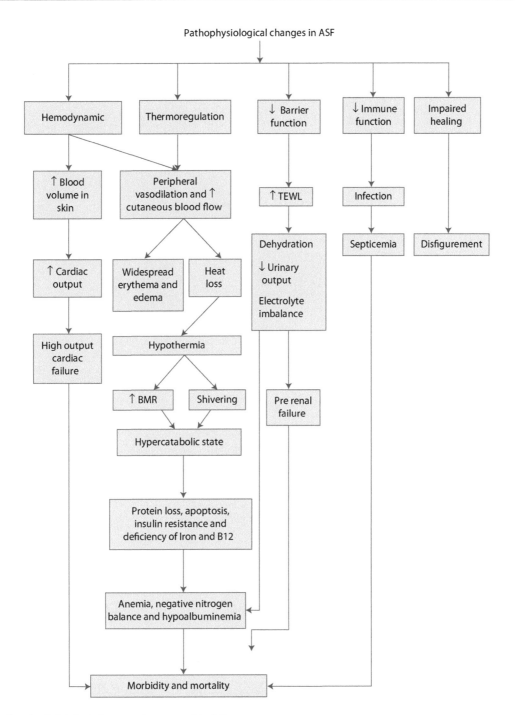

Figure 2.1 Pathophysiological changes in acute skin failure.

- Blood sugar
- Liver function test
- Blood urea and serum creatinine
- Serum electrolytes (Na+, K+, Cl⁻, Po4³⁻)
- Arterial blood gas analysis
- Urine routine and microscopy
- Chest radiograph
- Electrocardiogram (ECG)
- Skin swab culture
- Blood culture
- Other investigations specific for different conditions

TREATMENT OF ACUTE SKIN FAILURE

Initial assessment and supportive management

Prompt initiation of double-barrier nursing care and supportive pharmacotherapy are two equally important pillars of management that can salvage many lives. A flow chart of the steps of management is given in Figure 2.3.

The success of the above steps of treatment depends on the extent of the DICU and emergency care training of

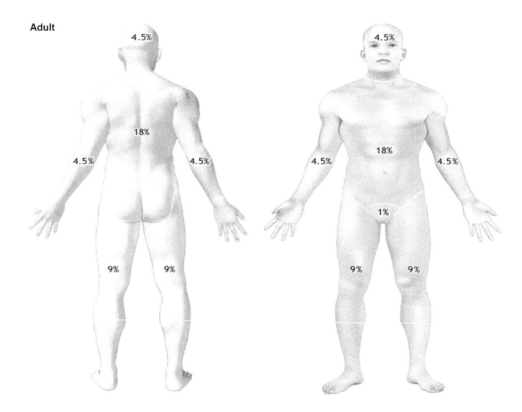

Figure 2.2 Rule of nine chart.

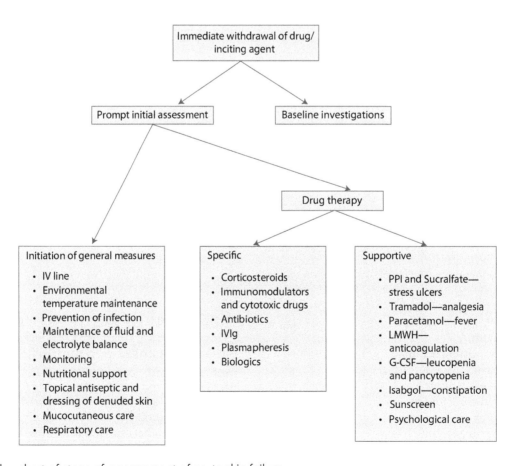

Figure 2.3 Flowchart of steps of management of acute skin failure.

dermatologists and paramedical workers. Displaying standard operative procedures pertaining to care of a patient with ASF is a must.

The important steps are as discussed in the following sections.

REMOVAL OF INCITING DRUG/AGENT/DISEASE CONDITION

We must observe prudence in prescribing and altering drug therapy in ASF.

- Immediate withdrawal of the suspected drug/inciting agent is of supreme importance (especially in SJS/TEN). Stoppage of the offending drug will slow or abort the process of ASF and allow skin epithelialization in a shorter period of time.
- If the reaction has been caused by drugs with longer half-lives, the pathological processes may continue for a longer duration [19].
- If administration of a class of drug is absolutely essential for the health of the patient, then the culprit medication should be substituted with a structurally unrelated molecule.
- It is of prime importance to restrict drug intake to the minimum possible. Drugs such as antibiotics, nonsteroidal anti-inflammatory drugs (NSAIDS), corticosteroids, vitamins, etc., should be given only on specific indications.
- Any other agent concerned with the etiology of ASF should be removed/avoided and the underlying condition should be treated aggressively.

OTHER IMPORTANT MEASURES

After evaluation of airway, breathing, circulation, and vitals, an IV line should be inserted and fluids should be initiated. The patient and the caregivers should then be asked history of the following:

- Onset, duration, and progression of the disease process.
- A detailed history of drug intake must be elicited (including ayurvedic/homeopathic/indigenous medicines or health supplements) prior to the onset of the eruptions, and efforts should be made to identify the likely offending drug.
- Personal or family history of drug reactions.
- Any prior disease comorbid condition.
- Any contact agent, sudden withdrawal of therapy, etc.

A thorough general, systemic, and cutaneous examination should be done including the following:

- Level of consciousness.
- Any clinical evidence of septicemia.
- Percentage of BSA involved, extent of erythema, and epidermal detachment should be recorded.

Counseling

Counseling of the patient and the family is an important but often overlooked part of "holistic" management. Counseling must be done frequently depending on the condition of the patient.

General measures

1. *Intravenous line*
   - Insert an IV line immediately on admission in DICU over uninvolved skin. If such an area is not identifiable, a central venous line should be considered. If both procedures are not possible, then venesection is the last resort.
   - The IV line should not be replaced before 96 hours unless there is evidence of phlebitis, local infection, or malfunction [20,21].
2. *Ambient temperature maintenance*
   - Room temperature should be maintained between 30°C and 32°C, which reduces caloric loss through the skin [22].
   - Alternatively, heated-air body warmers may be used to reduce shivering and the associated energy loss.
3. *Prevention of infection*
   The following measures are important to prevent sepsis:
   - The patient should ideally be treated in the DICU. Double-barrier nursing and sterile handling of the patient are of paramount importance.
     Barrier nursing techniques include the following [23]:
     - Enter DICU after washing hands and wearing protective clothing (such as masks, gloves, gowns, and goggles).
     - Limit movement of the patient, health-care worker, and attendants to and from the DICU.
     - Use masks, inclusive of patient.
     - Display instructions outside the DICU regarding precautions and measures to be taken by everyone before entering the room.
     - Strictly follow infection control measures (such as complete equipment sterilization and routine use of disinfectant).
     - Remove protective clothing after leaving the room and a new set of clothing should be worn before reentering the DICU.
   - Judicious use of antibiotics (details covered in specific section later).
   - For cultures, it is preferable to obtain the swab for culture and sensitivity from three lesional sites, particularly sloughed or crusted areas, on alternate days throughout the acute phase. Blood cultures are to be done at admission and then every 48 hours [24].
4. *Maintenance of fluid and electrolyte balance*
   - Fluid therapy during first 24 hour is of utmost importance. Optimum and rapid restoration of intravascular volume holds the key to rapid recovery.

- The Parkland formula (used for burns) helps us to calculate the replacement fluid [25].
- *Calculation of replacement fluid during first 24 hours*
  Resuscitation volume = 4 mL×Total body weight X% of BSA involved
  - This formula can sometimes overestimate replacement fluid during the first 24 hours [26]. In SJS/TEN and blistering disorders (where fluid loss is much more than other causes of ASF), it is calculated as one-half to three-quarters of value obtained by the Parkland formula, while in other conditions (psoriasis, erythroderma, DRESS, etc.), fluids are to be given at one-quarter to one-half the volume of the Parkland formula [27].
  - Half of this calculated volume is administered in the first 8 hours and the remaining half in subsequent 16 hours [25].
  - Isotonic solutions such as Normal saline (NS) and Ringer lactate (RL) are given as replacement therapy. Colloids are not preferred during the first 24 hours because of a risk of capillary leak [2].
  - If the BSA involvement is greater than 40%, colloidal resuscitation with 5% albumin followed by NS is recommended [25]. It is calculated as 0.3–0.4 mL/kg per % of BSA, given 6–8 hourly [28].
- *Calculation of replacement fluid volume after 24 hours*
  - Maintenance fluid is titrated so as to maintain ideal urine output of 1 mL/kg/h (approximately 1500 mL/day) [27,29].
  - *Maintenance fluid* = Input (Oral feeds + IV fluids) of previous day + (1500 mL – Urine output of previous day)
  - If urinary output is more than 1500 mL, then the corresponding amount is reduced from the calculated maintenance fluid.
  - NS is the fluid of choice.
  - If urine output is very low and not improving, then the volume of maintenance fluid should be reduced to 50% [30].
  - In bedridden patients, transurethral catheterization or condom drainage (in male patient) may be considered.
  Template of fluid therapy in ASF is given in Table 2.1.
- *Hyponatremia (<135 mEq/L)*
  - If serum Na >125 meEq/L, then 0.9% NaCl is recommended to correct the deficit [5].
  - If serum Na falls below 125 mEq/L, neurological symptoms may appear. Then 3% NS at 100 mL/h should be given until serum Na reaches 125 meq/L [31].
  - However, serum sodium correction should not exceed 6 meq/L/day.
- *Hypokalemia (<3.5 meq/L)*

Table 2.1 Template for fluid therapy in ASF (In a 60 kg adult with 20% BSA involvement)

Initial 24 hour	After 24 hour
Parkland formula	Urine output 1000 mL
(4 mL × wt kg × %BSA)	500 mL less than normal
4 × 60 × 20 = 4800 mL	hence to be added
Requirement in	2400 + 500 = 2900 mL
ASF1/2 = 2400 mL	
3/4 = 3600 mL	3600 + 500 = 4100 mL

Input = oral feeds + IV fluids
Output = urine output + vomitus + stools

  - Injectable potassium chloride (40 mmol/L) in 5% dextrose/NS, 6–8 hourly until corrected.
  - Milk, coconut water, banana, and potassium chloride syrup can be given [8].
- *Hypophosphatemia (2.5–4.5 mg/dL)*
  - Potassium phosphate may be added in IV fluids to prevent insulin resistance [8].
5. *Monitoring*
- Frequent monitoring of vital signs is essential to detect the first signs of a worsening systemic condition.
- *Clinical*
  - Pulse rate (1/2–1 hour initially and later 2 hourly)
  - Blood pressure (1/2–1 hour initially and later 2 hourly)
  - Respiratory rate (1/2–1 hour initially and later 2 hourly)
  - Anorectal temperature recording (perirectal thermometer must be used)
  - Maintenance of fluid intake and urinary output chart
- *Signs of sepsis* [24]
  - Sudden hypothermia with tachycardia and hypotension
  - Fever or shivering after the fourth day in a euthermic patient
  - Diminishing level of consciousness
  - Change in mental status
  - Falling urinary output
  - Deterioration of respiratory status
  - Loss of diabetic control
  - Failure of gastric emptying
  - Malena and hematemesis
  - Any sudden change in the condition
  Note: Systemic steroids may mask the signs of sepsis.
- *Periodicity of investigations*:
  - Complete blood count, daily
  - Blood glucose, 12 hourly
  - Serum electrolytes, 6 hourly
  - Serum creatinine, daily
  - Arterial blood gas analysis, 12 hourly
  - Specific cultures, as mentioned earlier
- If facilities are available, septicemia and disseminated intravascular coagulation can be monitored

by specialized tests such as coagulation assays, D-dimer assay, and fibrin degradation products.

6. *Nutritional support*
   - Aggressive nutritional support must be initiated early in order to
     - Avoid metabolic disturbances
     - Correct protein loss
     - Promote healing
     - Compensate the hypercatabolic state
   - If oral intake is poor, nasogastric feeding is a preferred way of giving adequate nutrition [24].
   - In ASF, gastric emptying may be delayed, resulting in regurgitation and inhalation; hence, feeding is given in small amounts, frequently. If the residual gastric aspirate is more than 50 mL, feeding scheduled at that time should be withheld [8].
   - *Caloric requirements*
     - Curreri formula is used to know caloric requirement, which is calculated as 25 Kcal/kg + 40 Kcal per % BSA involved to be given daily [32].
     - Energy supplementation should be started with 1500–2000 kcal/day in early catabolic phase, which is increased gradually by 500 kcal/day up to 3500–4000 kcal/day in recovery/anabolic phase [3].
   - *Protein requirements*: Davies formula is used to calculate protein requirement, which is 1 g/kg + 3 g per % BSA involved given daily [33].
   - *Others*: Vitamins (B complex and C), iron, and zinc after stabilization.
   - A detailed nutrition plan is provided in Chapter 3.
7. *Topical antiseptics and dressings*
   - Burn-cage must be used since it gives protection from houseflies and dust and permits the patient to stay without tight dressings. An air-fluidized bed prevents bed sores and increases patient comfort. However, some people feel that it increases evaporative loss and should be used only after stabilization of the patient [34].
   - Non infected detached epidermis and roof of deflated bullae serve as a biological dressing and hence should be retained.
   - NS/potassium permanganate (PP) bath/soaks are recommended (2 gPP in 200 L of water to make 1:10,000 solution) to remove crust and reduce chances of infection.
   - The following medicaments can be applied:
     - *Topical antibiotic*: Silver nitrate 0.5% cream is preferred. Fusidic acid, nadifloxacin, and mupirocin cream can also be used.
     - *Emollient*: 50% white soft paraffin with 50% liquid paraffin in soaked gauze pieces [22].
     - Silver sulfadiazine should be avoided in SJS/TEN andDRESS [35].
     - Adhesive dressings should be avoided [24].
   - *Biological dressings*: Sterile banana leaves, potato peels, and amnion can be used. Collagen-based skin substitutes can also be used; however, they are expensive with limited availability.
   - *Nanocrystalline silver dressings* (Figures 2.4 and 2.5): The advantages of using this dressing are as follows:
     - Silver has antimicrobial activity against a wide variety of microorganisms.
     - Anti-inflammatory properties.
     - A dressing once done can be continued for 3–7 days (depending on the type of nanosilver dressing used), reducing patient discomfort, pain, and handling, and hence the chances of cross infections. The secondary dressing needs to be changed due to soakage (generally in 2–3 days).
     - Found to be less painful than silver sulfadiazine cream dressings.
     - This dressing is available in various sizes including rolls to facilitate easier dressing.

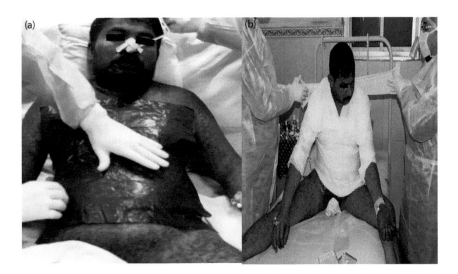

Figure 2.4 Nanocrystalline silver dressing being applied as a primary dressing, followed by secondary dressing.

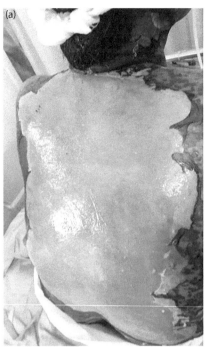 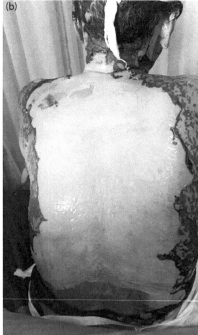 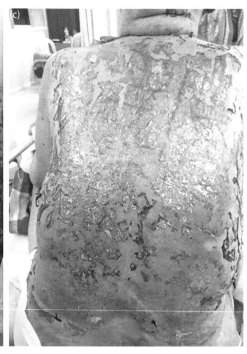

Figure 2.5 Case of toxic epidermal necrolysis (TEN) with nanocrystalline dressing. (a) Back of TEN patient on day 1. (b) Day 4, after removal of the first nanosilver dressing, a thin layer of newly formed epidermis is visible. (c) Day 10, after removal of the third nanosilver dressing, the epidermis is completely healed. No oozing or moist areas are seen. This is the end point of dressing. The thin film of the nanosilver dressing that is seen exfoliates on its own.

- In circumferential erosions on the extremities, the nanosilver dressings can be kept in place by stapling the dressing together but not directly to the wound.
- "Flex" forms are available for a snug fit.
- Administer injectable tramadol 50–100 mg IV over 2–3 minutes, 30 minutes before starting the dressing. Injectable ondansetron 4–8 mg IV is routinely administered to prevent nausea and vomiting associated with tramadol.
- Newer modalities include cadaveric allografts, cultured human allogeneic or autologous epidermal sheets, and human newborn fibroblasts cultured on a nylon mesh of Biobrane [36]. These are likely to be available in the near future.

8. *Mucocutaneous care*
  - Regular cleaning of mucous membranes prevents secondary infection and synechiae formation.
  - *Eye care*
    - For lid hygiene, regular normal saline wipes should be used to clean the eyelids while eyes are closed, from medial to lateral in a single stroke.
    - Lubrication of the ocular surfaces with preservative-free artificial tears and ointments should be done regularly to prevent exposure keratopathy and formation of synechiae.
    - Daily inspection and sweeping of the superior and inferior fornices should be done using a glass rod or cellulose sponge spears (Figure 2.6).

This is a painful procedure; hence, topical anesthetics like 0.5% proparacaine hydrochloride should be used. Instill 1 or 2 drops to the eye 2 or 3 minutes before the procedure. With a single drop, the onset of anesthesia begins within 30 seconds and persists for 15 minutes or longer.
    - An important point to note is that if a systemic drug has caused a reaction, the same molecule should not be used as an eye drop to take care of the eye complaints.
  - *Care of the oral cavity*
  Conscious patients
    - For cleaning, use a pediatric toothbrush and fluorinated toothpaste twice daily.
    - For rinsing, use a 10 mL syringe and equal quantity of 0.12% chlorhexidine mouthwash twice daily.
    - For pain relief, use benzydamine hydrochloride mouthwash every 3 hours.
  Unconscious patients
    - Clean the teeth with gauze soaked in 0.12% chlorhexidine mouthwash, followed by suction, twice daily. Chlorhexidine may also be administered by using sprays.
  Lips
    - *Fissuring of lips*: Apply white soft paraffin over the lips thrice daily.
    - *Crusting*: Normal saline compresses.
  Clotrimazole mouth paint prevents candidal infection in the oral cavity.

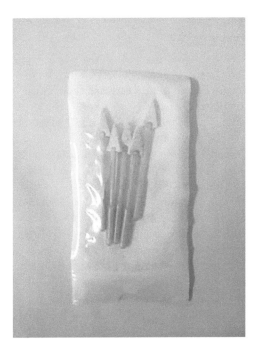

Figure 2.6 Cellulose sponge spears for prevention of synechiae.

- Nasal crusts can be loosened with normal saline nasal drops.
- *Care of genitalia*
  - The genitalia, especially in case of females who have erosions on the opposing surfaces should be examined regularly. Apply white soft paraffin ointment twice daily to prevent the formation of synechiae and late sequelae such as scarring and fibrosis.
  - Consider catheterizing the urethra to prevent urethral strictures.
9. *Respiratory care*
- Lung involvement may be complicated by pulmonary edema due to overzealous fluid replacement.
- Pooling of saliva and secretions may predispose to aspiration and therefore needs to be cleared frequently.

10. *Antibiotics*
- There is a definite possibility of development of sepsis in most cases of ASF, and antibiotics form an essential part of management. But pre-emptive antibiotic therapy without indication should be avoided [24]. They are the drugs of choice where infection is the primary cause of ASF such as in staphylococcal scalded skin syndrome.
- *Staphylococcus aureus*, gram-negative bacilli, and anaerobes may invade. Antibiotics that are commonly used are as follows [24]:
  - *Antistaphylococcal activity*: Amoxicillin + clavulanic acid/tetracyclines/vancomycin/clindamycin/teicoplanin/linezolid
  - *Gram-negative activity*: Amikacin/piperacillin + tazobactam/cefoperazone + sulbactam/imipenem)
  - *Anaerobic activity*: Metronidazole/tinidazole Doses of different antibiotics that can be used are given in Table 2.2.
11. *Other supportive measures* [37–62]
- *Stress ulcers*
  - IV injectable pantoprazole 40 mg 12 hourly, reduces the incidence of stress-related gastric and duodenal ulcers.
  - Sucralfate suspension coats gastric mucosa and prevents further harm.
- *Analgesics and antipyretics*
  - Standard NSAIDS have been implicated in various causes of ASF. Hence, paracetamol is first choice.
  - IV Injectable tramadol 50 mg, 6–8 hourly may be used when more analgesia is needed.
  - Benzodiazepines like alprazolam 0.5 mg may supplement the above drugs in pain management and alleviate anxiety.
- *Anticoagulation*
  - Deep vein thrombosis is a known complication in bedridden, old, debilitated, or obese patients.

Table 2.2 Doses of different antibiotics

Antibiotics	Dose
Amoxicilin + Clavulanic acid	1.2 gm IV 8 hourly
Vancomycin	45–60 mg/kg/day 6–12 hourly
Clindamycin	10–20 mg/kg/day PO 6–8 hourly
Linezolid	10 mg/kg PO/IV 8 hourly
Teicoplanin	10 mg/kg 12 hourly for 3 loading dose followed by once daily
Tetracycline	25–50 mg/kg/day 6 hourly, not to exceed 3 gm/day
Amikacin	15 mg/kg/day IV 8 hourly
Piperacillin + Cazobactum	100 mg/kg IV 8 hourly
Imipenem	10–15 mg/kg IV 6 hourly
Metronidazole	7.5 mg/kg PO/IV 6 hourly
Cefoperazone + Sulbactam	40–80 mg/kg/day, in two equally divided doses (1–2 gm IM/IV 12 hourly)

- Low molecular weight heparin (LMWH) 60 mg S/C OD for 3 days can be given as prophylactic therapy, if no contraindications exist [19].
- *Leukopenia*
  - Administration of G-CSF (Filgrastim 300 mg S/C OD) has been used to resist infectious complications like septicemia by improving neutropenia [63,64].
- *Prevention of constipation*
  - Isabgol/enema/glycerine pessary can be used.
- *Photoprotection*
  - Should be advised for a few months to prevent chances of cutaneous pigmentary changes.
- *Prevention of trophic/decubitus ulcers*
  - Examine the trophic ulcer prone sites—sacrum, ischial tuberosities, greater trochanters, and heels.
  - Synthetic fiber sheets are preferred over standard hospital sheets as they have lower coefficient of friction and reduce shearing forces, thus reducing the risk of pressure ulcers.
  - Prophylactic dressings like polyurethane foams are recommended to prevent pressure sores.
- *Physiotherapy*
  - Physiotherapy is important to prevent deep venous thrombosis, help loosening of secretions in the respiratory tract, prevention of skeletal muscle weakness, and to facilitate early mobilization.
  - Physiotherapy is carried out for 30 minutes in twice daily sessions. The position of the patient is changed every 2 hours.
- *Psychological care*
  - Providing emotional support and maintaining a continual dialogue with the patient and his/her family is a vital part of supportive care and addresses the patient's fears/anxieties and improves compliance.

Specific medication

The treatment of specific conditions causing ASF is provided in respective chapters and will not be discussed here.

CONCLUSION

ASF is the endpoint of all dermatological emergencies and needs to be managed as energetically as failure of other organ systems. A dedicated team of nursing staff, dermatologists, and cross consultation with other specialities are cornerstones for managing the acute failure of skin.

KEY POINTS

- ASF is a pan systemic disorder, which if not diagnosed and treated early may have grave consequences.
- There is a need to establish a DICU, at least in tertiary care centers.
- Immediate stoppage of the offending drug/agent and treatment of the underlying condition are the keys for survival.
- Irrational, unwanted, and empirical use of drugs may further complicate the condition.
- General measures and drug therapy are equally important in the management.
- Prudence is needed in the use of antibiotics and other symptom-relieving drugs.
- Adequate hydration along with double-barrier nursing in a warm environment is the cornerstone of supportive management.
- Steroids, other immunosuppressants, and biologics do not have a specific role in the management of ASF per se, but these are indicated for specific underlying diseases.
- Biological dressings that may be available in the future will reduce the use of antibiotics and reduce infections.

REFERENCES

1. Irvine C. "Skin failure"—A real entity: Discussion paper. *J R Soc Med* 1991;84:412–3.
2. Inamadar AC, Ragunatha S, Palit A. Acute skin failure. In: Wolf R, Parish LC, Parish JL (Eds), *Emergency Dermatology*. 2nd ed. New York: CRC Press, Taylor and Francis Group; 2017:52–64.
3. Vaishampayan SS, Sharma YK, Das AL, Verma R. Emergencies in dermatology: Acute skin failure. *Med J Armed Forces India* 2006;62:56–9.
4. Irvine C. "Skin failure"—A real entity: Discussion paper. *J R Soc Med* 1991;84:413–4.
5. Roujeau JC, Revuz J. Intensive care in dermatology. In: Champion RH, Pye RJ (Eds), *Recent Advances in Dermatology*. Edinburgh: Churchill-Livingstone; 1990:85–90.
6. Palit A, Inamadar AC. Acute skin failure: Myth or reality? *Al Ameen J Med Sci* 2013;6:193–4.
7. Nikolaus RP, Brunner M, Stingl G. Changing views of the role of Langerhans cells. *J Invest Dermatol* 2012;132(3):872–81.
8. Inamadar AC, Palit A. Acute skin failure: Concept, causes, consequences and care. *Ind J Dermatol Venereol Leprol* 2005;71:379–85.
9. Revuz J, Roujeau JC, Guillaume JC, Penso D, Touraine R. Treatment of toxic epidermal necrolysis, Créteil's experience. *Arch Dermatol* 1987;123:1156–58.

10. Luger TA, Stadler BM, Katz SI, Oppenheim JJ. Epidermal cell (keratinocyte) derived thymocyte activating factor (ETAF). *J Immunol* 1981;127:1493–8.

11. Holden CA, Berth-Jones J. Eczema, lichenification, prurigo and erythroderma. In: Burns T, Breathnach S, Cox N, Griffiths C (Eds). *Rook's Textbook of Dermatology*. 7th ed. Oxford: Blackwell-Science; 2004:17.1–17.25.

12. Kimgai-Asadi A, Freedberg IM. Exfoliative dermatitis. In: Freedberg IM, Eisen AZ, Wolff K, Austen KF, Goldsmith LA, Katz SI (Eds), *Fitzpatrick's Dermatology in General Medicine*. 6th ed. New York: McGraw-Hill; 2003:436–41.

13. Valeyrie-Allanore L, Oro S, Roujeau JC. Acute skin failure. In: Revuz J, Roujeau JC, Kerdel F, Valeyrie-allanore L (Eds), *Life-Threatening Dermatosis and Emergencies in Dermatology*. Berlin: Springer-Verlag; 2009:37–42.

14. Creamer D, Allen MH, Groves MW, Barker JN. Circulating vascular permeability factor/vascular endothelial growth factor in erythroderma. *Lancet* 1996;348:1101.

15. Yurt RW, Howell JD, Burns, electrical injury and smoke inhalation. In: Heliaer MA, Nichols DC (Eds), *Rogers Handbook of Pediatric Intensive Care*. 4th ed. New Delhi: Lippincott Williams and Wilkins; 2009:59–66.

16. Grant-Kels Fedeles F, Rothe MJ. Exfoliative dermatitis. In: Goldsmith LA et al. (Eds), *Fitzpatrick's Dermatology in Internal Medicine*. Vol. I, 8th ed. New York: McGraw-Hill; 2012:266–78.

17. Rothe MJ, Bialy TL, Grant-Kels JM. Erythroderma. *Dermatol Clin* 2000;18:405–15.

18. Vaishampayan SS, Das AL, Verma R. SCORTEN: Does it need modification? *Indian J Dermatol Venereol Leprol* 2008;74:35–7.

19. Garcia-Doval I, LeCleach L, Bocquet H, Otero XL, Roujeau JC. Toxic epidermal necrolysis and Stevens-Johnson syndrome: Does early withdrawal of causative drugs decrease the risk of death? *Arch Dermatol* 2000;136:323–7.

20. Committee for the development of guidelines for the prevention of vascular catheter associated infection; Indian society of critical care medicine. Epidemiology. *Indian J Crit Care Med* 2003;7(Suppl S1):6.

21. Ahmed KN. Procedures and techniques in dermatological emergencies. In: Inamadar AC, Palit A (Eds), *Care Dermatology*. New Delhi: Jaypee, Brothers Medical Publishers; 2013:125–55.

22. Inamdar AC, Palit A. Acute skin failure. In: Parikh D, Dhar S (Eds), *Perspectives in Clinical Dermatology*. Vol. 14. Mumbai: Galderma India; 2015:16–25.

23. [Online].Available:https://www.uhcw.nhs.uk/client-files/File/Isolation_and_Barrier_Nursing_2010.pdf

24. Gupta LK et al. Guidelines for the management of Stevens-Johnson/toxic epidermal necrolysis: An Indian perspective. *Indian J Dermatol Venerol Leprol* 2016;82:603–25.

25. Tyler M, Ghosh S. Burns. In: William NS, Bulstrode CJK, O'Connell PR (Eds), *Bailey and Love's Short Practice of Surgery*. 25th ed. London: Hodder Arnold; 2008:378–93.

26. Csontos C, Foldi V, Fischer T, Bogar L. Factors affecting fluid requirement on the first day after severe burn trauma. *ANZ J Surj* 2007;77:745–8.

27. Shiga S, Cartotto R. What are the fluid requirements in toxic epidermal necrolysis? *Burn Care Res* 2010;31:100–4.

28. Finkelstein JL et al. Pediatric burns. An overview. *Pediatr Clin N Am* 1993;39:1145–64.

29. Siegel NS, Lattazi WE. Fluid and electrolyte therapy in children. In: Arieff AI, DeFronzo RA (Eds), *Fluid, Electrolyte and Acid-Base*. New York: Churchill Livingstone; 1985:1211–30.

30. Holiday MA, Ray PE, Friedman AL. Fluid therapy for children: Facts, fashions and questions. *Arch Dis Child* 2007;92:546–50.

31. Spasovski G et al. Clinical practice guideline on diagnosis and treatment of hyponatremia. *Nephrol Dial Transplant* 2014;29(1):i1–i39.

32. Turner WW Jr., Ireton CS, Hunt JL, Baxter CR. Predicting energy expenditures in burned patients. *J Trauma* 1985;25(1):11–6.

33. Inamandar AC. Fluid, electrolyte andnutrition therapy in dermatological emergencies. In: Inamadar AC, Palit A (Eds),*Critical Care in Dermatology*. New Delhi: Jaypee Brothers Medical Publishers; 2013:177–85.

34. Inamdar AC. Dermatology intensive care unit (DICU). In: Inamadar AC, Palit A(Eds), *Critical Care in Dermatology*. New Delhi: Jaypee Brothers Medical Publishers; 2013:177–85.

35. Sharma VK, Jerajani HR, Srinivas CR, Valia A, Khandpur S. IADVL consensus guidelines 2006: Management of Stevens-Johnson syndrome and toxic epidermal necrolysis. In: Sharma VK (Ed), *Guidelines for Vitiligo, Stevens-Johnson Syndrome, Toxic Epidermal Necrolysis and Psoriasis*. 2nd ed. New Delhi: IADVL's Therapeutic Guidelines Committee; 2008.

36. Ghislain PD, Roujeau JC. Treatment of severe drug reactions: Stevens-Johnson syndrome, toxic epidermal necrolysis and hypersensitivity syndrome. *Dermatol Online J* 2002;8:5.

37. Griffiths CEM, Barker J, Bleiker T, Chalmers R, Creamer D (Eds). *Severe Cutaneous Adverse Reaction to Drugs. Rook's Textbook of Dermatology*. 9th ed. Edinburgh: Wiley Blackwell; 2016:119.20.

38. Chrousos GP. Adrenocorticosteroids and adrenocortical antagonists. In: Katzung BG (Ed), *Basic and Clinical Pharmacology*. 9th ed. New York: Lange Medical Books/McGraw-Hill; 2004:641–60.

39. Tripathi A et al. Corticosteroid therapy in an additional 13 cases of Stevens-Johnson syndrome:

A total series of 67 cases. *Allergy and Asthma Proc* 2000;21:101–5.

40. Kardaun SH, Jonkman MF. Dexamethasone pulse therapy for Stevens-Johnson syndrome/toxic epidermal necrolysis. *Acta Derm Venereol* 2007;87:144–8.

41. Kakourou T, Klontza D, Soteropoulou F, Kattamis C. Corticosteroid treatment of erythema multiforme major (Stevens-Johnson syndrome) in children. *Eur J Pediatr* 1997;156:90–3.

42. Das S, Roy AK, Biswas I. A six month prospective study to find out the treatment outcome, prognosis and offending drugs in toxic epidermal necrolysis from an urban institution in Kolkata. *Indian J Dermatol* 2013;58:191–3.

43. Pasricha JS, Khaitan BK, Shantharaman R, Mital A, Girdhar M. Toxic epidermal necrolysis. *Int J Dermatol* 1996;35:523–7.

44. Dhar S. Systemic corticosteroids in toxic epidermal necrolysis. *Indian J Dermatol Venereol Leprol* 1996;62:270–1.

45. Hirahara K et al. Methylprednisolone pulse therapy for Stevens-Johnson syndrome/toxic epidermal necrolysis: Clinical evaluation and analysis of biomarkers. *J Am Acad Dermatol* 2013;69:496–8.

46. Arévalo JM, Lorente JA, González-Herrada C, Jiménez-Reyes J. Treatment of toxic epidermal necrolysis with cyclosporin A. *J Trauma* 2000;48:473–8.

47. Valeyrie-Allanore L, Wolkenstein P, Brochard L, Ortonne N, Maître B, Revuz J, Bagot M, Roujeau JC. Open trial of ciclosporin treatment for Stevens-Johnson syndrome and toxic epidermal necrolysis. *Br J Dermatol* 2010;163(4):847–53.

48. Reese D, Henning JS, Rockers K, Ladd D, Gilson R. Cyclosporine for SJS/TEN: A case series and review of the literature. *Cutis* 2011;87:24–9.

49. Hewitt J, Ormerod AD. Toxic epidermal necrolysis treated with cyclosporin. *Clin Exp Dermatol* 1992;17:264–5.

50. Singh GK, Chatterjee M, Verma R. Cyclosporine in Stevens Johnson syndrome and toxic epidermal necrolysis and retrospective comparison with systemic corticosteroid. *Indian J Dermatol Venereol Leprol* 2013;79:686–92.

51. Viard I et al. Inhibition of toxic epidermal necrolysis by blockade of CD95 with human intravenous immunoglobulin. *Science* 1998;282:490–3.

52. Prins C et al. Treatment of toxic epidermal necrolysis with high-dose intravenous immunoglobulins: Multicenter retrospective analysis of 48 consecutive cases. *Arch Dermatol* 2003;139:26–32.

53. Trent JT, Kirsner RS, Romanelli P, Kerdel FA. Analysis of intravenous immunoglobulin for the treatment of toxic epidermal necrolysis using SCORTEN: The University of Miami Experience. *Arch Dermatol* 2003;139:39–43.

54. Mangla K, Rastogi S, Goyal P, Solanki RB, Rawal RC. Efficacy of low dose intravenous immunoglobulins in children with toxic epidermal necrolysis: An open uncontrolled study. *Indian J Dermatol Venereol Leprol* 2005;71:398–400.

55. Al-Mutairi N et al. Prospective, noncomparative open study from Kuwait of the role of intravenous immunoglobulin in the treatment of toxic epidermal necrolysis. *Int J Dermatol* 2004;43:847–51.

56. Shortt R, Gomez M, Mittman N, Cartotto R. Intravenous immunoglobulin does not improve outcome in toxic epidermal necrolysis. *J Burn Care Rehabil* 2004;25:246–55.

57. Bachot N, Revuz J, Roujeau JC. Intravenous immunoglobulin treatment for Stevens-Johnson syndrome and toxic epidermal necrolysis: A prospective noncomparative study showing no benefit on mortality or progression. *Arch Dermatol* 2003;139:33–6.

58. Schneck J, Fagot JP, Sekula P, Sassolas B, Roujeau JC, Mockenhaupt M. Effects of treatments on the mortality of Stevens-Johnson syndrome and toxic epidermal necrolysis: A retrospective study on patients included in the prospective EuroSCAR Study. *J Am Acad Dermatol* 2008;58:33–40.

59. Kamanabroo D, Schmitz-Landgraf W, Czarnetzki BM. Plasmapheresis in severe drug-induced toxic epidermal necrolysis. *Arch Dermatol* 1985;121:1548–9.

60. Egan CA, Grant WJ, Morris SE, Saffle JR, Zone JJ. Plasmapheresis as an adjunct treatment in toxic epidermal necrolysis. *J Am Acad Dermatol* 1999;40:458–61.

61. Paradisi A, Abeni D, Bergamo F, Ricci F, Didona D, Didona B. Etanercept therapy for toxic epidermal necrolysis. *J Am Acad Dermatol* 2014;71:278–83.

62. Fischer M, Fiedler E, Marsch WC, Wohlrab J. Antitumour necrosis factor-alpha antibodies (infliximab) in the treatment of a patient with toxic epidermal necrolysis. *Br J Dermatol* 2002;146:707–9.

63. Mahajan R, Kanwar AJ. Use of granulocyte colony-stimulating factor in the treatment of toxic epidermal necrolysis—Experience with 3 patients. *Skinmed* 2013;11:269–71.

64. Goulden V, Goodfield MJ. Recombinant granulocyte colony-stimulating factor in the management of toxic epidermal necrolysis. *Br J Dermatol* 1996;135:305–6.

3

Dermatology intensive care unit: Concept and requirements

SUKRITI BAVEJA AND ANWITA SINHA

INTRODUCTION

The first ever dermatology intensive care unit (DICU) was set up by Rene Touraine in the year 1974 for cases of acute skin failure who required specialized care. Despite this being a felt need by dermatologists and rapid advances happening in our specialty, this concept has failed to gain widespread acceptance and implementation.

DERMATOLOGY INTENSIVE CARE UNIT: THE CONCEPT

There are many advantages of managing dermatological emergencies in an independent DICU rather than a general ICU. They include the following:

- The major indication of admission into a DICU is acute skin failure. The majority of such cases are noninfectious and require reverse-barrier nursing in a rigorously maintained aseptic environment. A general ICU treats cases belonging to both infectious and noninfectious spectrums (mostly multiresistant), and there is a higher potential for cross infections. There is increased turnover of patients and increased traffic of the medical staff in the conventional ICU, which increases the chances of inducing infection. A stand-alone DICU provides a relatively better aseptic environment with a smaller number of patients who are generally noninfectious and only a limited number of people visiting the ICU.
- The ambient temperature of a conventional ICU is lower than the ideal range of temperature at which a patient of skin failure must be nursed.
- The noise levels in a conventional ICU are higher than in a DICU due to the increased number of patients, staff, and equipment.
- Nursing care in a case of acute skin failure is the cornerstone of management, requiring hours of meticulous skin care and monitoring that has to be backed up by the technical expertise of a nursing staff specifically trained in dermatology. Expecting the same level of skills, dedication, and time from the staff in the conventional ICU may be unfair considering their limited knowledge regarding dermatological diseases.
- Having a DICU in the department increases the ownership of the patient by the treating dermatologist, effectively making him or her accountable and eliminating "shared responsibility" among different specialties. This results in an increased level of care, decision-making, and motivation to acquire the required knowledge and skills. The knowledge gained about the nitty-gritty of basic practical management like care of the skin, fluid-calorie-protein calculation, and management of complications equips the dermatology team with valuable training and experience leading to a better standard of DICU care.

DERMATOLOGY INTENSIVE CARE UNIT: PHYSICAL SETUP

The DICU should be structurally and functionally a separate entity in the dermatological setup and should be specifically designed, staffed, furnished, equipped, and dedicated to the management of a patient with acute skin failure. It should have defined protocols and have its own quality control and training program. In concurrence with layout of ideal ICU guidelines laid out by the Indian Society of Critical Care Medicine (ISCCM) [1], and the European Society of Critical Care Medicine (ESCCM) [2], the following specifications are recommended for a standard DICU.

Location

A DICU should ideally be set up in a dermatology ward where separate rooms can be earmarked for the ICU setting.

Structure

Materials used for walls, roof, and floors should be easy to maintain and clean to prevent growth and spread of pathogens [3,5].

- *Floor*: Vitrified nonslippery tiles that are easy to clean and stain proof are a good option.
- *Walls*: Walls should be finished with similar vitrified tiles upto a height of 1.2–1.5 meters (4–5 feet).
- *Ceiling*: Material used should be smooth, nonfriable and free from fissures, joints, and crevices to prevent lodgment of dust particles. The materials should ideally absorb sound.

Layout and space requirement

A two- to four-bed DICU is an ideal proposition [3,4,8].

Bed space: Bed space should be a minimum of 14 m²(150 ft²) for comfortably working with a critically sick patient. In addition, there should be an extra space of 100%–150% to accommodate other equipment including a crash cart trolley, x-ray view box, portable bedside x-ray, ultrasound, and ventilator. Beds should be arranged in a fashion to enable adequate visibility from the nursing station. Separate cubicles or aluminium partitions with sliding doors for patients are better in terms of patient safety and privacy.

Bed type: A waterbed, water mattress, or flotation bed made up of polyvinyl chloride with interconnected flow chambers is ideal [4]. Air mattresses are a suitable alternative to avoid pressure sores. Beds should be motorized with facility for position changes (chair or Trendelenburg). The alpha bed is the other option.

Services per patient bed

- A multipara monitor per bed having facility for recording pulse, blood pressure, electrocardiogram (ECG), temperature, SpO_2 and respiratory rate [3].

- A ventilator, defibrillator, and bronchoscope in common and one to two infusion pumps per ICU bed.
- One oxygen outlet and 12 electrical outlets with pins to accommodate all standard electric pin sockets should be catered for each bed. Outlets should be connected to an uninterrupted power supply.
- A telephone outlet and alarm system.
- Bedside crash cart trolleys stocked with all emergency drugs and sterile instruments and disposables.
- Every bed should have a mounted hand disinfection system.

Individual workstations and central nursing station

Individual workstations for separate cubicles are recommended in an ideal setting to minimize cross infections [5]. These workstations are utilized for nutrition preparation, sterile dressings, and drug preparation.

A central nursing station from where all patients and monitors are observable is recommended. A handwashing facility should be located near the nursing station.

Entry and exit points, corridors, and doorways

There should preferably be a single entry or exit point to the ICU to avoid a thoroughfare (Figure 3.1) [1]. A

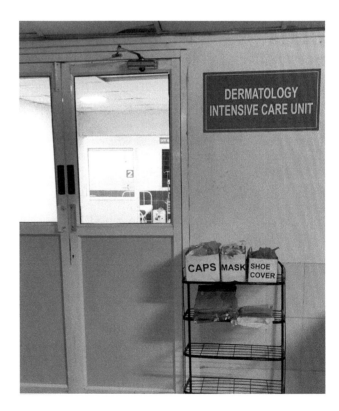

Figure 3.1 The entry door with station for cap, gown, mask, and disinfection hand-rub.

separate entrance for supplies and housekeeping staff can be designed. An emergency exit point should be in place for emergencies and disasters. Doorways to the bed spaces/rooms should be wide enough and appropriately placed to allow an ICU bed along with any attached equipment to pass easily.

Ancillary rooms/areas

- *Assisted shower rooms/patient toilet*: One shower room (8 m²) and a toilet (4.5 m²) should be designed having space for wheelchair movement [5]. A hydraulically operated tilt-table shower trolley for efficient and safe patient handling can be used for showering, dressing, and nursing.
- *Storage area/room*: The storage rooms should be easily accessible for nursing and medical staff to ideally have approaches from both the patient area and the supply route.
- *Laboratory area*: An enclosed area inside the ICU for point-of-care laboratory testing (e.g., arterial blood gas, blood sugars, urine strip tests, peripheral blood smears, etc.) should be available with adequate bench space. It should be equipped with 10–12 electric outlets, a sink, storage space for consumables, and sharp disposal apparatus.
- *Nourishment preparation area*: An identified enclosed area inside the ICU that should have a food preparation surface, sink, microwave oven, and a refrigerator.
- *Doctor's room*: A separate room adjoining the ICU should be earmarked for the treating doctor. It should be equipped with telephone, intercom, and alarm. A computer terminal with access to patient monitoring systems is desirable. Counseling of family members should be done here.
- *Visitor's room*: Should have seating facilities (one to two seats per bed) for the visitors with comfortable seating. Patient educational materials should be displayed here.

Environmental requirements

- *Heating, ventilation, and air conditioning (HVAC) of the ICU*: The ICU should be fully air conditioned, which allows control of temperature, humidity, and air exchange. Temperature should be maintained at 30°C–32°C, keeping in mind the poikilothermic patient [6]. Humidity of the room should be maintained at 70%. It is recommended to have six air exchanges per hour [1]. Central air-conditioning systems and recirculated air must pass through high-efficiency particulate air (HEPA) filters that can filter air with 99% efficiency down to 0.3 microns (Figure 3.2) as part of the HVAC system [9].
- *Electricity supply*: The ICU should have its own uninterrupted power backup system in place.

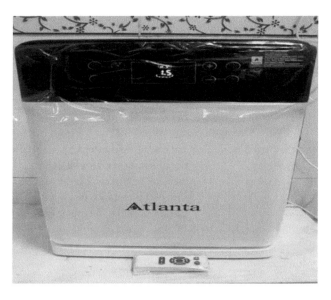

Figure 3.2 Commercially available air purifier with high-efficiency particulate air filter installed in the dermatology intensive care unit.

- *Light recommendations*: Access to natural light is recommended by regulatory authorities in the United States to improve patient outcomes. Spotlighting with high illumination is recommended for nursing procedures. Recommended spotlighting should be shadow-free 150 foot-candles (fc) strength. General overhead lighting should be at least 20fc [1].
- *Noise recommendations*: Noise levels should be under 45 dBA during the day and under 20 dBA at night [1].
- *Disaster preparedness*: There must be an emergency exit in the ICU to rescue patients in times of internal disaster. There should be adequate firefighting equipment inside the ICU.

STAFF AND MANPOWER REQUIREMENT

The DICU team has to be headed by a dermatologist. Nursing staff, with a nurse-to-patient ratio of 1:1 [3], with full-time presence by rotation in ICU is recommended for around-the-clock monitoring. The dermatologist as well as the nursing staff should be trained in aseptic reverse barrier nursing, dressings including advanced dressings, catheterization, Ryle tube insertion, basic and advanced cardiac life support, management of electrolyte abnormalities, and fluid and calorie requirements of the patient [4]. Cross referrals from the other specialties should be available around the clock.

EQUIPMENT AND EMERGENCY DRUGS

Instruments, equipment, and drugs required to set up a DICU are listed in Table 3.1 [4]. In addition it is recommended to group and label drugs and instruments by

Table 3.1 Equipment and drugs required in the dermatology intensive care unit

Vital parameters monitoring	Bedside tests and procedures	Resuscitation equipment	Patient comfort
Thermometer	Glucometer	Defibrillator	Air conditioner
Pulse oximeter	Kits for various diagnostic tests	Intubation equipment: Laryngoscope, endotracheal tube, mask, and resuscitation bag	Room humidifier and room heater
Electrocardiogram machine	IV canula, IV fluid transfusion and blood transfusion sets, central venous catheter, tourniquets, venesection sets, IV fluid stand, disposable syringes, sterile Vacutainers	Nebulizer	Air fluidized bed
Blood gas analyzer	Ryle tube, condom catheter, Foley catheter	Suction machine	Burn cage
Multipara monitor	Portable x-ray machine and view box	Mechanical ventilator	

Crash cart trolley with the following drugs:
- *Anaphylactic tray*: Adrenaline, hydrocortisone, pheniramine maleate
- *Cardiovascular drugs*: Dopamine, dobutamine, atropine, noradrenaline, furosemide, streptokinase
- *Crystalloids and colloids*: Normal saline, Ringer lactate, 5% dextrose, human albumin, dextran
- *Anticoagulants*: Low molecular weight heparin
- *Bronchodilators*: Aminophylline, salbutamol
- *Electrolyte corrections*: Potassium chloride, sodium bicarbonate, calcium gluconate

activity, like chest tray, central line tray, skin care tray, catheterization tray, Ryle tube insertion tray, etc. [4].

PROTOCOLS AND CHARTS

Protocols to deal with life-threatening emergency situations and also protocols for management of acute skin failure should be displayed in the form of charts as a ready reckoner [7]. A sample ready reckoner is provided at the end of the chapter (Chart 3.1). A list of topics for which ready reckoners can be displayed is given in Table 3.2. Nutrition and fluid requirement charts are also provided as ready reckoners (Charts 3.2 through 3.8).

ASEPSIS IN THE INTENSTIVE CARE UNIT

Strict asepsis in the DICU is the single most important step to avoid transmission of nosocomial infections to a patient with a compromised skin barrier [8]:

- *Universal precautions*: Should be practiced at all places and at all times.
- *Scrub station*: Should be in the anteroom of the ICU with written protocol on display for all visitors. The importance of handwashing in preventing methicillin-resistant *Staphylococcus aureus* infections cannot be overemphasized in the ICU setting. Use hand-rubs with 2% chlorhexidine between patient visits and clinical handwash solution (4% chlorhexidine) prior to invasive procedures and dressings. Handwashing should be done after handling any blood, body fluids, secretions, excretions, and contaminated items, between contact with different patients and between tasks and procedures on the same patient to prevent cross contamination between different body sites.
- *Gowns, gloves, caps, masks, shoe covers*: Personal protective equipment in the form of gowns, gloves, caps, masks, and shoe covers is of utmost importance in the

Table 3.2 List of topics whose ready reckoners can be made available

Life threatening emergencies	Acute skin failure
Management of anaphylaxis	SCORTEN
Cardiopulmonary resuscitation	Indications of antibiotics in acute skin failure
Heparinization	Fluid and calorie calculation
Management of cardiac failure	Diet chart
Management of respiratory failure	Naranjo adverse drug score
	Rule of 9 for calculating body surface area
	Drug dosage in adults and children
	Complications of Acute skin failure

setting of a reverse barrier nursing setting in a DICU. Remove and discard them into the appropriate bins immediately after visiting each patient.

- *DICU entry drill*: The first step before entering a DICU should be an antiseptic hand-wash followed by wearing of the cap, mask, and shoecovers. The DICU door should be pushed open with the help of the shoulders to prevent contamination of hands. Gown and gloves should be worn inside the DICU. The time during which gloves and gown are being worn is utilized in assessing the look of the patient. After wearing the gloves and gown, the hands should be kept in "Namaskar" position (Figure 3.3) to prevent inadvertent touching of unsterile surfaces. Inside the DICU all sterility measures are to be followed:

- *Waste disposal*: It is mandatory to have three covered bins (yellow, red, and black) in the DICU to dispose different grades of wastes. In addition, a white puncture-proof container for sharps disposal is mandatory. Wastes are to be disposed of in accordance with each country's respective regulations (in India, with Bio-Medical Waste Management Rules 2016 [10]).

- *Routine cleaning procedure in ICU*
  - Remove all portable equipment.
  - Scrub floor using detergent and water.
  - After washing floors, allow disinfectant solution in the form of 0.5% chlorine solution to remain on the floor for 5 minutes to ensure destruction of bacteria.
  - Wipe down walls with clean cloth and detergent.

- *Fumigation of ICU*: Fumigation should be undertaken when the ICU is not in use or between transfers-in of patients [9]. Formalin fumigation overnight using either a fumigator or formalin in galipot is sufficient. The ideal concentration is 500 mL of 40% formalin in 1000 mL of water for ~28 m³(1000 ft³)

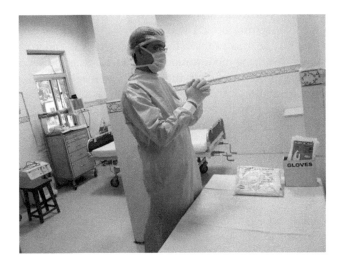

Figure 3.3 Entry drill: Gloves, gown, head cover, mask, and shoe cover to be worn before seeing the patient.

of ICU in an electric boiler/fumigator. This requires the sealing of windows and doors overnight while fumigating.

Recommendations for disinfecting various equipment in ICU: These are provided in Table 3.3 [8].

TRAINING

The philosophy of "treat-learn-treat" is to be followed. The hands-on management of patients in the DICU presents unique practical problems that can be solved by a motivated treating team. The skills learned need to be passed on to the junior members of the team who join the dermatology department subsequently.

CHALLENGES LIKELY TO BE FACED

Development of infrastructure: Dermatology and ICU is an oxymoron for nondermatologists. The projection for a stand-alone DICU requires convincing the hospital administration. Building a DICU from scratch requires planning, construction or modification of existing structure, and procurement of equipment.

Change of "our" mind-set: Acknowledging the importance and the will to establish a DICU by our own fraternity is also a huge challenge. But once cases are managed successfully in such DICUs, this issue may solve itself.

Maintaining strict asepsis: Training skin personnel to follow aseptic precautions starting from the entry drill to the nursing management of the skin requires efforts. The importance of reverse barrier nursing has to be reinforced, and this in itself can lead to very gratifying results.

Reducing crossreferrals: Relearned simple bedside procedures like insertion of a nasogastric tube, catheterization of urinary bladder, and dressing of pressure sores by the resident doctors and paramedics can reduce cross referrals. Other procedures like sweeping of the fornices of the eyes with sterile glass rod, once learned from the ophthalmologists, can be done by the DICU staff. Reducing cross referrals helps to minimize the number of personnel involved in direct contact with the patient and hence contributes to maintenance of asepsis.

Change of mind-set of other specialists: Initial resistance for consultation from the nondermatologists to see the patient at a place different than that of the conventional ICU may present itself, but better survival rates at the DICU can convince them of the concept.

CONCLUSION

A DICU is a new concept. Such a setup is important for better management of all dermatological emergencies. With increasing knowledge about pathogenesis, laboratory parameters, and newer treatment modalities, a DICU is the ideal place for treating acute skin failure and other

Table 3.3 Recommendations for disinfecting equipment

Equipment	Recommendation
Oral Thermometer	After each use, the thermometer is disinfected by wiping with a swab saturated with 70% isopropyl alcohol. Separate thermometer for individual patients should be used.
Sphygmomanometer Cuffs	Change covers regularly (1 per week) and wash inflatable section in detergent and water. Dry thoroughly or use 70% alcohol.
Bed ends, frames, Bedside locker, Cardiac table, Curtain rails	Mop with 1% sodium hypochlorite. Allow to dry.
Bowls-Bedpans/Urinals	Heat disinfection in a rinse temperature of minimum 82°C for 2 minutes. If not possible, bed pans, urine pots, and kidney trays should be kept in 7% Lysol for 24 hours or 3%–5% sodium hypochlorite solution for 30 minutes. Thereafter they are washed with soap and water and dried in sunlight.
Mattresses and Pillow	All should be covered with an impervious plastic cover. Plastic and rubber covers of mattresses and pillows should be washed with soap and water, cleaned with a suitable disinfectant, for example, 7% Lysol. Mattresses should be cleaned regularly. If possible keep in sunlight for 24 hours.
Toilet Bowls	Daily cleaning with a commercial bowl cleanser.
Bathrooms	Cleaned regularly and disinfected with phenol.
Ampoules/vials	Wipe neck (ampoule) or top surface of rubber cap (vials) with a 70% isopropyl alcohol impregnated swab and allow to dry before opening or piercing.
Soiled linen	Linen should be stripped off from the bed, taking care not to shake the linen during this action. The linen should be bagged properly before being sent to the laundry in a leak-proof bag. Washing with hot water and detergent has been shown to result in adequate cleaning of laundry. If needed for other reasons, bleach or ironing will reduce microbial contamination. Only linen used in procedures requiring sterile technique should be sterilized.

skin emergencies with a multidisciplinary and multiprong approach.

CASE STUDY: SETTING UP OF DERMATOLOGY INTENSIVE CARE UNIT IN A RESOURCE-POOR SETTING

The guidelines presented have been recommended for setting up a standard DICU, which in a resource-poor setting is generally not feasible. However, having a separate DICU facility with a less than ideal infrastructure is, in the author's experience, a better option than treating dermatology patients in a general ICU. The setting up of such a facility is much easier than it seems and is achievable even in an institution with availability of moderate resources.

Structure

A 6 × 6 meter (20 × 20 feet) room with one attached toilet, sufficient enough to place two beds can be selected to be set up for the DICU. All of the equipment and drugs listed earlier except portable x-ray machine and ventilator can be placed here.

A few adjustments that can be made in setting up a resource-constraint ICU are as given in Table 3.4.

While setting up a DICU in a resource-poor setting, there may be constraints in the space, equipment, and manpower, requiring modification of the ideal setup. However, maintenance of asepsis in the DICU is nonnegotiable. The basic structure of the DICU needs to be as sealed as possible from the outer environment. Fumigation of the DICU is done in the same manner as in the operating room and in

Table 3.4 Adjustments which can be done for a practical DICU

	Ideal ICU	Practical ICU
Space	5 rooms (for patients, doctors, waiting room with lockers for attendants, store room and toilet)	1 room
Number of beds	5 or more	2
Manpower	Exclusively for DICU	From existing manpower

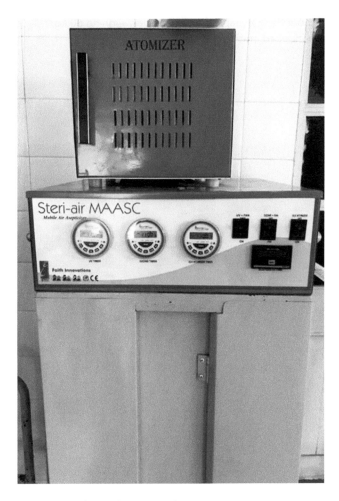

Figure 3.4 Ultraviolet air sterilizer.

a general ICU. To maintain sterility, install commercially available portable air purifiers that have HEPA filters that remove airborne particles of 0.3 microns with a minimum efficiency of 99.9% (Figure 3.4). These are much cheaper than the HVAC system.

KEY POINTS

- Dermatology ICU is a new concept.
- It is the ideal place for treatment of dermatological emergencies.
- 2-4 bed DICU with necessary equipment and staff are an essential requirement for management of dermaological emergency patients.
- Proper hygiene practises, protocols and training are cornerstones for managing patients successfully.

REFERENCES

1. Rungta N et al. ICU planning and designing in India. *Guidelines* 2010.
2. Valentin A et al. ESICM Working Group on Quality Improvement. Recommendations on basic requirements for intensive care units: Structural and organizational aspects. *Intensive Care Med* 2011;37:1575.
3. Arora MK et al. Minimum standards for ICU to be adopted throughout the country. *Draft prepared by the committee at AIIMS.* May 2012.
4. Inamadar AC. Dermatology intensive care unit (DICU). In: Inamadar AC (Ed). *Critical Care in Dermatology.* New Delhi: Jaypee Brothers Medical Publishers; 2013: 177–85.
5. Guideline for Intensive Care Unit Design Faculty of Critical Care Medicine College of Anaesthesiologistsand Intensivists of Sri Lanka. November 2016.
6. Gupta LK et al. Guidelines for the management of Stevens-Johnson syndrome/toxic epidermal necrolysis: An Indian perspective. *Indian J Dermatol Venereol Leprol* 2016;82(6):603–25.
7. Inamadar AC, Palit A. Acute skin failure: Concept, causes, consequences and care. *Indian J Dermatol Venereol Leprol* 2005;71:379–85.
8. NABH guidelines for hospital infection control manual for small healthcare organizations. New Delhi: National Accreditation Board for Hospitals and Healthcare Providers.
9. Omprakash HM. *Setting up a DermatosurgeryUnit. In: Venkataram M; Association of Cutaneous Surgeons of India (Eds), ACS(I) Textbook on Cutaneous and Aesthetic Surgery.* 2nd ed., Volume 1, Section 1. New Delhi: Jaypee Brothers Medical Publishers; 2017.
10. Bio-MedicalWaste Management Guidelines. *Government of India Ministry of Environment, Forest and Climate Change Notification.* New Delhi. March 28, 2016.
11. Walsh S, Lee HY, Creamer D. Severe cutaneous adverse reactions to drugs. In: Griffiths CEM, Barker J, Bleiker T, Creamer CR (Eds), *Rook's Textbook of Dermatology.* 9th ed. Part 11, Section 119. Edinburgh: Wiley Blackwell; 2016;13–23.
12. Noor NM, Hussein SH. Transepidermal water loss in erythrodermic patient of various etiologies. *Skin ResTechnol* 2013;19:320–3.

Chart 3.1 Ready Reckoner: Toxic epidermal necrolysis (TEN)/erythroderma: 65-year-old male/female weighing 60 kg presenting with TEN of 50% body surface area involvement or drug-induced erythroderma

General measures

Admit in dermatology intensive care unit
Withdrawal of offending drug
Asepsis precautions, reverse barrier nursing
Room temperature: 30°C−32°C
Nurse in propped-up position
Frequent change of position
Chest and limb physiotherapy

Initial assessment

Assess the "look of the patient"
Consciousness and orientation
Interest or disinterest of patient in the activities going on in the vicinity
Vital parameters
Area and severity of skin involvement
Systemic examination
Go through previous case notes for details:
- Course of the illness
- Comorbidities
- Previous admissions
- Treatment history and response
- Investigations carried out
- Drug reactions

Investigations

Confirming the diagnosis: Skin biopsy (in case the diagnosis is in doubt, or for medicolegal purposes)
Rule out comorbidities and complications
Workup for therapy

Investigations chart

	Baseline/On admission	Daily	Every 3 days	When indicated
Complete blood count	+	+	−	−
Peripheral blood smear (PBS) for sepsis, Sézary cells (in erythroderma)	+	+	−	−
Blood sugar	+	+	−	−
Liver function tests	+	+	−	−
Renal function tests	+	+	−	−
Serum electrolytes	+	+	−	−
Urine—routine microscopy	+	+	−	−
Bicarbonate levels (arterial blood gas analysis for severity of illness score for toxic epidermal necrolysis)	+	−	−	+
C-reactive protein	+	−	−	+
Erythrocyte sedimentation rate	+	−	−	+
Serum procalcitonin	+	−	−	+
Coagulation studies (especially when patient is expected to be bed bound for more than 3 days)	−	−	−	+
Chest x-ray and electrocardiogram	+	−	−	+
Blood culture	+	−	+	−
Urine culture	+	−	+	−
Skin swab culture minimum three sites	+	−	+	−
(Catheter tip culture IV and urine)	−	−	−	+, on removal
Anti- Hepatitis C virus (HCV) (risk due to oozing/bleeding from skin)	+	−	−	−
Enzyme-linked immunosorbent assay for HIV	+	−	−	−
HBsAg	+	−	−	−
Serum amylase	−	−	−	+
Skin biopsy	−	−	−	+
Lymph node biopsy	−	−	−	+

Chart 3.2 Fluid and nutrition requirements in adults (weight: 60 kg)

	Stevens-Johnson syndrome/toxic epidermal necrolysis (SJS/TEN)/TEN/Extensive erosions in vesicobullous disorders	Erythroderma
Fluid resuscitation in acute illness	Intravenous crystalloid fluid at 2 mL/kg body weight/% of body surface areaepidermal detachment [11]	Fluid intake of 2 L/day in addition to total urine output to replace increased transepidermal water loss [12] (approximately a total of 3–3.5 L/day)
Maintenance fluids	The maintenance fluid is titrated so as to maintain a urine output between 50–100 mL/h; shift gradually from IV to oral fluids	
Calorie requirement	1500–2000 Kcal on day 1; progressive increase of 500 Kcal/day to 3500–4000 Kcal	
Protein requirement	2–3 g/kg body weight per day (120–180 g/day)	

Chart 3.3 Fluid and nutrition requirements in a pediatric patient

	Stevens-Johnson syndrome/toxic epidermal necrolysis(SJS/TEN)/TEN/Extensive erosions in vesicobullous disorders	Erythroderma
Fluid resuscitation on day 1	Two-thirds of Parkland formula (4 mL/kg/% body surface area [BSA] involved); half of calculated volume given in first 8 hours and half in 16 hours; fluid of choice: N/3 normal saline	Resuscitate with IV fluids only if there is severe dehydration.
Maintenance fluids	100 mL/kg/day for first 10 kg(1000 mL);50 mL/kg/day for next 10 kg(1000 mL + 500 mL); 20 mL/kg/day above 20 kg (1500 mL + 20 mL/kg); fluid of choice:N/2 normal salinein 5% dextrose	As per daily requirement and increased fluid loss due to erythroderma.
Calorie requirement	Sutherland formula: 60 kcal/kg + 35 kcal/% BSA involved	As per daily requirement and existing deficit if erythroderma is chronic.
Protein requirement	Davies formula: 3 g/kg + 1g/% BSA involved	As per daily requirement and existing deficit if erythroderma is chronic.

Chart 3.4 Sample diet chart for Ryle tube feeds in dermatology intensive care unit (day 1)[a] (nonvegetarian) (for toxic epidermal necrolysis patient weighing 60 kg with 50% involvement of body surface area)

Sr No.	Time	Food products	Total calories (kcal)	Total proteins (g)
1.	0700 H	200 mL of milk	120	7
		02 eggs	140	12
		02 scoops Proteinex (50 g)	180	16
		Total	440	35
2.	1030 H	01 cup cooked pulses	90	6
		01 banana	80	1
		Total	170	7
3.	1400 H	200 mL of milk	120	7
		02 eggs	140	12
		01 scoop Proteinex (25 g)	90	8
		Total	350	27
4.	1730 H	Chicken soup (200 mL)	60	7
		1 cup cooked pulses	90	6
		Total	150	13
5.	2100 H	1 cup rice porridge (100 g)	120	4
		02 eggs	140	12
		Total	260	16
6.	0030 H	100 mL of milk	60	3
		02 ×Proteinex serving (50 g)	180	16
		Total	240	19
7.		Total	1610	118

[a] For calorie and protein increments on subsequent days refer to chart 3.8 (Choose and pick).

Chart 3.5 Sample diet chart for Ryle tube feeds in dermatology intensive care unit (day 1) (vegetarian) (for toxic epidermal necrolysis patient weighing 60 kg with 50% involvement of body surface area)

S No.	Time	Food products	Total calories (kcal)	Total proteins (g)
1.	0700 H	250 mL of milk	150	8.5
		03 scoops Proteinex (75 g)	270	24
		Total	420	32.5
2.	1030 H	01 cup cooked pulses	90	6
		01 banana	80	1
		Total	170	7
3.	1400 H	250 mL of milk	150	8.5
		02 scoop Proteinex (50 g)	180	16
		Total	330	24.5
4.	1730 H	100 g of curd	70	6
		1 cup cooked pulses	90	6
		Total	160	12
5.	2100 H	2 cups rice porridge (200 g)	240	8
		Total	240	8
6.	0030 H	100 mL of milk	60	3
		03 ×Proteinex serving (75 g)	270	24
		Total	330	27
7.		*Total*	1650	111

Chart 3.6 Sample diet chart for oral feeds in dermatology intensive care unit (day 1) (nonvegetarian) (for toxic epidermal necrolysis patient weighing 60 kg with 50% involvement of body surface area or for erythroderma patient weighing 60 kg)

	Time	Food products	Total calories (kcal)	Total proteins (g)
1.	0730 H	02 slices of white bread	160	6
		01 glass of milk (200 mL)	120	7
		01 scoop Proteinex (25 g)	90	8
		02 eggs	140	12
		Total	510	33
2.	1030 H	01 cup of tea/coffee	30	1
		Total	30	1
3.	1300 H	02 chapati	130	5
		01 cup cooked pulses	90	6
		Cooked chicken (100 g boneless)	110	23
		Total	330	34
4.	1730 H	One glass of milk (200 mL)	120	7
		01 scoop Proteinex (25 g)	90	8
		02 eggs	140	12
		Total	350	27
5.	2100 H	02 × chapatis	130	5
		01 cup cooked pulses	90	6
		Cooked chicken (50 g boneless)	55	12
		01 egg	70	06
		Total	345	29
6.		*Total*	1565	124

Chart 3.7 Sample diet chart for oral feeds in dermatology intensive care unit (day 1) (vegetarian) (for toxic epidermal necrolysis patient weighing 60 kg with 50% involvement of body surface area or for erythroderma patient weighing 60 kg)

Sr No.	Time	Food products	Total calories (kcal)	Total proteins (g)
1.	0730 H	02 slices of white bread	160	6
		01 glass of milk (200 mL)	120	7
		02 scoops Proteinex (50 g)	180	16
		Total	460	29
2.	1030 H	01 cup of cooked red beans (150 g)	200	15
		Total	200	15
3.	1300 H	02 × chapatis	130	5
		Cooked cottage cheese (100 g)	250	18
		01 cup cooked vegetables	140	5
		Total	520	28
4.	1730 H	One glass of milk (200 mL)	120	7
		01 scoop Proteinex (25 g)	90	8
		Total	210	15
5.	2100 H	02 × chapatis	130	5
		01 cup cooked soyabeans (100 g)	175	16
		100 g of curd	60	6
		Total	365	27
6.		Total	1755	114

Chart 3.8 Calorie and protein content of common food items used for increments (Pick and choose)

Sr No.	Food products	Total calories (kcal)	Total proteins (g)
1.	01 egg	70	6
2.	01 glass milk (200 mL)	120	7
3.	25 g Proteinex	90	8
4.	1 tbsp ghee	112	0.04
5.	1 tbsp butter	102	0.12
6.	01 banana (large)	110	1.5
7.	01 cup cooked rice	204	4.2
8.	01 cup cooked vegetables	90	3
9.	01 tbsp sugar	48	0
10.	18 kernels of cashew nuts	156	5

PART 2

Severe Cutaneous Drug Reactions

SHEKHAR NEEMA AND RADHAKRISHNAN SUBRAMANIAN

Stevens-Johnson syndrome/toxic epidermal necrolysis

RAMESH BHAT AND MERYL SONIA REBELLO

INTRODUCTION

SJS/TEN is a rare dermatological emergency, but probably the most challenging. It is considered as a spectrum of diseases with overlapping conditions. It is characterized by severe mucocutaneous erosions complicated by systemic involvement, which is the main cause for mortality. SJS, first described by American pediatricians Albert Stevens and Frank Johnson in 1922, involves a macular rash with painful mucosal blistering and epidermal detachment less than 10% of body surface area (BSA) [1]. TEN, also known as Lyell's syndrome, is a more severe and life-threatening condition with epidermal detachment greater than 30% BSA [2]. SJS/TEN overlap occurs with features in between SJS and TEN with 10%–30% BSA involvement. Erythema multiforme (EM) major and minor are much less severe conditions usually caused by infections, especially viral.

Bastuji-Garin et al. in 1993 [3], and Roujeau in 1994 [4], have classified and differentiated SJS/TEN and EM. Bastuji-Garin et al. have classified bullous EM and SJS/TEN into five categories as shown in Table 4.1.

EPIDEMIOLOGY

Incidence of SJS/TEN is rare, accounting for around one to two cases per million per year [5,6]. SJS/TEN occurs in all age groups, but older adults are more affected, and there is increased incidence in women.

ETIOPATHOGENESIS

SJS/TEN is primarily drug induced, which accounts for approximately 85% cases. The risk of developing SJS/TEN depends on certain internal and external environmental factors. Internal factors are the genetic makeup or susceptibility of the patient and external causes, such as drug structure, as depicted in the Swiss cheese risk model (Figure 4.1) [7].

Genetic factors

Genetic susceptibilities to various drugs have been identified. Recognition of these culprit drugs is through specific human leukocyte antigen (HLA) molecules and cytochrome polymorphisms (CYPs), which are selectively seen in these patients. This phenomenon was first described by Roujeau et al., who found an association of HLA-B12 with oxicam- and sulfonamide-related TEN [8]. Similar association with HLA-B*1502 and carbamazepine has been described by Chung et al. [9] HLA associations with SJS/TEN have been found to be associated with ethnic origin. HLA-B*1502 and carbamazepine induced TEN has been seen in Han Chinese, Indians, Malaysians, and Thais [10,11], but not in Europeans [12]. CYP2C cytochrome polymorphism has been seen in phenytoin-related SJS/TEN [13].

Environmental factors

Drugs are the major cause of SJS/TEN. Some common drugs implicated in causation of SJS/TEN are presented in

Table 4.1 Classification of bullous erythema multiforme and Stevens-Johnson syndrome/toxic epidermal necrolysis

Category	Bullous EM	SJS	SJS/TEN overlap	TEN with spots	TEN without spots
Percentage of BSA detachment	–	<10%	10%–30%	>30%	>10%
Typical target lesions	Seen	Not seen	Not seen	Not seen	Not seen
Atypical target lesions	Raised can be seen	Flat	Flat	Flat	Not seen
Widespread involvement	Not seen	Erythematous or purpuric macules	Erythematous or purpuric macules	Erythematous or purpuric macules	Large epidermal sheets without targets

Source: Bastuji-Garin S et al. *Arch Dermatol* 1993;129:92–6.
Abbreviations: BSA, body surface area; EM, erythema multiforme; SJS, Stevens-Johnson syndrome; TEN, toxic epidermal necrolysis.

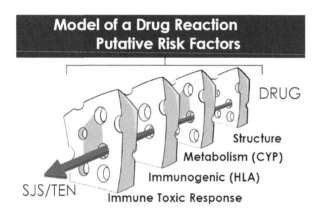

Model of a Drug Reaction Putative Risk Factors

DRUG
Structure
Metabolism (CYP)
Immunogenic (HLA)
Immune Toxic Response
SJS/TEN

Figure 4.1 Swiss cheese model for risk factors of Stevens-Johnson syndrome/toxic epidermal necrolysis.

Box 4.1. They can also occur secondary to infections like mycoplasma pneumonia, streptococcal infections, herpes simplex virus, cytomegalovirus, and live virus vaccinations [14–16].

Immunological mechanisms

SJS/TEN is a delayed-type hypersensitivity reaction with a latent period of 4–28 days. In rare cases, the latency period can be as long as 8 weeks [17]. The main mechanisms include the following:

- A drug is recognized as a foreign antigen by a T-cell receptor (TCR).
- The adaptive immune response is activated by the binding of the drug to antigen-presenting cells through HLA. This can occur in two ways:
  - p-i concept (pharmacological interaction of the drug with immune receptor): The drug directly binds to a TCR [18].
  - Hapten concept: The drug forms a complex with a peptide and then binds to TCR.
- This binding results in activation of CD8+ cytotoxic T cells and natural killer cell–mediated cytotoxicity.

BOX 4.1: Common drugs causing Stevens-Johnson syndrome/toxic epidermal necrolysis

- Allopurinol
- Carbamazepine
- Lamotrigine
- Nevirapine
- Oxicam nonsteroidal anti-inflammatory drugs
- Phenobarbital
- Phenytoin
- Sulfonamides

- A recent concept is also that HLA associated with carbamazepine can directly interact with a cytotoxic T-cell without any drug metabolism or antigen processing [19].
- The onset of the cytotoxic reaction leads to activation of cytotoxic signaling molecules, such as granulysin, perforin/granzyme B, and Fas/Fas ligand, resulting in keratinocyte apoptosis and epidermal detachment clinically [20–22].

CLINICAL FEATURES

Clinical signs and symptoms usually begin within 4 weeks (4–28 days) of drug intake [23].

Acute stage

Initially symptoms are nonspecific with painful mucous membranes, stinging of eyes, malaise, fever, and upper respiratory tract symptoms that precede the rash. In 1–3 days, mucocutaneous lesions develop, which are characterized by blistering and erosions with hemorrhagic crusting resulting in severe stomatitis (Figure 4.2) and purulent conjunctivitis. Extensive mucosal necrosis involving more than two mucosal sites is seen in 90% of cases.

Cutaneous lesions: Mainly manifest as dusky erythematous macular purpuric/flat lesions associated with pain and

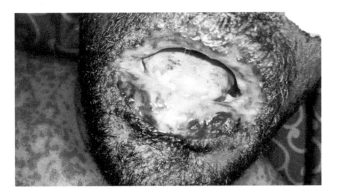

Figure 4.2 Severe mucositis in early phase.

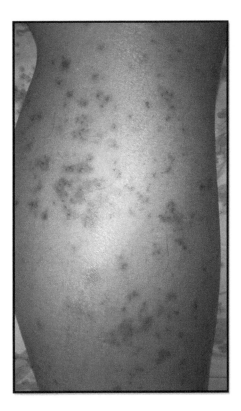

Figure 4.4 Targetoid lesions.

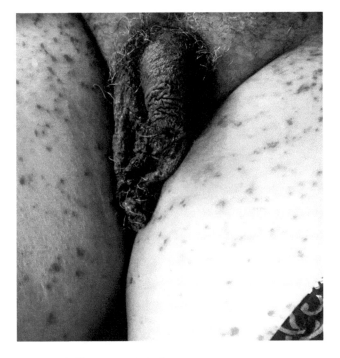

Figure 4.3 Flat purpuric lesions.

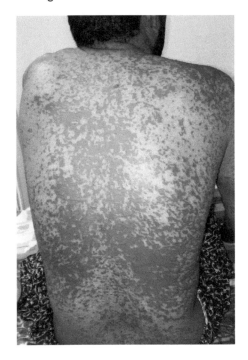

Figure 4.5 Lesions spread to trunk.

tenderness (Figure 4.3). Atypical target lesions having two concentric rings with a necrotic center are sometimes seen (Figure 4.4). Lesions start appearing over the presternal area, face, trunk, and proximal parts of limbs as shown in Figure 4.5. Over 2–3 days the lesions rapidly spread to involve the distal parts symmetrically (Figure 4.6 and 4.7). Flaccid blisters (Figure 4.8) that progress to sheet-like detachment is then classically seen (Figure 4.9). Pseudo-Nikolsky sign is positive (shearing tangential pressure over the affected skin leads to epidermal separation (Figure 4.10) [25]. Perilesional erythema is a sign of disease activity, and this is helpful in management and disease monitoring.

Mucous membranes: Involvement of mucous membranes is seen in more than 90% of cases of TEN [26–28]. Initially there is pain and burning sensation of the lips, oral cavity, conjunctivae, and genitalia, followed by development of flaccid hemorrhagic blisters as depicted in Figure 4.12. Blisters rupture and tend to extend. Erosions eventually get coated by grayish-white pseudomembranes in the oral cavity, and painful deglutition and increased salivation can occur. Involvement of mucosa of eyes leads to photophobia, pain, lacrimation, chemosis, and redness [29,30]. Severe involvement includes anterior uveitis, purulent conjunctivitis, and corneal ulcerations that can later cause blindness.

Genital erosions most often involve glans penis, scrotum (Figure 4.11), vulva, and vagina, which leads to burning

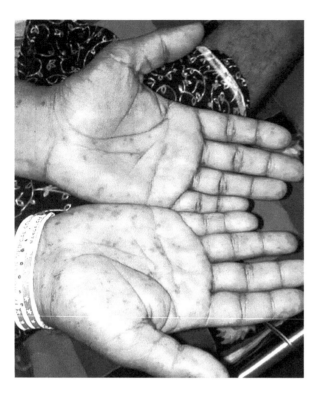

Figure 4.6 Acral involvement typically of hands and feet. Hand involvement being depicted in this image.

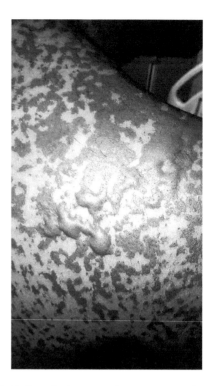

Figure 4.8 Bullous lesions overlying purpuric lesions.

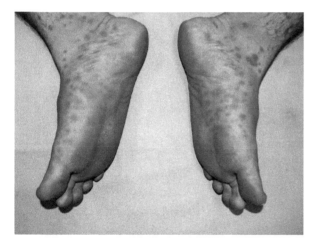

Figure 4.7 Acral involvement typically of hands and feet. Targetoid lesions on feet depicted in this image.

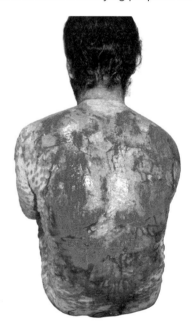

Figure 4.9 Sheet-like detachment.

micturition, urinary retention, and synechiae formation [31]. Anal lesions are less frequent (Figure 4.12).

Systemic manifestations: TEN results in acute skin failure [32]. Multiple internal organ system involvement and failure are seen as a result of extensive skin loss. Early features are barrier dysfunction with loss of water and electrolytes, thermal dysregulation, immune impairment, and infection. Hypovolemia is an early complication due to the fluid, electrolyte, and protein losses. This can result in reduced urinary outflow, and acute tubular necrosis can set in. Hypoproteinemia with daily losses of 150–200 g of protein due to increased catabolism and protein loss through the skin develops gradually.

Renal involvement is often present in TEN. Proteinuria, hematuria, and leukocyturia are seen [33]. Involvement of the gastrointestinal and respiratory tracts commonly occurs and may be caused by the release of massive amounts of pro-inflammatory cytokines into the systemic circulation. Specific involvement of bronchial epithelium must be suspected when dyspnea, bronchial hypersecretion, and marked hypoxemia are present during the early stages of TEN [7]. Delayed complications (pulmonary edema,

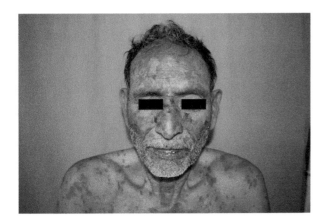

Figure 4.10 Pseudo-Nikolsky sign on forehead.

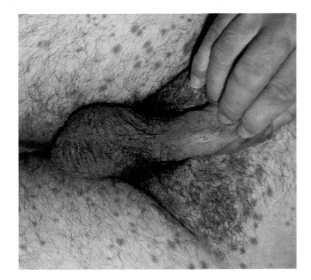

Figure 4.11 Scrotal erosions.

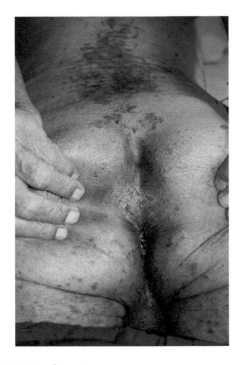

Figure 4.12 Anal erosions.

bacterial pneumonitis, and atelectasis) and long-term pulmonary function abnormalities (persistent reduction in carbon monoxide diffusing capacity) are often noted.

Esophageal erosions may result in dysphagia and bleeding. Intestinal erosions are usually asymptomatic but can manifest as bloody diarrhea, abdominal distension, and excretion of colonic intestinal epithelium, which can lead to bowel perforation [34,35].

Other metabolic complications like hyperglycemia and metabolic acidosis can occur secondary to the release of pro-inflammatory cytokines, thereby releasing stress hormones.

Skin lesions are usually colonized by *Staphylococcus aureus* during the first few days and later by *Pseudomonas aeruginosa* and other gram-negative bacilli. Extensive skin involvement with impaired immune function can increase the risk of bacteremia and sepsis [7].

In TEN, healing occurs by reepithelialization in 2 weeks with intertriginous areas, the back, pressure areas, and periorificial areas being the last to heal. Mucosal lesions can take even longer [24]. Cutaneous infections may delay healing.

Prognosis: Progression of disease lasts for about 4–5 days. After the acute phase, patients enter a plateau phase, which corresponds to progressive reepithelialization. Complete healing can take a few days to several weeks [7].

Chronic stage

Long-term sequelae can occur and should be assessed early to reduce morbidity [36]. Cutaneous sequelae frequently include hyper- and hypopigmentation (72%), scarring, nail dystrophies, and nail loss.

In around 70% of cases, late ocular complications are seen. They include dry eye syndrome, trichiasis, photophobia, symblepharon, corneal inflammation, and neovascularization. This can lead to reduced visual acuity and blindness [29,37].

Chronic inflammation, erosions, and ulcerations of genitalia lead to synechiae and stricture formation. Males may require circumcision. Strictures of vaginal mucosa can lead to dyspareunia and vaginal dryness [31]. Strictures of the birth canal can complicate vaginal delivery and cause birth complications.

MANAGEMENT

SJS/TEN is one of the true medical emergencies in dermatology. Early diagnosis and prompt treatment can be lifesaving and will yield a better prognosis. Management and prognosis depend on various factors including host factors and facilities with expertise. The most important steps of management include the following:

- Initial assessment of the patient
- Prompt withdrawal of drug
- Referral when necessary
- Supportive treatment and investigation
- Initiation of disease-modifying therapy
- Prevention of recurrence [24]

Initial assessment

To conduct the initial assessment the 5Ds as described by Shear are used: diagnosis, drug exposure, differential diagnosis, determining causality, and determining severity and mortality [7]:

- *Diagnosis*: This is based on identifying the three main features: classical cutaneous and mucous membrane involvement, systemic involvement, and histopathological findings. Histological assessment is an essential tool in the diagnosis of SJS/TEN and in ruling out diseases that mimic SJS/TEN. Characteristic features include keratinocyte destruction along the dermo-epidermal junction with perivascular mononuclear cell infiltrate in the papillary dermis with spongiosis and exocytosis. Close contact between dyskeratotic (necrotic) keratinocytes and sparse mononuclear cells ("satellite cell necrosis") is seen along with extensive keratinocyte necrosis and sometimes basal vacuolar degeneration leading to bulla formation at the dermoepidermal junction [38]. A skin biopsy for direct immunofluorescence (DIF) from perilesional skin is necessary, with a negative DIF confirming the diagnosis.
- *Drug exposure*: All medications taken 8 weeks prior to symptom development have to be taken into account [7].
- *Differential diagnosis*: This includes conditions mentioned in Box 4.2 [7,39].
- *Determining causality*: The most common cause of SJS/TEN is drug exposure [16]. Other causes include infection, contrast media, and vaccination [14,41–42].
- *Determining severity and mortality*: This is assessed by a scoring system called the *severity of illness score for toxic epidermal necrolysis* (SCORTEN) [43]. The first scoring is done within 24 hours of admission and then repeated again on the 3rd day. It consists of seven risk factors as shown in Box 4.3. Each is given a score of one and a total score is calculated by summing up the number of abnormal parameters. The prognostic value of SCORTEN is more accurate at day 3 of hospitalization [44]. Accordingly mortality rates are predicted as seen in Table 4.2 [24].

BOX 4.2: Differential diagnosis

- Erythema multiforme major
- Pemphigus vulgaris
- Mucous membrane and bullous pemphigoid
- Paraneoplastic pemphigus
- Staphylococcal scalded skin syndrome
- Generalized bullous fixed drug eruption
- Acute graft versus host reaction
- Toxic epidermal necrolysis (TEN)-like lupus erythematosus or lupus-associated TEN

BOX 4.3: Prognostic parameters of severity of illness score for toxic epidermal necrolysis (SCORTEN)

- Age older than 40 years
- Presence of malignancy
- Tachycardia (heart rate >120 beats/minutes)
- Initial percentage of epidermal detachment >10%
- Blood urea nitrogen >28 mg/dL
- Serum glucose >252 mg/dL
- Serum bicarbonate level 20 mmol/L

Table 4.2 Mortality rates according to severity of illness score for toxic epidermal necrolysis (SCORTEN)

SCORTEN	Mortality rate (%)
1	3.2
2	12.1
3	35.3
4	58.3
≥5	90

Investigations

Investigations are required to assess the degree of underlying damage to various organ systems and to determine prognosis along with further treatment. They include the following:

- Complete blood count
- Liver and renal function tests
- Blood electrolytes
- Blood sugar
- Urine—routine and microscopy
- Skin swab culture
- Blood culture
- Chest x-ray
- Mycoplasma serology
- Antinuclear antibody
- Skin biopsy

No standard confirmatory test has yet been found. But a rapid immunochromatographic test for serum granulysin has been found useful in predicting SJS/TEN [45].

Prompt withdrawal of drug

Immediate withdrawal of drug is of prime importance in controlling the disease process. Essential drugs have to be substituted in consultation with the treating physician.

Prompt referral

Early referral to centers with dermatology intensive care units, intensive care units, and burns units whenever necessary for a multidisciplinary approach will improve prognosis in these patients.

Supportive care

According to the Indian Association of Dermatology, Venereology, and Leprology (IADVL) consensus Guidelines, supportive care includes [46] the following:

Temperature regulation: Environmental temperature maintenance at 30°C–32°C helps to reduce catabolism and prevent caloric losses from the body.

Monitoring: Frequent monitoring of vital signs is important as they alert us of worsening systemic conditions. Monitoring is done initially at baseline and subsequently at periodic intervals. Parameters assessed include pulse rate, blood pressure, respiratory rate, fluid intake, urine output, blood glucose, serum electrolytes, serum creatinine, and specific cultures. Coagulation assays, D-dimer assays, and fibrin degradation products are monitored to look for septicemia and disseminated intravascular coagulation (DIC).

Prevention of infection: The following measures are important to prevent sepsis in patients with SJS/TEN:

- Barrier nursing and sterile handling of the patient
- Regular hand hygiene with chlorhexidine hand rubs and hand washes to be practiced by health-care workers and caregivers
- Avoid unnecessary insertion of urinary catheters, intravenous lines, or central lines
- If used, urinary catheters, intravenous lines, and central lines must be handled minimally and changed regularly
- Monitor for foci of sepsis in the body and for features of septicemia and DIC
- Environmental controls for dependency units (air exchanges, humidity and temperature control) and intensive care unit
- Activate sepsis protocols early
- Judicious use of antibiotics

Fluid and electrolyte balance: Fluid requirement is calculated by the Parkland formula:

- Fluid requirement = 4 mL/kg body weight × percentage of body surface area involved.
- The fluid requirement in TEN is only three-quarters of that required for burns as calculated. Of this half the fluid is administered in the first 8 hours and the other half in the next 16 hours. Fluid requirements beyond the first 24 hours should be managed according to the patient's condition (based on oral fluid intake and output).
- Input and output charting is useful to guide fluid administration. Urine output between 1000 and 1500 mL is maintained. Overcorrection may lead to pulmonary edema. Blood transfusion may be useful in some cases to dilute the drug metabolites, autoantibodies, and cytokines [47].

Feeding: Oral liquid diet, nasogastric tube, or total parenteral nutrition should be initiated. Caloric requirements are 30–35 kcal/kg/day and proteins of 1.5 g/kg/day have to be provided.

Care of skin and mucosa: Topical antiseptics after compression of denuded areas with normal saline-soaked gauze pieces. Detached skin has to be left in place. Adhesive dressings are to be avoided.

Oral care can be maintained by normal saline or antiseptic gargles. Saline compresses can be done for removing the lip crusting.

For eyes, lubricating and antibiotic eye drops are usually used. Lid adhesions are removed with glass rod sweeping of the fornices. Topical corticosteroids and cycloplegic eye drops are also advocated to prevent corneal scars and relieve pain, photophobia, and ciliary spasm [48]. Cyclosporine eye drops are also a useful adjunct. Bandage contact lenses and amniotic membrane grafting are done to facilitate reepithelialization of the ocular surface [49].

Genital mucosa can be treated by wet dressings or sitz baths, and lubrication with emollients is advised to avoid adhesions and stricture formation [50,51]. Intravaginal steroids and vaginal molds are used to prevent complications.

Respiratory care: Saline aerosols, bronchial aspiration, and postural drainage are methods to keep respiratory mucosa healthy.

Others: Antacids for gastrointestinal mucosa, analgesics and antipyretics to reduce the inflammatory process, anticoagulants in cases where there is risk for DIC, and psychological care by counseling the patient and family are other important measures [52].

Disease-modifying therapy

Disease-modifying therapy is aimed at halting the immunological processes that led to keratinocyte apoptosis. Various immunomodulating agents such as systemic corticosteroids, cyclosporine, intravenous immunoglobulin, plasmapheresis, tumor necrosis factor-α inhibitors, granulocyte colony-stimulating factor, and N-acetylcysteine have been used [24].

Systemic corticosteroids: These were the mainstay of therapy for SJS and TEN until recently. They work by both anti-inflammatory action and by inhibiting the immune-mediated process. A high dose at an early stage for a short duration is the ideal option [53,54].

Various authors have used corticosteroids in different protocols:

- Dexamethasone at a dose of 1 mg/kg. The corticosteroids are tapered and withdrawn within 5 days after the subsidence of erythema [54].
- Intravenous pulsed-dose methylprednisolone (three consecutive daily infusions of 20–30 mg/kg to a maximum of 500 mg given over 2–3 hours) [55].
- Hirahara et al. gave an infusion of methylprednisolone at 1000 mg/day for 3 consecutive days, followed by oral prednisolone at 0.8–1 mg/kg/day in tapering doses [56].
- Dexamethasone pulse therapy (1.5 mg/kg intravenous over 30–60 minutes on 3 consecutive days) to avoid long-term use of systemic corticosteroids [57].

Cyclosporine (CsA): Cyclosporine inhibits the activation of CD4+ and CD8+ (cytotoxic) T cells in the epidermis by suppressing interleukin-2 production. Cyclosporine is used in a dose of 3–5 mg/kg body weight, as oral capsules or solution for 7–10 days, or until resolution of skin lesions and reepithelization occurs [58]. It is presently one of the first-line drugs for use in SJS/TEN. Cyclosporine in combination with suprapharmacological doses of intravenous dexamethasone has been successfully used in the treatment of SJS/TEN [59].

Intravenous immunoglobulin: In 1998, Viard et al. demonstrated the reversal of Fas-mediated keratinocyte apoptosis by human immunoglobulin by *in vitro* studies [21]. The dose of IVIg used for treatment is 3 gm/kg. However, recent meta-analysis suggests that IVIg does not provide any mortality benefit as compared to supportive therapy.

TNF Inhibitors: Treatment with anti-TNF biologic agents seems to be very promising for the management of SJS/TEN [61,62]. In a recent study in 10 consecutive patients with TEN, 50 mg of etanercept was administered in a single subcutaneous injection. All patients responded promptly to treatment, reaching complete reepithelialization without complications or side effects [63].

Other therapies: Plasmapheresis, pentoxifylline, N-acetyl cysteine, and cyclophosphamide have been tried in cases of SJS/TEN with variable outcomes [64–67].

Prevention of recurrence

Cases should be notified to regulatory bodies. Patients should be advised to avoid reexposure to the suspect drug or related compounds [24].

STEVENS-JOHNSON SYNDROME/TOXIC EPIDERMAL NECROLYSIS IN PREGNANCY

Toxic epidermal necrolysis in pregnancy puts two lives at risk; hence, it requires the immediate attention of both dermatologist and gynecologist [68–70].

Management in pregnant women is not very different from nonpregnant patients. Systemic steroids are not favored in the first trimester but may be useful especially in the third trimester as they also help increase the lung maturity of the fetus. Intravenous immunoglobulin and cyclosporine can also be used in some cases [16].

STEVENS-JOHNSON SYNDROME/TOXIC EPIDERMAL NECROLYSIS IN CHILDREN

SJS/TEN in children occurs similarly as in adults, with respect to etiology and clinical features, and management also remains the same. Drugs are the most common etiology as seen in adults; however, the incidence of infections (*Mycoplasma* and *Cytomegalovirus*) inducing SJS/TEN is relatively higher in children as compared to adults [71]. Corticosteroids, intravenous immunoglobulin, and cyclosporine were therapies used for treatment of pediatric SJS/TEN in various studies [40,60].

SUMMARY OF THE INDIAN GUIDELINES AND RECOMMENDATIONS

For the management of SJS, SJS/TEN overlap, and TEN, the IADVL special interest group on cutaneous adverse drug reactions (SIG-CADR) recommends the following:

1. Immediately withdraw all suspected and offending drug(s) and related compounds.
2. Initiate supportive therapy as the primary measure to be undertaken in all patients of SJS/TEN presenting to a health-care provider.
3. If the rash has been identified at a primary or secondary health-care center, the treatment should be initialized and the patient referred to a tertiary care center for care by a dermatologist.
4. If resources are available, the treatment may be carried out in an intensive care setting or in an isolated room with maintenance of a sterile field.
5. A multidisciplinary approach involving dermatologist, physician/pediatrician, ophthalmologist, respiratory physician, intensivist, dietician, and any other specialist as per the need of the case should be adopted.
6. Disease-modifying treatment must be initiated as early as possible.
7. Systemic corticosteroids (preferably parenteral) were previously recommended as the disease-modifying treatment of choice. Prednisolone, dexamethasone, or methylprednisolone should be given early (preferably within 72 hours) in high dosage (1–2 mg/kg/day prednisolone or 8–16 mg/day of dexamethasone intravenous or intramuscular). A daily assessment of disease activity (such as the appearance of new lesions, perilesional erythema, and skin tenderness) should be done, and steroids should be maintained at the same dose until disease activity ceases. Thereafter, the dosage should be tapered quickly such that the total duration of steroid therapy is approximately 7–10 days. Steroids can also be administered in pulse form, employing slow intravenous infusion of methylprednisolone (500–1000 mg/day) or dexamethasone (100 mg) for 3 days.
8. Cyclosporine can also be employed alone (3–5 mg/kg/day for 10–14 days), especially in patients with relative contraindications to corticosteroid use (e.g., patients with tuberculosis and severe hyperglycemia). Presently it can also be used as a drug of first choice.
9. If both steroids and cyclosporine are used, steroids can be tapered even more quickly (2–3 days), and cyclosporine (3–5 mg/kg/day) can be continued for 7–10 days.
10. If a patient reports at a stage when the disease activity has already ceased, there is no need of any disease-modifying treatment. Such patients should be managed by supportive therapy alone.
11. Monitoring and management of complications (vital signs, signs of sepsis and systemic involvement) and sequelae with the help of a multidisciplinary team of specialists is important.

12. In patients with human immunodeficiency virus, children, and pregnant women in the first trimester, low-doses of intravenous immunoglobulin (cumulative dose 0.2–0.5 mg/kg) may be considered, given in the first 24–48 hours.
13. Strict avoidance of offending, suspected, or related drug(s) is absolutely necessary. A drug card should be issued to facilitate this.

CONCLUSION

SJS/TEN is one of the true dermatological emergencies. Though rare, risks of acute skin failure are high. Generally in dermatological practice, emergencies are not commonly encountered; hence, dermatologists are less acquainted with such scenarios, and treating these patients is more challenging. Due to the high mortality risks and long-term complications, early diagnosis with effective prompt treatment is necessary. Also, a multidisciplinary approach to the case will be beneficial to the patient and the doctor.

KEY POINTS

- SJS/TEN is one of the most important and common dermatological emergencies.
- SJS/TEN is caused mainly by drugs though infections s a cause may be more commoner in children.
- Targetoid skin lesions, purpura, skin detachment and mucosal erosions are the commonest cutaneous features.
- Multisystem involvement especially lungs, kidneys and hepatobiliary system are commonly involved.
- SCORTEN can be used to monitor patient prognosis.
- Systemic corticosteroids, Cyclosporine, IVIg, Etanercept are some of the mainline specific therapies.
- Supportive care is the cornerstone of therapy.

REFERENCES

1. Stevens A, Johnson F. A new eruptive fever associated with stomatitis and ophthalmia: Report of two cases in children. *Arch Pediatr Adolesc Med* 1922;24:526–33.
2. Lyell A. Toxic epidermal necrolysis: An eruption resembling scalding of the skin. *Br J Dermatol* 1956;68:355–61.
3. Bastuji-Garin S, Rzany B, Stern RS, Shear NH, Naldi L, Roujeau JC. Clinical classification of cases of toxic epidermal necrolysis, Stevens-Johnson syndrome, and erythema multiforme. *Arch Dermatol* 1993;129:92–6.
4. Roujeau JC. The spectrum of Stevens-Johnson syndrome and toxic epidermal necrolysis: A clinical classification. *J Invest Dermatol* 1994;102:28S–30S.
5. Roujeau J-C, Guillaume J-C, Fabre J-D, Penso D, Flechet ML, Girre JP. Toxic epidermal necrolysis (Lyell syndrome): Incidence and drug aetiology in France. *Arch Dermatol* 1990;126:37–42.
6. Rzany B et al. Epidemiology of erythema exudativum multiforme majus, Stevens-Johnson syndrome, and toxic epidermal necrolysis in Germany: Structure and results of a population based registry. *J Clin Epidemiol* 1996;49:769–73.
7. Dodiuk-Gad RP, Chung WH, Valeyrie-Allanore L, Shear NH. Stevens-Johnson syndrome and toxic epidermal necrolysis: An update. *Am J Clin Dermatol* 2015;16:475–93.
8. Roujeau JC, Huynh TN, Bracq C, Guillaume J-C, Revuz J, Touraine R. Genetic susceptibility to toxic epidermal necrolysis. *Arch Dermatol* 1987;123:1171–3.
9. Chung WH et al. Medical genetics: A marker for Stevens–Johnson syndrome. *Nature* 2004;428:486.
10. Mehta TY et al. Association of HLA-B*1502 allele and carbamazepine-induced Stevens-Johnson syndrome among Indians. *Indian J Dermatol Venereol Leprol* 2009;75:579–82.
11. Tangamornsuksan W, Chaiyakunapruk N, Somkrua R, Lohitnavy M, Tassaneeyakul W. Relationship between the HLA-B*1502 allele and carbamazepine-induced Stevens-Johnson syndrome and toxic epidermal necrolysis: A systematic review and meta-analysis. *JAMA Dermatol* 2013;149:1025–32.
12. Chung WH, Hung SI. Recent advances in the genetics and immunology of Stevens-Johnson syndrome and toxic epidermal necrosis. *J Dermatol Sci* 2012;66:190–6.
13. Chung WH et al. Genetic variants associated with phenytoin-related severe cutaneous adverse reactions. *JAMA* 2014;312:525–34.
14. Fournier S, Bastuji-Garin S, Mentec H, Revuz J, Roujeau JC. Toxic epidermal necrolysis associated with *Mycoplasma pneumoniae* infection. *Eur J Clin Microbiol Infect Dis* 1995;14:558–9.
15. Mulvey JM, Padowitz A, Lindley-Jones M, Nickels R. *Mycoplasma pneumoniae* associated with Stevens-Johnson syndrome. *Anaesth Intensive Care* 2007;35:414–7.
16. Harr T, French LE. Toxic epidermal necrolysis and Stevens-Johnson syndrome. *Orphanet J Rare Dis* 2010;5:39.
17. Lerch M, Pichler WJ. The immunological and clinical spectrum of delayed drug-induced exanthems. *Curr Opin Allergy Clin Immunol* 2004;4:411–9.
18. Pichler WJ. Pharmacological interaction of drugs with antigen-specific immune receptors: The p-i concept. *Curr Opin Allergy Clin Immunol* 2002;2:301–5.

19. Wei CY, Chung WH, Huang HW, Chen YT, Hung SI. Direct interaction between HLA-B and carbamazepine activates T cells in patients with Stevens-Johnson syndrome. *J Allergy Clin Immunol* 2012;129:1562–9.

20. Chung WH et al. Granulysin is a key mediator for disseminated keratinocyte death in Stevens-Johnson syndrome and toxic epidermal necrolysis. *Nat Med* 2008;14:1343–50.

21. Viard I et al. Inhibition of toxic epidermal necrolysis by blockade of CD95 with human intravenous immunoglobulin. *Science* 1998;282:490–3.

22. Nassif A et al. Drug specific cytotoxic T-cells in the skin lesions of a patient with toxic epidermal necrolysis. *J Investig Dermatol* 2002;118:728–33.

23. Mockenhaupt M et al. Stevens-Johnson syndrome and toxic epidermal necrolysis: Assessment of medication risks with emphasis on recently marketed drugs. The EuroSCAR-study. *J Investig Dermatol* 2008;128:35–44.

24. Gupta LK et al. Guidelines for the management of Stevens-Johnson syndrome/toxic epidermal necrolysis: An Indian perspective. *Indian J Dermatol Venereol Leprol* 2016;82(6):603–25.

25. Sachdev D. Sign of Nikolsky and related signs. *Indian J Dermatol Venereol Leprol* 2003;69:243–4.

26. Assier H, Bastuji-Garin S, Revuz J, Roujeau JC. Erythema multiforme with mucous membrane involvement and Stevens-Johnson syndrome are clinically different disorders with distinct causes. *Arch Dermatol* 1995;13:539–43.

27. Revuz J et al. Toxic epidermal necrolysis: Clinical findings and prognosis factors in 87 patients. *Arch Dermatol* 1987;123:1160–5.

28. Rajaratnam R et al. Toxic epidermal necrolysis: Retrospective analysis of 21 consecutive cases managed at a tertiary centre. *Clin Exp Dermatol* 2010;35:853–62.

29. Gueudry J, Roujeau JC, Binaghi M, Soubrane G, Muraine M. Risk factors for the development of ocular complications of Stevens-Johnson syndrome and toxic epidermal necrolysis. *Arch Dermatol* 2009;145:157–62.

30. Sotozono C et al. Diagnosis and treatment of Stevens-Johnson syndrome and toxic epidermal necrolysis with ocular complications. *Ophthalmology* 2009;116:685–90.

31. Meneux E, Wolkenstein P, Haddad B, Roujeau JC, Revuz J, Paniel BJ. Vulvovaginal involvement in toxic epidermal necrolysis: A retrospective study of 40 cases. *Obstet Gynecol* 1998;91:283–7.

32. Pereira FA, Mudgil AV, Rosmarin DM. Toxic epidermal necrolysis. *J Am Acad Dermatol* 2007;56:181–200.

33. Hung CC, Liu WC, Kuo MC, Lee CH, Hwang SJ, Chen HC. Acute renal failure and its risk factors in Stevens-Johnson syndrome and toxic epidermal necrolysis. *Am J Nephrol* 2009;29:633–8.

34. Michel P et al. Ileal involvement in toxic epidermal necrolysis (Lyell syndrome). *Dig Dis Sci* 1993;38:1938–41.

35. Powell N, Munro JM, Rowbotham D. Colonic involvement in Stevens-Johnson syndrome. *Postgrad Med J* 2006;82:10.

36. Fellahi A, Zouhair K, Amraoui A, Benchikhi H. Stevens-Johnson and Lyell syndromes: Mucocutaneous and ocular sequels in 43 cases. *Ann Dermatol Venereol* 2011;138:88–92.

37. Morales ME, Purdue GF, Verity SM, Arnoldo BD, Blomquist PH. Ophthalmic manifestations of Stevens-Johnson syndrome and toxic epidermal necrolysis and relation to SCORTEN. *Am J Ophthalmol* 2010;150:505–10.

38. Quinn AM et al. Uncovering histologic criteria with prognostic significance in toxic epidermal necrolysis. *Arch Dermatol* 2005;141:683–7.

39. Walsh S, Lee HY, Creamer D. Severe cutaneous adverse reactions to drugs. In: Griffiths CEM, Barker J, Bleiker T, Creamer CR (Eds), *Rook's Textbook of Dermatology*. 9th ed. Part 11, Section 119. Edinburgh: Wiley Blackwell; 2016; 13–23.

40. Kakourou T, Klontza D, Soteropoulou F, Kattamis C. Corticosteroid treatment of erythema multiforme major (Stevens-Johnson syndrome) in children. *Eur J Pediatr* 1997;156:90–3.

41. Baldwin BT, Lien MH, Khan H, Siddique M. Case of fatal toxic epidermal necrolysis due to cardiac catheterization dye. *J Drugs Dermatol* 2010;9:837–40.

42. Ball R, Ball LK, Wise RP, Braun MM, Beeler JA, Salive ME. Stevens-Johnson syndrome and toxic epidermal necrolysis after vaccination: Reports to the vaccine adverse event reporting system. *Pediatr Infect Dis J* 2001;20:219–23.

43. Bastuji-Garin S, Fouchard N, Bertocchi M, Roujeau JC, Revuz J, Wolkenstein P. SCORTEN: A severity-of-illness score for toxic epidermal necrolysis. *J Investig Dermatol* 2000;115:149–53.

44. Guegan S, Bastuji-Garin S, Poszepczynska-Guigne E, Roujeau JC, Revuz J. Performance of the SCORTEN during the first five days of hospitalization to predict the prognosis of epidermal necrolysis. *J Investig Dermatol* 2006;126:272–6.

45. Fujita Y et al. Rapid immunochromatographic test for serum granulysin is useful for the prediction of Stevens-Johnson syndrome and toxic epidermal necrolysis. *J Am Acad Dermatol* 2011;65:65–8.

46. Sharma VK, Jerajani HR, Srinivas CR, Valia A, Khandpur S. IADVL consensus guidelines 2006: Management of Stevens-Johnson syndrome and toxic epidermal necrolysis. In: Sharma VK (Ed), *Guidelines for Vitiligo, Stevens-Johnson Syndrome, Toxic Epidermal Necrolysis and Psoriasis*. 2nd ed. New Delhi: IADVL's Therapeutic Guidelines Committee; 2008.

47. Dhar S. Role of blood transfusion in the management of Stevens-Johnson syndrome (SJS) and toxic epidermal necrolysis (TEN). *Indian J Dermatol Venereol Leprol* 1998;64:250–1.

48. Fu Y, Gregory DG, Sippel KC, Bouchard CS, Tseng SC. The ophthalmologist's role in the management of acute Stevens-Johnson syndrome and toxic epidermal necrolysis. *Ocul Surf* 2010;8:193–203.

49. Kim KH, Park SW, Kim MK, Wee WR. Effect of age and early intervention with a systemic steroid, intravenous immunoglobulin or amniotic membrane transplantation on the ocular outcomes of patients with Stevens-Johnson syndrome. *Korean J Ophthalmol* 2013;27:331–40.

50. Mockenhaupt M. Stevens-Johnson syndrome and toxic epidermal necrolysis: Clinical patterns, diagnostic considerations, etiology, and therapeutic management. *Semin Cutan Med Surg* 2014;33:10–6.

51. Valeyrie-Allanore L, Ingen-Housz-Oro S, Chosidow O, Pierre W. French referral center management of Stevens-Johnson syndrome/toxic epidermal necrolysis. *Dermatol Sin* 2013;31:191–5.

52. Garcia-Doval I, LeCleach L, Bocquet H, Otero XL, Roujeau JC. Toxic epidermal necrolysis and Stevens-Johnson syndrome: Does early withdrawal of causative drugs decrease the risk of death? *Arch Dermatol* 2000;136:323–7.

53. Pasricha JS. Corticosteroids in toxic epidermal necrolysis. *Indian J Dermatol Venereol Leprol* 2008;74:493.

54. Das S, Roy AK, Biswas I. A six month prospective study to find out the treatment outcome, prognosis and offending drugs in toxic epidermal necrolysis from an urban institution in Kolkata. *Indian J Dermatol* 2013;58:191–3.

55. Martinez AE, Atherton DJ. High-dose systemic corticosteroids can arrest recurrences of severe mucocutaneous erythema multiforme. *Pediatr Dermatol* 2000;17:87–90.

56. Hirahara K et al. Methylprednisolone pulse therapy for Stevens-Johnson syndrome/toxic epidermal necrolysis: Clinical evaluation and analysis of biomarkers. *J Am Acad Dermatol* 2013;69:496–8.

57. Kardaun SH, Jonkman MF. Dexamethasone pulse therapy for Stevens-Johnson syndrome/toxic epidermal necrolysis. *Acta Derm Venereol* 2007;87:144–8.

58. Singh GK, Chatterjee M, Verma R. Cyclosporine in Stevens-Johnson syndrome and toxic epidermal necrolysis and retrospective comparison with systemic corticosteroid. *Indian J Dermatol Venereol Leprol* 2013;79:686–92.

59. Rai R, Srinivas CR. Suprapharmacologic doses of intravenous dexamethasone followed by cyclosporine in the treatment of toxic epidermal necrolysis. *Indian J Dermatol Venereol Leprol* 2008;74:263–5.

60. Brown KM, Silver GM, Halerz M, Walaszek P, Sandroni A, Gamelli RL. Toxic epidermal necrolysis: Does immunoglobulin make a difference? *J Burn Care Rehabil* 2004;25:81–8.

61. Scott-Lang V, Tidman M, McKay D. Toxic epidermal necrolysis in a child successfully treated with infliximab. *Pediatr Dermatol* 2014;31:532–4.

62. Gubinelli E, Canzona F, Tonanzi T, Raskovic D, Didona B. Toxic epidermal necrolysis successfully treated with etanercept. *J Dermatol* 2009;36:150–3.

63. Paradisi A, Abeni D, Bergamo F, Ricci F, Didona D, Didona B. Etanercept therapy for toxic epidermal necrolysis. *J Am Acad Dermatol* 2014;71:278–83.

64. Narita YM, Hirahara K, Mizukawa Y, Kano Y, Shiohara T. Efficacy of plasmapheresis for the treatment of severe toxic epidermal necrolysis: Is cytokine expression analysis useful in predicting its therapeutic efficacy? *J Dermatol* 2011;38:236–45.

65. Trautmann A, Klein CE, Kämpgen E, Bröcker EB. Severe bullous drug reactions treated successfully with cyclophosphamide. *Br J Dermatol* 1998;139:1127–8.

66. Walmsley SL, Khorasheh S, Singer J, Djurdjev O. A randomized trial of N-acetylcysteine for prevention of trimethoprim-sulfamethoxazole hypersensitivity reactions in *Pneumocystis carinii* pneumonia prophylaxis (CTN 057). Canadian HIV Trials Network 057 Study Group. *J Acquir Immune Defic Syndr Hum Retrovirol* 1998;19:498–505.

67. Revuz J. New advances in severe adverse drug reactions. *Dermatol Clin* 2001;19:697–709.

68. Goulden V, Goodfield MJ. Recombinant granulocyte colony-stimulating factor in the management of toxic epidermal necrolysis. *Br J Dermatol* 1996;135:305–6.

69. Niemeijer IC, van Praag MC, van Gemund N. Relevance and consequences of erythema multiforme, Stevens-Johnson syndrome and toxic epidermal necrolysis in gynecology. *Arch Gynecol Obstet* 2009;280:851–4.

70. Struck MF, Illert T, Liss Y, Bosbach ID, Reichelt B, Steen M. Toxic epidermal necrolysis in pregnancy: Case report and review of the literature. *J Burn Care Res* 2010;31:816–21.

71. Ferrandiz-Pulido C, Garcia-Patos V. A review of causes of Stevens-Johnson syndrome and toxic epidermal necrolysis in children. *Arch Dis Child* 2013;98:998–1003.

5

Drug-induced eosinophilia and systemic symptoms

RAJESH VERMA AND PRADEESH ARUMUGAM

INTRODUCTION

Drug reaction with eosinophilia and systemic symptoms (DRESS) is an idiosyncratic, potentially life-threatening, multisystem drug hypersensitivity disorder [1,2]. It is a peculiar syndrome historically described by various names such as phenytoin hypersensitivity, sulfone syndrome, anticonvulsant hypersensitivity syndrome, allopurinol hypersensitivity syndrome, drug-induced pseudolymphoma, drug-induced hypersensitivity syndrome (DIHS), hypersensitivity syndrome (HSS), and drug-induced delayed multiorgan hypersensitivity syndrome (DIDMOHS). The variable presentations that mimic many other diseases, prolonged latency period, and waves of the disease occurring over prolonged periods can make the diagnosis difficult. Early identification of this syndrome and active management are crucial in preventing serious complications and mortality.

EPIDEMIOLOGY

The incidence of DRESS is difficult to estimate due to inconsistencies in reporting. It is about 1 in 1000 to 1 in 10,000 [3]. A slight female preponderance exists with a male-to-female ratio of 0.8. There is no clear ethnic predisposition identified. Certain human leukocyte antigen (HLA) types have been identified that pose an added risk when particular medicines are administered (Table 5.1).

ETIOPATHOGENESIS

There is a complex interplay between the virus, the host immune response to the virus, and a drug-specific immune response, which produces the clinical picture in most cases [13].

Immune mechanisms

Based on several observations including the requirement for sensitization, positive skin tests for the culprit drug in some patients, and a shorter time to onset upon rechallenge; immune mechanisms can be a cause of DRESS [14]. Interleukin-5 (IL-5) plays a role in the generation of eosinophilia, and drug-specific T cells, activated in the skin and internal organs, serve to mediate the disorder. Drug-specific T-cell activation may be due to either haptenization or occur by pharmacological interaction of drugs with the immune receptor (p-i concept) [15].

Viral reactivation

Reactivation of human herpes viruses HHV-6, HHV-7, cytomegalovirus (CMV), and Epstein-Barr virus (EBV) leads to formation of activated circulating CD8+ T cells with cutaneous homing markers secreting large amounts of TNF-α and IFN-γ, seen especially in those with the most severe visceral involvement. Virus reactivation appears to occur in a sequential fashion, with HHV6 and EBV being detected earlier in the course of the disease, followed by HHV7 and CMV. In patients' EBV-transformed B cells, culprit drugs have been shown to trigger the production of EBV [16]. The fluctuation of viral loads gives rise to the "waves" of disease in DRESS, and the chronic phase of DRESS in some patients may be due to persistence of viral reactivation [14,15].

Table 5.1 List of drugs causing drug reaction with eosinophilia and systemic symptoms in corresponding population and human leukocyte antigen (HLA) alleles

Drug	High-risk population	HLA allele
Abacavir	Caucasian	B*5701[3,4]
Allopurinol	Han Chinese, Portuguese	B*5801[5]
Carbamazepine	European, Chinese	B*3101[6]
Dapsone	Chinese	B*1301[7]
Nevirapine	French	DRB1*01:01[8]
	Sardinian	Cw8-B14[9]
	Japanese	Cw8[10]
	Thai	B*3505[11]
	Caucasian	B*3501[12]
Phenytoin	Han Chinese	B*1301

Table 5.2 List of clinical features with corresponding frequency

Features	Frequency (%)
Exanthem	Ubiquitous
Eosinophilia	95
Visceral involvement	91
High fever	90
Atypical lymphocytes	67
Mucosal involvement (mild)	56
Lymphadenopathy	54

Source: Kardaun SH et al. Br J Dermatol 2013;169:1071–80.

Alteration in drug metabolism

1. *Anticonvulsants*: Genetic polymorphisms that affect detoxification of anticonvulsants could be a cause [14]. The inability to detoxify toxic arene oxide metabolites is probably a key factor for the cross-reactivity between phenytoin, oxcarbazepine, and phenobarbital [17].
2. *Sulfonamides*: Genetic polymorphisms that affect detoxification of sulfonamides have been identified in patients recovering from DRESS [18].

CLINICAL FEATURES

History

DRESS develops 2–6 weeks after initiation of the culprit drug on first exposure. The median time interval after drug intake is 22 days (interquartile range 17–31 days) [3]. With reexposure of the same drug there can be shorter latency. The patient may present with nonspecific symptoms in the early phase with asthenia, malaise, and fatigue. Rash and facial swelling are usually the presenting complaints. Fever and a cutaneous eruption are the most common symptoms, seen in 90% and 75% of patients, respectively [3]. Other symptoms related to the organ affected may be present at the time of presentation. Certain drugs have more propensities to affect particular organs. Phenytoin, minocycline, and dapsone can cause severe hepatic damage, while allopurinol causes renal damage. Chest pain and dyspnea should prompt detailed cardiological evaluation. Pulmonary and neurological symptoms are rarely reported. The cutaneous and visceral involvement may persist for months after drug withdrawal, and additional sites of involvement (e.g., cardiac, thyroid) may develop weeks or months later. Family history of similar rash for a similar drug can give a diagnostic clue of HLA polymorphism. Familial cases of DRESS to carbamazepine, linked to HLA-A3101, have been described [19]. The cutaneous and visceral involvement may persist for several weeks or months after drug withdrawal, and additional sites of involvement (e.g., cardiac, thyroid) may develop weeks or months later.

Clinical findings

The presenting feature is usually an exanthem. Table 5.2 gives the frequency of associated features in DRESS.

GENERAL EXAMINATION

Pallor may be seen due to pancytopenia. At least two groups of lymph nodes are enlarged in most of the cases.

VITAL SIGNS

Tachycardia and hypotension may be due to fever or cardiac involvement.

CUTANEOUS EXAMINATION

The most common finding is head and neck edema. Mucosal involvement is mild or absent. Various types of rash are seen in DRESS:
- *Urticated papular exanthema*: The most common variant, often accompanied by cutaneous edema and follicular accentuation (Figure 5.1)
- *Morbilliform eruption*: Resembling measles (Figures 5.2 and 5.3)
- *Erythroderma*: May be a presenting feature (Figures 5.4 and 5.5)

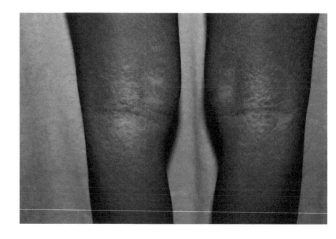

Figure 5.1 Urticated papular exanthema type of skin rash.

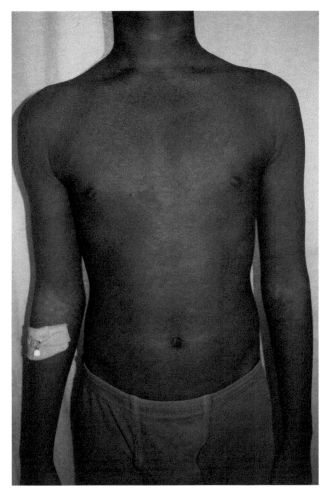

Figure 5.2 Morbilliform eruption resembling measles on the trunk.

- *Erythema multiforme-like rash*: Atypical targets not limited to acral sites, may be associated with a more severe systemic involvement [20]
- *Other less common manifestations*: Vesicles, follicular or nonfollicular pustules, purpuric lesions

FEATURES OF SPECIFIC ORGAN DAMAGE

1. *Liver*: The liver is the most common viscera to be involved and the primary cause of mortality from DRESS. Between 70% and 95% of cases of DRESS demonstrate liver abnormalities [3,21]. Any drug has the potential to cause liver dysfunction, especially phenytoin, minocycline, and dapsone [21]. Severity of involvement varies widely, from mild and transient hepatitis to fulminant hepatic failure requiring liver transplantation. Both hepatocellular and obstructive patterns of hepatitis have been reported. The presence of atypical targets and purpura at presentation indicate high risk for severe liver involvement [20].

2. *Hematological system*: The most common abnormality seen is that of eosinophilia. Pancytopenia is seen in some cases. IL-5, which stimulates eosinophil release, is elevated [22,23]. Lymphocytosis with levels

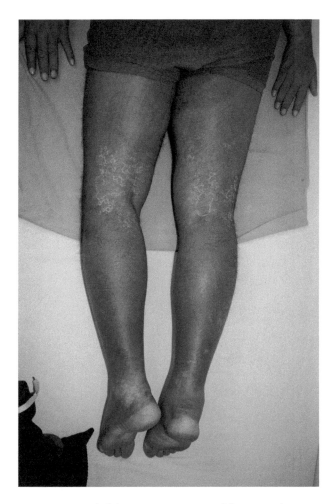

Figure 5.3 Morbilliform eruption resembling measles on the lower limbs.

up to >20 × 10⁹ leukocytes/L is seen. Atypical lymphocytes are frequently present in peripheral blood smear. Leukopenia, lymphopenia (possibly viral induced), and thrombocytopenia have been noted.

3. *Renal*: Renal involvement is seen in 12%–40% of patients [24]. Allopurinol is the most common

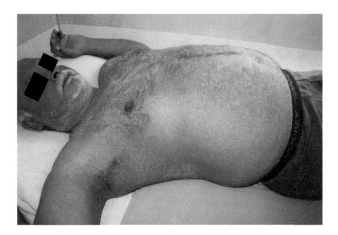

Figure 5.4 Erythroderma presentation in drug reaction with eosinophilia and systemic symptoms.

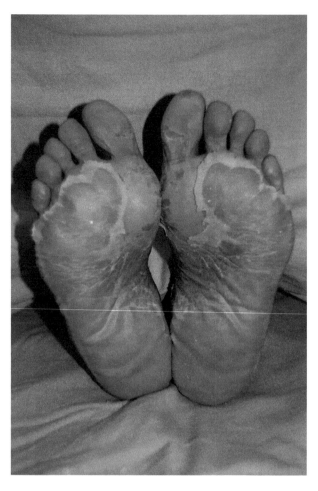

Figure 5.5 Drug reaction with eosinophilia and systemic symptoms with erythoderma patient having exfoliation of skin on soles.

offending drug. Any underlying renal dysfunction may be exacerbated by the syndrome. Prerenal acute kidney injury can be caused by dehydration from fever in the prodromal phase. Hematuria, proteinuria, and eosinophils are seen in the urine. Histologically, interstitial nephritis is seen. Severe renal impairment is exceptionally rare [24,25].

4. *Heart*: Pericarditis and myocarditis may be seen [26]. These are rare manifestations and usually have serious consequences. Chest pain and dyspnea should prompt for detailed evaluation. Tachycardia, hypotension, and signs of a pericardial and/or pleural effusion can be found on clinical examination. Electrocardiogram (ECG) may demonstrate T-wave abnormalities or other arrhythmias. Echocardiogram may demonstrate a pericardial effusion, or reduced ejection fraction. Cardiac enzymes such as CK-MB fraction and Trop-T may be elevated. Both pericarditis and myocarditis respond to standard therapy [27]. Acute necrotizing eosinophilic myocarditis (ANEM) is a severe form of myocarditis with extreme impairment of ejection fraction and major systolic dysfunction, carrying a high mortality (>50%) [28].

5. *Pulmonary*: Pleural effusion, pleuritis, or acute interstitial pneumonitis are infrequently reported [29]. Reduced diffusion gradient may be seen [30].

6. *Central nervous system*: Headache may indicate inflammation of the meninges. Few cases of seizures and cranial nerve palsies have been reported [30]. One case having symptoms of limbic encephalitis revealed symmetrical enhancement of the amygdala, cingulate gyrus and temporal lobes in brain shown by magnetic resonance imaging (MRI), with HHV-6 in the patient's cerebrospinal fluid (CSF) demonstrated by polymerase chain reaction (PCR) [31]. Another report of limbic encephalitis had syndrome of inappropriate antidiuretic hormone (SIADH) [32].

7. *Gastrointestinal*: Diarrhea or dysentery may point to an underlying ulcerative colitis [33]. Eosinophilic oesophagitis and dysphagia have also been reported [34].

8. *Endocrine system*: Usually affected in the later phase of DRESS. Both hyper- and hypothyroidism may be seen in the convalescent phase. Regular monitoring of thyroid function for a year after the acute event is advised [35]. Pancreatitis may progress to pancreatic insufficiency and type 1 diabetes [36]. However, the most common cause of diabetes is secondary to corticosteroid therapy.

Diagnostic criteria

Three criteria have been proposed:

1. *RegiSCAR DRESS scoring system* (Tables 5.3 and 5.4)
2. *J-SCAR criteria for DIHS (Japanese consensus group's criteria)* (Table 5.5)
3. *Bocquet et al. criteria* (Table 5.6) [37]: Bocquet criteria are simple to use and appropriate for the diagnosis of DRESS syndrome in clinical practice. Bocquet and RegiSCAR criteria should be complementary for the diagnosis of DRESS syndrome in suspected patients [38]. Several herpesviruses (including EBV, HHV-6, HHV-7, and CMV) may play a critical role in the pathogenesis of DRESS, while the Japanese criteria include only HHV-6 reactivation. Japanese DIHS may represent a severe subgroup of DRESS syndrome [39].

Clinical variants

Mini-DRESS is a term used for those who do not completely fulfill the criteria of DRESS. Overlap syndromes (i.e., simultaneously meeting criteria for two diagnoses) with acute generalized exanthematous pustulosis (AGEP) or Stevens-Johnson syndrome/toxic epidermal necrolysis (SJS/TEN) have also been reported [40].

DIFFERENTIAL DIAGNOSIS

The skin rash in DRESS is highly variable and dynamic as the disease progresses or fluctuates. The following differential

Table 5.3 RegiSCAR scoring for drug reaction with eosinophilia and systemic symptoms (DRESS) (abbreviated version)

RegiSCAR scoring for DRESS (simplified version)		
Sl. No	Findings	Maximum points
1	Extent of rash >50% of body surface area	1
2	Rash suggestive of DRESS (any two of edema/infiltration/purpura/scaling)	1
3	≥3 negative serological tests (hepatitis A, B, and C; mycoplasma/chlamydia; antinuclear antibody; blood culture)	1

4	Systemic involvement
	    i. Lymphadenopathy (≥2 sites, >1 cm): 1 point
	    ii. Atypical lymphocytosis: 1 point
	    iii. Eosinophilia
	        a. 10%–19% of TLC
	           (0.7–1.5×10^9 if TLC $<4 \times 10^9$): 1 point
	        b. ≥20% of TLC
	           ($>1.5 \times 10^9$ if TLC $<4 \times 10^9$): 2 points
	    iv. Organ involvement (Liver/heart/kidney/lung/pancreas/others [spleen/thyroid/gastrointestinal]): 1 point for each organ
		6

Table 5.4 RegiSCAR scoring system for drug reaction with eosinophilia and systemic symptoms (DRESS)

Criteria	No	Yes	Unknown/unclassifiable
Fever >38.5°C	−1	0	−1
Lymphadenopathy	0	1	0
Atypical lymphocytosis	0	1	0
Eosinophilia	0	–	0
750–1499/mm³ (10%–19.9%)	–	1	–
>1500/mm³ (>20%)	–	2	–
Rash >50% of BSA	0	1	0
Rash suggestive of DRESS	−1	1	0
Biopsy suggests DRESS	−1	0	0
Internal organ involvement	0	–	0
One	–	1	–
Two or more	–	2	–
Resolution in ≥15 days	−1	0	−1
Lab test done within 3 days of index date and negative for at least three (ANA, blood culture, HAV/HBV/HCV, mycoplasma/chlamydia)	0	1	0

Interpretation

<2 points: no case
2–3 points: possible case
4–5 points: probable case
5–9 points: definite case

Abbreviations: ANA, antinuclear antibody; BSA, body surface area; HAV, hepatitis A virus; HBV, hepatitis B virus; HCV, hepatitis C virus.

diagnosis should be kept in mind while investigating and managing a suspected DRESS:

1. Other cutaneous drug eruptions
2. Acute viral infections
3. Hypereosinophilic syndrome
4. Other causes of erythroderma
5. Systemic vasculitis (especially Churg-Strauss syndrome)
6. Angioimmunoblastic lymphoma

One of the most helpful features in distinguishing DRESS from the other severe cutaneous adverse reaction

Table 5.5 J-SCAR criteria for drug reaction with eosinophilia and systemic symptoms/drug-induced hypersensitivity syndrome (DIHS)

1. Maculopapular rash developing >3 weeks after starting with the suspected drug
2. Prolonged clinical symptoms 2 weeks after discontinuation of the suspected drug
3. Fever >38°C
4. Liver abnormalities (ALT >100U/L)/any other organ involvement
5. Leukocyte abnormalities
   a. Leukocytosis (>11 × 10⁹/L)
   b. Atypical lymphocytosis (>5%)
   c. Eosinophilia (>1.5 × 10⁹/L)
6. Lymphadenopathy
7. Human herpes 6 reactivation

Note: Typical DIHS: Presence of all seven criteria. Atypical DIHS: Only first five criteria.

Table 5.6 Bocquet et al. criteria for drug reaction with eosinophilia and systemic symptoms

1. Skin eruption
2. Blood eosinophilia (>1.5 × 10³/μL) or the presence of atypical lymphocytes
3. Internal organ involvement
   Lymphadenopathy (>2 cm in diameter)
   With one or more of the following organs involved
   a. Hepatitis (liver transaminases > twice the upper normal limit)
   b. Interstitial nephritis
   c. Interstitial pneumonia
   d. Carditis

Note: All three criteria should be fulfilled for diagnosis.

Table 5.7 Suggested panel of initial investigations (not limited to this list)

Category	Tests
Hematological	Full blood count, AEC
	Peripheral blood smear for atypical lymphocytes
Hepatic	Liver function tests
	Serum LDH
	Ferritin, CRP
	PT/INR/PTT
	Serum albumin
	Hepatitis B, C
	EBV, CMV, HHV-6, HHV-7 titers
Cardiac	Electrocardiogram
Pulmonary	Chest x-ray
Autoimmune	ANA, extractable nuclear antigens
	Complement
	Antineutrophil cytoplasmic antibody (If rash is petechial)
Renal	Urea and creatinine, calcium
	Urinalysis
	Spot urine protein: creatinine
Endocrine	Thyroid-stimulating hormone, free T3/T4
	Blood glucose
Infection	Blood cultures
Gastrointestinal	Amylase

Abbreviations: ANA, antinuclear antibody; CRP, C-reactive protein; INR, international normalized ratio; LDH, lactate dehydrogenase; PTT, partial thromboplastin time.

test are two clinical tests that may benefit patients. Overall positive rates for DRESS patch tests are diverse, ranging from 32.1% to 64% [42,43]. In the case of allopurinol-induced DRESS, patch tests always yield negative results.

Table 5.8 Further investigations (if warranted clinically)

Category	Tests
Hematological	Bone marrow examination
Cardiac	Echocardiogram
	Cardiac enzymes (creatine kinase, troponin)
Pulmonary	Pulmonary function tests
Renal	Wright stain of urine (for eosinophilia)
	Renal ultrasound
Neurological	CSF examination CT/MRI head
	Electroencephalogram
Infection	Mycoplasma serology
	PCR for herpes simplex virus
Gastrointestinal	Lipase
	Triglycerides
	Colonoscopy

Abbreviations: CT, computed tomography; MRI, magnetic resonance imaging; PCR, polymerase chain reaction; CSF, cerebrospinal fluid.

(SCAR) syndromes is latency of onset of the eruption; this is classically shorter in AGEP (<5 days) and SJS/TEN (7–10 days) than in DRESS, where the latency may be 2–6 weeks after drug ingestion. Where exfoliative erythroderma is the presenting cutaneous feature of DRESS, this may mimic the presentation of an acute severe eczema or psoriasis, or a cutaneous lymphoma. Where purpura and targets are present, the differential diagnosis of a systemic vasculitis should be considered. Angioimmunoblastic lymphoma is a rare differential of DRESS and may mimic its presentation [41].

INVESTIGATIONS

Investigations to be done in a case of DRESS are provided in Tables 5.7 and 5.8. The drug provocation test is not helpful because of the latency and should not be tried since it can be fatal in some. Patch testing and lymphocyte transformation

The optimal time for performing a patch test is 2–6 months after recovery from the adverse reaction [44]. The lymphocyte transformation test (LTT) detects drug-specific T cells by measuring the proliferation of T cells after encountering the antigens. The specificity of LTT is 85%, and sensitivity is 64% [45]. The optimal time to perform LTT for DRESS patients is 5–8 weeks after acute episodes [46].

Histopathology

No pathological finding is specific to diagnose DRESS. The skin biopsy helps to rule out other diseases like lymphoma or infections. Various inflammatory patterns can be seen, including eczematous, interface dermatitis, AGEP-like, and erythema multiforme-like [47]. Diffuse or superficial perivascular lymphocytic infiltration is a frequent finding.

TREATMENT

The most important initial management is identifying the culprit drug and early withdrawal. Culprit drugs can be identified using Naranjo scale and the World Health Organization-Uppsala Monitoring Center (WHO-UMC) classification [48,49]. Possible or more probable drugs are to be considered as culprits to induce DRESS syndrome.

There are no definite guidelines or evidence for the treatment of DRESS. Active management is based on previously published case series and case reports. The mainstay of active treatment is systemic corticosteroid therapy. Because relapse can occur when the dosage is reduced, a slow tapering of corticosteroids over a period of several weeks to months is often required [50]. In milder cases of DRESS, even in the setting of mild hepatitis, topical high-potency corticosteroids may be helpful and may lead to less viral reactivation. In refractory cases, or chronic disease, cyclosporine may be required. Supportive care should be given, which may include IV fluids, thermoregulation, catheterization, and supplemental oxygen. Extracorporeal membrane oxygenation (ECMO) may be required in cases of cardiac insufficiency secondary to myocarditis [27]. In the absence of indicators of infection, no empiric antibiotic therapy should be given. Topical emollient and topical corticosteroid therapy are to be applied. Management of organ-specific involvement should be done in consultation with respective specialities.

First line

In cases of limited severity with minimal cutaneous involvement, the application of highly potent topical steroids may suffice as treatment. The majority of patients require oral or intravenous corticosteroid therapy. A dose of oral prednisolone of 1 mg/kg/day is recommended as initial treatment, with a tapering off period varying from 1 to 3 months [50]. Where intravenous therapy is required, or where institution of oral therapy has failed to produce a satisfactory clinical improvement, methylprednisolone is indicated. One study using 1 g/day methylprednisolone for 3 days IV demonstrated safety and improved clinical outcome with this dose [51].

Second line

Cases of DRESS refractory to steroid treatment require alternative treatment. Cyclosporine can be used in persistent liver dysfunction or a chronic exfoliative dermatitis [52]. Intravenous immunoglobulin (IVIg) can be used [53–55]. However, severe adverse reactions have been observed [56].

Third line

The literature contains a number of case reports of other treatments used in refractory cases of DRESS. Plasmapheresis has been used [57]. Alternative immunosuppressants, such as cyclophosphamide, may be used in steroid-resistant cases [58]. Valganciclovir has been used, in theory to combat virus reactivation described in this syndrome. In cases of severe liver involvement, N-acetylcysteine has been used as an adjunct to other treatments [59].

A stepladder management of DRESS is provided in Table 5.9.

PROGNOSIS

DRESS syndrome is a severe adverse drug reaction that may be fatal in 10% of patients [60]. Poor prognostic factors include eosinophilia, pancytopenia, leukocytosis, thrombocytopenia, a history of chronic renal insufficiency, multiorgan involvement, tachycardia, tachypnea, coagulopathy, gastrointestinal bleeding, systemic inflammatory response syndrome, and raised creatinine and ferritin levels at initial presentation [61].

CONCLUSION

DRESS is an autoimmune reaction with cutaneous features ranging from maculopapular exanthem to erythroderma. Systemic involvement, especially liver involvement, may result in mortality. Early diagnosis is therefore of paramount importance, and systemic steroids over a prolonged duration is the treatment of choice.

Table 5.9 Suggested treatment ladder for DRESS

Treatment Ladder	
First Line	i. Oral corticosteroid
	ii. IV corticosteroid
Second line	i. Cyclosporine
	ii. IVIg
Third Line	i. Cyclophosphamide
	ii. Plasmapheresis

KEY POINTS

- DRESS is a common dermatological emergency due to drugs and drug latency of 4-6 weeks is a prominent feature.
- Skin rash, liver involvement, lymphadenopathy, eosinophilia and atypical lymhocytes in periheral blood are characteristic features.
- Multiple organ involvement and fatality may occur in severe cases.
- Oral Corticosteroids are the drugs of choice. Cyclosporine, IVIg are second line therapies.

REFERENCES

1. Roujeau JC, Stern RS. Severe adverse cutaneous reactions to drugs. *N Engl J Med* 1994;331:1272–85.
2. Newell BD, Moinfar M, Mancini AJ, Nopper AJ. Retrospective analysis of 32 pediatric patients with anticonvulsant hypersensitivity syndrome (ACHSS). *Pediatr Dermatol* 2009;26:536–46.
3. Kardaun SH et al. Drug reaction with eosinophilia and systemic symptoms (DRESS): An original multisystem adverse drug reaction. Results from the prospective RegiSCAR study. *Br J Dermatol* 2013;169:1071–80.
4. Orkin C et al. An epidemiologic study to determine the prevalence of the HLA-B*5701 allele among HIV-positive patients in Europe. *Pharmacogenet Genomics* 2010;20:307–14.
5. Hung S-I et al. HLA-B*5801 allele as a genetic marker for severe cutaneous adverse reactions caused by allopurinol. *Proc Natl Acad Sci USA* 2005;102:4134–9.
6. Genin E et al. HLA-A*31:01 and different types of carbamazepine-induced severe cutaneous adverse reactions: An international study and meta-analysis. *Pharmacogenomics J* 2014;14:281–8.
7. Wang H et al. Association between HLA-B*1301 and dapsone-induced hypersensitivity reactions among leprosy patients in China. *J Invest Dermatol* 2013;133:2642–4.
8. Martin AM et al. Predisposition to nevirapine hypersensitivity associated with HLA-DRB1*0101 and abrogated by low CD4 T-cell counts. *AIDS Lond Engl* 2005;19:97–9.
9. Littera R et al. HLA-dependent hypersensitivity to nevirapine in Sardinian HIV patients. *AIDS Lond Engl* 2006;20:1621–6.
10. Gatanaga H et al. HLA-Cw8 primarily associated with hypersensitivity to nevirapine. *AIDS* 2007;21:264.
11. Chantarangsu S et al. HLA-B*3505 allele is a strong predictor for nevirapine-induced skin adverse drug reactions in HIV-infected Thai patients. *Pharmacogenet Genomics* 2009;19:139–46.
12. Phillips EJ, Chung W-H, Mockenhaupt M, Roujeau J-C, Mallal SA. Drug hypersensitivity: Pharmacogenetics and clinical syndromes. *J Allergy Clin Immunol* 2011;127(3 Suppl):S60–66.
13. Shiohara T, Inaoka M, Kano Y. Drug-induced hypersensitivity syndrome (DIHS): A reaction induced by a complex interplay among herpesviruses and antiviral and antidrug immune responses. *Allergol Int Off J Jpn Soc Allergol* 2006;55:1–8.
14. Tas S, Simonart T. Drug rash with eosinophilia and systemic symptoms (dress syndrome). *Acta Clin Belg* 1999;54:197–200.
15. Pichler WJ, Adam J, Daubner B, Gentinetta T, Keller M, Yerly D. Drug hypersensitivity reactions: Pathomechanism and clinical symptoms. *Med Clin North Am* 2010;94:645–64.
16. Picard D et al. Drug reaction with eosinophilia and systemic symptoms (DRESS): A multiorgan antiviral T cell response. *Sci Transl Med* 2010;2:46ra62.
17. Pirmohamed M, Lin K, Chadwick D, Park BK. TNF-α promoter region gene polymorphisms in carbamazepine-hypersensitive patients. *Neurology* 2001;56:890–6.
18. Vaillant L. Drug hypersensitivity syndrome: Drug rash with eosinophila and systemic symptoms (DRESS). *J Dermatol Treat* 1999;10:267–72.
19. Anjum N, Polak ME, Ardern-Jones M, Cooper HL. Presence of the HLA-A*3101 allele in a familial case of drug reaction with eosinophilia and systemic symptoms, secondary to carbamazepine. *Clin Exp Dermatol* 2014;39:307–9.
20. Walsh S et al. Drug reaction with eosinophilia and systemic symptoms: Is cutaneous phenotype a prognostic marker for outcome? A review of clinicopathological features of 27 cases. *Br J Dermatol* 2013;168:391–401.
21. Husain Z, Reddy BY, Schwartz RA. DRESS syndrome: Part I. Clinical perspectives. *J Am Acad Dermatol* 2013;68:693. e1–14; quiz 706–8.
22. Mikami C et al. Eosinophil activation and in situ interleukin-5 production by mononuclear cells in skin lesions of patients with drug hypersensitivity. *J Dermatol* 1999;26:633–9.
23. Musette P, Janela B. New insights into drug reaction with eosinophilia and systemic symptoms pathophysiology. *Front Med [Internet]* December 4, 2017 [cited March 27, 2018];4. Available from: https://www.ncbi.nlm.nih.gov/pmc/articles/PMC5722807/
24. Augusto J-F et al. A case of sulphasalazine-induced DRESS syndrome with delayed acute interstitial nephritis. *Nephrol Dial Transplant Off Publ Eur Dial Transpl Assoc–Eur Ren Assoc* 2009;24:2940–2.
25. Savard S, Desmeules S, Riopel J, Agharazii M. Linezolid-associated acute interstitial nephritis and drug rash with eosinophilia and systemic symptoms (DRESS) syndrome. *Am J Kidney Dis Off J Natl Kidney Found* 2009;54(6):e17–20.

26. Bourgeois GP et al. Fulminant myocarditis as a late sequelae of DRESS-2 cases. *J Am Acad Dermatol* 2011;65:889–90.

27. Lo M-H et al. Drug reaction with eosinophilia and systemic symptoms syndrome associated myocarditis: A survival experience after extracorporeal membrane oxygenation support. *J Clin Pharm Ther* 2013;38:172–4.

28. Arsenovic N, Sheehan L, Clark D, Moreira R. Fatal carbamazepine induced fulminant eosinophilic (hypersensitivity) myocarditis: Emphasis on anatomical and histological characteristics, mechanisms and genetics of drug hypersensitivity and differential diagnosis. *J Forensic Leg Med* 2010;17:57–61.

29. Ang C-C, Wang Y-S, Yoosuff E-LM, Tay Y-K. Retrospective analysis of drug-induced hypersensitivity syndrome: A study of 27 patients. *J Am Acad Dermatol* 2010;63:219–27.

30. Ushigome Y, Kano Y, Ishida T, Hirahara K, Shiohara T. Short- and long-term outcomes of 34 patients with drug-induced hypersensitivity syndrome in a single institution. *J Am Acad Dermatol* 2013;68:721–8.

31. Fujino Y, Nakajima M, Inoue H, Kusuhara T, Yamada T. Human herpesvirus 6 encephalitis associated with hypersensitivity syndrome. *Ann Neurol* 2002;51:771–4.

32. Sakuma K, Kano Y, Fukuhara M, Shiohara T. Syndrome of inappropriate secretion of antidiuretic hormone associated with limbic encephalitis in a patient with drug-induced hypersensitivity syndrome. *Clin Exp Dermatol* 2008;33:287–90.

33. Atkinson RJ, Dennis G, Cross SS, McAlindon ME, Sharrack B, Sanders DS. Eosinophilic colitis complicating anti-epileptic hypersensitivity syndrome: An indication for colonoscopy? *Gastrointest Endosc* 2004;60:1034–6.

34. Schwartz RA, Husain Z, Reddy BY. Drug reaction with eosinophilia and systemic symptoms (DRESS) syndrome and dysphagia: A noteworthy association. *J Am Acad Dermatol* 2013;69:1058.

35. Cookson H, Creamer D, Walsh S. Thyroid dysfunction in drug reaction with eosinophilia and systemic symptoms (DRESS): An unusual manifestation of systemic drug hypersensitivity. *Br J Dermatol* 2013;168:1130–2.

36. Chiou C-C, Chung W-H, Hung S-I, Yang L-C, Hong H-S. Fulminant type 1 diabetes mellitus caused by drug hypersensitivity syndrome with human herpesvirus 6 infection. *J Am Acad Dermatol* 2006;54(2 Suppl):S14–17.

37. Bocquet H, Bagot M, Roujeau JC. Drug-induced pseudolymphoma and drug hypersensitivity syndrome (Drug Rash with Eosinophilia and Systemic Symptoms: DRESS). *Semin Cutan Med Surg* 1996;15:250–7.

38. Kim D-H, Koh Y-I. Comparison of diagnostic criteria and determination of prognostic factors for drug reaction with eosinophilia and systemic symptoms syndrome. *Allergy Asthma Immunol Res* 2014;6:216–21.

39. Shiohara T, Iijima M, Ikezawa Z, Hashimoto K. The diagnosis of a DRESS syndrome has been sufficiently established on the basis of typical clinical features and viral reactivations. *Br J Dermatol* 2007;156:1083–4.

40. Toxic epidermal necrolysis, DRESS, AGEP: Do overlap cases exist? [Internet]. [cited 2018 March 27]. Available from: https://www.ncbi.nlm.nih.gov/pmc/articles/PMC3517389/

41. Mangana J et al. Angioimmunoblastic T-cell lymphoma mimicking drug reaction with eosinophilia and systemic symptoms (DRESS Syndrome). *Case Rep Dermatol* 2017;9:74–9.

42. Barbaud A et al. A multicentre study to determine the value and safety of drug patch tests for the three main classes of severe cutaneous adverse drug reactions. *Br J Dermatol* 2013;168:555–62.

43. Santiago F, Gonçalo M, Vieira R, Coelho S, Figueiredo A. Epicutaneous patch testing in drug hypersensitivity syndrome (DRESS). *Contact Dermatitis* 2010;62:47–53.

44. Elzagallaai AA, Knowles SR, Rieder MJ, Bend JR, Shear NH, Koren G. Patch testing for the diagnosis of anticonvulsant hypersensitivity syndrome: A systematic review. *Drug Saf* 2009;32:391–408.

45. Nyfeler B, Pichler WJ. The lymphocyte transformation test for the diagnosis of drug allergy: Sensitivity and specificity. *Clin Exp Allergy J Br Soc Allergy Clin Immunol* 1997;27:175–81.

46. Kano Y, Hirahara K, Mitsuyama Y, Takahashi R, Shiohara T. Utility of the lymphocyte transformation test in the diagnosis of drug sensitivity: Dependence on its timing and the type of drug eruption. *Allergy* 2007;62:1439–44.

47. Ortonne N et al. Histopathology of drug rash with eosinophilia and systemic symptoms syndrome: A morphological and phenotypical study. *Br J Dermatol* 2015;173:50–8.

48. Naranjo CA et al. A method for estimating the probability of adverse drug reactions. *Clin Pharmacol Ther* 1981;30:239–45.

49. standardised-case-causality-assessment.pdf [Internet]. [cited March 27, 2018]. Available from: https://www.who-umc.org/media/2768/standardised-case-causality-assessment.pdf

50. Shiohara T, Kano Y. Drug reaction with eosinophilia and systemic symptoms (DRESS): Incidence, pathogenesis and management. *Expert Opin Drug Saf* 2017;16:139–47.

51. Natkunarajah J et al. Ten cases of drug reaction with eosinophilia and systemic symptoms (DRESS) treated with pulsed intravenous methylprednisolone. *Eur J Dermatol* 2011;21:385–91.

52. Zuliani E, Zwahlen H, Gilliet F, Marone C. Vancomycin-induced hypersensitivity reaction with acute renal failure: Resolution following cyclosporine treatment. *Clin Nephrol* 2005;64:155–8.

53. Santhamoorthy P, Alexander KJ, Alshubaili A. Intravenous immunoglobulin in the treatment of drug rash eosinophilia and systemic symptoms caused by phenytoin. *Ann Indian Acad Neurol* 2012;15:320–2.

54. Fields KS, Petersen MJ, Chiao E, Tristani-Firouzi P. Case reports: Treatment of nevirapine-associated dress syndrome with intravenous immune globulin (IVIG). *J Drugs Dermatol* 2005;4:510–3.

55. Kito Y, Ito T, Tokura Y, Hashizume H. High-dose intravenous immunoglobulin monotherapy for drug-induced hypersensitivity syndrome. *Acta Derm Venereol* 2012;92:100–1.

56. Joly P et al. Poor benefit/risk balance of intravenous immunoglobulins in DRESS. *Arch Dermatol* 2012;148:543–4.

57. Alexander T et al. Severe DRESS syndrome managed with therapeutic plasma exchange. *Pediatrics* 2013;131:e945–9.

58. Laban E et al. Cyclophosphamide therapy for corticoresistant drug reaction with eosinophilia and systemic symptoms (DRESS) syndrome in a patient with severe kidney and eye involvement and Epstein-Barr virus reactivation. *Am J Kidney Dis Off J Natl Kidney Found* 2010;55:e11–4.

59. Moling O et al. Treatment of DIHS/DRESS syndrome with combined N-acetylcysteine, prednisone and valganciclovir—A hypothesis. *Med Sci Monit Int Med J Exp Clin Res* 2012;18:CS57–62.

60. Chiou C-C et al. Clinicopathological features and prognosis of drug rash with eosinophilia and systemic symptoms: A study of 30 cases in Taiwan. *J Eur Acad Dermatol Venereol* 2008;22:1044–9.

61. Wei C-H et al. Identifying prognostic factors for drug rash with eosinophilia and systemic symptoms (DRESS). *Eur J Dermatol* 2011;21:930–7.

Acute generalized exanthematous pustulosis

SOUMYA JAGADEESHAN

INTRODUCTION

Acute generalized exanthematous pustulosis (AGEP), also known as toxic pustuloderma, is a rare cutaneous pustular eruption, classified as a severe cutaneous adverse reaction (SCAR), caused in more than 90% of cases by drugs. Though the clinical picture of drug-induced pustular eruptions in patients was described by Baker and Ryan in 1968 [1], it was Beylot et al., in 1980, who proposed the name for this disease [2]. It is characterized by the sudden eruption of nonfollicular sterile pustules, in a generalized distribution. AGEP has distinct clinical and histological features, thereby differentiating it from other conditions like pustular psoriasis or other drug eruptions. Due to the sudden, generalized nature of the eruption and the accompanying signs of acute systemic inflammation, this entity often presents in the emergency department and is considered a dermatological emergency.

EPIDEMIOLOGY

It is a rare disorder, with incidence being about one to five cases/million/year. However, this could be lower than the actual incidence due to underdiagnosis as the eruptions could be transient and misdiagnosed. It can affect all age groups. The EuroSCAR study revealed a mean age of occurrence of 56 ± 21 years and a female preponderance, with a male:female ratio of 0.8 [3]. The female preponderance is in accordance with the general trend in drug reactions. Seasonality has also been suggested, with a few studies reporting increased incidence during summer.

ETIOLOGY

In at least 90% of the cases, AGEP is caused by drugs. As per the EuroSCAR study, drugs with high risk to trigger AGEP were identified as ampicillin/amoxicillin, pristinamycin, quinolones, chloroquine, sulfonamides, terbinafine, and diltiazem. Less strong association was recorded for corticosteroids, macrolides, nonsteroidal anti-inflammatory drugs of the oxicam type, and antiepileptics. The time of onset after drug intake could depend on the drug concerned and its mechanism of action, and is therefore variable. It could range from 24 hours to 1–2 weeks. Rapid onset following the intake of certain drugs could be due to rechallenge to the drug to which there has been a prior exposure, or due to some mechanism that has so far not been elucidated.

Contact sensitivity and infectious agents have also been implicated in the causation of AGEP. The agents described include Coxsackie B4, Cytomegalovirus, Parvovirus B19, *Chlamydia pneumoniae*, *Escherichia coli*, etc. However, there was no significant risk associated with any particular infection in AGEP. Spider bites, venom, certain food items, and xenobiotics have also been reported to trigger AGEP [4].

PATHOGENESIS

AGEP is a T-cell-mediated disease; characterized by the activation, expansion, and subsequent migration of the drug-specific CD4+ and CD8+ T cells into the skin. The initial stages of pathogenesis consist of the exposure to the antigen, following which it is presented by the antigen-presenting cells to the major histocompatibility complex molecules, causing activation of CD4+ and CD8+ T cells. The drug-specific cytotoxic T cells and the proteins such as perforin and granzyme B cause apoptosis of keratinocytes and subcorneal vesicle formation. CD4+ T cells release CXCL-8, which recruits neutrophils and converts vesicles to pustules.

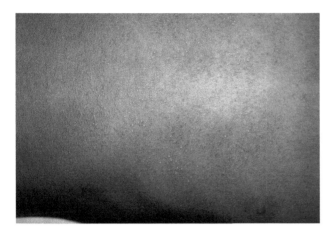

Figure 6.1 Tiny pustules over trunk in a case of acute generalized exanthematous pustulosis.

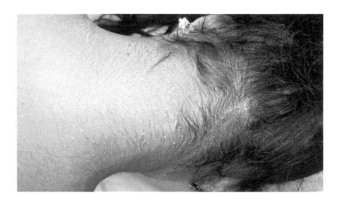

Figure 6.3 Nape of neck involvement in acute generalized exanthematous pustulosis.

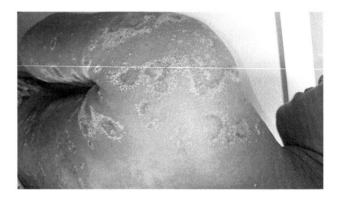

Figure 6.4 Grouped pustules on the back.

CLINICAL FEATURES

AGEP is characterized by the rapid appearance of dozens to hundreds of small, pinhead-sized, nonfollicular sterile pustules, often preceded by erythema and edema (Figure 6.1). Patients often describe a pruritic or burning sensation accompanying the eruption. There is usually accentuation in the intertriginous areas (Figure 6.2), nape of neck (Figure 6.3), and the face. Other areas may also be involved (Figures 6.4 through 6.6). Sometimes, the pustules may coalesce, and Nikolsky sign may be falsely positive. Other skin manifestations like purpuric lesions, atypical target-like lesions, marked facial edema, blisters, and vesicles have also been described with AGEP [5]. The eruption usually occurs a few hours to a few days after the administration of the offending drug. A localized variant also has been described. Besides the classical skin eruption, atypical cases with overlap with drug hypersensitivity syndrome and toxic epidermal necrolysis have also been reported.

Accompanying the skin eruption, fever above 38°C is almost always present. Other signs of systemic inflammation like leukocytosis (>10,000/mL), elevated levels of C-reactive protein, and mostly increased levels of neutrophils (>7000/mL) can be seen. Eosinophilia may be seen. Hypoalbuminemia and hypocalcemia may also be seen. Internal organ involvement can be seen in a few cases, including liver, renal, and pulmonary involvement, but is rather uncommon [6].

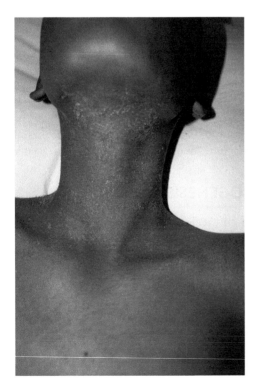

Figure 6.2 Involvement of front of neck.

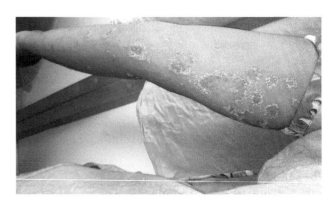

Figure 6.5 Lesions on the arm.

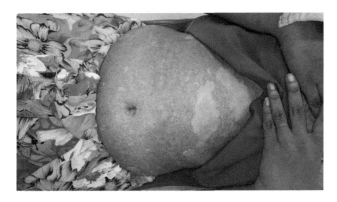

Figure 6.6 Similar lesions on the abdomen.

DIFFERENTIAL DIAGNOSIS OF AGEP

The most important differential diagnosis of AGEP is pustular psoriasis. The important differentiating features are given in Table 6.1. Other important differential diagnoses include pustular variant of drug hypersensitivity syndrome, subcorneal pustular dermatosis, pustular vasculitis, and Stevens-Johnson syndrome/toxic epidermal necrolysis.

DIAGNOSIS

Diagnosis of AGEP is usually with the help of clinical findings, histopathological findings, and patch tests.

1. *Histopathological features of AGEP*: Neutrophilic spongiotic pustules are the most striking feature of AGEP. There is spongiosis with minimal acanthosis of the epidermis. Apoptotic keratinocytes are seen in the adjacent epidermis. The main dermal features are papillary edema, mixed superficial, interstitial and mid-/deep-dermal infiltrates containing neutrophils and eosinophils.
2. *Patch test*: A patch test is conducted to confirm the offending agent causing AGEP. It should be conducted a month after resolution of skin lesions. Development of

a pustule at the site of application of the drug is considered a positive reaction in the case of AGEP. It can identify the culprit drug in almost 50% of cases. The risk of development of AGEP to a patch test is low and is generally considered safe. Other tests that can be done but are not widely available are lymphocyte transformation test (LTT) and lymphokine macrophage migration inhibition factor release assay.
3. *AGEP validation score*: The EuroSCAR study group presented a standardized scoring system in 2001 called the AGEP validation score. This scoring system takes into account the clinical pattern (presentation, evolution), biological data, and histological findings. The scale is used retrospectively by consensus groups to classify cases as definitive (8–12), probable (5–7), possible (1–4), or excluded. The details are given in Table 6.2.

MANAGEMENT

AGEP is generally a self-limiting disease. Management strategies include the following.

Immediate withdrawal of the offending drug

In patients taking multiple drugs, the drugs suspected to be the cause of AGEP should be discontinued, and patients should be counseled to avoid reexposure to the same drug.

Supportive care

Patients with severe forms of the disease are hospitalized and care should be given to maintain thermoregulation, fluid-electrolyte balance, nutritional support, avoidance of infections, and other supportive measures. In the pustular phase, moist dressings and antiseptic solutions may be used for relief of pruritus and prevention of bacterial superinfection. In the desquamation phase, emollients may be helpful in restoring skin barrier function.

Table 6.1 Differentiating features of acute generalized exanthematous pustulosis (AGEP) and pustular psoriasis

	AGEP	Pustular psoriasis
Age	Mostly adults, can occur in any age	Mostly adults
History of drug intake	Almost always present	Usually not present
History of psoriasis	Possible	Usually present
Clinical characteristics	Rapid development of dozens to hundreds of nonfollicular, sterile, pinhead-sized pustules on a background of edematous erythema with flexural accentuation	Discrete scaly plaques or generalized scaling with pustules may be seen; lakes of pus may be seen; more prolonged course
Fever	High, acute	Prolonged
Arthritis	Rare	Frequent
Histology	Spongiform subcorneal and/or intraepidermal pustules, edema of papillary dermis, vasculitis, exocytosis of eosinophils, single-cell necrosis of keratinocytes; psoriasiform acanthosis not seen	Subcorneal and/or intraepidermal pustules, papillomatosis, acanthosis; psoriasiform epidermal hyperplasia is a distinguishing feature

Table 6.2 Diagnostic criteria of acute generalized exanthematous pustulosis

Morphology	Features	Score
Pustules	Typical/compatible with disease/insufficient	+2/+1/0
Erythema	Typical/compatible with disease/insufficient	+2/+1/0
Distribution	Typical/compatible with disease/insufficient	+2/+1/0
Postpustular desquamation	Yes/no	+1/0
Mucous membrane involvement	Yes/no	−2/0
Course		
Acute onset	Yes/no	0/−2
Resolution	Yes/no	0/−4
Fever >38°C	Yes/no	+1/0
Polymorphonuclear cells >7/µL	Yes/no	+1/0
Histology	Other disease	−10
	Nonrepresentative	0
	Exocytosis of polymorphonuclear cells	+1
	Subcorneal and/or intraepidermal nonspongiform pustules	+2
	Spongiform subcorneal and/or intraepidermal pustules with papillary edema	+3
Score	8–12: Definite	
	5–7: Probable	
	1–4: Possible	
	0: Excluded	

Symptomatic treatment of pruritus and skin inflammation

Medium-potency topical corticosteroids are preferred along with oral antihistamines [7].

Severe cases

Only in severe cases, some authors consider systemic corticosteroids/other immunomodulators. A short course of corticosteroids (1–2 weeks) would be enough to manage most cases. Where the course is protracted, systemic steroids are indicated for a slightly longer duration.

CONCLUSION

Though this condition can often present in the emergency department, it is generally not a life-threatening one. However, it is important to identify the condition at the right time to avoid complications. Other physicians must also be sensitized regarding the existence of such a condition in order to prevent underdiagnosis and underreporting.

> ### KEY POINTS
>
> - AGEP is a less severe drug reaction compared to others though it can rarely present as emergency.
> - Pustules on skin and blood neutrophilia are characteristic features.

- Differentiating it from pustular psoriasis is difficult and drug history is important.
- Oral corticosteroids are the drugs of choice in severe cases.

REFERENCES

1. Baker H, Ryan TJ. Generalised pustular psoriasis. A clinical and epidemiological study of 104 cases. *Br J Dermatol* 1968;80:771–93.
2. Beylot C, Bioulac P, Doutre MS. Pustuloses exanthematiques aigues generalisees. A propos de 4 cas. *Ann Dermatol Venereol* 1980;107:37–48.
3. Sidoroff A et al. Risk factors for acute generalised exanthematous pustulosis (AGEP)—Results of a multinational case-control study (EuroSCAR). *Br J Dermatol* 2007;157:989–96.
4. Calistru AM, Lisboa C, Cunha AP, Bettencourt H, Azevedo F. Acute generalised exanthematous pustulosis to amoxicillin associated with parvovirus B19 reactivation. *Cutan Ocul Toxicol* 2012;31:258–61.
5. Roujeau JC et al. Acute generalised exanthematous pustulosis. Analysis of 63 cases. *Arch Dermatol* 1991;127:1333–8.
6. Hotz C et al. Systemic involvement of acute generalised exanthematous pustulosis: A retrospective study on 58 patients. *Br J Dermatol* 2013;169:1223–32.
7. Szatkowski J, Schwartz RA. Acute generalised exanthematous pustulosis (AGEP): A review and update. *J Am Acad Dermatol* 2015;73:843–8.

7

Drugs causing cutaneous necrosis

K. P. ANEESH AND P. VIJENDRAN

INTRODUCTION

Cutaneous necrosis is defined as skin disease with sudden onset of tissue death that results in significant morbidity and mortality and is usually, but not always, excruciatingly painful [1–4]. Cutaneous necrosis is a relatively rare complication of systemic drugs and can be mediated by various pathogenetic mechanisms. The clinical patterns and prognosis also vary depending upon the causative drug.

PATHOPHYSIOLOGY OF DRUG-INDUCED CUTANEOUS NECROSIS

Drug-induced cutaneous necrosis can be caused due to the following mechanisms [5]:

- Hypoxia
- Free radicals and proteases
- Chemical injury
- Secondary injury by infectious agents

Anticoagulants such as warfarin and heparin are the leading cause of drug-induced cutaneous necrosis. In 0.01%–0.1% of patients, warfarin is associated with warfarin-induced skin necrosis (WISN), a catastrophic complication that may even lead to death [6,7]. Warfarin induces a transient protein C deficiency, prior to reductions in the procoagulant factors. The resultant transient imbalance in the anticoagulant and procoagulant pathways leads to an initial paradoxical hypercoagulable state resulting in microvascular thrombosis and cutaneous necrosis [8,9].

Heparin-induced cutaneous necrosis is a rare but serious complication of administration of low molecular weight heparin (LMWH) or unfractionated heparin (UFH). It is associated with formation of immunoglobulin G (IgG) antibodies against the heparin-PF4 complex (platelet factor-4), leading to paradoxical intravascular thrombosis and thrombocytopenia [10]. Poor IV or subcutaneous injection technique is another proposed etiology of the condition as the lesions tend to occur at injection sites [11].

CLASSIFICATION OF DRUGS CAUSING CUTANEOUS NECROSIS

Depending on the underlying pathogenic mechanisms, drugs and chemicals causing cutaneous necrosis can be broadly classified into three groups: primary, secondary, and those aggravated by predisposing conditions as depicted in Box 7.1. A proposed classification of drugs causing cutaneous necrosis based on the primary or secondary pathogenic mechanisms and underlying aggravating factors is depicted in Table 7.1.

CLINICAL FEATURES OF CUTANEOUS NECROSIS

History

A thorough history to elucidate the possible causes of the necrosis of skin has to be taken. This should include history of recent travel and history of underlying illnesses such as diabetes, renal disease, AIDS, autoimmune diseases, inflammatory bowel disease, and malignancies. History of recent surgeries and prolonged bedridden states may also be contributory [4]. A thorough history would generally be able to identify the cause of the symptoms and the causative drug if implicated. The Naranjo adverse drug reaction probability score may be employed to assess the temporal association of the drug with the symptoms of the patients [14].

BOX 7.1: Proposed etiological classification of drug-induced cutaneous necrosis

Primary (Direct injury to keratinocytes)
  Immunological
  Nonimmunological

Secondary
  Vasculitis
  Disseminated intravascular coagulation
  Purpura fulminans
  Cryoglobulinemic
  Neutropenia

Aggravated by other predisposing factors
  Protein C and protein S deficiency
  Antiphospholipid antibody syndrome
  Antithrombin deficiency
  Factor V Leiden mutation

Clinical patterns

The clinical pattern of appearance of the cutaneous lesions may vary according to the underlying mechanism of injury to the cells.

MICROVASCULAR THROMBOSIS AND VASCULOPATHY

The term *vasculopathy* or *pseudovasculitis* is used to describe certain degrees of vascular alterations and injuries that fail to satisfy the criteria of vasculitis. Some instances of drug-induced vasculopathic reactions may manifest as cutaneous necrosis. Vasopressin and its analogues are known to cause peripheral vasoconstriction leading to cutaneous necrosis. Terlipressin, an arginin-vasopressin analogue with high V1-receptor affinity, when used in treatment of hepatorenal syndrome and esophageal varices has been reported to cause cutaneous necrosis in several case reports [15–22]. Skin lesions most commonly involve the thighs and abdomen followed by scrotum in men [23]. Use of vasopressin has been associated with cutaneous

Table 7.1 Proposed classification of drugs causing cutaneous necrosis

Primary mechanism	Secondary mechanism	Causes/predisposing factors	Example
Hypoxia	Thromboembolism		Transcatheter arterial thromboembolization
	Microvascular thrombosis	Protein C and protein S deficiency	Warfarin
		DIC	
		Thrombocytopenia	LMW heparin
		Cryoglobulinemia	
		APLA syndrome	
	Vasculitis	Antihistone ab	
		Antiphospholipid ab	
		ANCA-associated vasculitis	Antithyroid drugs, cefotaxime, minocycline, clozapine, allopurinol, TNF-α inhibitors
		Polyarteritis nodosa	Minocycline
	Vasculopathy		Levamisole
		Arterial vasoconstriction	Vasopressin, terlipressin
	Cholesterol embolism		Anticoagulants and thrombolytics
	Calciphylaxis		Iron dextran, immunosuppressants, corticosteroids, insulin injection, vitamin D, warfarin
	Pyoderma gangrenosum		Isotretinoin, propylthiouracil, tyrosine kinase inhibitor (sunitinib, imatinib, geftinib), G-CSF, TNF-α inhibitor (infliximab, adalimumab)
Chemical/traumatic injury	Altered tissue pH/osmolality		Injection arginine [12], injection hydroxyzine [13], oily substances, mustard
Infective	Necrotizing fasciitis due to neutropenia		NSAIDs, rituximab
Unknown			Interferon-α

Abbreviations: ANCA, antineutrophil cytoplasmic antibody; APLA, antiphospholipid antibody syndrome; DIC, disseminated intravascular coagulation; G-CSF, granulocyte colony-stimulating factor; LMW, low molecular weight; NSAIDs, nonsteroidal anti-inflammatory drugs; TNF, tumor necrosis factor.

necrosis and bullous lesions along with rhabdomyolysis in another case report [24].

Alternatively, drug-induced vascular injury may be associated with livedoid skin lesions. The red or hyperpigmented cutaneous streaks are subtle and are referred to as *micro-livedo* and are clinically different from the full-blown net-like hyperpigmentation in livedo reticularis. Microvascular occlusion due to cryofibrinogenemia, antiphospholipid antibody syndrome and hypercoagulable states from protein C and S deficiency have to be considered as differentials in such a clinical scenario [25].

WISN tends to occur in middle-aged obese females being treated for deep venous or pulmonary thrombosis for 3–6 days without bridging with heparin therapy [6]. Predisposing factors like protein C and protein S deficiency, antithrombin deficiency, or factor V Leiden mutation may be present. The lesions start initially as an acute-onset, poorly demarcated, erythematous flush of the affected area with associated paresthesia and edema. They later evolve into painful, well-demarcated lesions as fluid accumulates in the dermis and subcutaneous tissue [6]. Clinically this may result in peau d'orange appearance. Later inevitable full-thickness skin necrosis extending into the subcutaneous tissue ensues, which manifests clinically as petechiae and hemorrhagic bullae (Figure 7.1). These painful plaques evolve into necrotic and hemorrhagic blisters or ulcers as a consequence of occlusive thrombi in the skin and subcutaneous vessels [26]. Areas with extensive subcutaneous fat, such as abdomen, buttocks, thighs, legs, and mammary tissue in females are commonly affected. Though symptoms generally start within 10 days of introducing warfarin, delayed onset of lesions occurring up to 15 years after initiation of therapy have also been reported [27].

Heparin-induced skin necrosis (heparin-induced thrombocytopenia and thrombosis syndrome [HITT]) is commonly seen in middle-aged women 5–10 days of initiation of LMWH therapy [10]. In patients previously sensitized to heparin, sudden onset of skin necrosis may occur [28]. It may also have a delayed presentation several months after starting the therapy in naïve patients. Painful erythematous plaques appear at the injection site initially, which later progress to purpuric plaques with bullae formation and necrosis. The lesions are generally small and well circumscribed with a diameter of only a few centimeters [11,29].

DISSEMINATED INTRAVASCULAR COAGULATION AND PURPURA FULMINANS

Purpura fulminans is a rapidly progressing thrombotic disorder characterized by skin necrosis and disseminated intravascular coagulation (DIC) [30]. The clinical presentation of purpura fulminans is with acute-onset purpuric rash that rapidly progresses to large ecchymotic areas with sharp, irregular borders (Figure 7.2). In severe cases, gangrene and necrosis of the extremities may be observed [31]. Various drugs have been implicated in the causation of purpura fulminans. Individuals with protein C and protein S

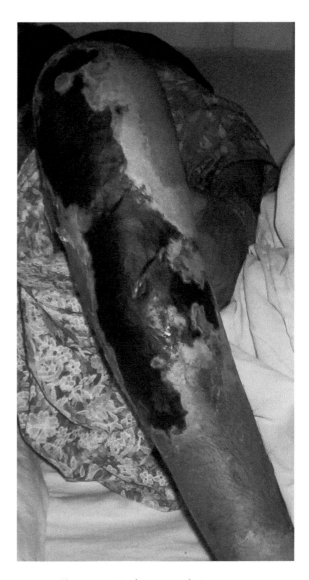

Figure 7.1 Skin necrosis due to warfarin.

deficiencies are predisposed to development of purpura fulminans, including the drug-induced ones. In a study by Bonaldo et al., analyzing the World Health Organization's Global Individual Case Safety Report (ICSR) database, the common drugs implicated in causation of purpura fulminans were antineoplastic agents, antithrombotic agents, and antibacterials for systemic use. Other drugs that were most frequently reported were paracetamol, dabigatran, oxaliplatin, and bevacizumab [32].

VASCULITIS

Vasculitis is the type of vascular injury characterized by perivascular inflammatory infiltrate and fibrinoid necrosis of the vessel wall. The clinical presentation varies based on the size of blood vessels primarily affected in the vasculitis process. Involvement of the small dermal vessels results in superficial palpable purpura, vesicobullous lesions, and superficial ulcers. These ulcers generally have regular borders. When the predominant vessels involved are the deeper intramuscular arteries, they present as

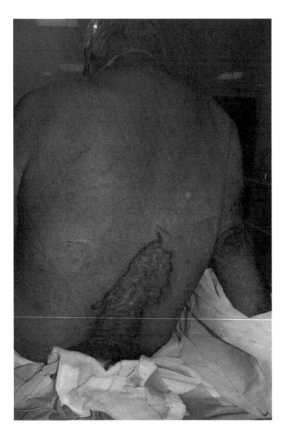

Figure 7.2 Violaceous plaque with ulceration in a case of heparin necrosis.

painful red nodules, punched-out irregularly shaped ulcers (Figure 7.3), or gangrene [33]. The lower extremities are most commonly affected, and involvement of upper parts of body indicates more severe disease [34]. Systemic symptoms of fever, malaise, and joint pains when present may require workup for a connective tissue disease before a final diagnosis of drug-induced ulceration is made [35,36].

Drug-induced leukocytoclastic vasculitis may present as superficial ulcerations and hemorrhagic bullae on the lower portion of the leg and is generally devoid of any systemic involvement.

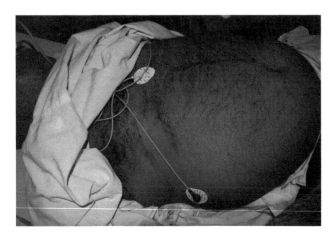

Figure 7.3 Vasculitic ulcer on abdomen.

Drug-induced C-ANCA- and P-ANCA-mediated cutaneous vasculitis affects small to medium-sized vessels and presents with deep painful ulcerations that may mimic pyoderma gangrenosum. Hydralazine, minocycline, propylthiouracil (PTU), penicillamine, allopurinol, and sulfasalazine have all been implicated in causation of ANCA-associated vasculitis [37–41].

PTU is implicated for 80%–90% of ANCA-associated vasculitides (AAV) due to antithyroid drugs. The increasing use of anti-tumor necrosis factor-α (anti-TNF-α) agents have resulted in increasingly higher incidence of AAV vasculitis induced by such agents. The pathogenetic mechanisms of drug-induced AAV are proposedly distinct from other forms of AAV. Drugs like minocycline have also been implicated in causation of polyarteritis nodosa–like lesions in the form of painful nodules progressing to cutaneous necrosis and ulceration [42,43].

FACTITIOUS DERMATITIS CAUSING NECROSIS BY INJECTION OF MEDICATIONS

This group is characterized by self-inflicted skin necrosis caused by injecting various medications. Factitious dermatitis is becoming increasingly common in clinical practice [44,45]. The behavior is not better explained by another mental disorder such as a delusional disorder or another psychotic disorder. Histopathology may show acute inflammation with increased polymorphonuclear leukocytes, scattered erythrocytes, areas of necrosis, and areas of healing with fibrocystic reaction [46].

FACTITIOUS PANNICULITIS DUE TO MEDICATIONS

Factitious or artefactual panniculitides result from external injury to subcutaneous fat [47]. The widespread use of injectable fillers in aesthetic dermatology and plastic surgery for the treatment of wrinkles and soft tissue augmentation has increased the incidence of drug-induced panniculitis causing cutaneous necrosis. Biodegradable or temporary fillers induce severe complications but are generally self-limiting when compared to semipermanent or permanent fillers. Cosmetic fillers currently used for tissue augmentation, such as bovine collagen, silicone, polymethyl methacrylate (PMMA) microspheres, polymethylsiloxane, and hydroxyethylmethacrylate particles in hyaluronic acid may sometimes induce factitious panniculitis [48–51]. Injections having phosphatidylcholine for the treatment of localized fat accumulation and lipomas may cause factitious panniculitis of the injected fat tissue. Other causes of factitious panniculitis causing cutaneous necrosis include subcutaneous injection of oily materials including mineral oils like paraffin or vegetable oils like cotton seed or sesame oils for augmenting the size of breasts or genitalia [52]. These substances induce a subcutaneous foreign body reaction known as sclerosing lipogranuloma or paraffinoma and may be associated with cutaneous necrosis [53]. Panniculitis and subsequent tissue necrosis have been reported at the sites of injection of several therapeutic drugs and have been listed in

Box 7.2. Extravasation of cytostatic agents during antineoplastic chemotherapy and acupuncture techniques also may induce panniculitis with skin necrosis. Clinical lesions show red-brown painful edema which evolves into necrotic plaques that heal with sclerotic, indurated scars (Figure 7.4) [54–57].

INVESTIGATIONS

Investigations relevant to arrive at the diagnosis, identify the underlying cause, and assess the response to treatment have to be employed on a case-by-case basis.

A properly done skin biopsy almost always yields diagnostic information. The site and technique of biopsy have to be chosen carefully. Histopathology sections may reveal evidence of vasculitis, intravascular thrombosis, or signs of arteritis as in drug-induced polyarteritis nodosa. The characteristic finding in WISN is diffuse microthrombi within dermal and subcutaneous capillaries, venules, and deep veins, with endothelial cell damage resulting in ischemic skin necrosis and marked extravasation of red blood cells. Vascular inflammation and arterial involvement can differentiate a primary vasculitic process from WISN [71,72]. Calcium deposits in dermis and subcutaneous vessels highlighted by von Kossa stain point to the possibility of calciphylaxis. Intravascular cholesterol clefts are characteristic of cholesterol microemboli [71]. Multiple swabs for culture of bacteria and fungi have to be obtained from appropriate sites and antibiotic therapy modified accordingly. A purulent, culture-positive, rapidly progressive ulcer is characteristic of necrotizing fasciitis [73].

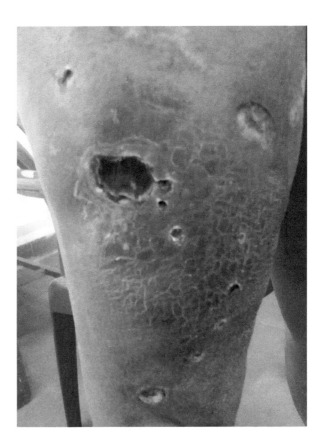

Figure 7.4 Factitious panniculitis due to Fortwin injection.

Protein C and protein S deficiency and prolonged platelet time (PT) may be found in WISN, whereas heparin– PF4 IgG antibodies may be positive in heparin-induced thrombocytopenia and thrombosis syndrome (HITT). Even though thrombocytopenia with more than 50% reduction in platelet count is a feature of HITT, platelet count may be normal when only skin necrosis is present. Other relevant biochemical investigations have to be chosen based on clinical suspicion. The available battery of investigations is listed in Table 7.2.

MANAGEMENT

The management of conditions causing cutaneous necrosis requires a multipronged approach. The primary aim should be to identify the culprit drug in cases of drug-induced cutaneous necrosis. Early diagnosis can allow for early treatment and can decrease the chance of morbidity and mortality. A temporal association between drug intake and appearance and aggravation of the symptoms needs to be considered prior to making a diagnosis. Once the causative drug is identified, immediate withdrawal of the same has to be done. The management of drug-induced cutaneous necrosis due to various causes is discussed under the following headings:

- General Management Principles
- Specific Management Aspects

Table 7.2 Battery of investigations

Confirmation of diagnosis	Routine investigations	To rule out underlying cause
Skin biopsy	CBC with platelet count	c-ANCA, p-ANCA
Swab for culture	ESR	APLA
	Blood urea, serum creatinine	Rheumatoid factor
	Serum bilirubin, liver enzymes	Antinuclear antibodies
	C-reactive protein	Serum complement levels (CH50, C3, C4)
	PT, aPTT	Protein C and protein S levels
		Serum cryoglobulin and cryofibrinogen levels
		Serum amylase and lipase
		Serum parathormone level
		Hepatitis C antibodies
		Hepatitis B surface antigen
		Fibrinogen levels
		Antithrombin III
		FDP
		D-dimer

Abbreviations: ANCA, antineutrophil cytoplasmic antibody; APLA, antiphospholipid antibody syndrome; aPTT, activated partial thromboplastin time; CBC, complete blood count; ESR, erythrocyte sedimentation rate; FDP, fibrin degradation product; PT, prothrombin time.

General management principles

DÉBRIDEMENT

Controlled débridement of necrotic tissue is the cornerstone of treatment and can increase patient survival and outcome [74]. Patients who underwent surgical débridement more than 12 hours after hospital admission had higher amputation and mortality rates in a series [75–78].

WOUND DRESSING AND CARE

Even though traditionally wet and dry gauze has been used as wound dressing, dressings that create a moist environment are now considered to provide the optimal conditions for wound healing [79]. Occlusive dressings are thought to increase cell proliferation and activity by retaining an optimum level of wound exudate. Various biomaterials that can be used as dressing materials to provide fast and efficient healing are enumerated in Box 7.3 [80–82].

BOX 7.3: Classification of biomaterials

Temporary impervious dressing materials

(a) *Single-layer materials*
Naturally occurring or biological dressing substitute, e.g., amniotic membrane, potato peel
Synthetic dressing substitute, e.g., synthetic polymer sheet (Tegaderm®, Opsite®), polymer foam or spray

(b) *Bilayered tissue-engineered materials*, e.g., TransCyte

Single-layer durable skin substitutes

(a) *Epidermal substitutes*
Cultured epithelial autograft (CEA)

(b) *Dermal substitutes*
Bovine collagen sheet, e.g., Kollagen®
Porcine collagen sheet
Bovine dermal matrix, e.g., Matriderm®
Human dermal matrix, e.g., AlloDerm®

Composite skin substitutes

(a) *Skin graft*
Xenograft
Allograft
Autograft

(b) *Tissue-engineered skin*
Apligraf®
Dermal regeneration template, e.g., Integra®
Biobrane®

Source: Anish S. *Indian J Dermatol Venereol Leprol* 2015; 81(2):175; Singh A, Shenoy Y. *Indian J Plast Surg* 2012;45(2):388; Halim A, Khoo T, Shah JY. *Indian J Plast Surg* 2010;43(3):23.

PREVENTION OF INFECTIONS AND TREATMENT OF EXISTING INFECTIONS

Prevention of contamination of the site and subsequent infections is pivotal in the management of acute skin necrosis. Empiric antibiotic therapy can be employed until definite culture results are obtained. The selection of antibiotics can further be modified based on the culture and sensitivity report. Culture reports obtained from superficial swabs are occasionally erroneous and should be avoided.

Broad-spectrum antibiotics are preferred as most of the infections are polymicrobial. Options include combinations such as ampicillin, gentamicin, and clindamycin or metronidazole. Ampicillin-sulbactam, ticarcillin-clavulanate potassium, and piperacillin-tazobactam also provide adequate anaerobic and aerobic coverage. Piperacillin-tazobactam or ticarcillin-clavulanate potassium therapy has the advantage of providing gram-negative and pseudomonas coverage. Nafcillin plus agents with anaerobic and gram-negative coverage has also been used in the treatment of such infections

Table 7.3 Management and treatment options to be considered

Condition	Considerations for management
Warfarin necrosis	Immediate discontinuation of warfarin
	VitaminA
	Fresh-frozen plasma
	Protein C concentrate
	Unfractionated heparin at therapeutic dose
	Antibiotic therapy if secondary infections present
Heparin necrosis	Immediate discontinuation of heparin
	Antithrombin (danaparoid sodium or hirudin)
	Systemic steroids
	Surgical débridement
	Contraindication: warfarin
Calciphylaxis secondary to drugs (in the setting of end-stage renal disease)	Hemodialysis
	Intravenous sodium thiosulfate
	Bisphosphonates
	Cinacalcet
	Paricalcitol
	Hyperbaric oxygen
	Analgesia for pain
	Surgical wound débridement
	Contraindication: systemic steroids
	Parathyroidectomy
	Hyperbaric oxygen
	Analgesia for pain
	Surgical wound débridement
	Contraindication: systemic corticosteroids
Calciphylaxis secondary to drugs (in the setting of primary hyperparathyroidism)	Parathyroidectomy
	Hyperbaric oxygen
	Analgesia for pain
	Surgical wound débridement
	Contraindication: systemic corticosteroids
Purpura fulminans due to drugs	Heparin
	Protein C and antithrombin III replacement
	Tissue plasminogen activator
	Systemic steroids
	Surgical débridement or amputation

Source: Karimi K et al. *J Cutan Med Surg* 2017;21:425–37 [88].

[83–86]. Skin necrosis may be due to necrotizing infections secondary to neutropenia caused by various drugs.

OTHER TREATMENT OPTIONS

Other less commonly used treatment options like hyperbaric oxygen therapy have been used as adjunctive therapy in the management of infections in necrotic tissues and necrotizing infections [87].

Specific management aspects

Discontinuation of the causative agent is the initial step of specific management. Contact with the etiological agent has to be interrupted as early as possible in cases of necrosis due to direct application of the incriminating substance. Further management options have to be carefully decided on a case-by-case basis. Management options to be considered based on the causative drug and various underlying pathogenic mechanisms are enumerated in Table 7.3 [88].

CONCLUSION

Although rare, drug-induced cutaneous necrosis is a serious adverse reaction associated with use of certain drugs. Early recognition of the condition with identification and discontinuation of the incriminating drug and implementation of therapeutic intervention including surgical débridement are essential in improving patient outcome. A thorough clinical history, along with relevant investigations, including a timely skin biopsy, are crucial for early diagnosis. The treating physician has to bear in mind the possibility of a factitious cause when approaching such cases presenting with cutaneous necrosis.

KEY POINTS

- Drug induced cutaneous necrosis is a rare severe drug reaction caused by drugs like heparin and warfarin mostly.
- Factitious causes need to be ruled out.
- Drug induced vasculitis and purpura fulminans contribute to the incidence.
- Identifying the condition early is very important to prevent further damage.
- Debridement, antibiotics to prevent secondary infection and supportive care are cornerstones in treatment.

REFERENCES

1. Grover S. Severe cutaneous adverse reactions. *Indian J Dermatol Venereol Leprol* 2011;77(1):3.
2. Wiffen P, Gill M, Edwards J, Moore A. Adverse drug reactions in hospital patients. A systematic review of the prospective and retrospective studies. *Bandolier Extra* 2002;2:1–16.
3. Gruchalla R. Understanding drug allergies. *J Allergy Clin Immunol* 2000;105:637–44.
4. Wallace JS, Hall JC. Use of drug therapy to manage acute cutaneous necrosis of skin. *J Drugs Dermatol* 2010;9:4.
5. Kumar V, Abbas AK, Aster JC. Chapter 1: Cell injury, cell death and adaptations. In: *Robbins Basic Pathology.* 9th ed. Philadelphia: Saunders; 2012: 6.
6. Chan YC, Valenti D, Mansfield AO, Stansby G. Warfarin induced skin necrosis. *Br J Surg* 2000;87(3):266–72.
7. Ad-El DD et al. Warfarin skin necrosis: Local and systemic factors. *Br J Plast Surg* 2000;53(7):624–6.
8. Grenier N, Chen-Tsai C. Nonpalpable purpura within a setting of anticoagulant therapy and metastatic carcinoma. *Int J Low Extrem Wounds* 2006;5(3):200–3.
9. Harenberg J, Hoffmann U, Huhle G, Winkler M, Bayerl C. Cutaneous reactions to anticoagulants: Recognition and management. *Am J Clin Dermatol* 2001;2(2):69–75.
10. Warkentin TE, Roberts RS, Hirsh J, Kelton JG. Heparin- induced skin lesions and other unusual sequelae of the heparin-induced thrombocytopenia syndrome: A nested cohort study. *Chest* 2005;127(5):1857–61.
11. Katsourakis A, Noussios G, Kapoutsis G, Chatzitheoklitos E. Low molecular weight heparin-induced skin necrosis: A case report. *Case Rep Med* 2011;1–2.
12. Amano H, Nagai Y, Kowase T, Ishikawa O. Cutaneous necrosis induced by extravasation of arginine mono-hydrochloride. *Acta Derm Venereol* 2008;88(3):310–1.
13. Chikako Kishi HA, Du J, Hwang SK, Zhang J. Cutaneous necrosis induced by extravasation of hydroxyzine. *Eur J Dermatol* 2014;24(1):130–1.
14. Naranjo CA et al. A method for estimating the probability of adverse drug reactions. *Clin Pharmacol Ther* 1981;30(2):239–45.
15. Di Micoli A et al. Terlipressin infusion induces ischemia of breast skin in a cirrhotic patient with hepatorenal syndrome. *Dig Liver Dis* 2008;40:304–5.
16. Posada C et al. Cutaneous necrosis secondary to terlipressin therapy. *Acta Derm Venereol* 2009;89:434–5.
17. Herrera J et al. Extensive cutaneous necrosis due to terlipressin use. *Gastroenterol Hepatol* 2015;38(1):12–3.
18. Bañuelos Ramírez DD, Sánchez Alonso S, Ramírez Palma MM. Sildenafil in severe peripheral ischemia induced by terlipressin. A case report. *Reumatol Clin* 2011;7(1):59–60.
19. Taşliyurt T et al. Ischemic skin necrosis following terlipressin therapy: Report of two cases and review of the literature. *Turk J Gastroenterol* 2012;23(6):788–91.
20. Lee HJ, Oh MJ. A case of peripheral gangrene and osteomyelitis secondary to terlipressin therapy in advanced liver disease. *Clin Mol Hepatol* 2013;19:179–84.
21. Lu YY, Wei KC, Wu CS. Terlipressin-induced extensive skin necrosis: A case report and published work review. *J Dermatol* 2012;39:866–8.
22. Yefet E et al. Extensive epidermal necrosis due to terlipressin. *Isr Med Assoc J* 2011;13:180–1.
23. Iglesias Julián E, Badía Aranda E, Bernad Cabredo B, Corrales Cruz D, Romero Arauzo MJ. Cutaneous necrosis secondary to terlipressin therapy. A rare but serious side effect. Case report and literature review. *Rev Esp Enfermedades Dig [Internet].* 2017 [cited September 29, 2017];109. Available from: https://online.reed.es/fichaArticulo.aspx?iarf=683767745233-413277197160
24. Koremberg R, Landau-Price D, Penneys M. Vasopressin induced bullous disease and cutaneous necrosis. *J Am Acad Dermatol* 1986;15:393–8.
25. Panuncialman J, Falanga V. Unusual causes of cutaneous ulceration. *Surg Clin North Am* 2010;90(6):1161–80.
26. Roujeau JC, Roujeau JC, Revuz J. Intensive care in dermatology. In: Champion RH, Pye RJ (Eds), *Recent Advances in Dermatology.* Edinburgh: Churchill-Livingstone; 1990:85–99.
27. Jorg I, Fenyvesi T, Harenberg J. Anticoagulant-related skin reactions. *Expert Opin Drug Saf* 2002;1(3):287–94.

28. Warkentin TE. Heparin-induced thrombocytopenia: A clinicopathologic syndrome. *Thromb Haemost* 1999;82(2):439–47.

29. Toll A, Gallardo F, Abella ME, Fontcuberta J, Barranco C, Pujol RM. Low-molecular-weight heparin-induced skin necrosis: A potential association with pre-existent hypercoagulable states. *Int J Dermatol* 2005;44(11):964–6.

30. Chalmers E et al. Purpura fulminans: Recognition, diagnosis and management. *Arch Dis Child* 2011;96(11):1066.

31. Kosaraju N, Korrapati V, Thomas A, James BR. Adult purpura fulminans associated with non-steroidal anti-inflammatory drug use. *J Postgrad Med* 2011;57(2):145–6.

32. Bonaldo G et al. Drugs-induced disseminated intravascular coagulation: A pharmacoepidemiological study based on WHO database of adverse drug reactions. *Clin Ther* 39(8):e31–2.

33. Chen KR CJ. Clinical approach to cutaneous vasculitis. *Am J Clin Dermatol* 2008;9(2):71–92.

34. Ioannidou DJ, Krasagakis K, Daphnis EK, Perakis KE, Sotsiou F, Tosca AD. Cutaneous small vessel vasculitis: An entity with frequent renal involvement. *Arch Dermatol* 2002;138(3):412–4.

35. Carlson JA, Cavaliere LF, Grant-Kels JM. Cutaneous vasculitis: Diagnosis and management. *Clin Dermatol* 2006;24(5):414–29.

36. Carlson JA, Ng BT, Chen KR. Cutaneous vasculitis update: Diagnostic criteria, classification, epidemiology, etiology, pathogenesis, evaluation and prognosis. *Am J Dermatopathol* 2005;27(6):504–28.

37. Choi HK. Drug-associated antineutrophil cytoplasmic antibody-positive vasculitis: Prevalence among patients with high titers of antimyeloperoxidase antibodies. *Arthritis Rheum* 2000;43:405–13.

38. Cambridge G, Wallace H, Bernstein RM. Autoantibodies to myeloperoxidase in idiopathic and drug-induced systemic lupus erythematosus and vasculitis. *Br J Rheumatol* 1994;33:109–14.

39. Choi HK, Slot MC, Pan G, Weissbach CA, Niles JL, Merkel PA. Evaluation of antineutrophil cytoplasmic antibody seroconversion induced by minocycline, sulfasalazine, or penicillamine. *Arthritis Rheum* 2000;43:2488–92.

40. Sato H et al. High prevalence of antineutrophil cytoplasmic antibody in childhood onset Grave's disease treated with propylthiouracil. *J Clin Endocrinol Metab* 2000;85:4270–3.

41. Sera N et al. Treatment with propylthiouracil is associated with appearance of antineutrophil cytoplasmic antibodies in some patients with Graves' disease. *Thyroid* 2000;10:595–9.

42. Culver B, Itkin A, Pischel K. Case report and review of minocycline-induced cutaneous polyarteritis nodosa. *Arthritis Care Res* 2005;53(3):468–70.

43. Tehrani R, Nash-Goelitz A, Adams E, Dahiya M, Eilers D. Minocycline-induced cutaneous polyarteritis nodosa. *J Clin Rheumatol Pract Rep Rheum Musculoskelet Dis* 2007;13(3):146–9.

44. Griffiths EM, Barker J. Psychodermatology and psychocutaneous disease. In: Griffiths CEM, Barker J, Bleiker T, Creamer CR (Eds), *Rook's Textbook of Dermatology*. 9th ed. Part 7, Section 86. Edinburgh: Wiley Blackwell; 2016; 22.

45. Choudhary SV, Choudhary SV, Khairkar P, Singh A, Gupta S. Dermatitis artefacta: Keloids and foreign body granuloma due to overvalued ideation of acupuncture. *Indian J Dermatol Venereol Leprol* 2009;75:606–8.

46. Antony SJ, Antony SJ, Mannion SB. Dermatitis artefacta revisited. *Cutis* 1995;55:362–4.

47. Requena L, Requena L, Sanchez Yus E. Panniculitis. Part II. Mostly lobular panniculitis. *J Am Acad Dermatol* 2001;45:325–61.

48. Garcia-Domingo MI et al. Disseminated and recurrent sarcoid-like granulomatous panniculitis due to bovine collagen injection. *J Investig Allergol Clin Immunol* 2000;10:107–9.

49. Requena C et al. Adverse reactions to injectable aesthetic microimplants. *Am J Dermatopathol* 2001;23:197–202.

50. Requena L, Cerroni L, Kutzner H. Histopathologic patterns associated with external agents. *Dermatol Clin* 2012;30:731–48.

51. Sanmartín O, Requena C, Requena L. Factitial panniculitis. *Dermatol Clin* 2008;26:519–27.

52. Darsow U et al. Subcutaneous oleomas induced by self-injection of sesame seed oil for muscle augmentation. *J Am Acad Dermatol* 2000;42:292–4.

53. Achauer BM, Achauer BM. A serious complication following medical-grade silicone injection of the face. *Plast Reconstr Surg* 1983;71:251–4.

54. Alfaro-Rubio A et al. Extravasación de agentescitostáticos: Unacomplicaciónseria del tratamientooncológico. *Actas Dermosifiliogr* 2006;97:169–76.

55. Goolsby TV, Lombardo FA. Extravasation of chemotherapeutic agents: Prevention and treatment. *Semin Oncol* 2006;33:139–43.

56. Lee JS, Ahn SK, Lee SH. Factitial panniculitis induced by cupping and acupuncture. *Cutis* 1995;55:217–18.

57. Jeong KH, Lee MH. Two cases of factitial panniculitis induced by electroacupuncture. *Clin Exp Dermatol* 2009;34:e170–3.

58. Gandhi V et al. Pentazocine-induced cutaneous sclerosis and panniculitis in an Indian male. *Int J Dermatol* 2004;43:516–17.

59. Farrant P, Creamer D, Fuller C. Extensive cutaneous fibrosis and ulceration caused by methadone injection. *Clin Exp Dermatol* 2005;30:87–8.

60. McCain J et al. Intramuscular aurothioglucose (Solganal) leading to panniculitis. *J Rheumatol* 1993;20:1632–3.

61. Pang BK, Munro V, Kossard S. Pseudoscleroderma secondary to phytomenadione (vitamin K1) injections: Texier's disease. *Australas J Dermatol* 1996;37:44–7.

62. Laws JW. Pyrexia of unusual origin. *BMJ* 1951;2:157–8.

63. Vetter WL, Weiland AJ, Arnett FC. Factitious extension contracture of the elbow: Case report. *J Hand Surg [Am]* 1983;8:277–9.

64. Kossard S, Ecker RI, Dicken CH. Povidone panniculitis. Polyvinylpyrrolidone panniculitis. *Arch Dermatol* 1980;116:704–6.

65. Soares Almeida LM, Requena L, Kutzner H, Angulo J, de Sa J, Pignatelli J. Localized panniculitis secondary to subcutaneous glatiramer acetate injections for the treatment of multiple sclerosis: A clinicopathologic and immunohistochemical study. *J Am Acad Dermatol* 2006;55:969–75.

66. Chong H et al. Persistent nodules at injection sites (aluminium granuloma)—Clinicopathological study of 14 cases with a diverse range of histological reaction patterns. *Histopathology* 2006;48:182–8.

67. O'Sullivan SS et al. Panniculitis and lipoatrophy after subcutaneous injection of interferon beta-1b in a patient with multiple sclerosis. *J Neurol Neurosurg Psychiatry* 2006;77:1382–3.

68. Kaufman HL et al. Panniculitis after vaccination against CEA and MUC1 in a patient with pancreatic cancer. *Lancet Oncol* 2005;6:62–3.

69. Prendiville J, Thiessen P, Mallory SB. Neutrophilic dermatoses in two children with idiopathic neutropenia: Association with granulocyte colony-stimulating factor (G-CSF) therapy. *Pediatr Dermatol* 2001;18:417–21.

70. Baars JW et al. Lobular panniculitis after subcutaneous administration of interleukin-2 (IL-2), and its exacerbation during intravenous therapy with IL-2. *Br J Cancer* 1992;66:698–9.

71. Miura Y, Ardenghy M, Ramasastry S, Kovach R, Hochberg J. Coumadin necrosis of the skin: Report of four patients. *Ann Plast Surg* 1996;37:332–7.

72. Nalbandian RM, Mader IJ, Barrett JL, Pearce JF, Rupp EC. Petechiae, ecchymoses, and necrosis of skin induced by coumarin congeners: Rare, occasionally lethal complications of anticoagulant therapy. *J Am Med Assoc* 1965;192:107–12.

73. Nazarian RM, Van Cott EM, Zembowicz A, Duncan LM. Warfarin-induced skin necrosis. *J Am Acad Dermatol* 2009;61(2):325–32.

74. Gray D et al. Consensus guidance for the use of debridement techniques in the UK. *Wounds UK* 2011;7(1):77–84.

75. Sudarsky LA, Laschinger JC, Coppa GF, Spencer FC. Improved results from a standardized approach in treating patients with necrotizing fasciitis. *Ann Surg* 1987;206:661–5.

76. NHS Wirral. Procedure for Conservative Sharp Debridement. 2009. Available at: http://www.wirral.nhs.uk/document_uploads/Policies_Nursing/ProcedureConservativeSharpDebridementJune09.pdf (accessed December 2, 2012).

77. Leaper D. Sharp technique for wound debridement. 2002. Available at: http://www.worldwidewounds.com/2002/december/Leaper/Sharp-Debridement.html (accessed December 2, 2012).

78. Vowden K, Vowden P. Wound debridement Part 1: Non-sharp techniques. *J Wound Care* 1999a;8(5):237–40.

79. Jones V, Grey JE. ABC of wound healing, wound dressings. *BMJ* 2006;332.

80. Anish S. Skin substitutes in dermatology. *Indian J Dermatol Venereol Leprol* 2015;81(2):175.

81. Singh A, Shenoy Y. Skin substitutes: An Indian perspective. *Indian J Plast Surg* 2012;45(2):388.

82. Halim A, Khoo T, Shah JY. Biologic and synthetic skin substitutes: An overview. *Indian J Plast Surg* 2010;43(3):23.

83. Hill MK, Sanders CV. Necrotizing and gangrenous soft tissue infections. In: Sanders CV, Nesbitt LT Jr (Eds). *The Skin and Infection: A Color Atlas and Text*. Baltimore: Williams & Wilkins, 1995:62–75.

84. Bosshardt TL, Henderson VJ, Organ CH Jr. Necrotizing soft-tissue infections. *Arch Surg* 1996;131:846–52.

85. Elliott D, Kufera JA, Myers RA. The microbiology of necrotizing soft tissue infections. *Am J Surg* 2000;179:361–6.

86. Chapnick EK, Abter EI. Necrotizing soft-tissue infections. *Infect Dis Clin North Am* 1996;10:835–55.

87. Moses AE. Necrotizing fasciitis: Flesh-eating microbes. *Isr J Med Sci* 1996;32:781–4.

88. Karimi K, Odhav A, Kollipara R, Fike J, Stanford C, Hall JC. Acute cutaneous necrosis: A guide to early diagnosis and treatment. *J Cutan Med Surg* 2017;21:425–37.

8

Approach to severe cutaneous adverse drug reactions

SHEKHAR NEEMA

INTRODUCTION

Adverse drug reaction (ADR) occurs in up to 15% of hospitalized patients resulting in extended hospital stay and increased economic burden [1]. Skin is one of the most common organs involved in ADR and consists of 15% of all ADR. Cutaneous adverse drug reactions (CADRs) have varied manifestations and can vary from urticaria and morbilliform exanthem to severe conditions such as toxic epidermal necrolysis. More than 90% of all CADRs are mild in nature, and urticaria and exanthema form the majority of CADRs. Severe cutaneous adverse reactions (SCARs) form 2% of CADR and can be life threatening [2,3]. SCAR includes Stevens-Johnson syndrome/toxic epidermal necrolysis (SJS/TEN), drug reaction with eosinophilia and systemic symptoms (DRESS), and acute generalized exanthematous pustulosis (AGEP). These three entities are classically considered part of the SCAR spectrum; however, other entities like exfoliative dermatitis, drug-induced vasculitis, generalized fixed drug eruption, anaphylaxis, anticoagulant-induced skin necrosis, and angioedema can sometimes be severe enough to cause life-threatening illness and are considered SCAR by some authorities.

APPROACH TO A CASE OF SEVERE CUTANEOUS ADVERSE REACTION

1. The first step in any case of CADR is to define whether the adverse reaction is mild or severe. The presence of extensive skin involvement; bullous or pustular skin lesions; positive Nikolsky sign; mucosal involvement; ocular discomfort; systemic symptoms or signs like abdominal pain, jaundice, fever, hepatomegaly, facial swelling, and lymphadenopathy are red flag signs for diagnosis of severe ADR. Laboratory abnormalities like leukocytosis, eosinophilia, atypical lymphocytes, and altered renal or liver function tests also suggest the severe nature of CADR.

2. The next step after severity assessment is to diagnose the exact nature of SCAR. The exact diagnosis of SCAR requires experience and keen clinical sense, as decision about treatment has to be taken at the earliest even before investigation results are available. Diagnosis of SCAR remains clinical and requires clinicians to make quick and dramatic decisions based on clinical judgement. Thus, it is important for clinicians to be aware of clinical features and differential diagnosis of SCAR. In this section, we discuss important clinical features, diagnostic criteria, and the differential diagnoses of SCARs.

    a. *Toxic epidermal necrolysis (TEN)*

        TEN generally occurs 7–21 days after starting the offending drug. It starts with nonspecific symptoms of fever, redness, or discomfort in eyes; pain during swallowing; and skin tenderness. These symptoms are followed by development of erythematous macules or targetoid lesions that coalesce and form bullae, and these bullae coalesce and form large areas of epidermal detachment. Sometimes sheets of epidermal detachment can occur without any preceding macules in what is known as TEN without spots. Mucosal involvement occurs in more than 90% cases and involves oral, ocular, or genital mucosa. Respiratory and gastrointestinal tracts can also be involved in some cases. Nikolsky sign is a clinical sign to demonstrate detachable skin, where tangential pressure leads to the separation of detachable skin [4]. Histopathologic examination of affected skin shows subepidermal bullae, widespread epidermal necrosis, apoptotic keratinocytes, and lymphocytic perivascular and dermal infiltrate.

TEN needs to be differentiated from other conditions, as untreated TEN can result in high mortality. Histopathologic examination (HPE) can be useful whenever there is clinical confusion. It is good practice to perform HPE of skin tissue even in cases where diagnosis is not in doubt, as some of these cases may have legal issues later on. Direct immunofluorescence (DIF) needs to be done to differentiate it from closely mimicking conditions such as paraneoplastic pemphigus and pemphigus vulgaris. Differential diagnoses and their differentiating features are discussed in Table 8.1.

b. *Drug reaction with eosinophilia and systemic symptoms*

DRESS is a rare, delayed drug-induced reaction characterized by skin and systemic involvement. There is a latency period of weeks between starting a drug and developing a rash, which results in delayed diagnosis. Mortality in DRESS is approximately 10% with most people dying from acute liver failure [5].

It is characterized by fever, rash, lymphadenopathy, leukocytosis, and abnormal liver tests. The rash is generally maculopapular or urticarial; however, a vesiculobullous, erythrodermic, purpuric, or targetoid appearance of rash has been described. Facial edema is a common feature of this condition. Hematologic abnormalities include leukocytosis and eosinophilia. Systemic involvement includes liver (most commonly), kidney, lung, and heart. There are three commonly used diagnostic criteria for diagnosis of DRESS, which are RegiSCAR criteria, Japanese consensus criteria, and Bocquet criteria.

DRESS needs to be differentiated from drug-induced maculopapular exanthem. Maculopapular exanthem can be differentiated by the absence of systemic symptoms; however, in some cases it becomes difficult to differentiate these cases from DRESS as they may show leukocytosis, lymphadenopathy, and single organ involvement. These kinds of reactions may be a severe form of drug-induced exanthem or milder variant of DRESS; they fall in the same spectrum and should be treated as such.

c. *Acute generalized exanthematous pustulosis*

AGEP is a rare drug-induced disorder, characterized by fever and generalized sterile pustules, 3–5 days after starting an offending drug. It is associated with drugs in almost 90% of cases [6]. Infections have been implicated in a minority of cases [7].

The patient presents with fever and generalized erythema, followed by development of sterile nonfollicular pustules. Mucous membrane and systemic involvement is uncommon. Investigations show neutrophilic leukocytosis, while histopathology shows subcorneal or intradermal pustules, papillary dermal edema, and perivascular neutrophilic infiltrate. Patch testing can be done to confirm the offending drug and should be done 1 month after resolution of skin lesions [8].

Differential diagnosis of AGEP includes conditions that manifest as pustules like bacterial folliculitis or acneiform eruption, though in AGEP, the pustules are nonfollicular. Microscopic examination of pus should always be performed in AGEP to rule out infectious etiology. Generalized pustular psoriasis (GPP) is most difficult to differentiate from AGEP. Prior or family history of psoriasis, psoriatic nail changes, and histopathological examination of skin can differentiate GPP from AGEP. Rarely, AGEP can also be a manifestation of DRESS. Diagnostic criteria have been developed for diagnosis of AGEP and to differentiate it from other conditions [9].

3. After determining the nature of CADR, the next step is to find out the causative agent of CADR. A complete drug history is very important and should include all drugs taken by the patient during last 2 months, both prescription as well as nonprescription drugs, such as oral contraceptives, laxatives, natural remedies, and ayurvedic or homeopathic drugs. Many patients consider these drugs to be free of adverse effects and do not give history unless specifically asked. A drug chart should be made for all patients that should have a timeline on one axis and all the drugs with date of introduction before development of rash on the other axis. Finding a culprit drug becomes easy if a drug is a high-risk drug known to cause a particular adverse reaction, is the only drug introduced before development of rash, and its temporal profile matches with development of rash. However, more often than not the algorithm to find the culprit drug becomes complicated by various other factors like polypharmacy, concomitant viral illness, comorbidities that may mimic drug reactions, and use of new drugs during the prodrome phase. The time relationships of drugs with various types of drug reactions are mentioned in Table 8.2.

There is no laboratory test available to determine causality in CADR, and assessment of causality remains clinical. Causality assessment after any ADR is of paramount importance as it helps in stopping the offending drug, continuing the essential drugs, and determining the future use of the drug. In case causality assessment is not done and the risk is not assigned, it leads to unnecessary stoppage of essential drugs and affects the management of comorbid conditions. The most common methods used in determining causality are expert judgement, World Health Organization-Uppsala Monitoring Center (WHO-UMC) causality assessment criteria, and the Naranjo scale. Details of these scales are given in Tables 8.3 and 8.4.

Most of the SCARs are in the probable category as rechallenge is not performed. Sometimes inadvertently, a patient gets exposed to the same drug again and

Table 8.1 Differentiating features of toxic epidermal necrolysis

Condition	Clinical features	Investigations	How to differentiate?
Erythema multiforme major [16]	Prodromal symptoms: Fever, sore throat, diarrhea; oral, ocular, genital mucosal involvement; target-shaped purpuric macule starts acrally and spreads centripetally	HPE: Subepidermal bulla, full-thickness epidermal necrosis, and lymphocyte-rich dermal infiltrate	Target-shaped lesions that are acrally distributed; BSA involvement is generally less than 10%, and HPE shows lichenoid dermal infiltrate in EM, while it is cell-poor in case of TEN
Pemphigus vulgaris	Oral ulcers, presence of flaccid bullae that rupture giving rise to widespread erosions	HPE: Suprabasal blister; DIF: Intercellular immune complex deposits (chicken wire pattern)	Absence of purpuric macule before development of bullae, ocular mucosa is generally not involved in pemphigus, and it has slower progression; HPE and DIF are diagnostic
Paraneoplastic pemphigus [17]	Recalcitrant stomatitis; polymorphous cutaneous eruption—pemphigus like, pemphigoid like, lichen planus like, graft versus host disease like, or erythema multiforme like	HPE: Suprabasal blister, dyskeratosis, interface dermatitis; DIF: Intercellular and basement membrane immune complex deposition; indirect immunofluorescence for confirmation	Prolonged illness; polymorphous rash; DIF suggests diagnosis; investigations to detect underlying malignancy
Generalized bullous fixed drug eruption [18]	Widespread, well-demarcated, dusky red patches with blisters and erosions	HPE: Subepidermal blisters, basal vacuolation, superficial perivascular infiltrate, apoptotic keratinocyte	Mucosal involvement is uncommon (10%), ocular involvement is not seen; HPE shows widespread distribution of apoptotic keratinocyte (in TEN, it is seen on edge), eosinophils and melanophages are more prominent
TEN-like acute cutaneous lupus erythematosus [19]	Clinical features similar to TEN with underlying SLE, triggered by excessive UV exposure; may not have any drug history	HPE: Similar to TEN; DIF: Immune complex deposition in vessel wall	Underlying lupus with positive serology (ANA, anti-dsDNA); DIF: Immune complex deposition
AGVHD [20]	Occurs in setting of bone marrow transplant, stage IV or severe AGVHD shows generalized TEN-like rash with mucosal involvement	HPE: Similar to TEN	Palms and soles are involved, systemic involvement with pain in abdomen and raised serum bilirubin
Staphylococcal scalded skin syndrome [21]	Prodrome: Fever, skin tenderness, irritability; diffuse erythema followed by development of flaccid bullae and erosions	HPE: Intraepidermal cleavage, no epidermal necrosis or apoptotic keratinocyte	Epidermal peeling is more superficial and no mucous membrane involvement, HPE is characteristic

Abbreviations: AGVHD, acute graft versus host disease; ANA, antinuclear antibody; anti-dsDNA, anti-double-stranded DNA; BSA, body surface area; DIF, direct immunofluorescence; EM, erythema multiforme; HPE, histopathologic examination; SLE, systemic lupus erythematous; TEN, toxic epidermal necrolysis; UV, ultraviolet.

Table 8.2 Temporal relationship of drugs with various types of drug eruptions

Eruption	Timeline
Exanthem	4–14 days
Urticaria	Minutes to hours
Drug-induced vasculitis	Variable
TEN	7–21 days
AGEP	Less than 4 days
DRESS	15–40 days
Anticoagulant induced skin necrosis	3–5 days
Exfoliative dermatitis	Days to weeks

Abbreviations: AGEP, acute generalized exanthematous pustulosis; DRESS, drug reaction with eosinophilia and systemic symptoms; TEN, toxic epidermal necrolysis.

develops an adverse event a second time, making the culprit drug evident.

The Naranjo scale is the most widely accepted algorithmic method to determine whether the adverse event is due to a drug or to other factors. Belhekar et al. studied agreement between the Naranjo algorithm and the WHO-UMC criteria for causality assessment and concluded that there is a poor agreement between the two methods of causality assessment, and the Naranjo algorithm was found to be more time consuming [10].

4. After confirmation of diagnosis and causality assessment, the next step is to perform investigations. Investigations are done for prognostication, systemic involvement, and secondary complications that can occur due to widespread skin denudation. Suggested investigations in a patient with SCAR are given in Table 8.5.

Table 8.3 World Health Organization-Uppsala Monitoring Center causality assessment scale

Causality assessment is based on four criteria

a. Time relationship between drug use and adverse event
b. Absence of other competing causes (medication, disease process)
c. Response to drug withdrawal or dose reduction (de-challenge)
d. Response to drug readministration (rechallenge)

The causal association is grouped into four categories depending on the criteria:

Certain	When all four criteria are met
Probable	When criteria a, b, c are met
Possible	When only criteria a is met
Unlikely	When criteria a and b are not met

Source: Tantikul C, Asian Pac J Allergy Immunol 2008;26:77.

Leukocytosis can be seen in DRESS and AGEP. Eosinophilia also may be present in DRESS. Leukocytosis or leukopenia in TEN may suggest super-added infection, and the focus of infection should be looked for. Thrombocytopenia can be a result of sepsis, and other features of sepsis should be looked for in the presence of thrombocytopenia. Raised blood urea and a mild increase in creatinine can be because of prerenal azotemia, as these patients have increased transepidermal water loss and oral mucosal involvement. However, persistently raised serum creatinine not responding to adequate fluid challenge suggests acute kidney injury, and nephrologist opinion

Table 8.4 Naranjo probability scale

Questions	Yes	No	Do not know
1. Are there previous conclusive reports on this reaction?	+1	0	0
2. Did the adverse event occur after the suspect drug was administered?	+2	−1	0
3. Did the adverse reaction improve when the drug was discontinued or a specific antagonist was administered?	+1	0	0
4. Did the adverse reaction reappear when the drug was readministered?	+2	0	0
5. Are there alternative causes that could have caused the reaction?	−1	+2	0
6. Did the reaction reappear when placebo was given?	−1	+1	0
7. Was the drug detected in blood in a concentration known to be toxic?	+1	0	0
8. Was the reaction more severe when the drug was increased or less severe when the dose was decreased?	+1	0	0
9. Did the patient have a similar reaction to the same or similar drugs in previous exposure?	+1	0	0
10. Was the adverse event confirmed by any objective evidence?	+1	0	0

Total score
0: Doubtful
1–4: Probable
5–8: Possible
>9: Definite

Source: Naranjo CA et al. Clin Pharmacol Ther 1981;30:239–45.

Table 8.5 Suggested investigations in case of severe cutaneous adverse reaction

- Hemoglobin, total leukocyte count, differential leukocyte count, platelets
- Urine routine and microscopic examination
- Blood urea, serum creatinine
- Liver function tests including transaminase level
- Blood sugar random
- HIV and hepatitis serology
- Chest x-ray posteroanterior view
- Electrocardiogram
- Serum electrolytes
- Histopathological examination of skin

should be sought at the earliest. Transaminitis is a part of DRESS, and mild transaminitis can also be seen in AGEP.

Other investigations that are specific to various SCARs are discussed below:

a. *TEN*: In a patient with TEN, the skin is denuded and a baseline surface swab should be performed in all cases. Apart from this, arterial blood gas should

Table 8.6 Supportive measures in case of severe cutaneous adverse reaction

- Patient should be nursed in a room with ambient temperature between 30°C and 32°C.
- Prevention of sepsis: Barrier nursing, handwashing, and prophylactic antibiotics should be used.
- Use an air-fluidized bed.
- Maintain fluid and electrolyte balance—IV fluid, monitor urine output, pulse, blood pressure, and, if required, central venous pressure.
- Nutrition—Nasogastric tube feeding may be necessary in case of oral mucosal involvement; a high-protein diet is recommended.
- Anticoagulant therapy or mobilization to prevent deep vein thrombosis and H2 blockers to prevent stress ulcers can be considered.
- Care of skin—Detached skin should be left in place; paraffin gauze dressing, nanosilver dressing, or amnion dressing can be used for denuded skin.
- Care of mucosa—Oral mucosal care includes removing crust with normal saline compresses and maintaining good oral hygiene by frequent cleaning of oral cavity.
- Eyes—Should be seen by ophthalmologist, as in patients with TEN, it can lead to permanent sequelae. Frequent instillation of artificial tear drops, removal of crust, and measures to prevent synechiae formation should be instituted.
- Vaginal mucosal involvement can lead to adhesion formation and permanent problems like dyspareunia if not treated during an acute episode. Formation of the adhesion should be prevented by use of tampons and daily change of tampons.

also be done, which helps in the calculation of the severity of illness score for toxic epidermal necrolysis (SCORTEN). SCORTEN is a validated predictor of mortality in patients with TEN [11].

b. *DRESS*: In patients with DRESS, human herpesvirus-6 (HHV-6) serology can be performed. Apart from this, organ-specific investigations depending on organ involvement should be performed. Ultrasound of the abdomen in case of liver involvement, contrast-enhanced computed tomography of the abdomen in case of pancreatic involvement, and computed tomography of the chest in case of lung involvement can be done depending on specific indications.

c. *AGEP*: In AGEP, Gram stain of pus should be performed in all cases to see whether the pustule is sterile or of infective etiology. Patch testing can be performed 1 month later to confirm the offending drug causing SCAR.

In patients with SCAR, especially in TEN, sepsis remains the most important concern and is a major cause of mortality, while in DRESS organ involvement, especially the liver, is a major cause of mortality. All dermatologists should be aware of features of sepsis and investigations to be performed in case of sepsis, to identify this complication early. Patients with fever, hypothermia, low blood pressure, tachypnea, and altered sensorium should be evaluated for sepsis. Investigations should include blood culture, urine culture, culture from surface swab and central line or endotracheal tube, serum procalcitonin level, and arterial blood gases apart from investigations that have already been discussed.

5. Once the diagnosis has been established, the next step is to start treatment. Treatment consists of supportive treatment, specific treatment, and treatment of complications. Treatment steps in case of SCAR are as follows:

a. *Stopping the offending drug*: This is the most important step in management of SCAR. However, at times it is not possible to identify the culprit drug, and then it becomes important to stop all the drugs. It is equally important to make all efforts to identify the offending agent and continue essential drugs.

b. *Supportive therapy*: As SCARs have large body surface area involvement and these patients develop acute skin failure, there is a high risk of development of sepsis and multiorgan involvement. Supportive therapy measures should be undertaken at the earliest in these patients. These measures are directly proportional to degree of involvement of body surface area and should be most stringently followed in patients with TEN, who have denudation of skin [12]. These measures are tabulated in Table 8.6.

c. *Specific therapy*: Specific therapy is discussed in respective chapters and tabulated in Table 8.7.

6. As we know that SCARs are life-threatening dermatoses, it is important to counsel the patient about the use of

Table 8.7 Specific therapy for management of severe cutaneous adverse reaction

Drug	Dose	Remarks
Toxic epidermal necrolysis		
Cyclosporine	3 mg/kg for 7 days; taper over 7 days	Has become drug of first choice in management of TEN
Corticosteroids	1–2 mg/kg or equivalent prednisolone for 3–5 days	Effective, however increased risk of sepsis
IV Immunoglobulin	0.6–1 gm/kg/day for 4 days	Equivocal or ineffective; not preferred
Etanercept	50 mg single dose	Found to be effective in many case series
Drug reaction with eosinophilia and systemic symptoms		
Corticosteroid	Prednisolone 1 mg/kg for 4–6 weeks and tapering	First choice
Cyclosporine	5 mg/kg for 7 days	Has been described in various case reports with successful outcome
Acute generalized exanthematous pustulosis		
Emollient and topical steroids		Generally sufficient with stopping offending drug
Oral steroids	Prednisolone 0.5–1 mg/kg for 5–7 days	

Source: Creamer D et al. *J Plast Reconstr Aesthet Surg* 2016;69:e119–53; Shiohara T, Kano Y. *Expert Opin Drug Saf* 2017;16:139–47; Kirchhof MG et al. *JAMA Dermatol* 2016;152:1254–7.

drugs after recovery to prevent future episodes. At the same time, it is also important to tell the patient which drugs are safe for him or her, or else the patient and physicians become too fearful of drugs. It is important to give a list of drugs that should not be consumed by the patient and list which can be safely consumed, in case a clinical situation demands their use. It is better to give an entire list of drugs from the same and related class which caused the reaction, and the list should be updated periodically as new drugs get approved. These reactions are idiosyncratic reactions, and the patient may have a genetic predisposition to develop CADR to a class of drug; therefore, the same predisposition may also be present in close relatives, and they also should be warned about possible ADRs in case they need to take the drug. Human leukocyte antigen (HLA) associations of various CADRs are being discovered which can help in the prevention of adverse reactions but can also help in confirming diagnoses in patients who developed CADR and in genetic counseling of family members. HLA associations of various CADRs are given in Table 8.8.

Table 8.8 HLA association of CADR

HLA	CADR
HLA B*1502	Carbamazepine-induced SJS/TEN
HLA B*5801	Allopurinol-induced TEN and DRESS
HLA B*5701	Abacavir-induced DRESS

Abbreviations: CADR, cutaneous adverse drug reaction; DRESS, drug reaction with eosinophilia and systemic symptoms; HLA, human leukocyte antigen; SJS, Stevens-Johnson syndrome; TEN, toxic epidermal necrolysis.

CONCLUSION

Severe CADRs are fortunately not common; however, on occurrence, they can result in morbidity and mortality. This has economic and legal ramifications, too. Systemic involvement is frequent, and a multidisciplinary approach to treatment is required in most cases. It is important to identify these conditions promptly and institute lifesaving treatment at the earliest.

KEY POINTS

- SCAR is an acronym for Severe cutaneous drug reactions.
- SJS/TEN, DRESS and AGEP are the common SCARs.
- Drug induced vasculitis, drug induced necrosis and drug induced erythroderma may also be considered part of SCAR in severe cases.
- Good history taking, clinical examination and thorough investigations can help differentiate theses conditions so that early specific management and supportive measures can be instituted.

REFERENCES

1. Koelblinger P, Dabade TS, Gustafson CJ, Davis SA, Yentzer BA, Kiracofe EA, Feldman SR. Skin manifestations of outpatient adverse drug events in the United States: A national analysis. *J Cutan Med Surg* 2013;17:269–75.

2. Alanko K, Stubb S, Kauppinen K. Cutaneous drug reactions: Clinical types and causative agents. A five-year survey of in-patients (1981–1985). *Acta Derm Venereol* 1989;69:223–6.

3. Chavda DA, Suthar SD, Singh S, Balat JD, Parmar SP, Mistry SD. A study of cutaneous adverse drug reactions in the outpatient department of Dermatology at a tertiary care center in Gujarat, India. *Int J Basic Clin Pharmacol* 2017;6:1115–22.

4. Lim VM et al. A decade of burn unit experience with Stevens-Johnson syndrome/toxic epidermal necrolysis: Clinical pathological diagnosis and risk factor awareness. *Burns* 2016;42:836–43.

5. Walsh SA, Creamer D. Drug reaction with eosinophilia and systemic symptoms (DRESS): A clinical update and review of current thinking. *Clin Exp Dermatol* 2011;36:6–11.

6. Sidoroff A et al. Risk factors for acute generalized exanthematous pustulosis (AGEP)—Results of a multinational case-control study (EuroSCAR). *Br J Dermatol* 2007;157:989–96.

7. Birnie AJ, Litlewood SM. Acute generalized exanthematous pustulosis does not always have a drug-related cause. *Br J Dermatol* 2008;159:492–3.

8. Fernando SL. Acute generalised exanthematous pustulosis. *Australas J Dermatol* 2012;53:87–92.

9. Sidoroff A et al. Acute generalized exanthematous pustulosis (AGEP)—A clinical reaction pattern. *J Cutan Pathol* 2001;28:113–19.

10. Belhekar MN, Taur SR, Munshi RP. A study of agreement between the Naranjo algorithm and WHO-UMC criteria for causality assessment of adverse drug reactions. *Indian J Pharmacol* 2014;46:117.

11. Bastuji-Garin S, Fouchard N, Bertochi M, Roujeau JC, Revux J, Wolkenstein P. SCORTEN: A severity of illness score for toxic epidermal necrolysis. *J Invest Dermatol* 2000;115:149–53.

12. Inamadar AC, Palit A. Acute skin failure: Concept, causes, consequences and care. *Indian J Dermatol Venereol Leprol* 2005;71:379–85.

13. Creamer D et al. UK guidelines for the management of Stevens-Johnson syndrome/toxic epidermal necrolysis in adults 2016. *J Plast Reconstr Aesthet Surg* 2016;69:e119–53.

14. Shiohara T, Kano Y. Drug reaction with eosinophilia and systemic symptoms (DRESS): Incidence, pathogenesis and management. *Expert Opin Drug Saf* 2017;16:139–47.

15. Kirchhof MG, Wong A, Dutz JP. Cyclosporine treatment of drug-induced hypersensitivity syndrome. *JAMA Dermatol* 2016;152:1254–7.

16. Huff JC, Weston WL, Tonnesen MG. Erythema multiforme: A critical review of characteristics, diagnostic criteria, and causes. *J Am Acad Dermatol* 1983;8(6):763–75.

17. Anhalt GJ. Paraneoplastic pemphigus. In: *Journal of Investigative Dermatology Symposium Proceedings* 2004 January 1 (Vol. 9, No. 1, pp. 29–33). Elsevier.

18. Cho YT, Lin JW, Chen YC, Chang CY, Hsiao CH, Chung WH, Chu CY. Generalized bullous fixed drug eruption is distinct from Stevens-Johnson syndrome/toxic epidermal necrolysis by immunohistopathological features. *J Am Acad Dermatol* 2014;70:539–48.

19. Cetin GY, Sayar H, Ozkan F, Kurtulus S, Kesici F, Sayarlıoglu M. A case of toxic epidermal necrolysis-like skin lesions with systemic lupus erythematosus and review of the literature. *Lupus* 2013;22:839–46.

20. Couriel D, Caldera H, Champlin R, Komanduri K. Acute graft-versus-host disease: Pathophysiology, clinical manifestations, and management. *Cancer* 2004;101:1936–46.

21. Handler MZ, Schwartz RA. Staphylococcal scalded skin syndrome: Diagnosis and management in children and adults. *J Eur Acad Dermatol Venereol* 2014;28:1418–23.

22. Tantikul C, Dhana N, Jongjarearnprasert K, Visitsunthorn N, Vichyanond P, Jirapongsananuruk O. The utility of the World Health Organization-The Uppsala Monitoring Centre (WHO-UMC) system for the assessment of adverse drug reactions in hospitalized children. *Asian Pac J Allergy Immunol* 2008;26:77.

23. Naranjo CA, Busto U, Sellers EM, Sandor P, Ruiz I, Roberts EA, Janecek E, Domecq C, Greenblatt DJ. A method for estimating the probability of adverse drug reactions. *Clin Pharmacol Ther* 1981;30:239–45.

Bullous Disorders

BIJU VASUDEVAN

9

Pemphigus vulgaris and foliaceus

RAGHAVENDRA RAO

INTRODUCTION

Pemphigus is a group of potentially life-threatening skin diseases contributing to significant morbidity and mortality among affected patients. It is considered as a dermatological emergency because of a plethora of complications, septicemia being the most prominent among them. Complications occur due to extensive denudation of the skin and also mainly due to the medications used in treating the condition, such as steroids and other immunosuppressive agents. Loss of fluid and electrolytes through the blisters may also affect health adversely. Early recognition of the disease and proper institution of treatment are necessary to achieve a better disease outcome.

Pemphigus vulgaris (PV) and pemphigus foliaceus (PF) are two major forms of pemphigus accounting for 80% and 18% of the total cases of pemphigus, respectively [1,2]. The term *pemphigus* is derived from the Greek word *pemphix*, which means "blister" or "bubble." It comprises a group of chronic blistering diseases affecting the skin and mucosae. It is characterized by the production of autoantibodies of the IgG class against extracellular domains of cell membrane proteins of keratinocytes, resulting in acantholysis (the loss of cell-cell adhesion between keratinocytes). Autoantibodies in pemphigus are characteristically directed against desmogleins (Dsg), which are part of the cadherin family of cell-cell adhesion molecules that are found in desmosomes [3].

EPIDEMIOLOGY

The incidence of pemphigus varies substantially around the world. PV is the most common subtype of pemphigus in Europe, the United States, Japan, and India. The incidence of PV ranges from 0.5 to 16.2 per million individuals per year. PF is less common in most populations, and the estimated incidence ranges from 0.5 to 6.7 per million individuals per year [1,2]. The highest incidence of PV was observed in some ethnic groups, namely, Ashkenazi Jews and those of Mediterranean origin. PF is the most common type of pemphigus in certain geographic regions of the world, such as South America (e.g., Brazil) and northern Africa (e.g., Tunisia) [4].

Onset of the disease is usually seen between 50 and 60 years of age, and the disease is more common among women. The endemic form of PF in Brazil (Brazilian pemphigus) affects mostly young adults, with a peak incidence between the second and third decades of life [4,5].

ETIOPATHOGENESIS

Pemphigus is an organ-specific autoimmune disease. Though the exact etiology is unknown, certain environmental factors such as drugs (e.g., penicillamine, captopril), viruses (such as herpes simplex virus), dietary factors, and physiological and psychological stressors might either initiate or aggravate the autoimmune process [6]. There is a strong association between human leukocyte antigen (HLA) class II alleles and PV; a meta-analysis demonstrated that DRB1*04, DRB1*08, and DRB1*14 increased susceptibility to the disease. Strong linkage disequilibrium is known to be present in the DRDQ loci in PV patients, such as DQB1*0503-DRB1*1401, DRB1*0402-DQB1*0302, and DRB1*0402-DQA1*0301.2 [7].

Both T-lymphocytes and B-lymphocytes play a critical role in the pathogenesis of pemphigus. CD4+ T cells regulate antibody production by interacting with B cells and directly infiltrate the tissue expressing the target antigen, where they modulate inflammation through cytokines and surface molecules. Evidence supports that autoreactive CD4+ T cells are involved in anti-Dsg3 antibody production. The finding that IgG4 is the predominant subclass of anti-Dsg3 antibodies suggests T-cell-dependent immunoglobulin class switching in pemphigus. Blister formation in pemphigus, as opposed to other autoimmune skin diseases (e.g., bullous pemphigoid and epidermolysis bullosa acquisita), does not require complement activation [3].

Autoantibodies in pemphigus are directed against the desmosomes components, especially desmogleins (Dsg) 1 and 3. The Dsg3:Dsg1 ratio in the oral mucosa is higher than that in the epidermis, which has high expression of Dsg1 [8]. The profile of autoantibodies against Dsg1 and Dsg3 largely corresponds to specific clinical features. Patients with PF have essentially only anti-Dsg1 autoantibodies. In the mucosal-dominant type of PV, patients have mostly, if not only, anti-Dsg3 autoantibodies, whereas those with the mucocutaneous type of PV have both anti-Dsg1 and Dsg3 autoantibodies [9]. Antidesmoglein autoantibodies are necessary and sufficient to generate the specific pathology of pemphigus.

Both the signaling-dependent pathway and signaling-independent pathway may contribute to the acantholysis (i.e., separation of the keratinocytes due to loss of cohesion) in pemphigus. Polyclonal PV autoantibodies induce clustering and endocytosis of Dsg3 with P38 mitogen-activated protein kinase (MAPK) activation, leading to collapse of the keratin filaments (i.e., the retraction of keratin filaments from desmosomes to the perinuclear area). In contrast, the loss of cell adhesion due to monoclonal anti-Dsg3 antibodies is not dependent on p38 MAPK activation; rather, it is likely to be caused by the direct inhibition of monoclonal antibodies against adhesive Dsg3 transinteraction (*steric hindrance*) [10].

Recently, non-Dsg autoantibodies such as antimuscarinic acetylcholine receptor (AchR) antibody titers have been reported in 100% of the cases. The levels of these antibodies correlated significantly with disease severity both at initial diagnosis and during follow-up [11].

CLINICAL FEATURES

Lesions in PV classically start in the oral mucosa and might then extend to the skin. Oral mucosa involvement consists of flaccid blisters that easily rupture, leaving behind painful erosions (Figure 9.1). This might potentially lead to weight loss and malnutrition. Though the buccal mucosa is commonly affected, lesions may also involve the gingiva, palate, and even oropharynx. Other mucosal surfaces, such as the larynx, esophagus, conjunctiva, nose, genitalia, and anus, might be less frequently affected. Cutaneous involvement usually occurs after a latent period of a few days to months; it is characterized by flaccid blisters (Figure 9.2) and partly crusted erosions (Figure 9.3) on healthy-appearing or erythematous skin, which show a tendency for peripheral extension (Figure 9.4). Areas of predilection include the head, upper trunk, and groin (Figure 9.5).

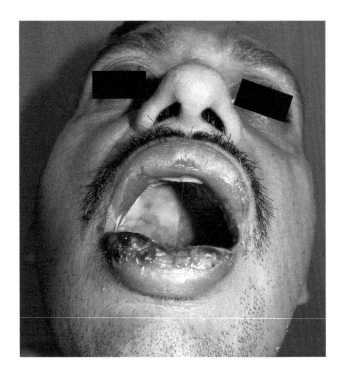

Figure 9.1 Lip and oral mucosal erosions as an early manifestation of pemphigus vulgaris.

Erosions of the intertriginous areas such as axillae and the groin might develop into vegetative plaques (pemphigus vegetans, Figure 9.6). Nikolsky sign (shearing pressure over the bony prominence at a distant site from the lesion results in appearance of blister or erosion) is often used to assess the clinical activity of the disease. A substantial number of

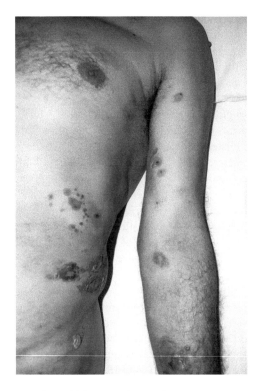

Figure 9.2 Flaccid blisters of pemphigus.

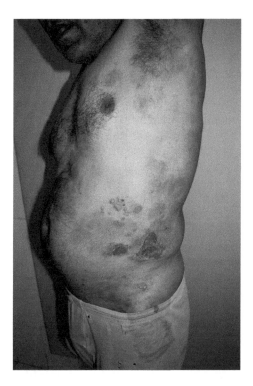

Figure 9.3 Flaccid blisters and crusted erosions of pemphigus vulgaris.

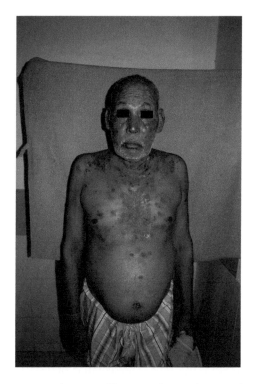

Figure 9.5 Distribution of lesions of pemphigus vulgaris on scalp, face, and upper trunk.

patients with PV can relapse with a PF clinical and histological phenotype, especially when the relapses occur after a long remission [3,12].

Unlike PV, PF typically does not affect mucosal sites; both endemic and sporadic PF share the same clinical,

histological, and immunological findings. Patients with PF usually present with multiple pruritic, scaly, and crusted erosions with flaky circumscribed patches in mostly seborrheic areas (Figure 9.7) that can extend, merge, and progress to exfoliative dermatitis (erythema and scaling that covers >90% of the body surface area); blisters are rarely

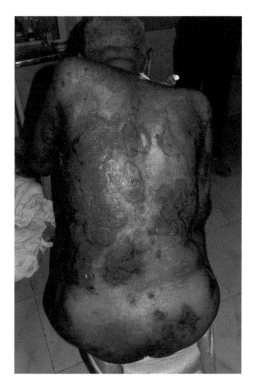

Figure 9.4 Expanding erosions of pemphigus vulgaris.

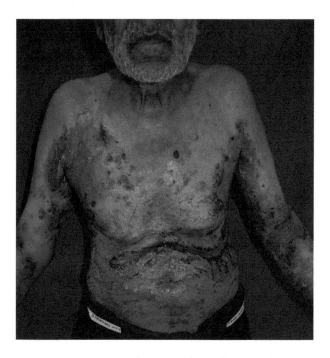

Figure 9.6 Vegetative plaques in the axilla: pemphigus vegetans.

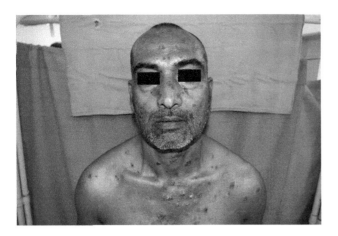

Figure 9.7 Seborrheic distribution of crusted plaques in pemphigus foliaceus.

seen owing to their superficial localization and consequent rupture. Occasionally, patients may present with erythematous, scaly, and crusted plaques in the butterfly area of the face, resembling the malar rash of systemic lupus erythematosus (SLE). This type of presentation of PF is designated as pemphigus erythematosus (Senear-Usher syndrome). Approximately 50% of these patients may show circulating antinuclear antibodies (ANAs).

DIAGNOSIS

The *acantholytic* cells can be demonstrated from a freshly erupted blister by Tzanck test; sensitivity and specificity of this test in pemphigus were found to be 100% and 43.4%, respectively [13]. Histopathological study of a fresh blister in pemphigus shows the presence of *acantholysis*, which can progress to the formation of intraepithelial blisters. In PF, a blister may occur subcorneally at the level of the granular cell layer. In PV, a suprabasal cleavage is encountered, often showing a "tombstone effect" (residual basal keratinocytes at the site of the floor of the blister are separated from each other but are still attached to the basement membrane zone through the hemidesmosomes). Although the epidermal blisters are classically noninflammatory, in both PV and PF, a slight eosinophilic or neutrophilic infiltration can be occasionally seen in the upper dermis and epidermis.

Direct immunofluorescence (DIF) microscopy of perilesional biopsy specimens is the most reliable and sensitive diagnostic test for all forms of pemphigus; it shows the intercellular staining (ICS) of IgG antibodies in a "fishnet" or "chicken wire" appearance. Approximately 50% of patients, especially those with active disease, will also show the deposition of C3. Other classes of immunoreactants will be encountered less frequently. In general, DIF is not useful to distinguish PV from PF; pemphigus erythematosus (PE) is an exception where one can find granular staining of a basement membrane zone in addition to an ICS pattern. DIF of lesional samples might yield false-negative results

owing to internalization of immune reactants on the cell surface by acantholytic keratinocytes [14].

Indirect immunofluorescence (IIF) microscopy using monkey esophagus or human skin as substrates enables a semiquantitative detection of serum IgG autoantibodies that bind to the epithelium in an intercellular pattern [15].

The molecular specificity of circulating pemphigus autoantibodies can be analyzed using highly sensitive and specific enzyme-linked immunosorbent assays (ELISAs) with recombinant autoantigens. The Dsg ELISA has 96%–100% sensitivity and specificity for disease diagnosis, indicating that nearly all patients with pemphigus have anti-Dsg antibodies [16]. In addition, biochips using tissue sections of monkey esophagus and cells transfected with recombinant autoantigens are available to detect anti-Dsg1 and anti-Dsg3 autoantibodies semiquantitatively by IIF microscopy [17]. Autoantibody levels often correlate with disease activity and are, therefore, an appropriate biomarker for monitoring disease activity. Anti-Dsg1 antibody titers tend to show a closer correlation with the course of the disease activity compared with anti-Dsg3 antibody titers [18]. Approximately 20%–40% of patients in clinical remission still have detectable levels of circulating autoantibodies, and low levels of anti-Dsg IgG autoantibodies are also occasionally detected among healthy individuals [19,20]. Though rare, relapse might occur even in patients who have undetectable anti-Dsg antibodies.

Complications

Since the introduction of corticosteroids in the treatment of pemphigus in the early 1950s, mortality rates have dramatically reduced, from 75% to 30%. The adjuvant use of immunosuppressants in the 1980s probably contributed to the further decrease in mortality from the disease itself to less than 5% [21]. Mortality in pemphigus is now mainly related to the adverse effects resulting from the therapy. Recent population-based studies using computerized databases has shown that the age- and gender-adjusted mortality in PV was estimated to be two- to threefold higher than the normal population [22,23].

Extensive cutaneous involvement can lead to features of acute skin failure. Infections are the most common complication. It can lead to sepsis, disseminated intravascular coagulation, and multiorgan dysfunction. There can be dehydration and electrolyte imbalance.

Mucosal involvement can be severe causing difficulty in swallowing and nutritional problems. Esophageal involvement can lead to severe malnutrition and stenosis at later stages. Laryngeal involvement can cause hoarseness and even breathing difficulties. Respiratory mucosal involvement can be fatal as respiratory failure may result. Genitourinary involvement can also lead to urinary retention, vaginal stenosis, and phimosis in few patients as a late sequelae.

The most frequent causes of death are due to infections (particularly pneumonia and septicemia), cardiovascular diseases, and peptic ulcer disease. Staphylococcus and pseudomonas account for a vast majority of infections in these patients. Rarely, deep venous thrombosis, pulmonary embolism, and myocardial infarction have also been reported.

Therapy-related common side effects include systemic infection, pneumonia, diabetes, arterial hypertension, cardiorespiratory diseases, and peptic ulceration. Hepatotoxicity, renal failure, pancytopenia, and occurrence of malignancies are other side effects of prolonged immunosuppressive therapy in pemphigus.

Patients receiving high-dose steroids may not show overt signs of septicemia. Subtle clinical signs such as high pulse rate and changes in the sensorium may indicate impending septicemia. Treatment with steroids may also predispose the patient to develop osteoporosis and cataract.

There is no difference in the mortality rates between those with PF and the general population, indicating that PF is a relatively mild disease [1]. Rarely, pemphigus foliaceus may go into erythroderma or Kaposi varicelliform eruption can develop in these patients leading to an emergency situation.

Treatment

Pemphigus is a serious, life-threatening condition and might lead to a great impact on the quality of life of affected patients. Ideally, these patients are better managed as inpatients. Baseline hematological and biochemical investigations should be done. Serial wound and blood culture should be sent, and infections should be treated aggressively with parenteral broad-spectrum antibiotics. It is also important to maintain fluid and electrolyte balance and barrier dressing.

There is a paucity of randomized clinical trials with large sample sizes and rigorous randomization methods in pemphigus. As a result, most of the published guidelines in the treatment of pemphigus rely on expert consensus.

Table 9.1 Various pharmacological agents used in the treatment of pemphigus

Suppressive therapy
- Corticosteroids: Oral or parenteral (in severe cases)
- Rituximab

Maintenance therapy
- Immunosuppressive agents: Azathioprine (1–2 mg/kg/day)
  - Mycophenolatemofetil (1.5–3 g/day)
- Cyclophosphamide, cyclosporine, methotrexate, dapsone, tetracycline/nicotinamide
- IV immunoglobulin

Refractory cases
- Plasmapheresis
- Photopheresis
- Immunoadsorption

Generally, patients with PV and PF respond to the same types of therapy [24,25].

Various therapeutic options are listed in Table 9.1. Corticosteroids with or without additional immunosuppressive agents are often used as the first line of treatment in many centers [26]. The treatment period can be roughly divided into three phases: initiation phase, consolidation phase, and remission phase. The goal for the initial phase of therapy is disease control, and it lasts until new blisters cease to appear for at least 2 weeks and most of the existing lesions show signs of reepithelization. Owing to their rapid effect (within days), high doses of corticosteroids (1–1.5 mg/kg/day) are often used in this phase, preferably as a single morning dose. Split-dose regimens (two to three times daily) have not been directly compared with once-daily regimens in pemphigus trials but are anecdotally associated with better therapeutic effect in refractory cases, at the potential expense of greater adrenal suppression.

The duration of the initiation phase varies from 3 to 8 weeks. In the consolidation phase (which lasts for 6–9 months approximately), most clinicians would start tapering the doses of steroids. Approximately half of patients will relapse during steroid taper; this can be tackled by adding steroid-sparing agents (such as mycophenolate mofetil and azathioprine). Some experts prefer to start them from day 1, while others initiate treatment with these agents when they begin to taper the dose of steroids. In the remission phase (approximate treatment duration of 2–3 years) steroids are completely stopped while the patient is maintained on immunosuppressive agents. The addition of immunosuppressive agents not only brings down the total cumulative dose of steroids, thereby reducing the side-effects related to long-term corticosteroid therapy, but also helps in maintaining remission [25]. Other maintenance treatment options are methotrexate, cyclosporine, IVIg, dapsone and tetracycline/nicotinamide. Cyclophosphamide is preferred only for severe recalcitrant cases owing to the unpredictable side effects.

IV corticosteroids (methylprednisolone or dexamethasone) may be used alternatively in patients who do not respond to conventional doses of steroids [3]. If the disease is not controlled with 1–1.5 mg/kg of steroids, then IV methylprednisolone at doses of 1 g daily for 5 days is preferred. Though dexamethasone-cyclophosphamide pulse (DCP) therapy was used extensively in the last two decades, many centers are giving it up.

Rituximab (a monoclonal antibody directed against CD20, a surface antigen on B lymphocytes) has revolutionized the treatment strategies in pemphigus. It is found to be efficacious in patients who are refractory with other systemic therapies [27]. Two protocols have been studied in pemphigus (Table 9.2). Both regimens have shown comparable results in terms of complete clinical remission, though the lymphoma protocol showed slightly higher rates of complete remission, shorter time to disease control, and longer duration of remission. Due to similar pathogenesis

Table 9.2 Dosing schedule of rituximab

Protocol	Regular dose	Low dose
Lymphoma	375 mg/m^2 weekly for 4 weeks	375 mg/m^2 weekly for 2 weeks
Rheumatoid arthritis	1000 mg on day 0 and day 15	500 mg day 0 and day 15

(autoimmune background) of rheumatoid arthritis (RA) and pemphigus, the RA protocol is now being preferred; this protocol is also found to be cost effective and requires fewer hospital visits. A lower-dose regimen has also been studied (Table 9.2). In the meta-analysis comparing the high versus low dosing RA protocol, higher-dose rituximab was found to be associated with a significantly longer duration of complete remission, a shorter time to disease control, and lower relapse rate [28]. A mean time to clinical remission of 3–6 months and a median remission duration of 15–19 months have been shown. Although some patients can sustain long-term remission of pemphigus after rituximab treatment, a significant proportion (40%–80%) of patients relapse, and the relapse rate generally increases with the length of the follow-up [28]. Hence, a single cycle of rituximab may not achieve a long-standing remission for pemphigus; regularly scheduled low-dose infusions have been suggested as maintenance therapy to prevent disease relapse. In a landmark study, Joly et al. compared treatment with a high dose of prednisone (1–1.5 mg/kg/day) alone given for 12–18 months with a regimen of rituximab plus lower initial doses of prednisone (0.5 mg/kg/day), rapidly tapered over 3–6 months in treatment naïve patients. At month 24, the number of patients who achieved complete remission in the latter group was almost three times compared with a corticosteroid-alone regimen. The findings showed that rituximab along with short-term prednisone can be used as the first-line treatment in pemphigus patients [29]. Severe side effects due to rituximab therapy can occur and include deep vein thrombosis, pulmonary embolism, hypogammaglobulinemia, neutropenia, progressive multifocal leukoencephalopathy, and severe infections. A meta-analysis of 153 patients treated with rituximab showed that 13% of patients developed serious adverse events, with three fatalities [30]. A fatal infection with *Pneumocystis jiroveci pneumonia* (PJP) was recently reported in patients who received rituximab therapy for pemphigus [31].

Plasmapheresis, extracorporeal photopheresis, and immunoadsorption can be considered in very refractory cases.

CONCLUSION

Pemphigus carries a high risk of morbidity and mortality and is one of the most common emergencies faced by dermatologists. Mucosal and systemic involvement can lead to various complications requiring emergent management. Extensive skin involvement is a common cause of acute skin failure. Immunosuppressants and rituximab form the major specific treatment modalities and along with supportive therapy form the cornerstone of treatment.

KEY POINTS

- Pemphigus is one of the commonest dermatological emergencies seen in practice.
- Pemphigus vulgaris is characterized by oral erosions, flaccid bullae on skin with Nikolsky positivity, other mucosal and systemic involvement.
- Infections are the commonest complication.
- Oral corticosteroids, Rituximab, other immunosuppressants like azathioprine and mycophenolate mainly as adjuvants are main therapeutic modalities.
- Pemphigus foliaceus is comparatively a milder disease than pemphigus vulgaris.

REFERENCES

1. Kridin K, Zelber-Sagi S, Bergman R. Pemphigus vulgaris and pemphigus foliaceus: Differences in epidemiology and mortality. *Acta Derm Venereol* 2017;97:1095–9.
2. Milinković MV, Janković, Medenica L, Nikolić M, Reljić V, Popadić S, Janković J. Incidence of autoimmune bullous diseases in Serbia: A 20-year retrospective study. *J Dtsch Dermatol Ges* 2016;14:995–1005.
3. Kasperkiewicz M, Ellebrecht CT, Takahashi H, Yamagami J, Zillikens D, Payne AS, Amagai M. Pemphigus. *Nat Rev Dis Primers* 2017;3:17026.
4. Alpsoy E, Akman-Karakas A, Uzun S. Geographic variations in epidemiology of two autoimmune bullous diseases: Pemphigus and bullous pemphigoid. *Arch Dermatol Res* 2015;307:291–8.
5. Bastuji-Garin S et al. Comparative epidemiology of pemphigus in Tunisia and France: Unusual incidence of pemphigus foliaceus in young Tunisian women. *J Invest Dermatol* 1995;104:302–5.
6. Ruocco V, Ruocco E, Lo Schiavo A, Brunetti G, Guerrera LP, Wolf R. Pemphigus: Etiology, pathogenesis, and inducing or triggering factors: Facts and controversies. *Clin Dermatol* 2013;31:374–81.
7. Yan L, Wang JM, Zeng K. Association between HLA-DRB1 polymorphisms and pemphigus vulgaris: A meta-analysis. *Br J Dermatol* 2012;167:768–77.
8. Furue M, Kadono T. Pemphigus, a pathomechanism of acantholysis. *Australas J Dermatol* 2017;58:171–3.
9. Amagai M. Autoimmunity against desmosomal cadherins in pemphigus. *J Dermatol Sci* 1999;20:92–102.
10. Vielmuth F, Waschke J, Spindler V. Loss of desmoglein binding is not sufficient for keratinocyte dissociation in pemphigus. *J Invest Dermatol* 2015;135:3068–77.

11. Lakshmi MJD et al. Correlation of antimuscarinic acetylcholine receptor antibody titers and antides-moglein antibody titers with the severity of disease in patients with pemphigus. *J Am Acad Dermatol* 2017;76:895–902.

12. Kimoto M, Ohyama M, Hata Y, Amagai M, Nishikawa TA. Case of pemphigus foliaceus which occurred after five years of remission from pemphigus vulgaris. *Dermatology* 2001;203:174–6.

13. Durdu M, Baba M, Seckin D. The value of Tzanck smear test in diagnosis of erosive, vesicular, bullous, and pustular skin lesions. *J Am Acad Dermatol* 2008;59:958–64.

14. Jindal A, Rao R, Bhogal B. Advanced diagnostic techniques in autoimmune bullous diseases. *Indian J Dermatol* 2017;62:268–78.

15. Shetty VM, Subramaniam K, Rao R. Utility of immunofluorescence in dermatology. *Indian Dermatol Online J* 2017;8:1–8.

16. Amagai M et al. Usefulness of enzyme-linked immunosorbent assay using recombinant desmogleins 1 and 3 for serodiagnosis of pemphigus. *Br J Dermatol* 1999;140:351–7.

17. van Beek N et al. Serological diagnosis of autoimmune bullous skin diseases: Prospective comparison of the BIOCHIP mosaic-based indirect immunofluorescence technique with the conventional multi-step single test strategy. *Orphanet J Rare Dis* 2012;7:49.

18. Belloni-Fortina A et al. Detection of autoantibodies against recombinant desmoglein 1 and 3 molecules in patients with pemphigus vulgaris: Correlation with disease extent at the time of diagnosis and during follow-up. *Clin Dev Immunol* 2009;2009:187864.

19. Kwon EJ, Yamagami J, Nishikawa T, Amagai M. Anti-desmoglein IgG autoantibodies in patients with pemphigus in remission. *J Eur Acad Dermatol Venereol* 2008;22:1070–5.

20. Torzecka JD et al. Circulating pemphigus autoantibodies in healthy relatives of pemphigus patients: Coincidental phenomenon with a risk of disease development? *Arch Dermatol Res* 2007;99:239–43.

21. Kridin K, Sagi SZ, Bergman R. Mortality and cause of death in patients with pemphigus. *Acta Derm Venereol* 2017;97:607–11.

22. Huang Y-H, Kuo C-F, Chen Y-H, Yang Y-W. Incidence, mortality, and causes of death of patients with pemphigus in Taiwan: A nationwide population-based study. *J Invest Dermatol* 2012;32:92–7.

23. Langan SM, Smeeth L, Hubbard R, Fleming KM, Smith CJP, West J. Bullous pemphigoid and pemphigus vulgaris—Incidence and mortality in the UK: Population based cohort study. *BMJ* 2008;337:a180.

24. Frew JW, Martin LK, Murrell DF. Evidence-based treatments in pemphigus vulgaris and pemphigus foliaceus. *Dermatol Clin* 2011;29:599–606.

25. Chams-Davatchi C et al. Randomized controlled open label trial of four treatment regimens for pemphigus vulgaris. *J Am Acad Dermatol* 2007;57:622–8.

26. Rosenbaum O, Mimouni D. Treatment of pemphigus vulgaris and pemphigus foliaceus: A systematic review and meta-analysis. *Am J Clin Dermatol* 2014;15:503–15.

27. Robinson AJ, Vu M, Unglik GA, Varigos GA, Scardamaglia L. Low-dose rituximab and concurrent adjuvant therapy for pemphigus: Protocol and single-centre long-term review of nine patients. *Australas J Dermatol* 2018;59:e47–52.

28. Wang HH, Liu CW, Li YC, Huang YC. Efficacy of rituximab for pemphigus: A systematic review and meta-analysis of different regimens. *Acta Derm Venereol* 2015;95:928–32.

29. Joly P, Maho-Vaillant M, Prost-Squarcioni C, Hebert V, Houivet E, Calbo S. First-line rituximab combined with short-term prednisone versus prednisone alone for the treatment of pemphigus (Ritux 3): A prospective, multicentre, parallel-group, open-label randomised trial. *Lancet* 2017;389:2031–40.

30. Feldman RJ, Ahmed AR. Relevance of rituximab therapy in pemphigus vulgaris: Analysis of current data and the immunologic basis for its observed responses. *Expert Rev Clin Immunol* 2011;7:529–41.

31. Wei KC, Wang YH, Wang WH, Chen W. Fatal infection of *Pneumocystis jiroveci* pneumonia in a pemphigus patient treated with rituximab. *J Eur Acad Dermatol Venereol* 2017;31:e350–1.

10

Paraneoplastic pemphigus

B. NIRMAL

INTRODUCTION

Paraneoplastic pemphigus (PNP) is a mucocutaneous blistering disease that is mostly fatal and is frequently induced by lymphoproliferative disorders. It can be considered as a paraneoplastic phenomenon that is caused by autoimmune disease but initiated by underlying lymphoproliferative disorder. The autoantibodies may deposit and damage skin, lungs, and other organs leading to the terminology *paraneoplastic autoimmune multiorgan syndrome* (PAMS) [1].

EPIDEMIOLOGY

PNP commonly affects adults between the ages of 45 and 70 years, though it has also been reported in children [2]. The disease has a wide geographic distribution and similar gender predisposition without clear racial and ethnic differences.

ETIOPATHOGENESIS

Etiology

PNP is mostly associated with lymphoproliferative disorders, and the most common association in children is Castleman disease. The most commonly found neoplastic conditions with PNP in decreasing order of frequency are as follows [3]:

- Non-Hodgkin lymphoma (39%)
- Chronic lymphocytic leukemia (18%)
- Castleman disease (18%)
- Carcinoma (9%)
- Thymoma (6%)
- Sarcoma (6%)

- Waldenström macroglobulinemia (1%)
- Hodgkin lymphoma (<1%)
- Monoclonal gammopathy (<1%)
- Melanoma (<1%)

The time when PNP develops with respect to the underlying malignancy is variable. In most patients PNP manifests after the detection of neoplasm [4]. Rarely, the underlying malignancy is not detected before the death of the patient [5].

Pathogenesis

The major pathogenic mechanisms of PNP include the following:

1. *Unmasking antigen targets*: The neoplastic process induces an autoimmune disorder in which both humoral and cell-mediated immunity are involved. Cell-mediated lichenoid interface dermatitis induced by the tumor uncovers previously hidden epithelial antigens through epitope spreading [6].
2. *Antigenic mimicry*: Cross-reactivity occurs between antibodies directed against tumor cells and epithelial antigens. First, damage to the cell membrane induced by antibodies directed against transmembrane desmoglein-3 initiates acantholysis and subsequently provides access to intracellular proteins. Antibodies to intracellular plakin proteins produce unique features of PNP like dyskeratosis.
3. *Cytokine dysregulation*: Dysregulation of cytokine production is induced by the tumor cells with massive secretion of IL-6. It promotes maturation of lymphocytes, activation of cytotoxic T cells, and antibody production [7].

CLINICAL FEATURES

Mucosa

Painful erosive mucositis is universally present, and a diagnosis of PNP should not be considered in its absence. Oral mucosal involvement is the initial manifestation in almost 50% of the patients. The buccal, labial, gingival, and lingual mucosae can all be involved. The lateral borders of tongue and vermilion are preferentially and characteristically involved. The mucosal involvement is much more severe than that of pemphigus and erythema multiforme (EM) (Figure 10.1). Mucosal lesions are persistent and resistant to therapy. Other mucosal involvement includes conjunctiva, nasopharynx, anogenital, and occasionally mucosa of esophagus, stomach, duodenum, or colon [8]. Eye involvement in PNP includes cicatrizing conjunctivitis, symblepharon, and corneal ulceration leading to visual impairment [9]. Nasal erosions can cause epistaxis.

Skin

Cutaneous lesions usually develop after the onset of mucosal lesions. Clinical variants that have been described include the following:

- Pemphigus like
- Pemphigoid like
- Lichen planus pemphigoides like
- Graft versus host disease (GVHD) like
- EM like
- Toxic epidermal necrolysis (TEN) like
- Cicatricial pemphigoid like
- Linear IgA dermatosis like

The lesions have variable morphology, and an individual patient can have more than one morphological type including flaccid bullae of pemphigus vulgaris, tense bullae

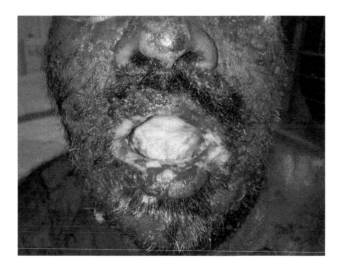

Figure 10.1 Severe oral mucosal involvement in paraneoplastic pemphigus.

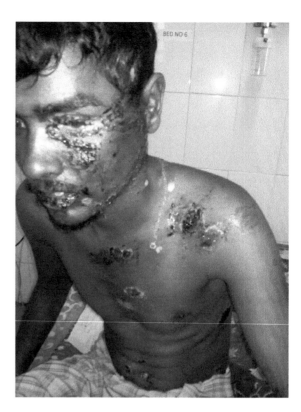

Figure 10.2 Progressive blister formation and erosions.

of bullous pemphigoid, inflammatory violaceous papules, and plaques resembling lichen planus or GVHD, targetoid lesions similar to those of EM or Stevens-Johnson syndrome (SJS), and extensive cutaneous desquamation resembling TEN. Less common variants include psoriasiform, pustular, vegetative lesions, alopecia, periungual, and palmoplantar involvement.

The blisters that occur are mostly flaccid except when they occur on lower limbs resembling bullous pemphigoid. The difference with other blistering disorders is that the blisters are persistent and keep forming erosions progressively (Figure 10.2). These blisters often present in waves. Another difference with pemphigus vulgaris is that the blisters in PNP typically arise on inflammatory macules or papules and do not develop on normal skin.

Some patients who develop PNP do not demonstrate circulating autoantibodies. These patients have predominantly lichenoid skin and mucosal lesions. They commonly develop bronchiolitis obliterans. These cases have been designated as lichenoid variants of PNP. The EM-like variant portends a very poor prognosis.

Lung

Approximately 30%–40% of patients develop lung involvement that is mostly fatal. Acantholysis of bronchial respiratory epithelium is demonstrable leading to restrictive bronchiolitis consistent with bronchiolitis obliterans, late in the course of the disease. Epiplakin antibodies are markers for lung involvement in PNP.

Other organs

Deposition of antibodies has been detected in renal glomeruli, urinary bladder, and muscle leading to renal failure, urinary retention, and muscle weakness.

INVESTIGATIONS

Laboratory diagnosis in PNP includes histopathology, direct immunofluorescence, indirect immunofluorescence, and serologic studies that detect antibodies.

Histopathology

Histopathologic findings are dependent on the type of clinical lesion morphology:

- *Noninflammatory cutaneous blisters*: Suprabasilar acantholysis predominant
- *Erythematous macules and papules*: Interface dermatitis predominant
- *Mixed clinical pattern*: Mixed histopathologic features of suprabasilar acantholysis and interface dermatitis

However, the most common histopathologic findings in PNP are suprabasal acantholysis, keratinocyte necrosis, and lichenoid interface dermatitis [10].

The spectrum of interface lichenoid dermatitis includes the following:

- *EM/GVHD like*: Individual keratinocyte necrosis and lymphocytic infiltration into the epidermis
- *Lupus erythematosus like*: Vacuolar interface change with sparse lymphocytic infiltrate
- *Lichen planus like*: Thick lichenoid band-like infiltrate along the dermoepidermal junction

Direct immunofluorescence (DIF)

Intercellular and/or basement membrane zone deposition of IgG or C3 is seen in many cases of PNP. Negative DIF studies are not uncommon. Sensitivity of DIF for PNP was found to be only 41% [11].

Indirect immunofluorescence (IIF)

Transitional epithelium of rat bladder is the preferred substrate for IIF studies in patients with PNP with sensitivity and specificity of 74%–86% and 83%–100%, respectively [12]. Rat bladder epithelium is particularly useful to differentiate PNP from pemphigus vulgaris.

Enzyme-linked immunosorbent assay (ELISA)

ELISA for antibodies against envoplakin has a sensitivity and specificity of 81% and 99%, respectively. The ELISA for periplakin had a sensitivity and specificity of 74% and 96%, respectively [13].

Other studies

Immunoprecipitation and immunoblotting are more sensitive and specific than IIF, but their availability is limited.

Evaluation for the underlying neoplasm

When PNP is suspected, it is of paramount importance to search for an occult neoplasm. Serologic evaluation may identify hematologic disorders such as chronic lymphocytic leukemia or Waldenström macroglobulinemia, while radiologic imaging can aid in the diagnosis of Castleman disease and lymphomas [14]. The various evaluations required include the following:

- History and physical examination for signs suggestive of malignancy or lymphoproliferative disease
- Complete blood count
- Serum protein electrophoresis
- Computed tomography scan of the chest, abdomen, and pelvis

DIAGNOSTIC CRITERIA

Though there are different criteria for PNP since 1990, there is still a lack of consensus. Anhalt criteria (Table 10.1) were the first criteria proposed for PNP in 1990. Three years later, Camisa and Helm [15] proposed a modification of the Anhalt et al. criteria. PNP was considered if all three

Table 10.1 Anhalt criteria

Clinical
Painful mucosal ulcerations and blisters and a polymorphous skin eruption, with papular lesions progressing to blisters and erosive lesions on the trunk, extremities, palms, and soles, in the context of occult neoplasm

Histologic findings
Vacuolar interface change, keratinocytes necrosis, and intraepidermal acantholysis

Direct immunofluorescence
Deposition of IgG and C3 in the intercellular spaces, and granular-linear complement deposition along the epidermal basement membrane zone

Indirect immunofluorescence
Serum antibodies that bind not only to cell surfaces of skin and mucosa in a pattern typical of pemphigus vulgaris, but also to simple, columnar, and transitional epithelia

Immunoprecipitation
Serum antibodies that recognize epidermal antigens of 250, 230, 210, 190 kDa

Table 10.2 Camisa and Helm criteria

Major criteria
Polymorphous mucocutaneous eruption
Concurrent internal neoplasia
Characteristic serum immunoprecipitation findings

Minor criteria
Positive cytoplasmatic staining of rat bladder by indirect
    immunofluorescence
Intercellular and basement membrane zone
    immunoreactants on direct immunofluorescence of
    perilesional tissue
Acantholysis in biopsy specimen from at least one
    anatomic site of involvement

Table 10.3 Joly et al. criteria

High specificity and sensitivity
1. Association with lymphoproliferative disorders
2. Indirect immunofluorescence positive on rat bladder
3. Immunoblotting detection of antibodies
    against envoplakin and periplakin

Low sensitivity and high specificity
1. Polymorphous eruption
2. Histology
3. Direct immunofluorescence
4. Immunoblotting detection of antibodies against
    desmoplakins and BPAG1

major or two major and two or more minor criteria are met
(Table 10.2). Joly et al. [11] evaluated the sensitivity and
specificity of the diagnostic criteria of PNP (Table 10.3).
One clinical and two biological criteria had high sensitivity (82%–86%) and specificity (83%–100%) for PNP. Four
other diagnostic features had high specificity (83%–100%)
but poor sensitivity (27%–59%).

DIFFERENTIAL DIAGNOSIS

Oral lesions

- Pemphigus vulgaris
- Lichen planus
- SJS
- Mucous membrane pemphigoid
- Major aphthous stomatitis

Cutaneous lesions

- Pemphigus vulgaris
- Bullous pemphigoid
- EM
- SJS/TEN
- Lichen planus
- GVHD

TREATMENT

The treatment of PNP includes treatment of the underlying
neoplasm, suppression of disease manifestations, and management of patient symptoms.

Treatment of neoplasm

Treatment of the underlying malignancy is beneficial in
some cases. In PNP associated with Castleman disease or
thymoma, resection of the tumor often results in disease
remission [16]. In PNP associated with other neoplastic disorders, the response of PNP to treatment of the underlying
neoplasm appears to be less favorable. Once initiated, PNP
often progresses relentlessly independent of the status of the
underlying neoplastic disease [17].

Suppression of disease

High-dose systemic glucocorticoids are often the first-line
therapy in patients with PNP. The cutaneous manifestations are more likely to respond to systemic glucocorticoids
than the oral mucosa [18]. Other immunosuppressives
such as cyclophosphamide, mycophenolate mofetil, azathioprine, and cyclosporine are often combined with systemic steroids for their glucocorticoid-sparing effects [19].
The response to rituximab therapy is highly variable [20].
The limited efficacy of rituximab may reflect the effect of
the drug on humoral immunity and the lesser effect on
cell-mediated immunity. Plasmapheresis [21], cyclophosphamide, IV immunoglobulin (IVIG), alemtuzumab, and
daclizumab have been reported to be effective in combination with other therapies (Table 10.4).

PROGNOSIS

Patients with EM-like skin lesions have the worst prognosis. Mortality rates of PNP vary between 75% and 90%. The
cause of death is usually sepsis, respiratory failure due to
pulmonary involvement, or underlying malignancy [22].

Table 10.4 Treatment of paraneoplastic pemphigus

First line
Steroids: Prednisolone 0.5–1 mg/kg, methylprednisolone
    1000 mg IV × 3 days
Rituximab: 375 mg/m² IV weekly × 4 weeks/1000 mg IV
    weekly × 2 weeks

Second line
Cyclosporine 5 mg/kg
Cyclophosphamide 2.5 mg/kg
Mycophenolate mofetil 1500 mg bid
High-dose IV immunoglobulin 2 g/kg IV q4 weeks
Plasmapheresis

KEY POINTS

- Paraneoplastic pemphigus (PNP) is a rare autoimmune blistering disorder most commonly associated with lymphoproliferative disorders.
- Antibodies against periplakin and envoplakin are strongly associated with PNP.
- Mucosal involvement universally occurs in all patients, if absent a diagnosis of PNP is not considered.
- The clinical features of PNP are widely variable—tense or flaccid bullae, lichenoid lesions, erosions, and targetoid lesions.
- Confirmation of PNP requires clinical, pathologic, and immunologic correlation.
- Surgical removal of the underlying tumor can be beneficial in patients with Castleman disease or thymoma, but not of value for other malignancies.

REFERENCES

1. Nguyen VT et al. Classification, clinical manifestations, and immunopathological mechanisms of the epithelial variant of paraneoplastic autoimmune multiorgan syndrome: A reappraisal of paraneoplastic pemphigus. *Arch Dermatol* 2001;137:193.
2. Czernik A, Camilleri M, Pittelkow MR, Grando SA. Paraneoplastic autoimmune multiorgan syndrome: 20 years after. *Int J Dermatol* 2011;50:905.
3. Kaplan I et al. Neoplasms associated with paraneoplastic pemphigus: A review with emphasis on non-hematologic malignancy and oral mucosal manifestations. *Oral Oncol* 2004;40:553.
4. Sehgal VN, Srivastava G. Paraneoplastic pemphigus/paraneoplastic autoimmune multiorgan syndrome. *Int J Dermatol* 2009;48:162.
5. Ohzono A et al. Clinical and immunological findings in 104 cases of paraneoplastic pemphigus. *Br J Dermatol* 2015;173:1447.
6. Billet SE, Grando SA, Pittelkow MR. Paraneoplastic autoimmune multiorgan syndrome: Review of the literature and support for a cytotoxic role in pathogenesis. *Autoimmunity* 2006;39:617.
7. Reich K et al. Graft-versus-host disease-like immunophenotype and apoptotic keratinocyte death in paraneoplastic pemphigus. *Br J Dermatol* 1999;141:739.
8. Wakahara M et al. Paraneoplastic pemphigus with widespread mucosal involvement. *Acta Derm Venereol* 2005;85:530.
9. Ahuero AE et al. Paraneoplastic conjunctival cicatrization: Two different pathogenic types. *Ophthalmology* 2010;117:659.
10. Weedon D. The vesicobullous reaction pattern. In: *Weedon's Skin Pathology*. 3rd ed. Edinburgh: Elsevier; 2010: 123.
11. Joly P et al. Sensitivity and specificity of clinical, histologic, and immunologic features in the diagnosis of paraneoplastic pemphigus. *J Am Acad Dermatol* 2000;43:619–26.
12. Poot AM et al. Laboratory diagnosis of paraneoplastic pemphigus. *Br J Dermatol* 2013;169:1016.
13. Probst C et al. Development of ELISA for the specific determination of autoantibodies against envoplakin and periplakin in paraneoplastic pemphigus. *Clin Chim Acta* 2009;410:13.
14. Coelho S, Reis JP, Tellechea O, Figueiredo A, Black M. Paraneoplastic pemphigus with clinical features of lichen planus associated with low-grade B cell lymphoma. *Int J Dermatol* 2005;44:366–71.
15. Camisa C, Helm TN. Paraneoplastic pemphigus is a distinct neoplasia-induced autoimmune disease. *Arch Dermatol* 1993;129:883–5.
16. Nikolskaia OV, Nousari CH, Anhalt GJ. Paraneoplastic pemphigus in association with Castleman's disease. *Br J Dermatol* 2003;149:1143.
17. Anhalt GJ. Paraneoplastic pemphigus. *J Investig Dermatol SympProc* 2004;9:29.
18. Frew JW, Murrell DF. Current management strategies in paraneoplastic pemphigus (paraneoplastic autoimmune multiorgan syndrome). *Dermatol Clin* 2011;29:607.
19. Williams JV, Marks JG Jr, Billingsley EM. Use of mycophenolate mofetil in the treatment of paraneoplastic pemphigus. *Br J Dermatol* 2000;142:506.
20. Anan T et al. Paraneoplastic pemphigus associated with corneal perforation and cutaneous alternariosis: A case report and review of cases treated with rituximab. *J Dermatol* 2011;38:1084.
21. Izaki S et al. Paraneoplastic pemphigus: Potential therapeutic effect of plasmapheresis. *Br J Dermatol* 1996;134:987.
22. Leger S et al. Prognostic factors of paraneoplastic pemphigus. *Arch Dermatol* 2012;148:1165.

11

Mucous membrane pemphigoid

DIPANKAR DE, SHEETANSHU KUMAR, AND SANJEEV HANDA

INTRODUCTION

Mucous membrane pemphigoid (MMP) consists of a group of autoimmune subepidermal bullous disorders characterized by predominant involvement of mucous membranes and occasional involvement of the skin [1]. The oral cavity is the most common mucosa involved, followed by conjunctiva, nasopharynx, anogenital region, larynx, and esophagus [2,3]. MMP can have a highly variable course ranging from mild disease localized to a single mucosal site to severe involvement of multiple mucosae. The disease is marked by bullae, erosions, and in later phases, scarring. Scarring of the esophageal and laryngeal mucosa can lead to strictures, a life-threatening complication. Conjunctival involvement also needs to be treated early, effectively, and urgently due to the probability of loss of vision [1]. Early diagnosis and initiation of treatment can prevent subsequent complications. However, the rarity of the disease along with a wide spectrum of clinical presentations makes MMP a diagnostic challenge, especially in the early stages [4].

Cicatricial pemphigoid was previously used synonymously with MMP. However, cicatricial pemphigoid is now defined as a clinical variant with predominantly skin involvement and excessive scarring.

EPIDEMIOLOGY

Traditionally, MMP is known to occur in elderly patients aged 60 years and above [5,6]. However, childhood-onset MMP is also reported. The youngest reported child with MMP was aged 10 months [7], with around 20 case reports of childhood onset MMP to date [4]. The incidence is nearly twice as high in females as compared to males [5,6]. There are no geographic or racial predilections reported for MMP. A retrospective study from India reported MMPs to constitute around 12% of subepidermal autoimmune blistering disorders. A female preponderance was reported in this study as well. Mean age of onset was reported around 60 years, slightly lower than in Europe. An associated malignancy was not reported in any of the patients in this series [8].

ASSOCIATED DISEASES

Malignancies and autoimmune disorders are the two disease entities that have been reported to have possible associations with MMP. Approximately 30% patients with anti-laminin-332 antibody-associated MMPs had solid cancers, as reported by a few cohort studies [9,10]. Various autoimmune disorders with reported association with MMP include rheumatoid arthritis, systemic lupus erythematosus, and vasculitis [11].

PATHOGENESIS

Molecular studies have identified six different target antigens in the pathogenesis of MMP, as summarized in Table 11.1 [12]. Antibodies against multiple target antigens in a single patient have been frequently reported in MMP cases.

Autoantibodies against BP180 antigen play a crucial role in the pathogenesis of bullous pemphigoid (BP) as well [13,14]. However, BP is caused by antibody formation against the NC16A domain of BP180, while the C-terminal epitopes induce the immune reaction in MMP [13,14]. Antibodies against $\alpha6$ integrin are commonly found in patients with

Table 11.1 Various target antigens implicated in pathogenesis of mucous membrane pemphigoid

Autoantigens	Location	Frequency
BPAG2 (180 Kd)	Transmembranous: hemidesmosome/ lamina lucida	75% [13,47]
BPAG1 (230 Kd)	Intracellular: hemidesmosome	25% [12]
Laminin-332 (Laminin-5/ Epiligrin)	Lamina lucida, lower part	20%–25% [64]
α6β4 integrin	Transmembranous: hemidesmosome	Rare
Laminin-6	Lamina lucida, lower part	Rare
Type VII collagen	Lamina densa or sublamina densa	Rare

Table 11.2 Frequency of involvement of mucosa and skin

Site	Frequency
Oral mucosa	85%
Frequency of involvement of different sites within oral cavity [24]	
Gingiva	
Palate	
Buccal mucosa	
Alveolar ridge	
Tongue	
Labial mucosa	
Conjunctiva	65%
Nasal mucosa	20%–40%
Skin	25%–30%
Anogenital area	20%
Pharynx	20%
Larynx	5%–15%
Esophagus	5%–15%

Source: Schmidt E, Zillikens D. Lancet 2013;381:320–32.

predominantly oral mucosal disease, while anti-β4 integrin antibodies are more commonly reported in patients with predominantly ocular involvement [15–17]. Cases with isolated anti-BP180 antibody-related MMPs are frequently reported; however, MMP with isolated anti-BP230 antibodies has only been reported in a single case [18].

When antibodies are formed against laminin-332 antigen, the α3 chain is a common target. Anti-laminin-332 antibodies are frequently associated with severe disease. Other factors known to be associated with severe disease include dual IgG/IgA positivity against laminin-332 [19–21], antibodies against multiple epitopes of BP180 antigen, as well as human leukocyte antigen (HLA) class II alleles [13].

CLINICAL PRESENTATION AND COMPLICATIONS

The frequency of area of involvement in MMP is presented in Table 11.2 [12], and site-specific clinical presentations are presented in Table 11.3.

Diseases limited to skin and oral mucosa are considered low risk as they incur a low risk of scarring. High-risk MMP involves other mucosal sites predisposed to scarring, including esophageal, ocular, laryngeal, or anogenital [1,22,23]. Affliction of these sites by fibrosis and strictures can result in morbidities like dysphagia, blindness, breathing difficulties, and trouble performing daily activities, respectively.

Oral involvement in mucous membrane pemphigoid

Oral mucosa is often the first and most common site of involvement by MMP, gingiva being the most common site in the oral cavity [1,2,4,24]. Typical lesions include diffuse erythema, blisters, erosion, and ulceration. Lesions usually appear on the attached gingiva. Desquamation of gingival tissue (called *desquamative gingivitis*) is the most common intraoral manifestation in MMP, which is also seen in

pemphigus vulgaris and lichen planus [25]. The frequency of involvement of gingiva and other sites within the oral cavity is presented in Table 11.2.

Erosions and ulcerations are the most common manifestations seen early in the course of the disease with intact vesicles encountered rarely. Pain, bleeding, and difficulty eating and swallowing are the common presenting complaints.

Although incidence of scarring in the oral cavity is less as compared to other sites [25], prolonged disease leads to scarring and a shiny glazed appearance of the oral mucosa. Submucosal fibrosis and scarring and adhesions of other tissues, such as the attached part of gingiva and tongue, are known complications that are seen later in the course of the disease.

Periodontitis has been commonly found to be present in patients of MMP with oral cavity involvement. Hence, all MMP patients should receive a dental consult [26].

Ocular involvement in mucous membrane pemphigoid

Patients with conjunctival involvement initially present with unilateral disease and mild, nonspecific symptoms, such as burning, dryness, and foreign-body sensation (Figure 11.1) [27]. Later the disease may progress to involve both eyes in a period of about 2 years [28]. Gradually, fibrosis, conjunctival scarring, forniceal shortening, and symblepharon occur, later progressing to ankyloblepharon. Up to 20% of MMP patients have disease limited to conjunctiva, called *ocular pemphigoid* [27].

Corneal involvement can result in corneal scarring, corneal neovascularization, opacification, and ulceration, all of which result in compromised vision [29]. Eyelid involvement results in entropion, lagophthalmos, notching of lid margin, and trichiasis. These can cause further corneal

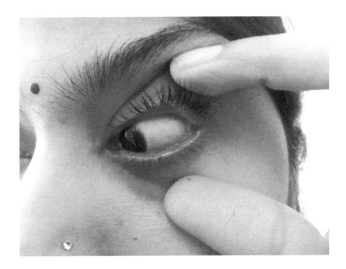

Figure 11.1 Conjunctiva congestion and early symblepharon formation.

damage, scarring, and secondary infectious keratitis [27]. Glaucoma is also known to occur in MMP patients, and is yet another cause of blindness [30].

Hence, all MMP patients should undergo a detailed ophthalmological evaluation with slit lamp examination and measurement of depth of fornix. Forniceal depth is an objective clinical parameter for measuring disease activity [31]. Patients who do not have ocular involvement at the time of initial disease diagnosis have a 5% annual risk of developing ocular lesions in the first 5 years [3].

Genital involvement in mucous membrane pemphigoid

Approximately 15% of MMP patients have genital mucosal involvement [32]. Erythema, edema, and erosions are among the early lesions seen. Vulva, vestibule, labia minora, and labia majora are the common sites involved in females [33]. The symptoms range from completely asymptomatic to dysuria, dyspareunia, or vulvar pain. Severe structural deformities can result from blistering and extensive scarring leading to partial to complete resorption of the labia minora, introital and urethral meatal stenosis, and clitoral phimosis. These changes can mimic genital lichen sclerosus et atrophicus posing a diagnostic difficulty [34]. Most women with vulvar disease have been reported to also show ocular involvement; however, isolated vulvar lesions in children have been described [35]. Male patients present with erosions on glans penis and prepuce, which may be later followed by phimosis or urethral meatal strictures [36].

Esophageal involvement in mucous membrane pemphigoid

Approximately 2%–13% patients with MMP have esophageal involvement [37]. Isolated involvement of esophageal mucosa has also been reported [38]. Fibrosis can result in

Table 11.3 Clinical presentations of mucous membrane pemphigoid based on site of involvement

Mucosa involved	Presentation
Skin	Predominant sites include head, neck, and upper trunk. Small vesicles or bullae on an erythematous urticarial base rupture to form crusted papules or plaques. Vegetative lesions are seen occasionally. Lesions heal with milia formation or atrophic scarring. Scarring results in cicatricial alopecia and other cosmetic issues.
Oral cavity	Desquamative gingivitis is the most common presentation. Erosions, ulcerations. Intact vesicles rarely. Pain, bleeding, and intolerance to spicy food. Mild scarring or atrophy, adhesions. Periodontitis.
Eye	Conjunctivitis, conjunctival scarring, shortened fornices, symblepharon, ankyloblepharon, entropion, lagophthalmos, trichiasis, scarring of lacrimal ducts, decreased tear secretion, corneal irritation, superficial punctate keratinopathy, corneal ulceration, corneal neovascularization, blindness.
Nasopharynx	Excessive nasal discharge, epistaxis, crusting, impaired airflow, chronic sinusitis, tissue loss, scarring.
Larynx	Hoarseness of throat, irritation of the throat, difficulty of phonation, supraglottic stenosis, compromised airway.
Esophagus	Stricture, difficult and painful swallowing, loss of weight, aspiration.
Anogenital region	Urethral stricture, vaginal stenosis, anal stenosis.

Source: Chan LS et al. Arch Dermatol 2002;138:370–9; Chan LS. Clin Dermatol 2001;19:703–11; Xu H-H et al. Dent Clin North Am 2013;57:611–30.

scarring and stenosis, which can cause dysphagia and odynophagia leading to weight loss. Esophageal fragility is common in these lesions and can be induced by endoscopy or even a food bolus [39,40].

Laryngeal involvement can lead to stenosis, which is a life-threatening complication, often requiring tracheostomy [41]. Deafness can result in patients with chronic MMP involving the middle ear [42]. Chronic oral and esophageal lesions are associated with a risk of malignancy.

The incidence of solid cancers has been found to be 30% in anti-laminin-332 antibody-associated MMP patients [9]. An association of MMP with hypothyroidism, especially in females, has also been reported [43].

DIAGNOSIS

The diagnosis of MMP rests on a combination of clinical presentation, histopathology, direct immunofluorescence (DIF) findings, and serology. Diagnostic delay in MMP is a common problem as the initial symptoms are subtle and early biopsies are not fruitful [44]. All patients with a clinical suspicion of MMP should undergo biopsy of lesional and perilesional skin, which should be sent for histopathological and DIF examination, respectively. Correct biopsy technique and careful tissue handling are of utmost importance in these cases, like other bullous disorders, due to the high propensity of the epidermis to separate and dislodge away from the underlying connective tissue.

Lesional tissue should be sent in formalin for histopathological examination. Perilesional tissue adjacent to a recently developed vesicle/bulla should be sent in Michel medium or buffered hypertonic saline for DIF examination [4]. Intact buccal mucosa is the preferred site of biopsy for DIF. If a buccal biopsy is negative and the clinical suspicion is high, a conjunctival biopsy is needed for which the patient should be referred to an ophthalmologist. However, conjunctival biopsies are not considered first-line as they confer a risk of disease exacerbation. A DIF sample sent from an old lesion is likely to be false negative [45].

Histopathology reveals a subepidermal split with inflammatory infiltrate similar to BP. A recent study reported that in ocular MMP, lesional neutrophils can serve as biomarkers of disease activity, fibrosis, and response to therapy. Lesional neutrophils may also be noted in lesions that appear noninflamed clinically [46].

Continuous linear deposits of IgG, IgA, and/or C3 are seen in the basement membrane zone (BMZ) on DIF. The amount of circulating and tissue bound autoantibodies is lower in MMP as compared to BP. Hence, the intensity of fluorescence is lower in MMP, leading to a difficulty in diagnosis [47,48]. A negative DIF in a setting of high clinical suspicion of MMP is an indication for repeat biopsy [49].

Circulating autoantibodies in serum are detected by indirect immunofluorescence (IIF). On salt-split IIF on human skin or other substrates, antibodies to BPAG2 and $\alpha6\beta4$ integrin bind on the epidermal side while antibodies against epiligrin and type VII collagen bind on the dermal side. Owing to the low levels of circulating antibodies in MMP patients, a positive IIF is noted in about 50%–80% patients with titers ranging from 1:10 to 1:40 [14,21]. Hence in patients with a strong clinical suspicion for MMP who test negative on IIF, further testing for serum autoantibodies is recommended using other antigen-specific testing systems. Soluble ectodomain of BP180 (LAD-1) is one such cell-derived fragment of BP180 used for testing [50–52]. Commercially available enzyme-linked immunosorbent assay and western blotting systems are used in conjunction with these antigens. An association of solid cancers with anti-laminin-332 antibody-associated MMP has made testing for laminin-332 antibodies pivotal [9,10].

Autoantibodies to BP180-NC16a are also secreted in saliva. IgG and IgA autoantibody testing in saliva has also been explored by researchers as a diagnostic modality for MMP. One study found a 30% increase in antibody detection upon testing both serum and saliva for autoantibodies [53].

DISEASE COURSE AND PROGNOSIS

The disease often follows a chronic progressive course. Periods of activity are interspersed with periods of quiescence. Rarely, cases go into spontaneous remission, predominantly those with disease localized to the oral cavity alone [54–56]. No definite criteria are currently accepted to predict the disease course. However, recent studies have evaluated the role of lesional neutrophils in ocular MMP as biomarkers of disease activity [46].

DIFFERENTIAL DIAGNOSIS

Various diseases enter the differential diagnoses of MMP depending on the mucous membrane involved. Early oral lesions of MMP may resemble pemphigus vulgaris, paraneoplastic pemphigus, oral lichen planus, Behcet disease, Stevens-Johnson syndrome, and bacterial gingivitis [3]. Ocular MMP needs to be differentiated from ocular rosacea, conjunctival lichen planus, Stevens-Johnson syndrome, toxic epidermal necrolysis, Sjögren syndrome, graft versus host disease, chronic allergic conjunctivitis, and infections [3].

While DIF is a helpful technique for diagnosis of the pemphigoid group of disorders, it is of little use in differentiating disorders within this group, including BP, epidermolysis bullosa acquisita, and bullous systemic lupus erythematosus. IIF on salt-split substrate is an important technique.

Differentiation from other mucocutaneous disorders, such as lichen planus and pemphigus vulgaris, can be done on histopathological examination of biopsy tissue. Table 11.4 shows the various features that may be helpful in differentiating MMP from other disorders.

MANAGEMENT

Sites involved and initiation of early therapy are among the major prognostic factors in MMP. Involvement of mucosae other than oral mucosa is associated with poor prognosis owing to development of scars.

The treatment goal is to avoid or delay scarring, hence avoiding life-threatening complications. Factors that make this goal difficult to achieve are the irreversible nature of fibrosis and scarring, poor response to immunosuppressive therapy especially in ocular lesions, paucity of randomized

Table 11.4 Differential diagnoses of mucous membrane pemphigoid

Disease	Mucous membrane pemphigoid (MMP)	Bullous pemphigoid (BP)	Epidermolysis bullosa acquisita	Bullous systemic lupus erythematosus
Clinical features	Multiple mucosal involvement, scarring, progressive	Rare mucosal involvement and scarring	Trauma-induced blisters, less scarring as compared to MMP	Lupus erythematosus symptoms, scarring rare
Direct immunofluorescence (all deposits along basement membrane zone)	Linear IgG, IgA and/ or C3	Linear IgG and/ or C3	Linear IgG	Linear or granular IgG, IgA, and C3
Indirect immunofluorescence on salt-split substrate (IgG antibody binding)	Either epidermal or dermal side	Either epidermal or dermal side	Dermal side	Dermal side
Immunoblotting	BPAG1, BPAG2, type VII collagen, laminin-5, integrin	BPAG1, BPAG2	Type VII collagen	Type VII collagen
Immunoelectron microscopy	Lamina lucida, sublamina densa	Intralamina lucida	Sublamina densa	Sublamina densa

Source: Xu H-H et al. Dent Clin North Am 2013;57:611–30.

controlled trials on disease therapy due to rarity of the disease itself, and persistence of the scarring process even after treatment of inflammation in conjunctival lesions. The treatment is usually individualized based on disease severity, patient age, general health status, and presence of medical comorbidities. A multidisciplinary approach is required in therapy and often requires involvement of dermatologists, otolaryngologists, dentists, ophthalmologists, and gastroenterologists.

Low-risk patients with involvement of oral mucosa with or without skin lesions are initially managed with topical therapy alone. Severe recalcitrant cases require systemic therapy. High-risk cases with involvement of mucosal sites like ocular mucosa, esophagus, and larynx should be treated with aggressive systemic therapy right from the beginning to prevent complications due to scarring [57]. Surgical interventions may also be required after development of cicatrix and stenosis.

Topical agents

High-potency topical corticosteroids are the mainstay of local therapy [1]. Gel-based topical corticosteroids can be used in oral cavity lesions, especially those with gingival involvement. Complications of therapy include local candidiasis, which can be avoided by maintaining good oral hygiene. Intralesional corticosteroids can be used in localized lesions. Triamcinolone injections in a dose of 0.1 mL/cm^2 in a strength of 10 mg/mL may be used for this purpose [4].

Apart from corticosteroids, the other topical agent that has been successfully used as reported by various case reports is topical tacrolimus. It is a safe, effective drug that has been used both as an alternative to and in conjunction with topical corticosteroids [58,59].

Benzocaine/lidocaine gel can be used as a local anesthetic to enable the patient to swallow food and enable oral hygiene procedures like brushing and cleaning the teeth.

Systemic therapy

Systemic therapy is usually advocated in high-risk patients or in low-risk patients with poor or no response to topical therapy. Multiple immunosuppressive anti-inflammatory medications have been used.

DAPSONE

The efficacy of dapsone in MMP has been reported by multiple studies. Dapsone has been found to be a relatively safe and effective modality and should be considered first-line treatment for MMP [60–62]. In cases with no response to dapsone therapy in 3 months, other agents like cyclophosphamide, azathioprine, and methotrexate should be considered.

CYCLOPHOSPHAMIDE

Traditionally used in severe disease or rapidly progressive disease, cyclophosphamide is generally administered in conjunction with systemic corticosteroids. It can be given orally (1–2.5 mg/kg/day or 50–200 mg/day) or as IV pulse therapy (0.5–1 g/m^2 monthly). Three-day pulse can be administered in patients where a rapid disease control is warranted, for example, before ocular surface surgery. There is some evidence to support that cyclophosphamide fares better than dapsone in control of disease progression [63]; however, large controlled studies supporting the same are lacking [57]. In a retrospective study on 115 patients with ocular MMP, cyclophosphamide was found to be the most efficacious drug, and the response was better than mycophenolate mofetil (MMF), azathioprine, and dapsone [65].

The side effects were reported to be minimum with MMF and maximum with azathioprine. Cyclophosphamide in combination with systemic corticosteroids has been recommended by international consensus as a first-line modality for treatment of "high-risk" MMP [1].

CORTICOSTEROIDS

Administered in cases with severe disease or rapid progression, systemic corticosteroids like prednisolone (dose 1–1.5 mg/kg/day) are the agent of choice for initial management. Once clinical remission is achieved, corticosteroids should be tapered, and steroid-sparing agents can be used for long-term disease control.

AZATHIOPRINE

Azathioprine has also been successfully used in MMP [23]. It usually takes around 8–12 weeks to produce an effect. Before initiating therapy, thiopurine S-methyltransferase levels should be checked and dose decided accordingly ranging from 1 to 4 mg/kg/day. Side effects include bone marrow suppression, gastrointestinal intolerance, and hepatotoxicity.

METHOTREXATE

Another steroid-sparing agent used in the therapy of MMP is methotrexate. McClusky et al. [66] used methotrexate in 17 patients with ocular MMP, of which 89% of patients achieved control of ocular inflammation.

MYCOPHENOLATE MOFETIL

MMF in conjunction with oral corticosteroids has been found to be an effective and safe option. Staines et al. performed a case series and reported control of inflammation in most of their patients [67].

RITUXIMAB

Rituximab is a promising agent for MMP therapy, especially in severe treatment-refractory disease. It shows dramatic efficacy in these cases. Better benefit is observed in oral disease as compared to ocular MMP [68]. In a recent review, 20 out of 28 patients of MMP showed complete response, while 3 patients had partial response [69]. However, owing to poor response or relapse, nearly half of the patients required a second cycle of rituximab therapy. In a series of 25 severe or refractory MMP patients, clinical improvement was reported after rituximab therapy [70]. A retrospective study concluded that rapid and prolonged disease control with fewer side effects would be observed if rituximab was added to conventional therapy [71]. Rituximab monotherapy or a combination of other immunomodulators with rituximab was used for treating ocular MMP in 32 patients, and rituximab was found to be an efficacious and well-tolerated drug for ocular MMP in another study [69]. In a single case series, three patients with recalcitrant isolated desquamative gingivitis were successfully treated with rituximab [72]. Hence, rituximab has emerged as a promising drug for therapy of MMP patients.

INTRAVENOUS IMMUNOGLOBULIN

High-dose IV immunoglobulin (IVIg) courses every 4 weeks is an effective modality for severe and treatment-refractory MMP. In a study on 13 patients of extensive or treatment-refractory MMP, significant clinical response and decline in autoantibody titers were noted posttherapy with IVIg [73]. In a review article that analyzed 13 studies on 70 patients given IVIg for MMP, 65 patients showed a complete response [74]. The adverse effects were mild and included headache and nausea. However, in patients in whom IVIg was discontinued before achieving complete clinical remission, the disease kept on progressing.

Surgical intervention

Surgical intervention is required in cases where scarring has occurred, to prevent and treat severe complications such as blindness, airway stenosis, and esophageal and anogenital strictures [74]. Ophthalmological surgical interventions include correction of entropion, tarsorrhaphy, corneal graft, amniotic membrane transplantation, and keratoplasty. Oral mucosal grafts can be used in patients with ocular lesions like lid margin keratinization, trichiasis, and conjunctival scarring [75]. Corneal transplant can be used to restore the clarity of visual axis in cases with severe conjunctival scarring. Surgical intervention should not be performed in active disease as it may lead to disease exacerbation. Patients with quiescent disease are candidates for surgical management.

Laser

Low-level laser therapy has shown promising results as an efficacious therapy for MMP. Predominantly used in oral mucosal lesions, it can be used in conjunction with topical corticosteroids [76].

Self-management strategies

Self-management strategies include maintenance of meticulous oral hygiene, avoidance of trauma, and avoidance of alcohol mouthwashes. Eye care includes use of artificial lubricants, gels, ointments, and artificial tears.

The treatment algorithm for MMP is provided in Table 11.5.

CONCLUSION

MMP is a subepidermal blistering disease affecting mucosa and skin with a chronic progressive course characterized by periods of exacerbations and quiescence. The diagnosis of MMP rests on a combination of clinical presentation, histopathology, DIF findings, and serology. As the initial findings may be subtle and biopsies may be nonconfirmatory, early diagnosis may be challenging. Initiation of treatment at an early stage is imperative to prevent scarring and

Table 11.5 Treatment algorithm

Low-risk patients	• Potent topical corticosteroids • Dapsone: 50–200 mg, incremental, as needed and tolerated • Tetracycline (up to 2000 mg/day) or minocycline • Prednisolone (0.5–1 mg/kg/day)
High-risk patients	• Prednisolone 1–2 mg/kg/day or IV steroid pulse therapy • Mycophenolate mofetil in standard dose • Azathioprine in standard dose • High-dose IV immunoglobulin • Cyclophosphamide in standard dose • Methotrexate 0.3–0.5 mg/kg/week • Rituximab in rheumatoid arthritis or lymphoma protocol

Source: Adapted from Xu H-H et al. Dent Clin North Am 2013;57:611–30.

complications. There is paucity of large, randomized controlled trials comparing the efficacy of different therapeutic modalities owing to rarity of disease. Therapy has to be individualized in each patient based on the disease characteristics and comorbidities of the patient. A multidisciplinary approach is desirable to improve outcome. Surgical interventions may be required for restoring function and improving quality of life.

KEY POINTS

- MMP is a debilitating disease primarily affecting mucosa and sometimes skin.
- A high index of suspicion may be required for diagnosis, as early findings may be subtle.
- Early diagnosis and management are imperative to prevent scarring and functional impairment, which may sometimes be life threatening.
- A multidisciplinary approach is required for prevention of progression and effective treatment of complications.

REFERENCES

1. Chan LS et al. The first international consensus on mucous membrane pemphigoid: Definition, diagnostic criteria, pathogenic factors, medical treatment, and prognostic indicators. Arch Dermatol 2002;138:370–9.
2. Chan LS. Mucous membrane pemphigoid. Clin Dermatol 2001;19:703–11.
3. Thorne JE, Anhalt GJ, Jabs DA. Mucous membrane pemphigoid and pseudopemphigoid. Ophthalmology 2004;111:45–52.
4. Xu H-H, Werth VP, Parisi E, Sollecito TP. Mucous membrane pemphigoid. Dent Clin North Am 2013;57:611–30.
5. Ahmed AR, Kurgis BS, Rogers RS. Cicatricial pemphigoid. J Am Acad Dermatol 1991;24:987–1001.
6. Laskaris G, Sklavounou A, Stratigos J. Bullous pemphigoid, cicatricial pemphigoid, and pemphigus vulgaris. A comparative clinical survey of 278 cases. Oral Surg Oral Med Oral Pathol 1982;54:656–62.
7. Kharfi M, Khaled A, Anane R, Fazaa B, Kamoun MR. Early onset childhood cicatricial pemphigoid: A case report and review of the literature. Pediatr Dermatol 2010;27:119–24.
8. De D et al. Clinical, demographic and immunopathological spectrum of subepidermal autoimmune bullous diseases at a tertiary center: A 1-year audit. Indian J Dermatol Venereol Leprol 2016;82:358.
9. Egan CA, Lazarova Z, Darling TN, Yee C, Cote T, Yancey KB. Anti-epiligrin cicatricial pemphigoid and relative risk for cancer. Lancet 2001;357:1850–1.
10. Leverkus M, Schmidt E, Lazarova Z, Brocker EB, Yancey KB, Zillikens D. Antiepiligrin cicatricial pemphigoid: An underdiagnosed entity within the spectrum of scarring autoimmune subepidermal bullous diseases? Arch Dermatol 1999;135:1091–8.
11. Matsushima S et al. A case of anti-epiligrin cicatricial pemphigoid associated with lung carcinoma and severe laryngeal stenosis: Review of Japanese cases and evaluation of risk for internal malignancy. J Dermatol 2004;31:10–5.
12. Schmidt E, Zillikens D. Pemphigoid diseases. Lancet 2013;381:320–32.
13. Oyama N et al. Bullous pemphigoid antigen II (BP180) and its soluble extracellular domains are major autoantigens in mucous membrane pemphigoid: The pathogenic relevance to HLA class II alleles and disease severity. Br J Dermatol 2006;154:90–8.
14. Murakami H et al. Analysis of antigens targeted by circulating IgG and IgA autoantibodies in 50 patients with cicatricial pemphigoid. J Dermatol Sci 1998;17:39–44.
15. Rashid KA, Gurcan HM, Ahmed AR. Antigen specificity in subsets of mucous membrane pemphigoid. J Invest Dermatol 2006;126:2631–6.
16. Bhol KC, Goss L, Kumari S, Colon JE, Ahmed AR. Autoantibodies to human α6 integrin in patients with oral pemphigoid. J Dent Res 2001;80:1711–5.
17. Tyagi S, Bhol K, Natarajan K, Livir-Rallatos C, Foster CS, Ahmed AR. Ocular cicatricial pemphigoid antigen: Partial sequence and biochemical characterization. Proc Natl Acad Sci USA 1996;93:14714–9.

18. Inoue T, Yagami A, Iwata Y, Ishii N, Hashimoto T, Matsunaga K. Mucous membrane pemphigoid reactive only with BP230. *J Dermatol* 2016;43:1228–9.

19. Bernard P et al. Prevalence and clinical significance of anti-laminin 332 autoantibodies detected by a novel enzyme-linked immunosorbent assay in mucous membrane pemphigoid. *JAMA Dermatol* 2013;149:533–40.

20. Setterfield J, Shirlaw PJ, Bhogal BS, Tilling K, Challacombe SJ, Black MM. Cicatricial pemphigoid: Serial titres of circulating IgG and IgA antibasement membrane antibodies correlate with disease activity. *Br J Dermatol* 1999;140:645–50.

21. Setterfield J et al. Mucous membrane pemphigoid: A dual circulating antibody response with IgG and IgA signifies a more severe and persistent disease. *Br J Dermatol* 1998;138:602–10.

22. Kourosh AS, Yancey KB. Therapeutic approaches to patients with mucous membrane pemphigoid. *Dermatol Clin* 2011;29:637–41.

23. Tauber J, Sainz de la Maza M, Foster CS. Systemic chemotherapy for ocular cicatricial pemphigoid. *Cornea* 1991;10:185–95.

24. Arduino PG et al. Describing the gingival involvement in a sample of 182 Italian predominantly oral mucous membrane pemphigoid patients: A retrospective series. *Med Oral Patol Oral Cir Bucal* 2017;22:e149–e52.

25. Petruzzi M. Mucous membrane pemphigoid affecting the oral cavity: Short review on etiopathogenesis, diagnosis and treatment. *Immunopharmacol Immunotoxicol* 2012;34:363–7.

26. Jascholt I, Lai O, Zillikens D, Kasperkiewicz M. Periodontitis in oral pemphigus and pemphigoid: A systematic review of published studies. *J Am Acad Dermatol* 2017;76:975–8.e3.

27. Kirzhner M, Jakobiec FA. Ocular cicatricial pemphigoid: A review of clinical features, immunopathology, differential diagnosis, and current management. *Semin Ophthalmol* 2011;26:270–7.

28. Foster CS. Cicatricial pemphigoid. *Trans Am Ophthalmol Soc* 1986;84:527–663.

29. Ahmed M, Zein G, Khawaja F, Foster CS. Ocular cicatricial pemphigoid: Pathogenesis, diagnosis and treatment. *Prog Retin Eye Res* 2004;23:579–92.

30. Tauber J, Melamed S, Foster CS. Glaucoma in patients with ocular cicatricial pemphigoid. *Ophthalmology* 1989;96:33–7.

31. Williams GP et al. Validation of a fornix depth measurer: A putative tool for the assessment of progressive cicatrising conjunctivitis. *Br J Ophthalmol* 2011;95:842–7.

32. Amber KT, Murrell DF, Schmidt E, Joly P, Borradori L. Autoimmune subepidermal bullous diseases of the skin and mucosae: Clinical features, diagnosis, and management. *Clin Rev Allergy Immunol* 2017;54:26–51.

33. Sand FL, Thomsen SF. Skin diseases of the vulva: Inflammatory, erosive-ulcerating and apocrine gland diseases, zinc and vitamin deficiency, vulvodynia and vestibulodynia. *J Obstet Gynaecol* 2018;38(2):149–60.

34. Goldstein AT, Anhalt GJ, Klingman D, Burrows LJ. Mucous membrane pemphigoid of the vulva. *Obstet Gynecol* 2005;105:1188–90.

35. Hoque SR, Patel M, Farrell AM. Childhood cicatricial pemphigoid confined to the vulva. *Clin Exp Dermatol* 2006;31:63–4.

36. Ramlogan D, Coulsom IH, McGeorge A. Cicatricial pemphigoid: A diagnostic problem for the urologist. *J R Coll Surg Edinb* 2000;45:62–3.

37. Trattner A, David M, Sandbank M. Esophageal manifestations in autoimmune bullous diseases. *Int J Dermatol* 1992;31:687–90.

38. Sallout H, Anhalt GJ, Al-Kawas FH. Mucous membrane pemphigoid presenting with isolated esophageal involvement: A case report. *Gastrointest Endosc* 2000;52:429–33.

39. Sawicka K et al. Mucous membrane pemphigoid as a cause of acute dysphagia—An endoscopic study. *Prz Gastroenterol* 2015;10:247–9.

40. Zehou O et al. Oesophageal involvement in 26 consecutive patients with mucous membrane pemphigoid. *Br J Dermatol* 2017;177:1074–85.

41. Nash R, Hughes J, Kuchai R, Sandison A, Sandhu G. Assessment and management of laryngeal mucous membrane pemphigoid: Our experience in six patients and a proposed severity scale. *Clin Otolaryngol* 2017;42:752–6.

42. Alexandre M et al. A prospective study of upper aerodigestive tract manifestations of mucous membrane pemphigoid. *Medicine (Baltim)* 2006;85:239–52.

43. Siassipour A, Katz J. Oral mucous membrane pemphigoid associated with hypothyroidism: A retrospective study and a case report. *Quintessence Int* 2017;48:569–73.

44. Radford CF, Rauz S, Williams GP, Saw VPJ, Dart JKG. Incidence, presenting features, and diagnosis of cicatrising conjunctivitis in the United Kingdom. *Eye* 2012;26:1199–208.

45. Labowsky MT, Stinnett SS, Liss J, Daluvoy M, Hall RP 3rd, Shieh C. Clinical implications of direct immunofluorescence findings in patients with ocular mucous membrane pemphigoid. *Am J Ophthalmol* 2017;183:48–55.

46. Williams GP et al. Conjunctival neutrophils predict progressive scarring in ocular mucous membrane pemphigoid. *Invest Ophthalmol Vis Sci* 2016;57:5457–69.

47. Schmidt E et al. Cicatricial pemphigoid: IgA and IgG autoantibodies target epitopes on both intra- and extracellular domains of bullous pemphigoid antigen 180. *Br J Dermatol* 2001;145:778–83.

48. Mehta M, Siddique SS, Gonzalez-Gonzalez LA, Foster CS. Immunohistochemical differences between normal and chronically inflamed conjunctiva: Diagnostic features. *Am J Dermatopathol* 2011;33:786–9.

49. Shimanovich I, Nitz JM, Zillikens D. Multiple and repeated sampling increases the sensitivity of direct immunofluorescence testing for the diagnosis of mucous membrane pemphigoid. *J Am Acad Dermatol* 2017;77:700–5.e3.

50. Bedane C et al. Bullous pemphigoid and cicatricial pemphigoid autoantibodies react with ultrastructurally separable epitopes on the BP180 ectodomain: Evidence that BP180 spans the lamina lucida. *J Invest Dermatol* 1997;108:901–7.

51. Kromminga A et al. Cicatricial pemphigoid differs from bullous pemphigoid and pemphigoid gestationis regarding the fine specificity of autoantibodies to the BP180 NC16A domain. *J Dermatol Sci* 2002;28:68–75.

52. Lee JB, Liu Y, Hashimoto T. Cicatricial pemphigoid sera specifically react with the most C-terminal portion of BP180. *J Dermatol Sci* 2003;32:59–64.

53. Ali S et al. Salivary IgA and IgG antibodies to bullous pemphigoid 180 noncollagenous domain 16a as diagnostic biomarkers in mucous membrane pemphigoid. *Br J Dermatol* 2016;174:1022–9.

54. Fleming TE, Korman NJ. Cicatricial pemphigoid. *J Am Acad Dermatol* 2000;43:571–91, quiz 91-4.

55. Brauner GJ, Jimbow K. Benign mucous membrane pemphigoid: An unusual case with electron microscopic findings. *Arch Dermatol* 1972;106:535–40.

56. Person JR, Rogers RS 3rd. Bullous and cicatricial pemphigoid. Clinical, histopathologic, and immunopathologic correlations. *Mayo Clin Proc* 1977;52:54–66.

57. Neff AG, Turner M, Mutasim DF. Treatment strategies in mucous membrane pemphigoid. *Ther Clin Risk Manag* 2008;4:617–26.

58. Assmann T, Becker J, Ruzicka T, Megahed M. Topical tacrolimus for oral cicatricial pemphigoid. *Clin Exp Dermatol* 2004;29:674–6.

59. Gunther C, Wozel G, Meurer M, Pfeiffer C. Topical tacrolimus treatment for cicatricial pemphigoid. *J Am Acad Dermatol* 2004;50:325–6.

60. Arash A, Shirin L. The management of oral mucous membrane pemphigoid with dapsone and topical corticosteroid. *J Oral Pathol Med* 2008;37:341–4.

61. Ciarrocca KN, Greenberg MS. A retrospective study of the management of oral mucous membrane pemphigoid with dapsone. *Oral Surg Oral Med Oral Pathol Oral Radiol Endod* 1999;88:159–63.

62. Rogers RS 3rd, Mehregan DA. Dapsone therapy of cicatricial pemphigoid. *Semin Dermatol* 1988;7:201–5.

63. Kirtschig G, Murrell D, Wojnarowska F, Khumalo N. Interventions for mucous membrane pemphigoid/cicatricial pemphigoid and epidermolysis bullosa acquisita: A systematic literature review. *Arch Dermatol* 2002;138:380–4.

64. Domloge-Hultsch N, Gammon WR, Briggaman RA, Gil SG, Carter WG, Yancey KB. Epiligrin, the major human keratinocyte integrin ligand, is a target in both an acquired autoimmune and an inherited subepidermal blistering skin disease. *J Clin Invest* 1992;90:1628–33.

65. Saw VP et al. Immunosuppressive therapy for ocular mucous membrane pemphigoid strategies and outcomes. *Ophthalmology* 2008;115:253–61.e1.

66. McCluskey P, Chang JH, Singh R, Wakefield D. Methotrexate therapy for ocular cicatricial pemphigoid. *Ophthalmology* 2004;111:796–801.

67. Staines K, Hampton PJ. Treatment of mucous membrane pemphigoid with the combination of mycophenolate mofetil, dapsone, and prednisolone: A case series. *Oral Surg Oral Med Oral Pathol Oral Radiol* 2012;114:e49–56.

68. Schmidt E, Seitz CS, Benoit S, Brocker EB, Goebeler M. Rituximab in autoimmune bullous diseases: Mixed responses and adverse effects. *Br J Dermatol* 2007;156:352–6.

69. You C, Lamba N, Lasave AF, Ma L, Diaz MH, Foster CS. Rituximab in the treatment of ocular cicatricial pemphigoid: A retrospective cohort study. *Graefes Arch Clin Exp Ophthalmol* 2017;255:1221–8.

70. Roux-Villet CL et al. Rituximab for patients with refractory mucous membrane pemphigoid. *Arch Dermatol* 2011;147:843–9.

71. Maley A, Warren M, Haberman I, Swerlick R, Kharod-Dholakia B, Feldman R. Rituximab combined with conventional therapy versus conventional therapy alone for the treatment of mucous membrane pemphigoid (MMP). *J Am Acad Dermatol* 2016;74:835–40.

72. Haefliger S, Horn MP, Suter VG, Bornstein MM, Borradori L. Rituximab for the treatment of isolated refractory desquamative gingivitis due to mucous membrane pemphigoid. *JAMA Dermatol* 2016;152:1396–8.

73. Yeh SW, Usman AQ, Ahmed AR. Profile of autoantibody to basement membrane zone proteins in patients with mucous membrane pemphigoid: Long-term follow-up and influence of therapy. *Clin Immunol* 2004;112:268–72.

74. Tavakolpour S. The role of intravenous immunoglobulin in treatment of mucous membrane pemphigoid: A review of literature. *J Res Med Sci* 2016;21:37.

75. Sotozono C et al. Visual improvement after cultivated oral mucosal epithelial transplantation. *Ophthalmology* 2013;120:193–200.

76. Cafaro A, Broccoletti R, Arduino PG. Low-level laser therapy for oral mucous membrane pemphigoid. *Lasers Med Sci* 2012;27:1247–50.

12

Bullous pemphigoid

DIPANKAR DE, SHEETANSHU KUMAR, AND SANJEEV HANDA

INTRODUCTION

Bullous pemphigoid (BP) is the most common subepidermal blistering disorder [1]. Few salient features that characterize the disease are incidence in elderly population, presence of tense blisters, relatively benign course and prognosis as compared to pemphigus, presence of subepidermal bulla, and antibody binding on histopathology and immunofluorescence, respectively [2]. BP is associated with autoantibody especially IgG directed against hemidesmosomal target proteins BP 180 (type XVII collagen, BPAG2) and against BP 230 (BPAG1-e).

EPIDEMIOLOGY

The incidence of BP has ranged from 2.5 to 71 per million population per year depending on the population on which the study was carried out [3,4].

Factors that may be playing a role in the surge in incidence of BP are (1) a rise in the proportion of the elderly population due to increased life expectancy [5]; (2) an increase in the use of diuretics, antipsychotics, and other drugs predisposing to BP [6,7]; (3) a rise in the prevalence of incapacitating neurological disorders as a result of increased survival of patients [8,9]; and (4) early and accurate diagnosis of BP owing to the availability of enhanced diagnostic modalities and sensitization of physicians to prodromal symptoms and atypical variants of BP that may have been missed in the past.

ASSOCIATED DISEASES

Multiple population- and hospital-based studies have confirmed the association of BP with various medical conditions and drugs. The associations with neurological disorders [10], psychiatric disorders [11], cardiovascular disease, diabetes, and other immunological diseases have been reported most frequently.

Neurological and psychiatric diseases

The prevalence of neurological disorders, chiefly Alzheimer disease and other forms of dementia, Parkinson disease, and cerebrovascular disease in patients of BP have ranged from 19.5% to 46% in different studies [9–15]. The expression of BP180 and BP230 antigens in the central nervous system and cross-reacting immune response between neural and cutaneous antigens have been hypothesized to play a role in the association of BP with neurological disorders [8,6,16,17].

Drugs

Drugs commonly associated with BP are phenothiazines, loop diuretics, spironolactone, and gliptins [5–7,18–20]. BP associated with drugs can be classified into drug-induced or drug-triggered BP [1,21]. A drug may act as a hapten and change the antigenic properties of proteins of lamina lucida after binding to them, or a drug may unmask the cryptic antigens by structurally modifying the molecules, thus creating an immune response [22]. The majority of drugs causing BP have been found to contain sulfhydryl groups (captopril, furosemide, penicillamine, penicillin and its derivatives, and some cephalosporins) or phenol groups (acetylsalicylic acid or cephalosporins) [22].

Malignancies

A significant association with hematological malignancies has been found in a meta-analysis of eight studies [28]. However, extensive malignancy screening in patients of BP apart from age-appropriate cancer screening is not indicated [23–27].

CLINICAL FEATURES

Prodrome

The onset of bullous lesions in BP is typically preceded by a prodromal phase lasting up to several weeks and even months [29,30]. This prodromal phase is characterized by nonbullous pruritic polymorphic lesions, such as eczematous or urticarial plaques, excoriated papules, and prurigo-like lesions [30].

Bullous stage

The bullous stage of BP manifests as tense serous or hemorrhagic bullae on a normal or erythematous base associated with moderate to severe pruritus (Figure 12.1) [31]. There is usually symmetrical distribution of the lesions (Figure 12.2). The size attained by the bulla can be up to several centimeters in diameter (Figure 12.3). Annular and figurate urticarial plaques can also be seen [31–33]. The lower abdomen, flexures of the limbs and abdomen, and intertriginous areas are the frequently affected sites (Figure 12.4) [29]. Oral involvement is seen in 10%–25% of cases [34]. Nikolsky sign is not seen [33]. The lesions heal without scarring unless secondarily infected. Erythema can be seen persisting at the site of previous blisters for even up to several weeks and months. Postinflammatory changes like hypo- or hyperpigmentation and milia can be seen sometimes. Bullous pemphigoid is characterized by a chronic course with waxing and waning. The disease is usually self-limiting after a course of a few years [2,35]. The cutaneous lesions are not life threatening in most cases, but there is up to six times higher mortality seen in BP patients as compared to age-matched controls [36]. Although the association of BP with malignancies is controversial, the

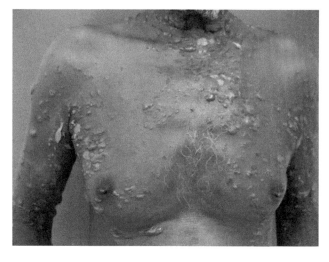

Figure 12.2 Symmetrical involvement of chest and flexures.

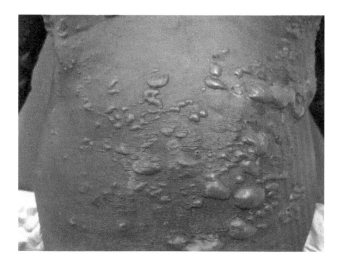

Figure 12.3 Involvement of lower abdomen with large bullae.

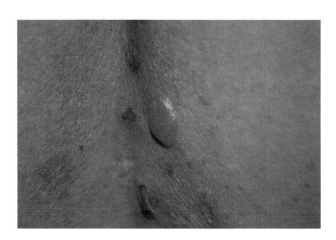

Figure 12.1 Tense bullae on the back.

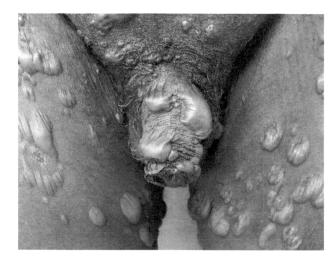

Figure 12.4 Involvement of groin.

presence of figurate erythematous lesions can be a sign of associated malignancy [37].

Nonbullous cutaneous pemphigoid

In up to 20% of BP cases, characteristic bullous lesions never develop during the entire course of disease. In these cases, nonspecific urticarial and eczematous lesions are the only manifestations throughout the entire course [38]. An eczematous variant is characterized by eczematous plaques, excoriated papules, and nodules associated with severe pruritus [39]. Similarly, an urticarial variant presents with pruritic urticarial lesions. Pemphigoid nodularis is another such variant characterized by prurigo-like nodules on distal extremities. Bullous lesions are present only occasionally in pemphigoid nodularis [31].

Erythrodermic bullous pemphigoid

Erythrodermic BP is one of the rare presentations of BP with only a few case reports available in the literature [40,41]. It is characterized by erythroderma with or without bullous lesions. Blisters when present may precede or follow the development of erythroderma [41,42]. A high index of suspicion is required for diagnosis in the absence of bullous lesions. The diagnosis relies on characteristic histopathological and direct immunofluorescence (DIF) findings.

Complications

Apart from the neurological, psychiatric, and other systemic associations of BP that were discussed earlier, the risk of pulmonary embolism and infection in patients of BP is around three times higher when compared to the general population [43,44].

Course of disease

BP is characterized by a chronic but usually self-limiting waxing and waning course lasting months to years. Relapses are common and encountered in up to half of the patients within 1 year after stopping treatment, with most relapses occurring within 3 months [32]. The factors found to be associated with relapse in different studies were older age, extensive disease at presentation, associated dementia, positive DIF, and higher titers of anti-BP180 NC16A antibodies after receiving treatment [45,46].

The first-year mortality rate for BP ranges from 10% to 40% in different studies and is around two to six times higher than the age- and sex-matched controls [32,47–52]. The presence of factors like extensive disease at presentation; age greater than 80 years; treatment with doses of prednisolone >35 mg/day; serum albumin values <3.6 g/dL; Karnofsky score ≤40; or comorbidities like cardiac disease, diabetes mellitus, or neurological diseases have been found to be associated with higher mortality and poor prognosis [48,51,52,54,55].

Diagnosis

The diagnosis of BP is based on the clinical, histopathological, and immunofluorescence and serological findings. An elaborate clinical history stressing the onset and evolution of symptoms; presence of pruritus; presence of associated neurological, psychiatric, and other systemic diseases and malignancies; and recent drug intake are of paramount importance. Comorbidities such as cardiovascular diseases, immunodeficiency, and diabetes also play a role in individualizing the treatment modalities in each patient. Detailed examination to determine the extent of involvement and morphology of lesions also aids in deciding the management strategy.

Histopathology

Subepidermal bulla with dense inflammatory infiltrate consisting primarily of eosinophils but also including neutrophils, macrophages, and T lymphocytes in the papillary dermis and basement membrane zone (BMZ) is seen typically on histopathology of a skin biopsy taken from the edge of a fresh bulla [1,56]. Differentiating among the subepidermal blistering disorders on the basis of histopathology alone is difficult, and immunofluorescence study is required.

Direct immunofluorescence

Perilesional DIF is the gold standard for the diagnosis of autoimmune bullous disorders [57]. Although not very specific, DIF has high sensitivity for subepidermal blistering disorders.

On DIF, bullous pemphigoid characteristically demonstrates the deposition of predominantly IgG (IgG4 and IgG1 subclass primarily) and/or C3 along the BMZ zone along with deposition of IgA and IgE to some extent. The sensitivity of DIF can be augmented further by performing salt-split immunofluorescence and n-serrated and u-serrated pattern analysis. On salt-split DIF, immunofluorescence is observed in the BMZ of the epidermal side of the salt-split tissue in BP. The n-serrated pattern in BP helps to differentiate it from epidermolysis bullosa acquisita in which the u-serrated pattern is observed [1,57].

Treatment

The treatment strategy in BP depends on extent of disease, presence of comorbidities, and general health condition of the patient. The goal of the treatment is to control the disease on minimum possible systemic or topical drugs in view of the fact that most of the patients are elderly with comorbidities and on multiple drugs already, thus prone to adverse effects and drug interactions. Ruling out drug-induced BP and stopping the causative drug is of utmost importance along with working up the patient for associated malignancies.

Currently, there is paucity of prospective controlled trials for the management of BP, and the treatment strategies are based mostly on treatment guidelines and clinical experience.

TREATMENT GUIDELINES

Although at least three guidelines exist for the management of BP proposed by French reference centers for autoimmune bullous diseases [58], British Association of Dermatologists [59], and the German Dermatological Society [60], universal consensus regarding treatment guidelines has still to be formulated.

Glucocorticoids have been suggested as the mainstay of treatment with supplementation by steroid-sparing agents in all of these guidelines. The grading of disease severity and activity is based on percentage of skin involvement or number of new blisters [60,61]. For mild disease (<10% body surface area [BSA]), topical therapy with clobetasol propionate 0.05% ointment combined with anti-inflammatory antibiotics, such as doxycycline, tetracycline, minocycline, and erythromycin, is indicated [59]. The recommendation for moderate (10%–30% BSA) and severe disease (>30% BSA) is systemic therapy with prednisolone at a dose of 0.5–1.0 mg/kg/day. Other modalities like dapsone, azathioprine, mycophenolate mofetil, and cyclosporine can be used either as monotherapy or in combination in case of comorbidities and contraindications to corticosteroids.

BIOLOGICS

Rituximab

Although large prospective studies are lacking, rituximab has been found to be effective for management of BP in several case reports [1,2]. In one retrospective study, it was concluded that first-line therapy with a combination of rituximab and prednisolone for BP is more effective than prednisolone monotherapy [62]. However, caution should be exercised in the use of rituximab in elderly patients, as its use can be associated with increased risk of mortality in this age group.

Omalizumab

Omalizumab, a monoclonal antibody against IgE binding, has been used with success in cases of refractory BP in a few of the case reports. Its success in BP is owing to the possible role of anti-BP180 IgE antibodies in the pathogenesis of BP. In a case series including six patients of BP treated with omalizumab, five out of six patients showed significant improvement in clinical features and serum IgE levels, favoring the fact that IgE can be a target of therapy in BP [53].

MANAGEMENT OF ERYTHRODERMIC OR EXTENSIVE BULLOUS PEMPHIGOID

Erythroderma secondary to any underlying cause is a dermatological emergency. Supportive care in the management of erythrodermic BP should be the same as the management of erythroderma in general. Maintaining hydration, ambient temperature, and nutritional requirements and correcting electrolyte imbalances are the mainstays of supportive

care. Owing to the presence of extensive bullae and erosions, barrier nursing care under aseptic precautions to prevent secondary infections is of importance. Extensive secondary infection poses a therapeutic challenge in view of the risk of flare of the infection prohibiting the use of immunosuppressive agents. Empiric broad-spectrum systemic antibiotics along with or prior to the use of immunosuppressive agents are required to control and prevent the progression of the underlying infections. Skin is the most common focus of secondary infections, and antibiotics with gram-positive coverage should be used as empiric treatment until blood and pus culture and sensitivity are available. Hospital-acquired gram-negative infections should also be considered and managed accordingly in case of onset of infection after prolonged hospital stay.

CONCLUSION

Bullous pemphigoid can manifest with emergency features, especially erythroderma and with extensive lesions, though rarely. Associations of old age, malignancy, and autoimmune disorders complicate the situation further in a few cases. Early diagnosis is the key, as treatment in early stages prevents these complications from occurring.

KEY POINTS

- Bullous pemphigoid is the commonest bullous disorder.
- It usually manifests in the elderly and can present rarely as an emergency especially when the lesions are extensive, in the erythrodermic variant and due to complications or comorbidities.
- Subepidermal bulla.

REFERENCES

1. Bagci IS, Horvath ON, Ruzicka T, Sardy M. Bullous pemphigoid. *Autoimmun Rev* 2017;16:445–55.
2. Bernard P, Antonicelli F. Bullous pemphigoid: A review of its diagnosis, associations and treatment. *Am J Clin Dermatol* 2017;18:513–28.
3. Baican A et al. Pemphigus vulgaris is the most common autoimmune bullous disease in Northwestern Romania. *Int J Dermatol* 2010;49:768–74.
4. Thorslund K, Seifert O, Nilzén K, Grönhagen C. Incidence of bullous pemphigoid in Sweden 2005–2012: A nationwide population-based cohort study of 3761 patients. *Arch Dermatol Res* 2017;309:721–7.
5. Bastuji-Garin S et al. Risk factors for bullous pemphigoid in the elderly: A prospective case-control study. *J Invest Dermatol* 2011;131:637–43.
6. Bastuji-Garin S et al. Drugs associated with bullous pemphigoid. A case-control study. *Arch Dermatol* 1996;132:272–6.

7. Lloyd-Lavery A, Chi CC, Wojnarowska F, Taghipour K. The associations between bullous pemphigoid and drug use: A UK case-control study. *JAMA Dermatol* 2013;149:58–62.

8. Langan SM, Groves RW, West J. The relationship between neurological disease and bullous pemphigoid: A population-based case-control study. *J Invest Dermatol* 2011;131:631–6.

9. Taghipour K, Chi CC, Vincent A, Groves RW, Venning V, Wojnarowska F. The association of bullous pemphigoid with cerebrovascular disease and dementia: A case-control study. *Arch Dermatol* 2010;146:1251–4.

10. Cordel N et al. Neurological disorders in patients with bullous pemphigoid. *Dermatology* 2007;215:187–91.

11. Försti A-K et al. Psychiatric and neurological disorders are associated with bullous pemphigoid: A nationwide Finnish care register study. *Sci Rep* 2016;6:37125.

12. Chen YJ et al. Comorbidity profiles among patients with bullous pemphigoid: A nationwide population-based study. *Br J Dermatol* 2011;165:593–9.

13. Tarazona MJ, Mota AN, Gripp AC, Unterstell N, Bressan AL. Bullous pemphigoid and neurological disease: Statistics from a dermatology service. *An Bras Dermatol* 2015;90:280–2.

14. Khosravani S, Handjani F, Alimohammadi R, Saki N. Frequency of neurological disorders in bullous pemphigoid patients: A cross-sectional study. *Int Sch Res Notices* 2017;6053267.

15. Brick KE et al. A population-based study of the association between bullous pemphigoid and neurologic disorders. *J Am Acad Dermatol* 2014;71:1191–7.

16. Seppanen A. Collagen XVII: A shared antigen in neurodermatological interactions? *Clin Dev Immunol* 2013;2013:240570.

17. Kunzli K, Favre B, Chofflon M, Borradori L. One gene but different proteins and diseases: The complexity of dystonin and bullous pemphigoid antigen 1. *Exp Dermatol* 2016;25:10–6.

18. Stavropoulos PG, Soura E, Antoniou C. Drug-induced pemphigoid: A review of the literature. *J Eur Acad Dermatol Venereol* 2014;28:1133–40.

19. Bene J et al. Bullous pemphigoid and dipeptidyl peptidase IV inhibitors: A case-noncase study in the French pharmacovigilance database. *Br J Dermatol* 2016;175:296–301.

20. Tan CW, Pang Y, Sim B, Thirumoorthy T, Pang SM, Lee HY. The association between drugs and bullous pemphigoid. 2017;176:549–51.

21. Vassileva S. Drug-induced pemphigoid: Bullous and cicatricial. *Clin Dermatol* 1998;16:379–87.

22. Ruocco V, Sacerdoti G. Pemphigus and bullous pemphigoid due to drugs. *Int J Dermatol* 1991;30:307–12.

23. Teixeira VB, Cabral R, Brites MM, Vieira R, Figueiredo A. Bullous pemphigoid and comorbidities: A case-control study in Portuguese patients. *An Bras Dermatol* 2014;89:274–9.

24. Lindelof B, Islam N, Eklund G, Arfors L. Pemphigoid and cancer. *Arch Dermatol* 1990;126:66–8.

25. Ogawa H et al. The incidence of internal malignancies in pemphigus and bullous pemphigoid in Japan. *J Dermatol Sci* 1995;9:136–41.

26. Ong E, Goldacre R, Hoang U, Sinclair R, Goldacre M. Associations between bullous pemphigoid and primary malignant cancers: An English national record linkage study, 1999–2011. *Arch Dermatol Res* 2014;306:75–80.

27. Schulze F, Neumann K, Recke A, Zillikens D, Linder R, Schmidt E. Malignancies in pemphigus and pemphigoid diseases. *J Invest Dermatol* 2015;135:1445–7.

28. Atzmony L et al. Association of bullous pemphigoid with malignancy: A systematic review and meta-analysis. *J Am Acad Dermatol* 2017;77:691–9.

29. Zenzo G D, Marazza G, Borradori L. Bullous pemphigoid: Physiopathology, clinical features and management. *Adv Dermatol* 2007;23:257–88.

30. Lamb PM, Abell E, Tharp M, Frye R, Deng J-S. Prodromal bullous pemphigoid. *Int J Dermatol* 2006;45:209–14.

31. Walsh SR, Hogg D, Mydlarski PR. Bullous pemphigoid: From bench to bedside. *Drugs* 2005;65:905–26.

32. Schmidt E, della Torre R, Borradori L. Clinical features and practical diagnosis of bullous pemphigoid. *Dermatol Clin* 2011;29:427–38.

33. Kippes W, Schmidt E, Roth A, Rzany B, Brocker EB, Zillikens D. Immunopathologic changes in 115 patients with bullous pemphigoid. *Hautarzt* 1999;50:866–72.

34. Di Zenzo G et al. Multicenter prospective study of the humoral autoimmune response in bullous pemphigoid. *Clin Immunol* 2008;128:415–26.

35. Korman N. Bullous pemphigoid. *J Am Acad Dermatol* 1987;16:907–24.

36. Joly P et al. Incidence and mortality of bullous pemphigoid in France. *J Invest Dermatol* 2012;132:1998–2004.

37. Graham-Brown RA. Bullous pemphigoid with figurate erythema associated with carcinoma of the bronchus. *Br J Dermatol* 1987;117:385–8.

38. Bakker CV, Terra JB, Pas HH, Jonkman MF. Bullous pemphigoid as pruritus in the elderly: A common presentation. *JAMA Dermatol* 2013;149:950–3.

39. Jeong SJ, Lee CW. Bullous pemphigoid: Persistent lesions of eczematous/urticarial erythemas. *Cutis* 1995;56:225–6.

40. Korman NJ, Woods SG. Erythrodermic bullous pemphigoid is a clinical variant of bullous pemphigoid. *Br J Dermatol* 1995;133:967–71.

41. Amato L, Gallerani I, Mei S, Pestelli E, Caproni M, Fabbri P. Erythrodermic bullous pemphigoid. *Int J Dermatol* 2001;40:343–6.

42. Tappeiner G, Konrad K, Holubar K. Erythrodermic bullous pemphigoid. *J Am Acad Dermatol* 1982;6:489–92.

43. Savin JA. The events leading to the death of patients with pemphigus and pemphigoid. *Br J Dermatol* 1979;101:521–34.

44. Langan SM, Hubbard R, Fleming K, West J. A population-based study of acute medical conditions associated with bullous pemphigoid. *Br J Dermatol* 2009;161:1149–52.

45. Bernard P et al. Risk factors for relapse in patients with bullous pemphigoid in clinical remission: A multicenter, prospective, cohort study. *Arch Dermatol* 2009;145:537–42.

46. Fichel F et al. Clinical and immunologic factors associated with bullous pemphigoid relapse during the first year of treatment: A multicenter, prospective study. *JAMA Dermatol* 2014;150:25–33.

47. Langan SM, Smeeth L, Hubbard R, Fleming KM, Smith CJ, West J. Bullous pemphigoid and pemphigus vulgaris—Incidence and mortality in the UK: Population based cohort study. *BMJ* 2008;337:a180.

48. Cortés B, Marazza G, Naldi L, Combescure C, Borradori L, the Autoimmune Bullous Disease Swiss Study Group. Mortality of bullous pemphigoid in Switzerland: A prospective study. *Br J Dermatol* 2011;165:368–74

49. Li J, Zuo YG, Zheng HY. Mortality of bullous pemphigoid in China. *JAMA Dermatol* 2013;149:106–8.

50. della Torre R et al. Clinical presentation and diagnostic delay in bullous pemphigoid: A prospective nationwide cohort. *Br J Dermatol* 2012;167:1111–7.

51. Roujeau J, Lok C, Bastuji-Garin S, Mhalla S, Enginger V, Bernard P. High risk of death in elderly patients with extensive bullous pemphigoid. *Arch Dermatol* 1998;134:465–9.

52. Joly P et al. Prediction of survival for patients with bullous pemphigoid: A prospective study. *Arch Dermatol* 2005;141:691–8.

53. Yu KK, Crew AB, Messingham KA, Fairley JA, Woodley DT. Omalizumab therapy for bullous pemphigoid. *J Am Acad Dermatol* 2014;71:468–74.

54. Parker SR et al. Mortality of bullous pemphigoid: An evaluation of 223 patients and comparison with the mortality in the general population in the United States. *J Am Acad Dermatol* 2008;59:582–8.

55. Rzany B et al. Risk factors for lethal outcome in patients with bullous pemphigoid: Low serum albumin level, high dosage of glucocorticosteroids, and old age. *Arch Dermatol* 2002;138:903–8.

56. Machado-Pinto J, McCalmont TH, Golitz LE. Eosinophilic and neutrophilic spongiosis: Clues to the diagnosis of immunobullous diseases and other inflammatory disorders. *Semin Cutan Med Surg* 1996;15:308–16.

57. Sardy M, Kostaki D, Varga R, Peris K, Ruzicka T. Comparative study of direct and indirect immunofluorescence and of bullous pemphigoid 180 and 230 enzyme-linked immunosorbent assays for diagnosis of bullous pemphigoid. *J Am Acad Dermatol* 2013;69:748–53.

58. Bernard P, Bedane C, Prost C, Ingen-Housz-Oro S, Joly P. [Bullous pemphigoid. Guidelines for the diagnosis and treatment. Centres de reference des maladies bulleuses auto-immunes. Societe Francaise de Dermatologie]. *Ann Dermatol Venereol* 2011;138:247–51.

59. Venning VA, Taghipour K, Mohd Mustapa MF, Highet AS, Kirtschig G. British Association of Dermatologists' guidelines for the management of bullous pemphigoid 2012. *Br J Dermatol* 2012;167:1200–14.

60. Eming R et al. S2k guidelines for the treatment of pemphigus vulgaris/foliaceus and bullous pemphigoid. *J Dtsch Dermatol Ges* 2015;13:833–44.

61. Joly P et al. A comparison of oral and topical corticosteroids in patients with bullous pemphigoid. *N Engl J Med* 2002;346:321–7.

62. Cho YT, Chu CY, Wang LF. First-line combination therapy with rituximab and corticosteroids provides a high complete remission rate in moderate-to-severe bullous pemphigoid. *Br J Dermatol* 2015;173:302–4.

Erythroderma

D. V. LAKSHMI

13

Approach to Erythroderma

D. V. LAKSHMI

INTRODUCTION

Erythroderma (ED) aptly fits into the Latin idiom *mille viae ducunt homines per saecula Romam,* meaning "All roads lead men forever to Rome," and connotes that different paths take one to the same goal. With a culminating clinical pattern of erythema and scaling as a presenting feature (Figure 13.1), secondary to an underlying cause in most scenarios, erythroderma constitutes a common encounter every clinician will face in practice, rightly demanding an evaluation with intensive care and thus a "dermatological emergency" status.

The controversy of terminology: Erythroderma or exfoliative dermatitis?

In 1868, the Greek term *erythroderma* was introduced by Ferdinand Von Hebra describing an exfoliative dermatitis involving more than 90% of the skin surface [1]. Erythroderma and exfoliative dermatitis are largely used synonymously; however, erythroderma is often the preferred term [2]. *Exfoliative dermatitis* refers to the presence of widespread erythema and marked scaling, while *erythroderma* is characterized by pronounced erythema and perceptible scaling. But the salient feature that clubs them as a single term is widespread involvement of the body surface area.

Definition

Erythroderma is defined as a generalized or nearly generalized sustained erythema of the skin, involving more than 90% of the body surface area with a variable degree of scaling [2]. It is essential to understand that erythroderma is a morphological reaction pattern and not a definitive disease; an interplay of inflammatory mediators triggers a cascade that eventually culminates in a clinical entity of widespread erythema and scaling. Thus, clinical recognition of the erythroderma is easy, but the diagnosis of the underlying systemic or cutaneous cause may be a very difficult and challenging aspect.

EPIDEMIOLOGY

The incidence of erythroderma varies widely among various surveys. Sehgal et al., in a study survey from India, recorded the incidence of 35 per 100,000 dermatologic outpatients, but a larger survey by Sigurdson et al. showed an annual incidence of 0.9 per 100,000 population [2–4].

The incidence as a function of age is usually variable, and any age group may be affected; however, affected patients are usually older than 45 years, with an average age of onset of 55 years [2]. In general, studies have shown a male predominance with the male-to-female ratio ranging from 2:1 to 4:1 [2].

In a retrospective Indian study by Sarkar et al. in the pediatric age group, neonatal and infantile erythroderma were found to be prominent contributors [5]. In another study by Sarkar et al., the incidence of childhood erythroderma was 0.11% out of 16,000 pediatric patients, with a male-to-female ratio of 0.89:1 and the mean age of onset being 3.3 years in their study [6].

CLASSIFICATION

Based on the clinical course, erythroderma was classified into three forms, a classification that is no longer employed and is now only of historic interest [7]:

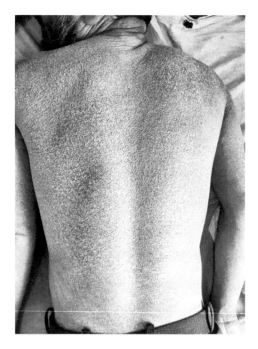

Figure 13.1 Clinical picture of erythroderma showing generalized scaling and erythema. (Photo courtesy of Dr. Shilpa K, BMC&RI, Bengaluru.)

1. *Wilson-Brocq type*: Chronically relapsing form
2. *Hebra type*: Chronically persisting form
3. *Savill type*: Self-limiting epidemic form

Erythroderma can be better classified depending on the cause [7]:

- *Primary form*: Where the underlying cause is not evident most of the time, e.g., Sézary syndrome, atopic dermatitis in elderly
- *Secondary form*: Where a preexisting skin condition is definitely identifiable most of the time, e.g., psoriasis, eczema

PATHOGENESIS

The exact mechanism is unclear (Figure 13.2). Adhesion molecules and their ligands play a significant role in endothelial-leukocyte interactions, which impact the binding, transmigration, and infiltration of lymphocytes and mononuclear cells during inflammation, injury, or immunological stimulation [8]. The rise in adhesion molecule expression (vascular cell adhesion molecule [VCAM]-1, intercellular adhesion molecule [ICAM]-1, E-selectin, and P-selectin) seen in exfoliative dermatitis stimulates dermal inflammation, which may lead to epidermal proliferation and increased production of inflammatory mediators. Thus, erythroderma develops secondary to an intricate interaction of cytokines (interleukin [IL]-1, IL-2, and IL-8), cellular adhesion molecules (mainly intercellular adhesion molecule 1), and the tumor necrotic factor [9]. These interactions result in increased epidermal turnover rate with decreased

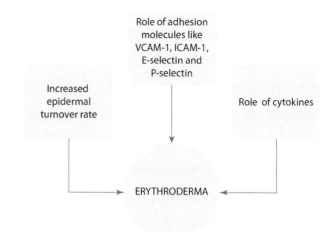

Figure 13.2 Pathogenesis of erythroderma.

transit time and accelerated mitotic rate and an increased absolute number of the germinative skin cells. This also causes a significant loss of protein and folate [10].

ETIOLOGY

A preexisting dermatosis is the most common cause of adult erythroderma. A number of dermatoses can progress to erythroderma, but the most common include psoriasis and eczema [11,12]. Primary dermatoses and other etiologies causing adult erythroderma are enumerated in Table 13.1.

Eczematous erythroderma

Eczematous erythroderma accounts for about 50% of all adult erythroderma cases. Eczematous erythroderma is often caused by contact dermatitis, seborrheic dermatitis, autosensitization dermatitis, and atopic dermatitis. Initially presenting as localized eczema, they then generalize to become erythroderma under the influence of intrinsic and extrinsic factors like dysfunction of T cells, preexisting liver or kidney disorder, inappropriate treatments for eczema (including home remedies), and environmental changes. Edematous redness and scaling are present over the entire body skin. This is accompanied by intense itching and, sometimes, indolent lymphadenopathy, particularly of the inguinal lymph nodes. Systemic symptoms such as fever, dehydration, protein loss, body temperature instability, and opportunistic infection may be found. Oral and topical steroids are extremely effective as a treatment modality.

Psoriatic erythroderma/erythrodermic psoriasis

Erythrodermic psoriasis (EP) is a severe variant of psoriasis, with an estimated prevalence among psoriatic patients ranging from 1% to 2.25% and constitutes ~25% of all cases of erythroderma [13,14]. The genetic basis of EP is not yet well known, though Class I antigens HLA-Cw6, HLA-B57,

Table 13.1 Causes of erythroderma in adults

Eczema	Papulosquamous disorders	Bullous dermatosis
Atopic dermatitis	Psoriasis	Pemphigus foliaceous
Seborrheic dermatitis	Pityriasis rubra pilaris	Paraneoplastic pemphigus
Contact dermatitis	Impetigo herpetiformis	Hailey-Hailey disease
Stasis dermatitis	Darier disease	Bullous pemphigoid
Connective tissue disorders	Photosensitive dermatosis	Infective causes
Dermatomyositis	Chronic actinic dermatitis	Viral
Subacute cutaneous lupus	Actinic reticuloid	HIV
erythematosis	Others	Human herpes virus
Systemic disease	Pseudolymphoma	Fungal
Sarcoidosis	Perforating folliculitis	Dermatophytosis
Acute graft versus host disease	Radiation recall dermatitis	Candidiasis
Postoperative transfusion induced	Senile erythroderma with hyper-IgE	Parasitic
Malignancy	Drugs	Norwegian scabies
Solid tumors	Thiazides, antimalarials, anti-epileptics,	Toxoplasmosis
Lymphoproliferative malignancies	nonsteroidal anti-inflammatory drugs	Leishmaniasis
	Penicillin group, terbinafine	Toxin mediated
	antitubercular drugs, dapsone	Staphylococcal scalded skin
		syndrome
		Toxic shock syndrome

HLA-B13, and HLA-B17 have been associated with psoriasis vulgaris (PV), and IL36RN mutations have been associated with pustular psoriasis [15,16].

It is one of the leading causes of erythroderma and is more common in men than women (3:1), and the majority of cases have a positive history of psoriasis with an identifiable trigger [14].

Histopathology may reveal clues to an underlying psoriatic pathology in some cases.

Drug-induced erythroderma

With the introduction of newer drugs in the field of medicine, the incidence of drug-induced erythroderma is also increasing. Systemic drugs, topical drugs, alternative medicinal preparations, and home remedies can all be responsible. Adverse drug eruptions may initially present as morbilliform, lichenoid, or urticarial forms and eventually progress to erythroderma. It may be associated with facial edema and become purpuric in dependent areas. Associated signs of possible drug etiology include fever, lymphadenopathy, organomegaly, edema, leukocytosis with eosinophilia, and liver and renal dysfunction.

The general rule in drug-induced erythroderma is as follows: "Onset in drug-induced erythroderma is rapid and resolution also faster with discontinuation."

Histopathology shows perivascular infiltrate with eosinophils, lichenoid infiltrate, necrotic keratinocytes, and vacuolar degeneration of basal layer.

Immunobullous disorders and erythroderma

Erythrodermic presentation is uncommon in bullous disorders, though, pemphigus foliaceus, bullous pemphigoid

(BP), paraneoplastic pemphigus, and epidermolysis bullosa acquisita have been reported to cause erythroderma [17–20].

Pemphigus foliaceus (PF) usually has a benign course and rarely leads to erythroderma. The prevalence is only 0.5% cases in PF [18]. Erythroderma may be preceded by moist crusted lesions on the face and upper trunk with conspicuous, moist, and adherent scales. Eventually, crops of thin-walled bullae may erupt. Triggering factors such as ultraviolet (UV) exposure, drugs, and various infections have been attributed to causing this exacerbated clinical form of erythroderma [17,18]. Histopathology showing acantholysis in the upper epidermis, within or adjacent to the granular layer, leading to a subcorneal bulla should arouse suspicion of underlying blistering dermatoses. In PF, direct immunofluorescence (DIF) shows IgG immunostaining on the epithelial cell surfaces, which can be granular and/or linear, resulting in a chicken wire pattern [17,18].

BP is notorious for protean forms of clinical presentations: classical generalized BP, localized, pemphigoid nodularis, lichen planus pemphigoides, seborrheic type, dyshidrosiform, figurative erythema like, erythema multiforme like, and also erythrodermic [19]. Erythrodermic bullous pemphigoid is an unusual manifestation of BP characterized by blistering, which may present prior to or following the onset of erythroderma. It is also found to be UV induced. Erythroderma as lichenoid or exfoliative form in the absence of blistering has also been reported [19]. Immunofluorescence microscopy plays a confirmatory role here. Circulating antibodies to the basement membrane zone, with an epidermal pattern on salt-split skin on DIF, and the presence of eosinophilic spongiosis in the skin biopsy specimen support the diagnosis of BP.

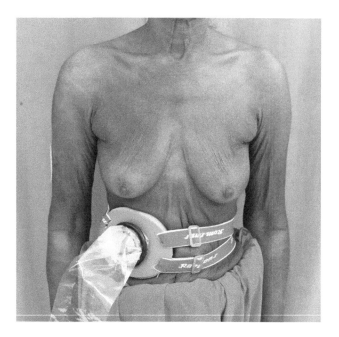

Figure 13.3 Erythroderma in a case of abdominal malignancy.

Paraneoplastic pemphigus (PNP) also can have polymorphous lesions like BP; diffuse erythema, vesiculobullous lesions, papules, scaly plaques, exfoliative erythroderma, erosions, or ulcerations. Initially erythema, which can be macular, urticarial, targetoid, or polymorphous, occurs, and then they develop bullae and erosions [21]. Painful

intractable oral mucositis involving vermilion border of lips, lateral borders of tongue, and oropharynx is a constant feature of PNP [21–23]. The most commonly associated neoplasms in PNP are lymphoproliferative or hematological neoplasms. When PNP is associated with an underlying malignancy, it is extremely resistant to treatment and carries a 90% mortality rate, independent of the course of malignancy. Refractoriness of the erythrodermic mucocutaneous lesions which presents along with blisters, to the standard immunosuppression therapy, should arouse suspicion of PNP, and screening for an underlying occult neoplasm is to be mandatorily done. A pan–computed tomography (CT) scan and flow cytometry on peripheral blood should be mandatory when PNP is confirmed by immunoprecipitation studies [21–23].

Malignancy and erythroderma

Erythroderma is found to be associated with an underlying malignancy in 1%–11% of patients (Figure 13.3) [24,25]. Figure 13.4 enumerates malignancies found in association with erythroderma. The most common malignancy is cutaneous T-cell lymphoma (CTCL) comprising mycosis fungoides and Sézary syndrome [25]. Reticuloendothelial neoplasms are more common causes of erythroderma compared to visceral neoplasms.

Erythroderma can be a part of a paraneoplastic state, occurring parallel to the malignancy or as a premonitory state occurring initially even before malignancy is diagnosed

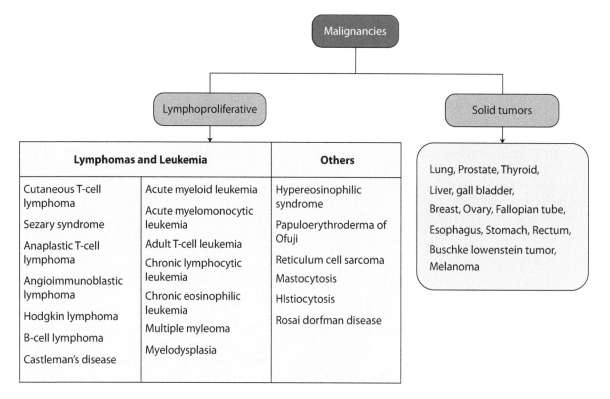

Figure 13.4 Malignancies found in association with erythroderma.

[26]. Malignancy-associated erythroderma is attributed to a complicated interaction of cytokines (IL-1, IL-2, and IL-8) and adhesion molecules (VCAM, ICAM, E-selectin) causing binding, transmigration, and infiltration of lymphocytes resulting in increased epidermal turnover. Alternatively, a tumor-induced host immune response or antigenic cross-reactivity between tumor and skin may cause these skin changes [27,28]. However, it is difficult to diagnose as it may not show neoplastic cells on histopathology for many of the initial years.

The International Society for Cutaneous Lymphomas has recognized variants of erythrodermic CTCL, which includes Sézary syndrome (SS), erythrodermic mycosis fungoides (lacks hematologic findings of SS), and erythrodermic CTCL, not otherwise specified [29]. Sézary syndrome is diagnosed by demonstration of a peripheral blood T-cell clone by molecular/cytogenetic methods: an expanded CD4+ population resulting in CD4:CD8 ratio >10%, absolute Sézary cell count of at least 1000 cells/mm³ and immunophenotypic abnormalities. Clinically it presents as intractable pruritus, erythroderma, and lymphadenopathy. Hematological involvement shows >5% atypical circulating lymphocytes [29]. The dermal infiltrate in Sézary syndrome mainly shows a T-helper-2 cytokine profile, whereas benign reactive erythroderma shows a T-helper-1 cytokine profile, indicating that, although clinically similar, they have different underlying pathogenic mechanisms [30,31]. Immunophenotype in Sézary syndrome is of a mature helper T cell with memory phenotype, viz., CD2, CD3, CD4, CD5, CD45R0+, and CD8–. CD4+ cells also lose the CD26 marker and when this CD26– subset exceeds 30% of CD4+ cells along with hematological involvement, a diagnosis of SS is made [32]. Two antigens P140 and SCS have been found in skin-infiltrating cells of patients with Sézary syndrome [32]. Resolution of the erythroderma can be seen with curative resection of the tumor, and its recurrence might indicate recurrence of the tumor. Absolute Sézary cell count and lymph node involvement are independent prognostic factors. In addition, development of skin tumors on a background of erythroderma, visceral involvement, advancing age, and presence of Ebstein-Barr virus genome in keratinocytes all have poor prognosis [32,33].

Papuloerythroderma of Ofuji is a disease of unknown etiology, a prelymphomatous condition characterized by the onset of disseminated brownish erythematous papules that converge to produce erythroderma that typically spares the major skin folds. It affects elderly men more often than women. Apart from cutaneous involvement, the most characteristic laboratory finding is peripheral eosinophilia with high levels of immunoglobulin E and lymphopenia. Liver function tests may be abnormal, with elevated alkaline phosphatase and γ-glutamyl transferase. It has also been reported to progress to T-cell lymphoma and is found in association with visceral neoplasms, Hodgkin lymphoma, acute myeloid leukemia, hypereosinophilic syndrome, AIDS, drug hypersensitivity, and biliary sepsis after cholecystectomy. Topical and systemic corticosteroids at low doses along with antihistamines, Psoralen plus ultraviolet A (PUVA), UV-B, retinoid-PUVA, and other treatments, such as cyclosporine, etretinate, azathioprine, and interferon-α, have been used successfully to treat this condition.

Idiopathic erythroderma (Red man syndrome)

In approximately one-third of erythrodermic patients, no underlying disease may be found, and this subset is termed *idiopathic erythroderma*. Ohga et al. considered erythroderma without any apparent cause and lasting more than 3 months as chronic idiopathic erythroderma (CIE) in their study and found that it is an independent condition likely to occur in the elderly [34]. Shift in immunity to Th2 type in CIE was described as one of the main mechanisms involved as elevated serum levels of thymus and activation-regulated chemokine (TARC), a T2 helper chemokine was found along with lower IgE levels unlike that occurring in atopic dermatitis [34].

Clinically this form presents as a chronic relapsing pruritic erythroderma in association with significant dermatopathic lymphadenopathy, peripheral edema, and extensive palmoplantar keratoderma more common than in other types of erythroderma (Figures 13.5 and 13.6), and

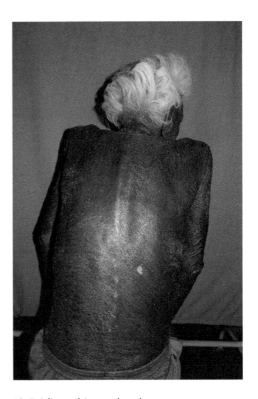

Figure 13.5 Idiopathic erythroderma.

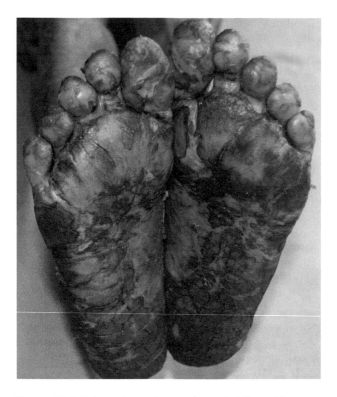

Figure 13.6 Palmoplantar keratoderma in idiopathic erythroderma.

hypothermia more than hyperthermia [35]. However, it is essential to follow up these patients regularly to identify any underlying cause in due course, as follow-up studies have shown conditions like atopic dermatitis and cutaneous T-cell lymphoma occurring in such cases [35–37].

Idiopathic erythroderma has been considered a distinctive form of prelymphomatous T-cell dyscrasia eventually causing Sézary syndrome in some cases. In histopathology, if dermal infiltrate shows atypical lymphoid cells, lymphomatoid drug eruption, idiopathic erythroderma and Sézary syndrome should be considered. Idiopathic erythroderma should be considered after three key procedures: biopsy of lesional skin, analysis of peripheral blood and lymph node biopsy. Each of these samples needs to be analyzed for morphology, immunophenotype, and the presence of a T-cell clone.

When the course of erythroderma is more recalcitrant and progressive, one must consider an evolving T-cell dyscrasia, whether in the context of idiopathic erythroderma or Sézary syndrome [38].

APPROACH TO A CASE OF ERYTHRODERMA

History

A detailed history is crucial for diagnosing the underlying etiology:

1. History of preexisting medical conditions, allergies, and skin diseases (atopic or other dermatitis, psoriasis, etc.).

2. A complete medication history and recent intake of drug. This must include details about all prescription, over-the-counter, naturopathic, and herbal medications.
3. The timing of symptoms is also essential. The onset of symptoms is usually acute, especially in drug-induced erythroderma, while those secondary to a primary skin disease may have a slower course [39]. Pruritus is the most commonly observed symptom in up to 90% of patients with erythroderma, and it is found to be most severe in patients with atopic dermatitis or Sézary syndrome [7]. In children, congenital onset is seen in ichthyosis and immunodeficiency states.
4. Family history of psoriasis, pityriasis rubra pilaris (PRP), and atopy.

Clinical examination

Physical examination is important to assess the underlying etiology and detect potential complications. Vitals should be checked. Generalized lymphadenopathy occurs in more than one-third of patients. Dermatopathic lymphadenopathy needs to be differentiated from lymphoma. If a lymph node is prominent, biopsy may be required. The patient should be palpated for any organomegaly (liver-spleen) and lymphadenopathy. Hepatomegaly is commonly seen in drug-induced erythroderma and splenomegaly with lymphoma. Systemic examination is a must. Lung fields and precordium should be auscultated for signs of congestive heart failure or consolidation. Because of continuous protein loss due to scaling and exudation, hypoalbuminemia sets in, and edema develops. Edema can be facial (drug induced), pedal, or in the form of anasarca. Protein loss and negative nitrogen loss may cause enteropathy and muscle wasting in long-standing cases of erythroderma [40]. The general cutaneous examination should include documentation of the total area of skin involved and if there are any islands of sparing (well-demarcated areas of spared skin).

Cutaneous clues

Features of the skin examination often help in arriving at an underlying cause:

1. *Scales*: It is one of the erythroderma-defining clinical signs. Scaling accompanies or follows erythema within a few days. The nature of scales may be fine or large and lamellar. In acute cases the scales are large, and with chronicity they appear smaller [41]. Their color varies from white to brown and can be associated with pruritus with a sense of tightness of skin.

Scaling is prominent with psoriasis. Scaling is thick and semiadherent in psoriasis. Furfuraceous or bran-like scales are characteristic of PRP, fine scales with atopic dermatitis/dermatophyte infection, bran-like scales with seborrheic dermatitis, and posterythema desquamation are common with drug reactions or bacterial infections and islands of sparing with PRP along with a yellow tinge to the skin and hyperkeratosis of *the palms and soles* [7,42].

2. *Blisters and crusting*: When any active bulla, crusting is noted amid erythrodermic arena or even in the noninvolved skin, secondary infection, autoimmune blistering disorders should be considered.

3. *Presence of specific lesions*: Keratotic follicular papules in PRP, well-defined erythematous scaly plaques in psoriasis, bulla in pemphigus and infections, erosions in pemphigus, and toxic epidermal necrolysis (TEN).

4. *Induration of skin*: It is seen in immunodeficiency states, atopic dermatitis, neuroichthyosis and mastocytosis (Darier sign seen) [43].

5. *Skin tenderness*: Staphylococcal scalded skin syndrome (SSSS), TEN, toxic shock syndrome.

6. *Spared areas*:
   a. *Nose sign* [44]: Sparing of the nose and the paranasal area as an island of normal skin has been described in exfoliative dermatitis (Figure 13.7). The possible mechanism of nose sparing may be relatively more sun exposure to this area, which might have some ameliorating effect due to its presumptive antimitotic action. It has also been described in airborne contact dermatitis, polymorphic light eruption, severe atopic dermatitis, and PRP. The cause is speculated to be the inability of physical, chemical, or airborne allergens to lodge at this site, due either to the anatomic peculiarity of the nose or to frequent scratching and relative vascular insufficiency that prevent the circulating antigens from reaching the skin.
   b. *Areolar sparing*: Areolar sparing has been noted in cases of CTCL, drug reactions, eczema, psoriasis, photosensitivity, and PRP.
   c. *Sparing of major flexures*: In papuloerythroderma of Ofuji, disseminated brownish erythematous papules converge to produce erythroderma that typically spares the major skin folds known as "deck-chair sign."

7. *Nail examination*: The nails can become dystrophic, ridged, or thickened and shed eventually. Nail changes such as onycholysis are most common with psoriasis but can be seen with any acute erythrodermic process and can result in the shedding of the nails that will regrow with recovery unless a scarring process (e.g., lichen planus) is involved. Shore-line nails with alternating bands of nail plate discontinuity represent drug-induced erythroderma reflecting the periods of time the drug was used.

8. *Mucosal examination*: Oral cavity and genital mucosa should always be examined (frequently involved in drug reactions, may show changes of lichen planus).

9. *Palms and soles*: Look for hyperkeratosis (keratoderma).

10. *Other features*: PRP has special features, including the presence of islands of spared skin called *nappes claires*, keratotic papules over the dorsum of fingers, and diffuse palmoplantar keratoderma known as *keratotic sandal*, which has a characteristic orange hue. Eczematous erythroderma is characterized by exudation, scaling, and crusting. Lichenification and involvement of the eyelids, retroauricular areas, and skin creases are seen in cases of airborne contact dermatitis. Cases of drug-induced erythroderma have facial edema and exfoliation [2].

Dermoscopy in erythroderma

Dermoscopy has become a useful bedside tool assisting the noninvasive diagnosis of various general dermatological disorders [45–48]. Even in erythroderma it can provide additional information at a submacroscopic level. Though it may not give definitive confirmation in all scenarios, few dermatoses can be distinguished. Thus, dermoscopic findings must be interpreted within the overall clinical context of the patient. By understanding vascular patterns and arrangements, scaling patterns, and follicular abnormalities, diagnostic clues can be obtained in erythroderma, too.

Table 13.2 enumerates dermoscopic features seen in few erythrodermic states.

Laboratory investigations

HEMATOLOGICAL

The changes in blood are as follows:

1. Anemia (due to iron and folate loss).

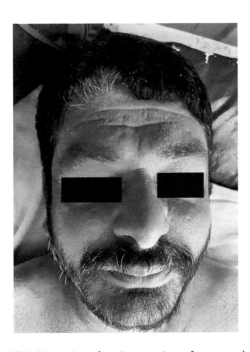

Figure 13.7 Nose sign showing sparing of nose and an island of paranasal area around in erythroderma. (Photo courtesy of Dr. Shilpa K, BMC&RI, Bengaluru.)

Table 13.2 Dermoscopy in erythroderma

Clinical entity	Features
Erythrodermic psoriasis	Monomorphous pattern of diffusely distributed whitish scales
	Regularly arranged dotted/glomerular vessels
	Homogenous reddish background
Erythrodermic atopic dermatitis	Yellowish scales/sero crusts
	Patchy distributed dotted vessels
	Unspecific sparse whitish scales may be seen
Erythrodermic pityriasis rubra pilaris	Orange blotches
	Islands of nonerythematous (spared) skin displaying reticular vessels
	Diffuse whitish scaling with scattered dotted vessels over reddish background
Erythrodermic scabies	Dark-brown triangular structures located at the end of whitish structureless wavy lines (delta-wing jets with contrail)
Erythrodermic mycosis fungoides	Linear vessels (including spermatozoon-like vessels) and dotted vessels

2. *Raised erythrocyte sedimentation rate (ESR)*: ESR is an acute phase reactant.
3. Hypoalbuminemia.
4. Serum electrolyte abnormalities.
5. *Elevated serum IgE and eosinophilia*: This is particularly of significance in atopic erythroderma and is also seen in Hodgkin disease.
6. *Sézary cells*: The blood should be examined for abnormal cells, especially Sézary cells. Large Sézary cells (15–20 μm in diameter, hyperconvoluted cerebriform nucleus) are diagnostic even in small numbers [49]. Greater than 20% count in circulating Sézary cells may be seen in Sézary syndrome [50]. The presence of clonal T cells in the peripheral blood by analysis of T-cell receptor genes using polymerase chain reaction is highly diagnostic of Sézary syndrome [49]. Actinic reticuloid is differentiated from Sézary syndrome by the increased CD8+ T cells in the latter with a nuclear contour index of 6.5 or more of peripheral blood lymphocytes.

Total and differential blood count, hemoglobin, serum electrolytes, renal and liver functions, electrocardiogram (ECG), skin swabs, and blood culture are other essential investigations.

HISTOPATHOLOGY

The histopathology often is nonspecific, composed of orthokeratosis (hyperkeratosis, parakeratosis), acanthosis, and a chronic perivascular inflammatory infiltrate with or without eosinophilia. Thus, clinicopathologic correlation in erythroderma is often difficult. In several case series, it was found that the biopsy helped diagnose primary disease in 30%–65% of the cases [51,52].

The specific pathological features of the underlying dermatosis are masked by the nonspecific features of erythroderma. The course and stage of erythroderma also can modify the histopathologic picture; like in the acute stage, spongiosis and parakeratosis are seen predominantly,

whereas in the chronic stage acanthosis and elongated rete ridges are seen.

Despite the uniformity of histological features, residual histological features may be retained that form main diagnostic histological clues in predicting the underlying cause. Subtle histopathologic features of the underlying disease are found to be present in about two-thirds to half of patients [53,54]. The diagnostic accuracy of histopathology has given promising results in psoriatic erythroderma and T-cell lymphoma in various studies [55,56]. The changes of early macular and squamous lesions of psoriasis were more often found than those of fully developed or late lesions [55].

Factors that can enhance the accuracy of clinicopathological correlation include the following:

1. If more than one clinical morphology is seen, like areas of predominant scales, plaques, follicular lesions, or bullae, then perform a biopsy on each different skin lesion.
2. Analyze sequential biopsy specimens during the course of the disease and follow-up.
3. If lymphadenopathy is found to be potentially abnormal and not merely reactive, then perform fine needle aspiration cytology and peripheral smear alongside skin biopsy as baseline investigation. This may prove helpful in suspected lymphomas and lymphoproliferative disorders.
4. Special stains (e.g., periodic acid-Schiff in dermatophytosis), DIF, immunohistochemistry, and immunophenotyping as adjuncts in relevant cases [57].

Table 13.3 enumerates histological features and possible underlying disease in erythroderma.

CULTURE

In erythroderma, swabs from skin, especially when SSSS, toxic shock syndrome (TSS), congenital cutaneous candidiasis, or secondary infection is suspected, need to be taken. A potassium hydroxide (KOH) mount is a simple bedside

Table 13.3 Histological clues in erythroderma

Condition	Histological clues
A. Psoriasiform pattern	
Psoriasis	Parakeratosis with regular acanthosis, Munro microabscess, suprapapillary thinning of epidermis with absent granular layer, squirting papillae
Actinic reticuloid	Hyperkeratosis, acanthosis, superficial and deep mixed dermal infiltrate with few atypical mononuclear cells
Pityriasis rubra pilaris	Alternating orthokeratosis and parakeratosis (vertical and horizontal checkerboard pattern with shoulder parakeratoses) with keratotic plugging, psoriasiform hyperplasia with normal granular layer
B. Eczematous pattern	
Contact dermatitis	Spongiosis, eosinophils within dermal infiltrate
Seborrheic dermatitis	Parakeratosis with neutrophils at follicular ostia
Atopic dermatitis	Spongiosis, acanthosis, parakeratosis, eosinophils within dermal edema and infiltrate
C. Atypical cellular pattern	
Cutaneous T-cell lymphoma	Exocytosis of mononuclear cells, epidermotropism, Pautrier microabscesses, tagging of atypical lymphocytes
Drug-induced erythroderma	Necrotic keratinocytes, presence of eosinophils, spongiosis
Sarcoidosis	Dermal noncaseating epithelioid "naked" cell granulomas; occasional giant cells surrounded by sparse lymphocytes
Dermatomyositis	Vacuolar change, colloid bodies increased dermal mucin
Scabies	Perivascular and interstitial infiltrates with eosinophils, scabetic mite/scybala/fecal pellets in stratum corneum
Dermatophytosis	Focal parakeratosis, hyphae in stratum corneum
Pemphigus foliaceus	Subcorneal intraepidermal cleavage, acantholytic keratinocytes, direct immunofluorescence depicting IgG-bound cell surface, circulating antibodies
Bullous pemphigoid	Subepidermal bulla with eosinophils
Acute graft versus host disease	Vacuolar change, satellite cell necrosis

laboratory investigation in candidiasis, to be done initially. Even cultures of urine, blood, and cerebrospinal fluid in candidiasis are beneficial [43].

WORKUP FOR OCCULT MALIGNANCY

If suspected, chest radiograph, computed tomography scan, ECG, ultrasonography of abdomen, stool for occult blood, mammography, sigmoidoscopy, prostate examination, and cervical smear are included in the workup. Immunophenotyping, flow cytometry, and, in particular, B-cell and T-cell gene rearrangement analysis are to be advised when lymphoma is strongly suspected.

Complications

The complications that can occur in erythroderma include secondary infection, septicemia, hypoalbuminemia, hyperpyrexia, hypothermia, electrolyte disturbances due to transepidermal water loss (hypernatremic dehydration), renal failure, dermatopathic enteropathy, and high-output cardiac failure. Erythrodermic patients are at a significantly increased risk for enhanced percutaneous absorption.

Due to the impaired barrier function, there is percutaneous water loss through areas of extensive scaling. This almost equals 3–4 liters per day; thus, adequate fluid replacement must be ensured. There is loss of essential nutrients, principally proteins and iron. Proteins are shed through the skin as scaling, which may exceed 9 g/m^2 body surface area (increases by 20%–30% in psoriatic erythroderma and 10%–15% in nonpsoriatic erythroderma) [16]. Decreased hepatic metabolism, protein-losing enteropathy, and increased basal metabolic rate (BMR) all contribute to hypoproteinemia. There occurs a state of negative nitrogen balance and severe protein wasting. Impaired absorption and loss through skin of iron and vitamin B12 contribute to anemia. Further, due to rapid turnover there is a state of relative folate deficiency.

Hemodynamic changes are marked due to severe peripheral vasodilatation and increased cutaneous blood flow leading to increased cardiac output. In the presence of preexisting comorbidities of valvular or hypertensive heart disease, it may lead to high-output cardiac failure. This increased blood flow leads to increased heat dissipation through convection and radiation leading to hypothermia. Compensatory mechanisms lead to uncontrolled shivering, and the patients often present with chills. Scaling causing blockage of sweat ducts might even lead to hyperthermia [13]. All of these compensatory mechanisms cause a rise in the BMR. There is altered glucose metabolism and a state of relative insulin resistance.

In due course, long-term complications include postinflammatory hypopigmentation or hyperpigmentation in darker skin types, alopecia, nail dystrophies, and rarely nevi and keloid formation. There are reports of occurrence of generalized vitiligo and pyogenic granuloma after exfoliative dermatitis [58,59].

Thus, once erythroderma is diagnosed, clinical diagnosis is complete only when underlying cause is identified and complications are recognized early.

Course and prognosis

The estimated death rate is 4.6%–64% in erythroderma, but this has since been reduced due to advancement in diagnosis and therapy [60–62]. The most common causes of death in patients with erythroderma are septicemia, lung infections such as pneumonia, and heart failure [56]. Elderly patients are at higher risk of mortality [61,63].

Treatment

These patients need hospitalization. Adequate bed rest and intensive care management are essential. The main principles in management of erythroderma include the following:

- *Correction of hematological, biochemical, and metabolic imbalance*: Periodically serum electrolytes should be monitored and corrected accordingly. The clinician needs to keep an eye on symptoms like muscle cramps, constipation, abnormal heart rhythms, numbness and weakness (for hypokalemia), and nausea, vomiting, headache, restlessness, decreased urine output, muscle twitching, irritability, and seizures (for hypo- or hypernatremia).

Table 13.4 Specific management in erythroderma

Condition	Line of management
Psoriasis	• Topically use medium-potency topical steroids, colloidal oatmeal baths, emollients, vitamin D analogs • Avoid coal tar preparations and phototherapy in acute, fulminant erythrodermic psoriasis due to risk of Koebnerization and rebound phenomenon • Systemic agents: Methotrexate, retinoids, azathioprine • Cyclosporine acts as a crisis buster, needs monitoring of blood pressure and renal parameters • Recalcitrant cases: Biologics—Tumor necrosis factor-α inhibitors (etanercept, adalimumab, infliximab, golimumab, and ustekimumab [IL-12/23 inhibitor], ixekizumab [IL17 inhibitors], brodalumab)
Atopic dermatitis and eczemas	• Systemic steroids • Emollients are mainstay • Antihistamines
Pemphigus and other bullous disorders	• Immunosuppressive therapy: Oral corticosteroids, cyclophosphamide, azathioprine • Rituximab • IVIg
Pityriasis rubra pilaris	• Retinoids, methotrexate
Scabies	• Permethrin 5% topically with oral ivermectin 200 μg/kg
Staphylococcal scalded skin syndrome, toxic shock syndrome	• IV antibiotics • Contact tracing (carriers of toxigenic strains)
Drugs	• Immediate withdrawal of drug • Oral corticosteroids
Photosensitive dermatoses	• Sun protection • Oral corticosteroids, azathioprine
Diffuse mastocytosis	• H1 and H2 antagonists • Avoidance of triggers for mast cell degranulation (e.g., codeine, opiates, aspirin, procaine, radiographic dyes, pancuronium)
Lymphoma	• Extracorporeal phototherapy, psoralen plus ultraviolet A, alkylating agents, Interferon-α, bexarotene • Biologicals: Alemtuzumab, daclizumab

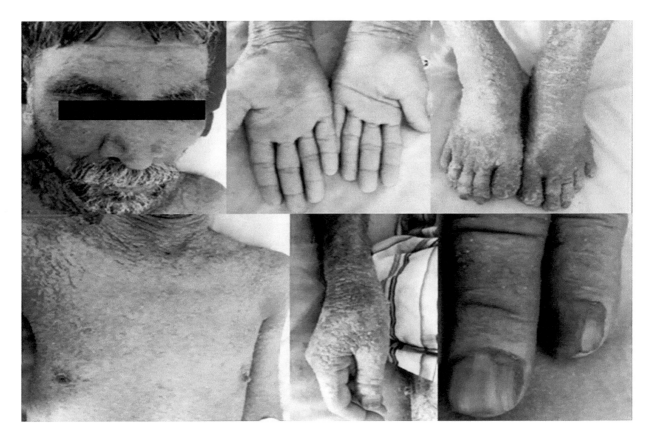

Figure 13.8 Case scenario of Darier induced erythroderma.

- *Maintenance of fluid and electrolyte balance*: Depending on the degree of dehydration, fluids need to be substituted. Normal saline is the recommended fluid. Maintenance fluid is also essential for which 5% dextrose is preferred. If volume overload is present, then fluid restriction is to be done. Sodium and potassium are to be added and serums levels periodically recorded. Both hypo- or hypernatremia states can occur. Hence, fluid supplementation and restriction should be done cautiously.
- *Prevention and treatment of infections*: Antibiotics are prophylactically initiated to curb the possibility of infection developing as a complication and also if preexisting infective states exist that can worsen the erythrodermic state. Secondary superinfection with *Staphylococcus aureus* or *Streptococcus* species is also possible. Skin swabs must be taken from the crusted lesions or any other open sites, and requisite oral antibiotics can be initiated.
- *Correction of caloric, protein, and nutrient intake*: Due to excess protein loss through scales, calorie intake should meet the demands of hypermetabolic state in erythroderma. A high-protein diet is essential. Iron and folate, if deficient, can be added to the diet.
- *Ambient humidity and temperature*: It is essential to maintain the environmental temperature at 30°C–32°C and record it every 4 hours. A daily intake-output chart is to be maintained.

- *Maintenance of skin barrier*: Maintain the skin barrier by topical application of bland emollients and wet dressings every 2–3 hourly. A daily tepid bath may be soothing.
- *Antihistamines*: Sedative antihistamines 25–50 mg orally every 4–6 h/day is advisable.
- *Treatment of specific disease* (Table 13.4): A short course of systemic steroids may be required for the treatment of atopic dermatitis, seborrheic dermatitis, and drug-induced erythroderma. Avoid steroids in cases of psoriasis, PRP, and malignancy-induced erythroderma. The dosage of steroids should be tapered down slowly. Acitretin may be useful in Darier's disease (Figure 13.8) and Pityriasis rubra pilaris.

An algorithmic approach is provided in Figure 13.9.

CONCLUSION

Erythroderma is a dermatological emergency requiring immediate attention. Every effort should be made to determine the underlying etiology and document complications during admission. Early diagnosis is of paramount significance as it allows early treatment and prevention of erythroderma-associated morbidity and mortality. Early initiation of treatment directed at both the complications and the underlying cause significantly improves the prognosis of patients with erythroderma.

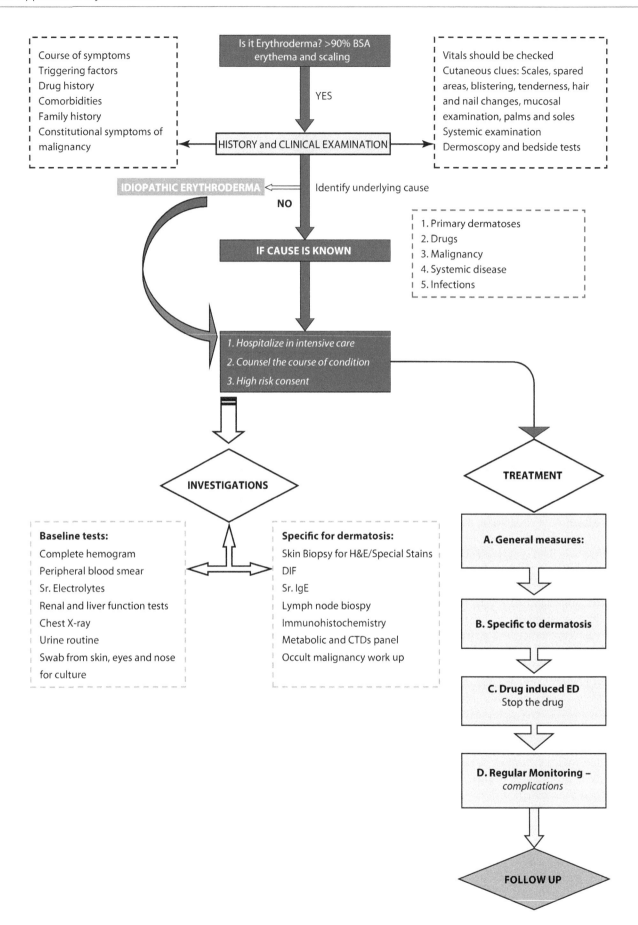

Figure 13.9 Algorithm for approach to a case of erythroderma.

KEY POINTS

- Erythroderma is a dermatological emergency that can cause significant mortality.
- A detailed history and early diagnosis are of paramount significance as identifying underlying cause is the key for reducing the sequelae of complications and morbidity.
- A high index of suspicion in patients with prolonged, rapidly extending erythema and scaling may facilitate early diagnosis of a potentially treatable malignancy and improve outcomes.
- Histopathology of serial biopsies can give promising results in many cases.
- Management is mainly supportive with correction of the hematological, biochemical, and metabolic imbalances and treatment of the underlying cause.

REFERENCES

1. Hebra F. *On Diseases of the Skin*. London: New Sydenham Society; 1868.
2. Sehgal VN, Srivastava G. Exfoliative dermatitis: A prospective study of 80 patients. *Dermatologica* 1986;173:278–84.
3. Sigurdsson V, Steegmans PH, van Vloten WA. The incidence of erythroderma: A survey among all dermatologists in the Netherlands. *J Am Acad Dermatol* 2001;45:675–8.
4. Morar N et al. Erythroderma: A comparison between HIV positive and negative patients. *Int J Dermatol* 1999;38:859–900.
5. Sarkar R. Neonatal and infantile erythroderma: 'The red baby'. *Indian J Dermatol* 2006;51:178–81.
6. Sarkar R, Sharma RC, Koranne RV, Sardana K. Erythroderma in children: A clinico-etiological study. *J Dermatol* 1999;26:507–11.
7. Sterry W, Steinhoff M. Erythroderma. In: Bolognia JL, Jorizzo JL, Schaffer JV (Eds), *Dermatology*. 3rd ed. Philadelphia: Elsevier Saunders; 2012:171–81.
8. Okoduwa C et al. Erythroderma: Review of a potentially life-threatening dermatosis. *Indian J Dermatol* 2009;54(1):1–6.
9. Moy AP, Murali M, Kroshinsky D, Duncan LM, Nazarian RM. Immunologic overlap of helper T-cell subtypes 17 and 22 in erythrodermic psoriasis and atopic Dermatitis. *JAMA Dermatol* 2015;151:753–60.
10. Hild DH. Folate loss from the skin in exfoliative dermatitis. *Arch Intern Med* 1969;123:51–7.
11. Sigurdsson V, Toonstra J, Hezemans-Boer M, van Vloten WA. Erythroderma. A clinical and follow-up study of 102 patients, with special emphasis on survival. *J Am Acad Dermatol* 1996;35:53–7.
12. Yates VM, Kerr RE, Frier K, Cobb SJ, MacKie RM. Early diagnosis of infantile seborrhoeic dermatitis and atopic dermatitis: Total and specific IgE levels. *Br J Dermatol* 1983;108:639–45.
13. Boyd AS, Menter A. Erythrodermic psoriasis. Precipitating factors, course, and prognosis in 50 patients. *J Am Acad Dermatol* 1989;21:985–91.
14. Burton J, Rook A, Wilkinson D. Eczema, lichen simplex, erythroderma and prurigo. In: Rook A, Wilkinson D, Ebling F (Eds), *Textbook of Dermatology*. 4th ed. Boston: Blackwell; 1986:367–418.
15. Liu Y, Krueger JG, Bowcock AM. Psoriasis: Genetic associations and immune system changes. *Genes Immun* 2007;8(1):1–12.
16. Bhalerao J, Bowcock AM. The genetics of psoriasis: A complex disorder of the skin and immune system. *Hum Mol Genet* 1998;7(10):1537–45.
17. Gopal V, Pinto M, Mala MS. Pemphigus foliaceus: A rare case of exfoliative dermatitis. *Clin Dermatol Rev* 2017;1:19–21.
18. Fariba G, Ayatollahi A, Hejazi S. Pemphigus foliaceus. *Indian Pediatr* 2012;49:240–1.
19. Papakonstantinou E, Raap U. Bullous pemphigoid challenge: Analysis of clinical presentation and diagnostic approach. *J Dermatol Clin Res* 2016;4(2):1068.
20. Hafliger S, Klotgen HW, Horn M, Beltraminelli H, Borradori L. Erythrodermic epidermolysis bullosa acquisita. *JAMA Dermatol* 2015;151(6):678.
21. Paolino G et al. Paraneoplastic pemphigus: Insight into the autoimmune pathogenesis, clinical features and therapy. *Int J Mol Sci* 2017;26:18(12).
22. Barnadas M et al. Therapy of paraneoplastic pemphigus with Rituximab: A case report and review of literature. *J Eur Acad Dermatol Venereol* 2006;20:69–74.
23. Anhalt GJ et al. Paraneoplastic pemphigus. An autoimmune mucocutaneous disease associated with neoplasia. *N Engl J Med* 1990;323:1729–35.
24. Montgomery H. Exfoliative dermatosis and malignant erythroderma: The value and limitations of histopathologic studies. *Arch Derm Syphilol* 1933;27(2):253–73.
25. Vamja CJ, Belgaumkar VA, Deshmukh NS, Tolat SN. Erythroderma: A marker for visceral malignancy: Rare case report. *Int J Res Dermatol* 2017;3:293–5.
26. Chung UQ, Moscella SL, Zembowicz A, Liu V. Clinical and pathological findings of paraneoplastic dermatoses. *J Am Acad Dermatol* 2006;54:745–62.
27. John N, Ahern E, Chakraborty A. Paraneoplastic rash as the presenting feature of squamous cell carcinoma of the lung. *Age Ageing* 2007;36(4):468–9.
28. Eltawansy SA, Agrawal A, Modi A, Hassanien S, Zhang B, Pei Z, Ghali W. Exfoliative erythroderma as a paraneoplastic presentation of adenocarcinoma of the gallbladder. *J Gastrointest Oncol* 2015;6(2):E26–9.
29. Strutton G. Cutaneous infiltrates: Lymphomatous and leukaemia. In: Weedon D (Ed), *Weedon Skin*

Pathology Ebook: Expert Consult. 3rd ed. Edinburgh: Elsevier; 2010: 980.

30. Abel EA et al. Benign and malignant forms of erythroderma: Cutaneous immunophenotypic characteristics. *J Am Acad Dermatol* 1988;19:1089–95.

31. Sigurdsson V et al. Interleukin-4 and interferon-gamma expression of the dermal infiltrate in patients with erythroderma and mycosis fungoides: An immunohistochemical study. *J Cutan Pathol* 2002;27:429–35.

32. Russell Jones R et al. Sezary syndrome. In: Philip E, Le Boit, Burg G, Weedon D, Sarasain A (Eds), *WHO Classification of Tumors. Pathology and Genetics of Skin Tumors.* Lyon: IARC Press; 2006: 175–7.

33. Russell Jones R. Diagnosing erythrodermic cutaneous T cell lymphoma. *Br J Dermatol* 2005;153:1–5.

34. Ohga Y, Bayaara B, Imafuku S. Chronic idiopathic erythroderma of elderly men in an independent entity that has a distinct TARC/IgE profile from adult atopic dermatitis. *Int J Dermatol* 2018;57(6):670–4.

35. Sigurdsson V, Toonstra J, van Vloten WA. Idiopathic erythroderma: A follow-up study of 28 patients. *Dermatology* 1997;194:98–101.

36. Botella-Estrada R et al. Erythroderma: A clinicopathological study of 56 cases. *Arch Dermatol* 1994;130:1503–7.

37. Cherny S, Mraz S, Su L, Harvell J, Kohler S. Heteroduplex analysis of T-cell receptor gamma gene rearrangement as an adjuvant diagnostic tool in skin biopsies for erythroderma. *J Cutan Pathol* 2001;28:351–5.

38. Magro CM, Crowson AN, Drysen ME. Histopathology of eczema. In: Rudikoff D, Cohen SR, Scheinfeld N (Eds), *Atopic Dermatitis and Eczematous Disorders.* Boca Raton, FL: CRC Press; 2014: 303.

39. Grant-Kels JM, Fedeles F, Rothe MJ. Exfoliative dermatitis. In: Goldsmith LA, Katz SI, Gilchrest BA, Paller AS, Leffell DJ, Wolff K (Eds), *Fitzpatrick's Dermatology in General Medicine.* 8th ed. New York: McGraw Hill Medical; 2012.

40. Inamadar AC, Palit A. Acute skin failure: Concept, cause, consequences and care. *Indian J Dermatol Venereol Leprol* 2005;71:379–85.

41. MM Karakayli G et al. Exfoliative erythroderma. *Am Fam Physician* 1999;59:625–30.

42. Mistry N, Gupta A, Alavi A, Sibbald GR. Review of the diagnosis and management of erythroderma (generalized red skin). *Adv Skin Wound Care* 2015;28:228–36.

43. Sarkar R, Garg S, Garg VK. Neonatal erythroderma (red baby). *Indian J Paediatr Dermatol* 2013;14(3):47–54.

44. Agarwal S, Khullar R, Kalla G, Malhotra YK. Nose sign of exfoliative dermatitis: A possible mechanism. *Arch Dermatol* 1992;128(5):704.

45. Errichetti E, Piccirillo A, Stinco G. Dermoscopy as an auxiliary tool in the differentiation of the main types of erythroderma due to dermatological disorders. *Int J Dermatol* 2016;55(12):616–8.

46. Campione E et al. Severe erythrodermic psoriasis in child twins: From clinical-pathological diagnosis to treatment of choice through genetic analyses: Two case reports. *BMC Res Notes* 2014;7:929.

47. Bollea Garlatti LA, Torre AC, Bollea Garlatti ML, Galimberti RL, Argenziano G. Dermoscopy aids the diagnosis of crusted scabies in an erythrodermic patient. *J Am Acad Dermatol* 2015;73:e93–5.

48. Errichetti E, Stinco G. Dermoscopy in general dermatology: A practical overview. *Dermatol Ther (Heidelb)* 2016;6:471–507.

49. Russel-Jones R, Whittaker S. T-cell receptor gene analysis in the diagnosis of Sézary syndrome. *J Am Acad Dermatol* 1999;41:254–9.

50. Mittal RR et al. Clinicopathological correlation: Erythroderma. *Indian J Dermatol Venereol Leprol* 1996;62:351–3.

51. Zhang P et al. Analysis of Th1/Th2 response pattern for erythrodermic psoriasis. *J Huazhong Univ Sci Technolog Med Sci* 2014;34(4):596–601.

52. Rosenbach M et al. Treatment of erythrodermic psoriasis: From the medical board of the National Psoriasis Foundation. *J Am Acad Dermatol* 2010;62(4):655–62.

53. Walsh NMG et al. Histopathology in erythroderma: Review of series of cases by multiple observers. *J Cutan Pathol* 1994;21:419–23.

54. Zip C, Murray S, Walsh NM. The specificity of histopathology in erythroderma. *J Cutan Pathol* 1993;20:393–4.

55. Tomasini C et al. Psoriatic erythroderma: A histopathologic study of forty–five patients. *Dermatology* 1997;194:102–6.

56. Hisatomi K et al. Post-operative erythroderma after cardiac operations. The possible role of depressed cell-mediated immunity. *J Thorac Cardiovas Surg* 1992;107:648–53.

57. Sentis HJ, Willemze R, Scheffer E. Histopathologic studies of Sezary syndrome and erythrodermic mycosis fungoides: A comparison with benign forms of erythroderma. *J Am Acad Dermatol* 1986;15:1217–26.

58. Mogavera HS. Exfoliative dermatitis. In: Provost TT, Farmer ER (Eds), *Current Therapy in Dermatology.* 2nd ed. Philadelphia: Dekker; 1988; 20–1.

59. Torres JE, Sanchez JL. Disseminated pyogenic granuloma developing after an exfoliative dermatitis. *J Am Acad Dermatol* 1995;32:280–2.

60. Karakayli G et al. Exfoliative dermatitis. *Am Fam Physician* 1999;59(3):625–30.

61. Sehgal VN, Srivastava G, Sardana K. Erythroderma/exfoliative dermatitis: A synopsis. *Int J Dermatol* 2004;43:39–47.

62. Wilson DC, Jester JD, King LE. Erythroderma and exfoliative dermatitis. *Clin Dermatol* 1993;11(1):67–72.

63. Pruszkowski A, Bodemer C, Fraitag S, Teillac-Hamel D, Amoric JC, de Prost Y. Neonatal and infantile erythrodermas: A retrospective study of 51 patients. *Arch Dermatol* 2000;136:875–80.

14

Psoriatic erythroderma

TARUN NARANG AND DIVYA KAMAT

INTRODUCTION

Psoriasis accounts for approximately 25% of all erythrodermas and is the most common cause of erythroderma in adults in India and second globally. Psoriatic erythroderma is one of the most severe forms of psoriasis, which causes significant morbidity and is also potentially life threatening. It occurs in 1%–2.25% of all of the psoriatic cases [1]. Erythroderma can occur because of progressive worsening of plaque psoriasis or can be aggravated due to certain precipitating factors. Rarely, it could be the initial manifestation of psoriasis [2,3].

PATHOGENESIS

The subtype that initially starts as plaque psoriasis and gradually progresses to erythroderma usually has good prognosis and is relatively stable. The other subtype is characterized by rapid development of generalized erythema, and the individual plaques are often not distinct.

Various triggering factors have been reported as given in Table 14.1 [2,4–6].

Pathogenesis in erythrodermic psoriasis slightly differs from chronic plaque psoriasis. The Th2 differentiation is favored in erythrodermic psoriasis (EP) with significantly higher levels of serum immunoglobulin E [7,8]. The levels of IL-4 and IL-10 were also found to be higher in erythrodermic psoriasis [9]. Higher levels of transcription factor GATA-3 (a key regulator of Th2 development from naïve Th cells) and IL-4 (a signature Th2 cytokine) are indicative of Th2 predominance in EP patients [9]. The Th17 pathway has also gained significance in erythrodermic psoriasis as it is the second most frequent T-cell subset found after Th2. Th17 cells secrete IL-17, IL-22, and IFN-gamma inducing production of inflammatory chemokines by T cells, dendritic cells,

and neutrophils, and thus contribute to pathogenesis in EP [10]. Rapid systemic release of TNF-α in EP may be responsible for disease onset and severity. TNF-α is also an important player in the pathogenesis of EP, especially given the documented efficacy of anti-TNF-α agents in disease treatment [11].

There is probably an immunological overlap between erythrodermic psoriasis and atopic dermatitis, too [12].

CLINICAL FEATURES

Erythrodermic psoriasis can present at any age, although it is most frequently seen between 45 and 60 years of age. Males are two to three times more commonly affected than females.

Patients usually present initially with fever with chills and generalized malaise. Generalized lymphadenopathy is a usual feature, especially in cases with severe pruritus. Pedal edema is often present due to significant loss of protein through scaling. This is common to all forms of erythroderma.

Cutaneous features are generalized redness, scaling, and infiltration involving more than 75% of body surface area [3]. Individual lesions reminiscent of plaque psoriasis can sometimes be identified in the evolving phase (Figures 14.1 and 14.2). The acute type of erythroderma often has diffuse erythema without any well-defined plaques (Figure 14.3). If 100% of the body is involved, it is often difficult to distinguish it from other causes of erythroderma. Subtle cutaneous features should be looked for closely, which could give a clue to the possible primary cause of erythroderma. The erythema in papulosquamous disorders is often bright red to salmon in color. Scaling is thick and semiadherent in psoriasis.

Table 14.1 Triggers in psoriasis

Triggers	Underlying condition/agent
Physiological state	Pregnancy
Environmental and psychological	Sunburn, skin trauma, emotional stress, alcoholism
Iatrogenic	Computed tomography contrast material
Rebound phenomenon	Withdrawal of topical and oral steroids, methotrexate, cyclosporine, coal tar, phototherapy
Systemic illnesses	HIV, leukemia, T-cell lymphoma, gout
Pharmaceutical drugs	Lithium, antimalarials, trimethoprim/ sulfamethoxazole, infliximab, β-blockers
Irritants	Coal tar, imiquimod, tazarotene, overuse of topical corticosteroids (i.e., use of more than 60 g per week of a high-potency topical corticosteroid), phototherapy

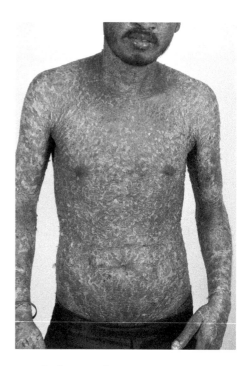

Figure 14.2 Thick semiadherent scales seen in erythrodermic psoriasis—chronic stable variant.

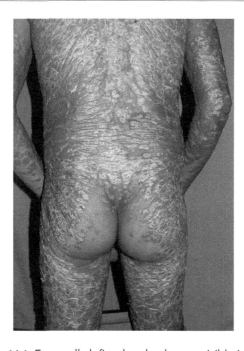

Figure 14.1 Few well-defined scaly plaques visible in a case of psoriatic erythroderma.

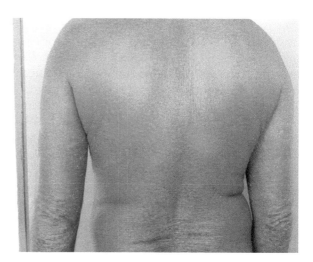

Figure 14.3 Diffuse erythema in acute type of erythrodermic psoriasis.

typical nail changes might not be present, and the nails might just show Beau lines (Figure 14.4) or onychomadesis [3].

Differential diagnosis

All causes of erythroderma form differential diagnosis. However, pityriasis rubra pilaris (PRP) is the closest, and a yellow hue may sometimes be the only differentiating feature (Figure 14.5).

Dermoscopy

The presence of regularly arranged monomorphic red dotted vessels with whitish scales has a sensitivity of 88% and

Nail changes

Dull nails, ridging, thickening, and distal onycholysis are seen. Sometimes shedding of the nails in the form of onychomadesis is also present. Nail pitting commonly seen in psoriasis can also be seen in reactive arthritis and other eczematous disorders like atopic dermatitis. Salmon patch or oil drop sign is fairly specific for psoriasis. In the acute type of erythroderma

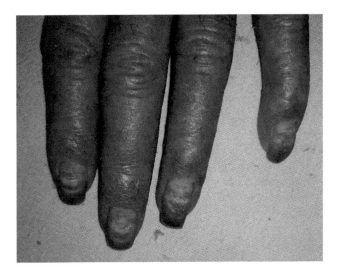

Figure 14.4 Beau lines in a case of psoriatic erythroderma.

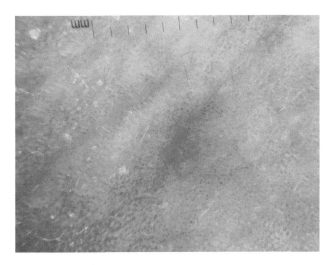

Figure 14.6 Dermoscopy of psoriatic erythroderma with regularly arranged red dotted vessels.

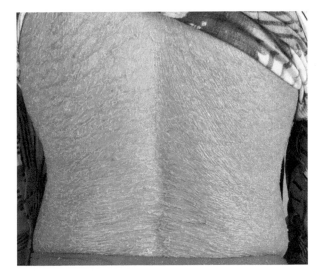

Figure 14.5 Pityriasis rubra pilaris with characteristic orange hue.

Figure 14.7 Dermoscopy of pityriasis rubra pilaris with orange blotchy areas with whitish scales.

specificity of 84.9% in the diagnosis of plaque psoriasis (Figure 14.6) [13]. Dermoscopy of other conditions that are the closest differentials are provided in Figures 14.7 through 14.9.

COMPLICATIONS

Acute respiratory distress syndrome (ARDS) has been known to occur in the setting of generalized pustular psoriasis and psoriatic erythroderma. Although the exact etiology is not known, the role of an increased level of pro-inflammatory cytokine storm has been implicated [14].

Erythrodermic psoriasis was found to be more prone to hyperuricemia and microalbuminuria. Since methotrexate is excreted mainly through the renal route, and cyclosporine itself has been known to alter the renal structure, it is imperative to closely monitor the renal function tests. Hyperuricemia can precipitate gout even in the absence of metabolic syndrome [15].

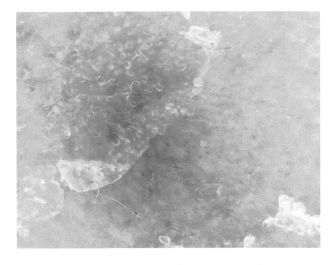

Figure 14.8 Dermoscopy of airborne contact dermatitis with yellowish scale crust with patchy dotted vessels.

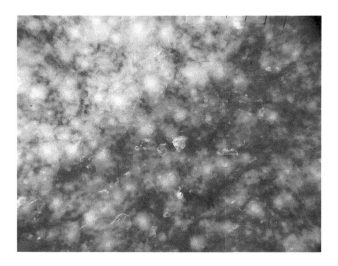

Figure 14.9 Dermoscopy of erythrodermic mycoses fungoides: Multiple polygonal structures of white storiform streaks with unevenly and intermittently distributed pigmented dots in the septa between the lobules.

Although rarely seen, Kaposi varicelliform eruption (KVE) has been described in erythrodermic psoriasis. The term *psoriasis herpeticum* has been used to describe this. Prompt recognition of grouped polycyclic ulcers, confirmation by Tzanck smear, and initiation of antiviral therapy is important so as to prevent systemic infection [16].

DIAGNOSIS

In acute-onset erythroderma, early changes of psoriasis are visible on biopsy, such as very slight epidermal hyperplasia and focal parakeratosis. The spongiosis is minimal with or without the presence of neutrophils. Papillary dermis shows dilated capillaries that are vertically oriented. More evolved lesions show a prominent psoriasiform hyperplasia with confluent parakeratosis. The granular layer is absent, and there is thinning of the suprapapillary plates. Papillary dermal changes like dilated and tortuous capillaries are more prominent. The epidermal changes are more variable, but the papillary dermal changes are more consistent and reliable in erythroderma [17].

MANAGEMENT

General management of erythroderma is to be followed as described in the previous chapter. Specific treatment for psoriatic erythroderma is described here.

Topical agents

- *Steroids*: Medium-potency steroids applied twice a day is useful as an adjunctive therapy. There are reports of topical corticosteroids, under whole-body occlusion, being used initially prior to initiating the definitive treatment [18].
- *Topical vitamin D analogues*: Calcitriol and calcipotriol are generally avoided in situations in which usage can lead to excessive systemic absorption, as in erythrodermic

psoriasis. However, there are reports of it being used in combination with other systemic agents, wherein a left-right comparison showed rapid improvement on the side where the combination was given. The dose used was 100 g/week of calcipotriol [19].

Phototherapy

Due to the risk of Koebnerization, the use of phototherapy has been discouraged or relatively contraindicated in cases of acute fulminant erythrodermic psoriasis. After initial stabilization, phototherapy can be used as a combination therapy when psoriasis is refractory to acitretin monotherapy [5].

Systemic therapy

The majority of cases of erythrodermic and pustular psoriasis are triggered by withdrawal of oral steroids that have been started erroneously. A common approach is to taper the systemic steroids very slowly while the patient is started on systemic psoriasis therapy. The recommended first-line therapy for severe acute erythrodermic psoriasis is cyclosporine or infliximab, which are rapid acting. Acitretin and methotrexate are preferred in subacute erythroderma. Second-line treatment options are etanercept and combination therapies. There are no head-to-head randomized trials comparing the efficacy of the various systemic agents. The choice depends on the individual patient characteristics and comorbidities.

Cyclosporine: Owing to its rapid onset of action, cyclosporine is often the preferred first-line drug for severe, acute, and unstable cases of erythroderma. In these situations, it is started at 5 mg/kg/day. It is slowly tapered by 0.5 mg/kg every 2 weeks after remission. As it is not recommended to give cyclosporine continuously for more than 1 year, a more definitive treatment must be initiated after initial remission. Nephrotoxicity and hypertension are the two most significant side effects; hence, treatment requires strict monitoring of blood pressure and serum creatinine. In order to reduce the dose, duration, and side effects of each drug, combination therapy with acitretin or methotrexate can also be used [2,3].

Infliximab: This is an anti-TNF-α, chimeric monoclonal antibody that has a rapid onset of action comparable to that of cyclosporine. It is given as an IV infusion at 5 mg/kg at 0, 2 and 6 weeks which is repeated every 8 weeks thereafter for maintenance. It is now recommended as a first-line therapy for erythrodermic psoriasis. It is notorious for causing reactivation of latent tuberculosis and is contraindicated in the presence of active infection. Over multiple infusions, the efficacy might be reduced due to development of anti-drug antibodies. Combination with conventional agents like methotrexate and acitretin has also been successful [2,3].

Methotrexate: This is the first-line agent of choice for the stable type of erythrodermic psoriasis. It is given at a dose of 0.3–0.4 mg/kg weekly, either orally or as a subcutaneous injection. Folic acid 1 mg daily on non methotrexate days or

5 mg weekly is usually supplemented along with it to reduce gastrointestinal side effects. Hepatotoxicity and bone marrow suppression are significant adverse effects that need to be monitored. It has a slower onset of action, like acitretin, and is therefore preferred for the stable type of erythrodermic psoriasis progressing from an initial plaque stage. It has been used as a combination therapy with cyclosporine, infliximab, and etanercept [2,3].

Acitretin: Like methotrexate, acitretin has a slower onset of action and is preferred for the stable type of erythrodermic psoriasis. It is given in the dose of 25–50 mg per day. It regularizes keratinocyte proliferation and differentiation and modulates the inflammatory response. Dose-dependent side effects include xerosis, cheilitis, and pruritus. It is best avoided in females of reproductive age as it requires strict contraception for 3 years after discontinuation because of its teratogenicity [2,3].

OTHERS

Apremilast: This is a selective phosphodiesterase 4 inhibitor that has been approved for moderate to severe psoriasis. There are no trials reporting its use in erythrodermic psoriasis. It is particularly useful when the patient has other comorbidities limiting the use of other conventional first-line drugs, and it does not require close laboratory monitoring [20,21].

Etanercept: It is administered as weekly or twice weekly subcutaneous injections of up to 50 mg. Few studies reported sustained remission on long-term monotherapy [22,23]. It has also been used in combination with methotrexate.

Adalimumab: It is a fully human monoclonal antibody against TNF-α given 80 mg subcutaneously at week 0 followed by 40 mg every other week. A multicenter study reported significant reduction in PASI at 12–14 weeks of treatment, which was also reported by Mumoli et al. [24,25]

Ustekinumab: It is a fully monoclonal antibody against the p40 subunit of IL-12 and IL-23 targeting the Th1 and Th17 pathways. It is given at a dose of 45 mg subcutaneously at weeks 0 and 4 and every 12 weeks thereafter. The lesser frequency of administration is its major advantage over other biologics [26]. In several reports in cases of recalcitrant erythrodermic psoriasis, where multiple TNF-α agents had failed, there was eventually a response with use of ustekinumab [27,28].

Secukinumab: This is a fully monoclonal IgG1 antibody against IL-17A. In a case series published by Tsai et al. consisting of a cohort of 10 patients, it was reported that although the response was suboptimal, it was still superior compared to their previous case series using ustekinumab [29]. In another series, quick and effective response to secukinumab was seen in all patients at week 16 [30].

A multicenter retrospective study evaluated the efficacy and safety of biologics in erythrodermic psoriasis, and it was found that overall, biologics have a good short-term efficacy. However, on long-term follow-up, only approximately one-third of patients were still receiving the same biologic, and in others it had to be changed due to lack of efficacy or adverse effects [24].

INFANTILE ERYTHRODERMIC PSORIASIS

Infantile psoriatic erythroderma is often a challenging diagnosis in the absence of clear-cut preexisting lesions. Differential diagnoses such as atopic dermatitis and seborrheic dermatitis often closely mimic psoriasis, as all of these can have a history of preceding diaper rash. Other causes of erythroderma including nonbullous ichthyosiform erythroderma (NBIE), staphylococcal scalded skin syndrome (SSSS), Netherton syndrome, and infantile PRP must also be considered [28]. Systemic therapy is challenging in the pediatric population and must be reserved for severe erythrodermic psoriasis. The continuous use of these agents must be limited to 6-month periods. Both methotrexate and acitretin can be given with regular laboratory monitoring. Acitretin might cause bony abnormalities on long-term use; hence, cyclical or rotational therapy is preferred. Cyclosporine can be used for acute disease control. Biologics that have been evaluated in the pediatric population are adalimumab, etanercept, infliximab, and ustekinumab, but long-term safety data are not available, and they must be reserved for recalcitrant cases [30]. As per the European Medicines Agency, adalimumab has been approved as first-line therapy for plaque psoriasis in children ≥4 years of age. Second-line biologics include etanercept and ustekinumab approved in children ≥6 years and ≥12 years, respectively [31]. Severe recalcitrant infantile pustular psoriasis must also raise suspicion of monogenic autoinflammatory syndromes including deficiency of IL-1 receptor antagonist (DIRA) and deficiency of IL-36 receptor antagonist (DITRA). Anakinra has been shown to benefit these cases [32].

HIV and psoriatic erythroderma

Psoriasis usually presents as severe recalcitrant disease in the presence of HIV infection. Atypical features and unresponsiveness to conventional therapy warrant investigations and HIV testing. A characteristic feature of HIV and psoriasis is the presence of multiple morphological types coexisting at a given point. Erythrodermic variant was the most common reported variant in one study. Other features include inverse pattern, rupoid-like scales, sebopsoriasis, and reactive arthritis-like psoriasis (Figure 14.10). Often very large scales resembling lamellar ichthyosis can be seen [33]. Initiation of HAART (highly active antiretroviral treatment) helps to clear psoriasis [34]. First-line therapies in erythrodermic psoriasis include phototherapy and retinoids. Combination therapies such as Re-UVB and Re-PUVA (retinoids and psoralen plus ultraviolet A) have also been tried [33]. Biologics that have been used in HIV coinfection are infliximab and etanercept. HIV testing usually forms the pre-TNF-α workup and is a relative contraindication. TNF-α is thought to be involved in HIV transcription and is involved in the pathogenesis of cachexia and fever; thus, the possible efficacy of TNF-α inhibitors may be explained [35].

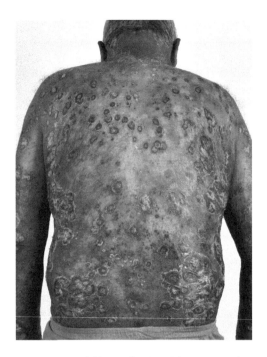

Figure 14.10 Rupoid-like scales in HIV-associated psoriatic erythroderma.

PROGNOSIS

The majority of erythrodermic psoriasis patients respond to one or more available treatment options; however, a subset of patients does not respond to the treatment and requires a combination of agents. The introduction of biologics has revolutionized the treatment of psoriasis. Recurrences can occur, and 10%–15% of patients relapse with erythrodermic psoriasis following abrupt cessation of treatment or infections [36]. The prognostic data for psoriatic erythroderma are deficient and highly variable, with mortality rates ranging anywhere from 9% to 64% [1,37]. The majority of deaths associated with erythrodermic psoriasis are attributed to bacterial infections, such as pneumonia or staphylococcal septicemia [38].

KEY POINTS

- Psoriasis is the second most common cause of erythroderma in adults globally.
- Recurrences and relapse can occur as erythrodermic psoriasis following abrupt cessation of treatment or infections.
- Histopathology is helpful in diagnosis in the early stages of psoriatic erythroderma.
- The recommended first-line therapy for severe acute erythrodermic psoriasis is cyclosporine or infliximab, which are rapidly acting.
- Methotrexate and acitretin are preferred in subacute erythroderma.
- Biologicals have shown promising results in psoriatic erythroderma.

CONCLUSION

Psoriatic erythroderma is a serious, potentially life-threatening condition with significant morbidity and increased risk of death compared with other forms of psoriasis. Management should include careful evaluation for triggering factors and managing them in addition to aggressive therapies or combination of therapies requiring close monitoring.

REFERENCES

1. Boyd AS, Menter A. Erythrodermic psoriasis. *J Am Acad Dermatol* 1989;21:985–91.
2. Liao W et al. Erythrodermic psoriasis: Pathophysiology and current treatment perspectives. *Psoriasis (Auckl)* 2016;6:93–104.
3. Rosenbach M et al. Treatment of erythrodermic psoriasis: From the medical board of the National Psoriasis Foundation. *J Am Acad Dermatol* 2010;62:655–62.
4. Tsutsumi R, Yoshida Y, Yamamoto O. Imiquimod-induced psoriatic erythroderma treated with infliximab. *Acta Derm Venereol* 2017;97:279–80.
5. Nguyen TV, Wu JJ, Lim HW, Koo JY. Acute exacerbation of erythrodermic psoriasis with phototherapy: Pathophysiology and results of a National Psoriasis Foundation survey regarding photo-management of erythrodermic skin. *J Psoriasis Psoriatic Arthritis* 2016;1:142–6.
6. Potter KA, Motaparthi K, Schoch JJ. Erythrodermic psoriasis after discontinuation of ixekizumab. *JAAD Case Rep* 2018;4:22–3.
7. Zheng Y. High serum IgE concentration in patients with psoriasis. *J Clin Res Dermatol* 2017;4:1–4.
8. Li L-F, Sujan SA, Yang H, Wang W-H. Serum immunoglobulins in psoriatic erythroderma. *Clin Exp Dermatol* 2005;30:125–7.
9. Zhang P et al. Analysis of Th1/Th2 response pattern for erythrodermic psoriasis. *J Huazhong Univ Sci Technolog Med Sci* 2014;34:596–601.
10. Singh RK et al. Erythrodermic psoriasis: Pathophysiology and current treatment perspectives. *Psoriasis (Auckl)* 2016;6:93–104.
11. Lee W-K et al. Erythrodermic psoriasis treated with golimumab: A case report. *Ann Dermatol* 2015;27(4):446–9.
12. Moy AP, Murali M, Kroshinsky D, Duncan LM, Nazarian RM. Immunologic overlap of helper T-cell subtypes 17 and 22 in erythrodermic psoriasis and atopic dermatitis. *JAMA Dermatol* 2015;151:753.
13. Lallas A et al. Accuracy of dermoscopic criteria for the diagnosis of psoriasis, dermatitis, lichen planus and pityriasis rosea: Dermoscopy of inflammatory skin diseases. *Br J Dermatol* 2012;166:1198–205.
14. Sadeh JS. Pustular and erythrodermic psoriasis complicated by acute respiratory distress syndrome. *Arch Dermatol* 1997;133:747–50.

15. Yin Z. Renal function of psoriatic patients: Erythrodermic psoriasis has more significant hyperuricemia. *Biomed Res* 2017;28:4.

16. Yeh Y-T, Ko J-H. Psoriasis herpeticum: Kaposi's varicelliform eruption in psoriasis. *Dermatologica Sinica* 2015;33:247–8.

17. Tomasini C, Aloi F, Solaroli C, Pippione M. Psoriatic erythroderma: A histopathologic study of forty-five patients. *Dermatol Basel Switz* 1997;194:102–6.

18. Prystowsky JH, Cohen PR. Pustular and erythrodermic psoriasis. *Dermatol Clin* 1995;13:757–70.

19. van der Vleuten CJ, Gerritsen MJ, Steijlen PM, de Jong EM, van de Kerkhof PC. A therapeutic approach to erythrodermic psoriasis: Report of a case and a discussion of therapeutic options. *Acta Derm Venereol* 1996;76:65–67.

20. Papadavid E, Kokkalis G, Polyderas G, Theodoropoulos K, Rigopoulos D. Rapid clearance of erythrodermic psoriasis with apremilast. *J Dermatol Case Rep* 2017;11:29–31.

21. Arcilla J, Joe D, Kim J, Kim Y, Truong VN, Jaipaul N. Erythrodermic psoriasis treated with apremilast. *Dermatology Reports* 2016;8.

22. Romero-Maté A, García-Donoso C, Martinez-Morán C, Hernández-Núñez A, Borbujo J. Long-term management of erythrodermic psoriasis with anti-TNF agents. *Dermatol Online J* 2010;16:15.

23. Fraga NA, de A, Paim M de F, Follador I, Ramos AN, Rêgo VRP, de A. Psoríase eritrodérmica refratária em criança com excelente resposta ao etanercepte. *An Bras Dermatol* 2011;86(4 suppl 1):144–7.

24. Viguier M et al. Efficacy and safety of biologics in erythrodermic psoriasis: A multicentre, retrospective study. *Br J Dermatol* 2012;167:417–23.

25. Mumoli N, Vitale J, Gambaccini L, Sabatini S, Brondi B, Cei M. Erythrodermic psoriasis. *QJM* 2014;107:315.

26. Pescitelli L et al. Erythrodermic psoriasis treated with ustekinumab: An Italian multicenter retrospective analysis. *J Dermatol Sci* 2015;78:149–51.

27. Buggiani G, Derme AM, Krysenka A, Pescitelli L, Lotti T, Prignano F. Efficacy of ustekinumab in sub-erythrodermic psoriasis: When TNF-blockers fail. *Dermatol Ther* 2012;25:283–5.

28. Santos-Juanes J, Coto-Segura P, Mas-Vidal A, Osuna CG. Ustekinumab induces rapid clearing of erythrodermic psoriasis after failure of antitumour necrosis factor therapies. *Br J Dermatol* 162:1144–6.

29. Weng H-J, Wang T-S, Tsai T-F. Clinical experience of secukinumab in the treatment of erythrodermic psoriasis: A case series. *Br J Dermatol* 2018;178:1439–40.

30. Mateu-Puchades A, Santos-Alarcón S, Martorell-Calatayud A, Pujol-Marco C, Sánchez-Carazo J-L. Erythrodermic psoriasis and secukinumab: Our clinical experience. *Dermatol Ther* 2018;31:e12607.

31. Fortina AB et al. Treatment of severe psoriasis in children: Recommendations of an Italian expert group. *Eur J Pediatr* 2017;176:1339–54.

32. Cowen EW. DIRA, DITRA, and new insights into pathways of skin inflammation: What's in a name? *Arch Dermatol* 2012;148:381.

33. Morar N, Willis-Owen SA, Maurer T, Bunker CB. HIV-associated psoriasis: Pathogenesis, clinical features, and management. *Lancet Infect Dis* 2010;10:470–8.

34. Chiricozzi A, Saraceno R, Cannizzaro MV, Nisticò SP, Chimenti S, Giunta A. Complete resolution of erythrodermic psoriasis in an HIV and HCV patient unresponsive to antipsoriatic treatments after highly active antiretroviral therapy (Ritonavir, Atazanavir, Emtricitabine, Tenofovir). *Dermatology* 2012;225:333–7.

35. Lernia V, Zoboli G, Ficarelli E. Long-term management of HIV/hepatitis C virus associated psoriasis with etanercept. *Indian J Dermatol Venereol Leprol* 2013;79:444.

36. Hawilo A et al. Erythrodermic psoriasis: Epidemiological clinical and therapeutic features about 60 cases. *Tunis Med* 2011;89:841–7.

37. Nicolis GD. Exfoliative dermatitis. *Arch Dermatol* 1973;108:788.

38. Green MS, Prystowsky JH, Cohen SR, Cohen JI, Lebwohl MG. Infectious complications of erythrodermic psoriasis. *J Am Acad Dermatol* 1996;34:911–4.

15

Eczema-induced erythroderma

MANJUNATH HULMANI AND N. SRILAKSHMI

INTRODUCTION

Eczematous dermatoses are globally the most common cause of erythroderma, though in India they are closely second in line to psoriasis [1–3]. Endogenous and exogenous eczemas collectively form a greater proportion of such cases. Eczematous erythroderma is often caused by atopic dermatitis, contact dermatitis, seborrheic dermatitis, and autosensitization dermatitis. An interplay between intrinsic and extrinsic factors masks the original dermatoses, which culminate in eczematous dermatoses, making diagnosis difficult. Thus, final diagnosis can only be made through clinicopathological and biochemical evaluation in each individual patient [4].

ETIOPATHOGENESIS

The pathogenesis of eczema-induced erythroderma is unclear. Currently, it is believed that the condition is secondary to an intricate interaction of cytokines and cellular adhesion molecules, which results in a breach of epidermal barrier function causing erythroderma. Atopic dermatitis, contact allergic or irritant dermatitis, seborrheic dermatitis, and autosensitization dermatitis (e.g., stasis dermatitis with secondary contact allergy) can lead to autosensitization or generalization of the reaction [5]. Another study found that

in erythrodermic atopic dermatitis, only VCAM-1 expression was significantly higher than in lesional skin of atopic dermatitis [6].

Lymphocytes sensitized in the skin (with the help of Langerhans cells) migrate to the regional lymph nodes where they sensitize other lymphocytes and then distribute themselves to distant skin sites where they elicit an allergic response that may lead to erythroderma. Generalized contact allergic dermatitis may occur at any age, with erythroderma developing more commonly in patients with moderate to severe atopic dermatitis. Common extrinsic factors resulting in erythroderma can be traced to inappropriate topical (heat rubs, certain herbal remedies) or systemic treatment of eczema and environmental changes [7].

CLINICAL PRESENTATION

A detailed history of the sequence of events leading to the development of erythroderma is crucial for diagnosing the underlying etiology and appropriate management. Patients must be asked about preexisting eczematous skin diseases (atopic or other dermatitis). Erythroderma developing in primary eczema is often sudden in onset. Generalization of venous eczema is frequent in the geriatric age group. However, atopic erythroderma may occur at any age [8].

Pruritus is observed in up to 90% of patients with erythroderma, and it is most severe in patients with atopic dermatitis [7]. Exacerbation of existing lesions usually precedes the generalization, which follows the usual pattern. Eczematous erythroderma may follow the pattern of the preexisting eczema, and pruritus is often intense [8]. The disease course is rapid if it results from contact allergens; it takes a gradual course if it results from the generalized spread of the primary skin disease (e.g., atopic dermatitis) [3].

A thorough physical examination is critical to assess the underlying etiology, to detect the potential complications, and to allow appropriate treatment. Features of the skin examination that may help diagnostically include the following:

- Blisters and crusting—think of secondary infection
- Fine scales with atopic dermatitis
- Bran-like scales with seborrheic dermatitis

In cases of preexisting dermatoses, nail changes, such as horizontal ridging in atopic dermatitis, may precede the erythroderma [7]. Other common nail changes observed are shiny nails, discoloration, brittleness, dullness, subungual hyperkeratosis, Beau lines, and paronychia [9].

The various causes of eczema-induced erythroderma are given in Box 15.1 and are discussed briefly in the following sections [8].

ALLERGIC CONTACT DERMATITIS

A history of previous contact allergies as well as eczematous lesions and severe oozing patches on body regions

exposed to allergens are important in establishing the diagnosis of erythroderma caused by allergic contact eczema (Figure 15.1). It can be confirmed by patch testing after resolution of the erythroderma [4]. Generalized allergic contact eczema 2 days after exposure to an iodine compound applied during wound care of a chronic venous leg ulcer is a well-known example [4]. Other agents responsible for allergic contact dermatitis leading to erythroderma commonly include topical benzocaine, tincture of benzoin, balsam under a cast, lanolin, paraphenylenediamine, thimerosal, and nickel [7,10].

IRRITANT CONTACT DERMATITIS

Irritant contact dermatitis usually manifests in the skin with inflammation, mild edema, and scaling. Excessive or repeated exposure to detergents can lead to irritant contact dermatitis. The diagnosis of irritant contact dermatitis is based on significant exposure to (known) irritants and a temporal relationship between exposure and the development of dermatitis, together with the exclusion of allergic contact dermatitis by patch testing.

ATOPIC ECZEMA

Although occurring at any age, atopic erythroderma is found most frequently in patients with a history of moderate to severe atopic dermatitis. As a result, well-established preexisting lesions can be found, especially when

---

BOX 15.1: Causes of eczematous erythroderma

Exogenous eczemas
- Irritant eczema
- Allergic contact eczema
- Photoallergic contact eczema
- Infective eczema
- Dermatophytide
- Post-traumatic eczema

Endogenous eczemas
- Atopic eczema
- Seborrheic eczema
- Asteatotic eczema
- Venous eczema
- Metabolic eczema or eczema associated with systemic disease
- Eczematous drug eruptions

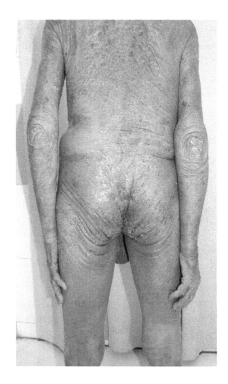

Figure 15.1 Oozing and crusting that characterize eczematous erythroderma.

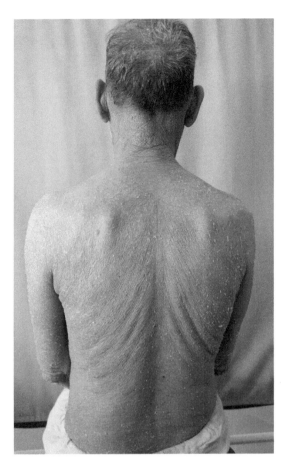

Figure 15.2 Lichenification and atrophy in atopic erythroderma.

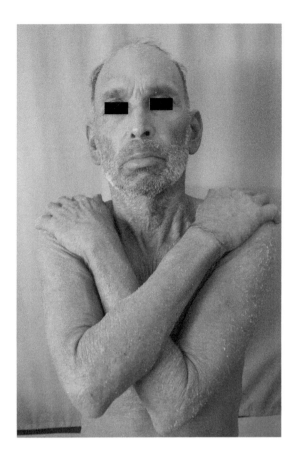

Figure 15.3 Mild scaling characteristic of asteatotic erythroderma.

the erythroderma is of recent onset. The pruritus is intense, and secondary excoriations or prurigo-like lesions are frequently observed. Lichenification is often prominent, and atrophy of the skin may be seen (Figure 15.2) [9].

These patients usually suffer from allergic rhinitis, asthma, food allergies, or allergic conjunctivitis. Typically, during the early stages of the erythroderma, these patients present with a characteristic flexural distribution of eczema lesions, and in some cases, infraorbital folds and palmar hyperlinearity are seen. These findings are important clues in establishing an exacerbation of atopic eczema as the cause of the erythroderma [4]. Past history of atopy and characteristic distribution pattern are suggestive of the disease. Pruritus is often severe; the presence of an atopic epicanthal fold of the lower eyelid and atopic cataract are other clues for diagnosis of erythroderma due to atopic dermatitis [10].

Increased serum IgE and eosinophilia may accompany other signs and symptoms of atopy [9].

XEROTIC ECZEMA

Very common in old age, it appears innocuous but can progress to erythroderma gradually (Figure 15.3).

SEBORRHEIC ECZEMA

The patient diagnosed with erythroderma associated with seborrheic eczema has a long-standing history of inflammatory scaly patches on the eyebrows, nasolabial folds, ears, chest, and back. The skin biopsy findings in these cases are consistent with an acute eczema [4].

STASIS ECZEMA

Autosensitization reaction due to acute exacerbation of stasis dermatitis or due to the contact allergy to the topical applications can occur leading to a state of erythroderma.

CHRONIC ACTINIC DERMATITIS

Chronic actinic dermatitis (CAD), an immune-mediated photodermatosis, comprises persistent light reactivity, actinic reticuloid, photosensitive eczema, and photosensitivity dermatitis. It is characterized by a persistent eczematous eruption of infiltrated papules and plaques, which predominantly affects exposed skin, sometimes extending to covered areas. Eczematous patches, which later become confluent, occur on exposed areas such as the back of the hands, face, scalp, neck, etc. Progression to erythroderma has been reported (Figure 15.4) [11].

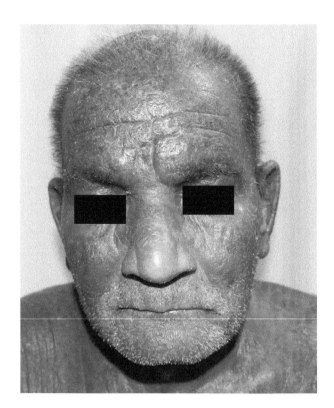

Figure 15.4 Photodermatitis causing erythroderma.

Figure 15.5 Airborne contact dermatitis causing erythroderma.

AIRBORNE CONTACT DERMATITIS (PHYTOPHOTODERMATITIS, PARTHENIUM DERMATITIS)

Airborne contact dermatitis (ABCD) is an inflammatory reaction caused by exposure to particles suspended in air. Many allergens and chemicals (plant origin and non-plant origin) have been documented as causative agents of ABCD. Two major families of plants are responsible for the vast majority of cases of ABCD: the Compositae family and the Anacardiaceae family. Well-known plants of the Compositae family include ragweed, goldenrod, sunflowers, and chrysanthemums. The flowers, leaves, stems, and pollens of these plants are coated with sesquiterpene lactones, which are the primary substances responsible for producing an allergic reaction upon airborne exposure [12,13]. *Parthenium hysterophorus* is a member of the Compositae family, it has spread all over India and has become the most common cause of plant dermatitis. Erythroderma is a rare manifestation of parthenium dermatitis. Parthenium dermatitis usually begins as an airborne contact dermatitis pattern or as a localized dermatitis. Repeated exacerbations occur because of continued exposure with seasonal variations (mostly in summer, sometimes in spring) and application of topical irritants prepared locally. This is further compounded by delayed presentation for treatment because of the mild nature of the initial dermatitis and later the inability to change the occupation or the place of living because of financial constraints. Thus, in untreated patients, the dermatitis

gradually spreads and eventually progresses to erythroderma over a variable period of time (Figure 15.5). Sparing of the nose is usually characteristic (Figure 15.6). Patch testing to establish the etiology is preferably undertaken

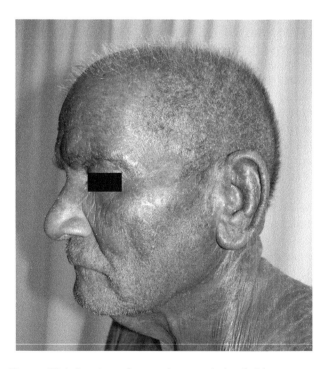

Figure 15.6 Sparing of nose characteristic of airborne contact dermatitis erythroderma.

after the skin lesions have subsided completely and immunosuppressive medications are stopped [14].

ERYTHRODERMA IN CHILDREN

In the pediatric age group, the common causes of eczematous erythroderma are atopic dermatitis and seborrheic dermatitis [15].

Atopic dermatitis

Some authors feel that there is a considerable clinical overlap between clinical features of infantile seborrheic dermatitis and atopic dermatitis. Although atopic dermatitis can present with skin symptoms in neonates, erythroderma is a rare manifestation of the disease in the neonatal period. A positive family history of atopy, the presence of dermatitis on the cheeks and flexural creases of the limbs, and itching that is apparent after 3 months of age would point to the diagnosis. In young infants, the primary lesions of atopic dermatitis are frequently vesicular, and exudation is common (Figure 15.7). Sparing of the napkin area and axilla is also characteristic [15]. Atopic dermatitis presenting as erythroderma is usually observed later, after the first

month of life, and hence is not a common differential for neonatal exfoliative dermatitis. Atopic dermatitis may have its onset in the first month; however, it is rarely erythrodermic in neonates [16].

Infantile seborrheic dermatitis

Infantile seborrheic dermatitis typically presents during the first months of life and is in the form of inflammatory, yellowish, greasy scaling on the scalp (cradle cap) with involvement of the skin folds of the neck, axillae, groin, and diaper areas (Figure 15.8) [15,17].

HISTOLOGICAL CLUES TO DIAGNOSIS OF ECZEMATOUS ERYTHRODERMA

It is advisable to take two or three simultaneous biopsies from different sites. Eczema is characterized by histological signs such as exocytosis, superficial lymphocytic infiltrate, spongiosis, irregular acanthosis, and the presence of eosinophils in the dermis [18]. Hyperkeratosis, spongiosis, perivascular lymphocytic infiltrate, and eosinophils indicate dermatitis [10]. Histopathology helps in about 60% of the cases to identify the etiology (Box 15.2) [18].

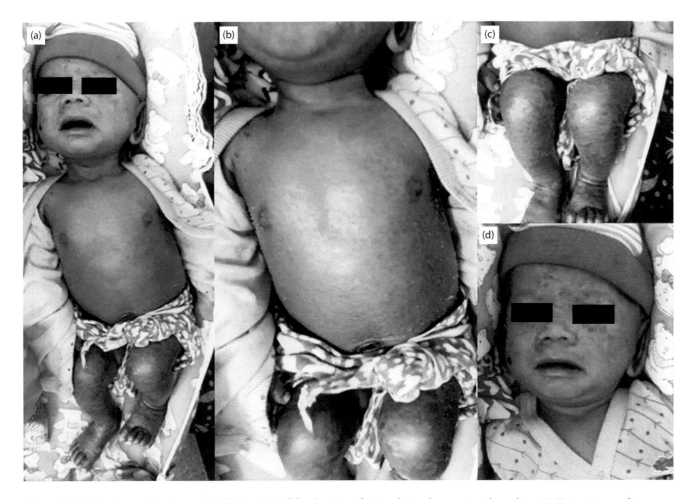

Figure 15.7 Atopic erythroderma in infants. (a) Full body view. (b) Trunk involvement with scaling. (c) Extensive scaling over extensors of lower limbs. (d) Facial involvement.

BOX 15.2: **Histopathology of various forms of eczema causing erythroderma**

- *Contact dermatitis*: Spongiosis, eosinophils within dermal infiltrate
- *Atopic dermatitis*: Spongiosis, eosinophils within dermal infiltrate
- *Seborrheic dermatitis*: Parakeratosis with neutrophils at lips of follicular ostia
- *Actinic reticuloid*: Hyperkeratosis, acanthosis, superficial and deep mixed dermal infiltrate with some atypical mononuclear cells [3]

Atopic dermatitis

A constant finding in atopic erythroderma is mild to moderate spongiosis, which is sometimes located in the follicular infundibulum. However, spongiosis is found in other forms of dermatitis, including contact dermatitis. Almost always, acanthosis and parakeratosis are additional histologic features. A perivascular, rarely epidermotropic infiltrate is observed in the upper dermis; it is accompanied by dermal edema and prominent dermal vessels. In one series, numerous eosinophils were found within the infiltrate in 77% of patients [9].

INVESTIGATIONS/DIAGNOSIS

- Patch test (after recovery during quiescent phase, for suspected allergic contact dermatitis, photoallergic contact dermatitis, airborne contact dermatitis) is to be done after erythroderma regresses.
- Serum IgE and absolute eosinophil count in atopic dermatitis.
- Raised titers of the squamous cell carcinoma–related antigens (SCC-RAg), which are significantly elevated in

cervical, lung, and esophageal SCC, particularly with internal metastasis of SCC, have been found in senile erythroderma following eczema and other benign dermatoses [19]. Elevated lactate dehydrogenase (LDH) has been observed in erythroderma and/or severe atopic dermatitis patients. Thus, changes in serum SCC-RAg and LDH levels serve as useful clinical markers for assessing the severity and clinical course of senile erythroderma following eczema [20,21].

TREATMENT

Treatment of dermatitis-related erythroderma

Topical steroids are effective treatment for localized eczema; however, oral steroids may be necessary for acute contact dermatitis with erythroderma. In general, a dose of 0.5–1 mg/kg needs to be administered each morning, and the systemic steroids need to be tapered slowly. Blood pressure should be monitored, and baseline documentation should include laboratory studies for diabetes (blood glucose, HbA1c) and a chest radiograph. After completion of an oral course of therapy, patch tests should be performed if the responsible allergen has not been identified. Antihistamines may be useful as they can relieve itch during relapses. In the treatment of severe atopic dermatitis, cyclosporine, methotrexate, azathioprine, and mycophenolate mofetil have been used with success [7]. Persons with severe atopic dermatitis may have hyperimmunoglobulin E (IgE) syndrome with high levels of IgE in the peripheral blood. These individuals often carry *Staphylococcus aureus* on their skin and nares. The staphylococcus acts as a superantigen, further increasing IgE levels. Treatment with anti-inflammatory antibiotics to control the staphylococcus on the skin (e.g., doxycycline, cotrimoxazole) may be necessary in addition to the use of topical emollients, topical steroids,

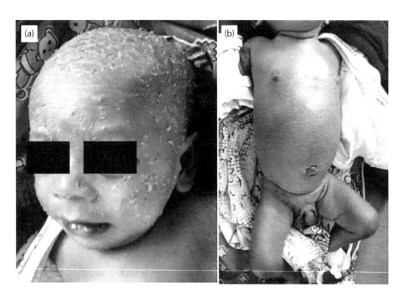

Figure 15.8 Seborrheic erythroderma in infants. (a) Greasy scaling over scalp. (b) Erythema and scaling over trunk.

topical immune response modifiers, and the systemic agents previously mentioned for severe atopic eczema [7].

COMPLICATIONS

Despite skilled efforts, exfoliative dermatitis can sometimes prove fatal, especially in elderly patients. Secondary infection, dehydration, electrolyte imbalance, temperature dysregulation, and high-output cardiac failure are potential complications in all cases [22,23]. Postinflammatory hypopigmentation or hyperpigmentation may occur, especially in individuals with dark skin. Generalized vitiligo or pyogenic granulomas have also been recorded after exfoliative dermatitis. Nevi and keloid formation are rare benign sequelae, as are alopecia and nail dystrophies [3].

PROGNOSIS

Eczematous erythroderma may continue for months or years, and tends readily to relapse. As the patients are often elderly, the prognosis must always be guarded. The metabolic disturbances involve a serious risk of hypothermia, cardiac decompensation, peripheral circulatory failure, and thrombophlebitis. Cutaneous, subcutaneous, and respiratory infections are common, and the majority of patients who die do so from pneumonia [8].

Careful monitoring of the patient and correction of the hematologic, biochemical, and metabolic imbalance when required will improve the final outcome in patients.

CONCLUSION

Eczematous erythroderma is characterized by pruritus, oozing, and lymphadenopathy in comparison to psoriatic erythroderma, which is the other common form. Delineating exact etiology is difficult, especially in cases of atopic erythroderma. Oral corticosteroids are the drugs of choice. A few key points to differentiate the various etiologies are provided in Box 15.3.

BOX 15.3: Differentiating features for various types of eczematous erythroderma

Underlying disease	Clinical clues	Histologic clues	Additional hints
Atopic dermatitis	• Preexisting lesions • Severe pruritus • Lichenification, including eyelids • Prurigo nodularis • In neonates and infants, crusted eczematous lesions on extensor surfaces, face, scalp; spares diaper area; pruritus; onset week 6–16; family history for atopy	• Mild to moderate acanthosis • Variable spongiosis • Dermal eosinophils • Parakeratosis	• Elevated serum IgE, eosinophilia • Personal or family history of atopy (e.g., asthma, allergic rhinitis) • Cataracts
Dermatitis (nonatopic), including contact and stasis with autosensitization	• Preexisting localized disease • Distribution of initial lesions	• Variable spongiosis	• Occupation and hobbies • Patch testing • Review oral medications (systemic contact dermatitis)
Chronic actinic dermatitis	• Initial lesions in photodistribution	• Lichenoid infiltrate of lymphocytes and exocytosis • Possible lymphocyte nuclear pleomorphism	• Drug history • UVA, UVB, and visible light phototesting • Photopatch testing
Seborrheic dermatitis	In neonates and infants: • Greasy, scaling plaques and satellite papules on scalp (cradle cap), and in skin folds of neck, axillae, and groin • Diaper area involvement • Nonpruritic • Early onset (week 2–12)		

KEY POINTS

- Eczema is the commonest cause of erythroderma globally.
- Contact dermatitis, Atopic dermatitis, Seborrheic dermatitis, and Stasis dermatitis are the commonest eczemas leading to erythroderma.
- Pruritus is characteristically severe in this type of erythroderma.
- Oral Corticosteroids are the drugs of choice.

REFERENCES

1. Sudho R, Hussain SB, Bellraj E, Frederick M, Mahalaxmi V, Sobhana S, Anandan S. Clinicopathological study of exfoliative dermatitis. *Indian J Dermatol Venereol Leprol* 2003;69:30–1.
2. Tan TL, Chung WM. A case series of dermatological emergencies—Erythroderma. *Med J Malaysia* 2017;72(2):141–143.
3. Sehgal VN, Srivastava G, Sardana K. Erythroderma/exfoliative dermatitis: A synopsis. *Int J Dermatol* 2004;43(1):39–47.
4. César A, Cruz M, Mota A, Azevedo F. Erythroderma. A clinical and etiological study of 103 patients. *J Dermatol Case Rep* 2016 31;10(1):1–9.
5. Groves RW, Kapahi P, Barker JN, Haskard DO, MacDonald DM. Detection of circulating adhesion molecules in erythrodermic skin disease. *J Am Acad Dermatol* 1995;32(1):32–6.
6. Sigurdsson V, de Vries IJ, Toonstra J, Bihari IC, Thepen T, Bruijnzeel-Koomen CA, van Vloten WA. Expression of VCAM-1, ICAM-1, E-selectin, and P-selectin on endothelium in situ in patients with erythroderma, mycosis fungoides and atopic dermatitis. *J Cutan Pathol* 2000;27(9):436–40.
7. Mistry N, Gupta A, Alavi A, Sibbald RG. A review of the diagnosis and management of erythroderma (generalized red skin). *Adv Skin Wound Care* 2015;28(5):228–36.
8. Jones JB. Eczema, lichenification, prurigo and erythroderma. In: Burns DA, Breathnach SM, Cox NH, Griffiths CM (Eds), *Rook's Textbook of Dermatology.* 8th ed. Hoboken, NJ: Wiley; 2010:23.1–23.51.
9. Sterry W, Assaf C. Erythroderma. In: Bolognia JL, Jorizzo JL, Rapini RP (Eds), *Dermatology.* 2nd ed. New York: Elsevier; 2008:149–58.
10. Hulmani M, NandaKishore B, Bhat MR, Sukumar D, Martis J, Kamath G, Srinath MK. Clinico-etiological study of 30 erythroderma cases from tertiary center in South India. *Indian Dermatol Online J* 2014;5:25–9.
11. Somani VK. Chronic actinic dermatitis—A study of clinical features. *Indian J Dermatol Venereol Leprol* 2005;71:40913.
12. Schloemer JA, Zirwas MJ, Burkhart CG. Airborne contact dermatitis: Common causes in the USA. *Int J Dermatol* 2015;54:271–4.
13. Swinnen I, Goossens A. An update on airborne contact dermatitis: 2007–2011. *Contact Dermatitis* 2013;68:232–8.
14. Agarwal KK, Nath AK, Jaisankar TJ, D'Souza M. Parthenium dermatitis presenting as erythroderma. *Contact Dermatitis* 2008;59(3):182–3.
15. Sarkar R, Garg VK. Erythroderma in children. *Indian J Dermatol Venereol Leprol* 2010;76:341–7.
16. Dhar S, Banerjee R, Malakar R. Neonatal erythroderma: Diagnostic and therapeutic challenges. *Indian J Dermatol* 2012;57:475–8.
17. Sehgal VN, Srivastava G. Erythroderma/generalized exfoliative dermatitis in pediatric practice: An overview. *Int J Dermatol* 2006;45(7):831–9.
18. Megna M, Sidikov AA, Zaslavsky DV, Chuprov IN, Timoshchuk EA, Egorova U, Wenzel J, Nasyrov RA. The role of histological presentation in erythroderma. *Int J Dermatol* 2017;56:400–4.
19. Charry S et al. Heteroduplex analysis of T-cell receptors gamma gene re-arrangement as an adjuvant tool in diagnosis in skin biopsies from erythroderma. *J Cutan Pathol* 2001;28:351–5.
20. Tsukahara T, Otoyama K, Horiuchi Y. Significance of elevated serum squamous cell carcinoma (SCC)-related antigen and lactate dehydrogenase (LDH) levels in senile erythroderma following eczema. *J Dermatol* 1993;20(6):346–50.
21. Horiuchi Y, Tsukahara T, Otoyama K. Immunohistochemical study of elevated expression of squamous cell carcinoma (SCC)-related antigens in erythrodermic epidermis. *J Dermatol* 1994;21(2):67–72.
22. Huygens S, Goossens A. An update on airborne contact dermatitis. *Contact Dermatitis* 2001;44(1):1–6.
23. Inamadar AC, Palit A. Acute skin failure: Concept, causes, consequences and care. *Indian J Dermatol Venereol Leprol* 2005;71:379–85.

16

Drug-induced erythroderma

ANUPAMA BAINS AND SAURABH SINGH

INTRODUCTION

Drug-induced exfoliative dermatitis (ED) is a form of severe adverse drug reaction (ADR) that may be immunologic and/or nonimmunologic resulting from administration of a particular drug at doses intended for prevention, diagnosis, or treatment of disease state or drug interactions [1]. They involve extensive body surface area greater than 90% with erythema and scaling, usually occurring from days to several weeks after drug exposure. In diagnosing a drug-induced ED, it is important to decide whether the eruption is due to the disease, primarily to the drug, or possibly to an interaction between the disease and the drug.

EPIDEMIOLOGY

Drugs are the second most common group of causes of erythroderma after preexisting dermatoses (psoriasis and eczema) [2]. The exact incidence and prevalence of drug-induced erythroderma are not known as most of the studies are retrospective. In a study from south India, drugs were implicated in 16.6% cases of erythroderma [3]. Sarkar et al. found that drugs were the most common cause of erythroderma in children and were implicated in 29% of them [4]. Among the different patterns of cutaneous ADRs, erythroderma is seen in 1.7%–3% of cases [5–7]. In a prospective study from India on cutaneous ADRs, erythroderma was observed in 2.5% patients [8].

ETIOLOGY

The various drugs implicated in erythroderma are shown in Table 16.1 [3,6,9–37]. Commonly implicated drugs include allopurinol, carbamazepine, phenytoin (antiepileptics), penicillin, amoxicillin, sulfonamides, dapsone (antibiotics), lithium, isoniazid, and antimalarials [3,6,9,14,17,34]. Sarkar et al. found that in cases of childhood erythroderma phenytoin, phenobarbitone, amoxicillin, and indigenous medicine were the main causative agents [4].

PATHOGENESIS

The underlying pathogenesis that leads to drug-induced erythroderma is still not well understood. Drug-induced erythroderma is an immunological reaction that depends on T-cell response elicited depending on the antigenic epitopes of the drug, its pharmacodynamics, and protein binding.

DRESS syndrome can also present with erythroderma. Pathogenesis of DRESS syndrome is multifactorial, which includes genetic predisposition, environmental factors, immunogenic properties of a drug, and dysregulation of immune system (Figure 16.1). In individuals with DRESS syndrome, mutation of genes encoding for oxidative enzymes leads to accumulation of toxic metabolites. According to Hapten hypothesis, these reactive metabolites bind to tissue macromolecules to form a complete antigen or neoantigen, which further initiates the immune response. Glutathione protects against these reactive metabolites. Reduced glutathione levels as seen in HIV patients predispose these patients to drug reaction [38–40]. Ceratin HLA haplotypes have also been implicated in the pathogenesis [41]. HLA-B*5801 has been associated with allopurinol-induced DRESS syndrome in the Han-Chinese population, Abacavir-induced

Table 16.1 Drugs associated with erythroderma [1,5,6,7,8,12,15–39]

Xanthine oxidase inhibitor	*Allopurinol*
Antieplileptics	Barbiturates
	Carbamazepine
	Phenytoin
	Phenobarbitone
	Sodium valproate
Antipsychotics	Chlorpromazine
Antitubercular drugs	*Isoniazid*
	Para-amino salicylic acid
	Rifampicin
	Streptomycin
Antibiotics	Aminoglycosides
	Aztreonam
	Cephalosporins
	Minocycline
	Nitrofurantoin
	Penicillins
	Sulfonamides
	Tetracyclines
	Trimethoprim
	Vancomycin
	Quinolones
Antimalarial	*Chloroquine*
	Hydroxychloroquine
	Mefloquine
	Quinacrine
Antileprosy drugs	Clofazimine
	Dapsone
Nonsteroidal anti-inflammatory drugs	Indomethacin
Opiates	Codeine
	Morphine
Chemotherapy	Actinomycin D
	Cisplatin
	Mitomycin-C
	Pentostatin
	Imatinib
Xanthine derivatives	Aminophylline
Proton pump inhibitors	*Omeprazole*
	Pantoprazole
H2 receptor blockers	Cimetidine
	Ranitidine
Antihypertensives	Calcium channel blockers
	Captopril
	Chlorothiazide
Antiarrhythmic drugs	Amiodarone
	Mexiletine
	Quinidine
Retinoids	Isotretinoin
	Acitretin
Sulfonylureas	Chlorpropamide
	Tolbutamide

(Continued)

Table 16.1 (*Continued*) Drugs associated with erythroderma [1,5,6,7,8,12,15–39]

Heavy metals	Arsenic
	Gold
	Mercury
Chelating agents	Dimercaprol
Others	Acetaminophen
	Chinese herbs
	Ethylenediamines
	Interleukin-2
	Interferon-α
	Interferon-ß
	Isosorbide dinitrate
	Lithium
	Thalidomide
	Silodosin
	Intravesical mitomycin-C
	Warfarin
	Leflunomide
	Escitalopram
	Nonionic contrast medium
	Iodixanol

Note: Commonly implicated drugs are shown in italics.

hypersensitivity and HLA-B*5701 have been noted in Caucasians, while high frequency of HLA-B*3505 has been noted in patients of Thailand with nevirapine-induced hypersensitivity syndrome [42]. There is also reactivation of herpesviruses, especially herpesviruses 6 and 7 (HHV-6, HHV-7), cytomegalovirus (CMV), and Ebstein-Barr virus (EBV), which modulate the immune response to drugs [38–40]. Other predisposing factors for hypersensitivity reactions include polypharmacy, advanced age, autoimmune disease, connective tissue disease, and renal or liver impairment [43,44].

CLINICAL FEATURES

The age of patients ranges from 30 to 76 years, and a male predominance is seen [10,11]. Indian data showed that the age of patients in drug-induced erythroderma ranged from 30 to 50 years [45]. The erythroderma is acute in onset. The latent period between intake of drug and onset of rash is usually 1–2 weeks [1]. However, in cases of DRESS syndrome, this period can be prolonged and is typically 2–6 weeks [38].

History of drug intake should be taken in detail and should be documented (Table 16.2). Type of drug, indication of drug intake, time period between onset of rash and initiation of drug, and whether the patient has discontinued the drug after onset of rash are important. Latent period between onset of rash and administration of drug helps to calculate the time required by the body to eliminate the drug. History regarding use of similar drug in the past, past history, and family history of drug rash should be noted.

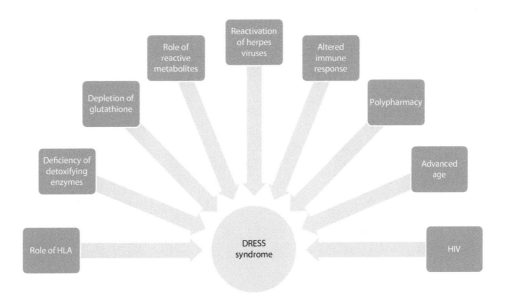

Figure 16.1 Pathogenesis of drug reaction with eosinophilia and systemic symptoms syndrome.

Table 16.2 Drug history in erythroderma

1. Drug X	Indication:..		
	Since................	Prescribed by Doctor/	
	Over the counter:......................		
Brand and/Generic name:	Date of initiation:	Date of stoppage:	Intermittent/ Continuous intake:
Manufacturer/Batch no./Expiry date: (If known)	Dosage/Frequency:		
	Route of administration:	Any increase in dose during treatment?	

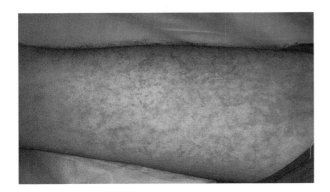

Figure 16.2 Morbilliform rash in drug reaction with eosinophilia and systemic symptoms.

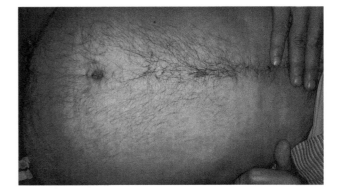

Figure 16.3 Urticarial rash in drug reaction with eosinophilia and systemic symptoms.

In drug-induced cases ED onset is acute, fever is common, and it resolves in a short period once the culprit drug is stopped. Patients may initially present with morbilliform (Figure 16.2), lichenoid, and urticarial rashes (Figure 16.3) [13]. Lesions usually start from flexures [1] and later on progress to involve most of the body surface area. Lesions are more florid, and scales are usually large in acute cases [10]. Alternating bands of nail plate discontinuity and leukonychia can be seen in drug-induced erythroderma,

also called *shoreline* nails [46]. Fever is a common feature in drug-induced erythroderma [10]. Erythroderma usually resolves in 2–6 weeks after stopping the offending drug [14].

Patients with DRESS syndrome can also present as having erythroderma (Figures 16.4 through 16.7) [7,47,48].

The differences between drug-induced and non-drug-induced erythroderma are enumerated in Table 16.3 [50].

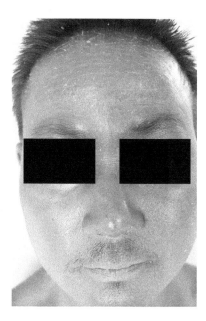

Figure 16.4 Face involvement in drug-induced erythroderma.

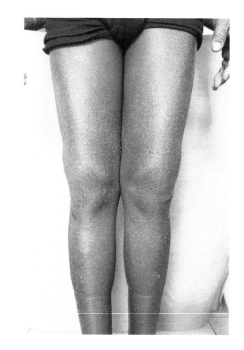

Figure 16.6 Involvement of anterior aspect of lower limbs.

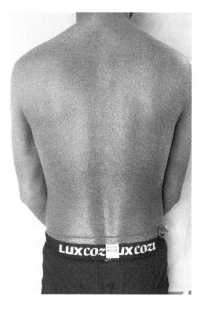

Figure 16.5 Truncal involvement in drug-induced erythroderma.

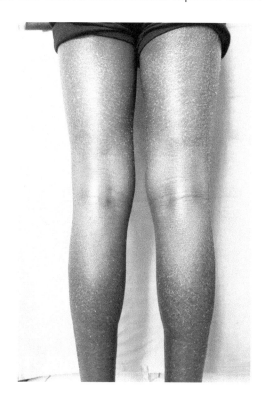

Figure 16.7 Involvement of posterior aspect of lower limbs.

METHODS TO CHECK FOR PROBABILITY OF DRUG REACTION (DRUG CAUSALITY ASSESSMENT)

Causality assessment determines the causal relation between the drug administered and the occurrence of an adverse event. Various algorithms used in decisions on causality of ADRs are Jones algorithm, Naranjo algorithm, Yale algorithm, Karch algorithm, Begaud algorithm, Australian Adverse Drug Reactions Advisory Committee and the World Health Organization-Uppsala Monitoring Center (WHO-UMC) criteria [51]. These algorithms reduce the variation in the evaluation of ADRs. However, none of these algorithms are gold standard [51–53].

DIFFERENTIAL DIAGNOSIS

It is known that certain drugs can precipitate psoriatic erythroderma [54]. So even if preexisting dermatoses are known, then every other cause of erythroderma should be ruled out.

Table 16.3 Differences between drug-induced and non-drug-induced erythroderma

	Non-drug-induced exfoliative dermatitis	Drug-induced exfoliative dermatitis
Onset and progression	Insidious and gradual	Acute and rapid
Morphology	Initially of primary dermatoses, later diffuse erythema and scaling	Pruritic maculopapular/lichenoid/urticarial rash, later generalized erythema and scaling
Sites involved	Predominantly skin	Skin and mucosal surfaces
Lymphadenopathy	Present	Present
Resolution	Slow	Rapid with drug discontinuation
Relapse	Seen	No relapse
Biopsy	Subtle changes of preexisting dermatosis may be seen	Epidermal necrosis with dense lymphocytic infiltrate with/without eosinophils
Systemic involvement	Usually secondary to erythroderma	In drug reaction with eosinophilia and systemic symptoms, systemic involvement is primary event with skin rash

The rash also needs to be differentiated from viral exanthem. Viral exanthem is commonly seen in children. It is characterized by rapidly spreading pink-red macules and papules that start from the head and neck followed by involvement of other body parts. Itching is absent or mild in comparison to drug rash. There is associated fever, conjunctivitis, malaise, and sore throat. The rash is self-limiting in nature [55].

Acute graft versus host disease usually occurs within 6 months after transplant and presents with nausea, vomiting and diarrhea, and jaundice with skin rash, and can mimic the early phase of ED. Diagnosis will require histological evaluation.

Drug-induced ED should be delineated from other severe cutaneous adverse reactions like Stevens-Johnson syndrome (SJS), Stevens-Johnson syndrome/toxic epidermal necrolysis (SJS-TEN) overlap, and toxic epidermal necrolysis (TEN) which are blistering states, unlike ED which is a desquamative condition.

INVESTIGATIONS

Peripheral eosinophilia is common in drug-induced erythroderma but is not specific as it can also be present in cases of erythroderma secondary to eczema, psoriasis, and cutaneous T-cell lymphoma [9,10].

Skin biopsy

Banerjee et al. observed clinicohistopathological correlation in 75% of cases with drug-induced erythroderma [11,45,56,57]. Lichenoid interface dermatitis on histopathology can give a clue to diagnosis of drug-induced erythroderma [45,58]. In an Indian study, parakeratoses, basal cell vacuolization, perivascular lymphocytic infiltrate, and eosinophils were common in cases of drug-induced erythroderma [9]. While in another study by Mathew et al., nonspecific dermatitis was seen in the majority of cases on histopathology [56].

In cases of DRESS syndrome, various histopathological patterns can be observed. These are eczematous, interface dermatitis, acute generalized exanthematous pustulosis like, and erythema multiforme like. Interface dermatitis is the most common pattern [59]. Walsh et al. found that the presence of apoptotic keratinocytes in histopathology was associated with erythema multiforme, such as lesions and liver injury in patients of DRESS syndrome [60].

A patient of drug-induced erythroderma should also be worked up for systemic involvement, particularly in patients of DRESS syndrome. So, complete hemogram, liver function tests, renal function tests, urine routine microscopy, chest X-ray, and electrocardiogram should be done in these patients.

DIAGNOSTIC TESTS TO IDENTIFY THE CULPRIT DRUG

These include *in vivo* skin testing, *ex vivo* tests, and drug provocation tests. *In vivo* tests include patch test, prick test, and intradermal test. *Ex vivo* tests are lymphocyte transformation test (LTT), enzyme-linked immunospot (ELISpot) assay, and intracellular cytokine staining.

In vivo skin tests

These include patch test, prick test, and intradermal test. Drug skin testing should be done 6 weeks to 6 months after complete subsidence of the adverse drug reaction. The patient should be off steroids and other immunosuppressives for at least 1 month [61].

PATCH TEST

The patch test is a noninvasive test, but the sensitivity is low [13]. In a prospective multicenter study, patch test was positive in 64% of cases with DRESS syndrome, and multiple drug reactivity was common in these patients. It helps to identify those drugs also which were least suspected [62].

PRICK TEST

The commercialized form of the drug is tested. If possible, pure drug and its vehicle should be tested separately. The test is performed on the volar aspect of the forearm. Readings are taken at 20 minutes and after 1 day. A wheal with a diameter larger than 3 mm than that of the negative control (0.9% saline) is taken as a positive test. For a positive control, codeine phosphate at 9% and/or with histamine (10 mg/mL) is used [61].

INTRADERMAL TEST

Indication: It is used only if a prick test is negative at 20 minutes.

Contraindication: It is not done in cases of erythema multiforme, SJS, and TEN.

Delayed positive results can be present in the prick test, but they are more frequent with the intradermal test. With intradermal tests, delayed positive results can be seen in maculopapular rash, eczema, erythroderma, and fixed drug eruption. *In vivo* skin tests can be negative in 30%–50% of patients. A negative test does not rule out an ADR. A positive test in the case of a patch test can be due to past history of contact dermatitis to a drug or its vehicle. So, proper relevance should be sought.

Ex vivo tests

LYMPHOCYTE TRANSFORMATION TEST

It is an *ex vivo* test that measures the proliferation of T cells to a drug by generating drug-specific T-cell clones. Its advantage is that it can be done with many drugs. However, a negative test does not exclude drug hypersensitivity, and the procedure is cumbersome and technically demanding [63].

ELISPOT AND INTRACELLULAR CYTOKINE STAINING

ELISpot assay and intracellular cytokine staining are *ex vivo* assays used to detect delayed-type hypersensitivity reactions. These tests measure the release of cytokine produced by a population of T cells that has been exposed to a particular concentration of the suspected drug. It is a rapid test and is currently being used in research settings [64].

Drug provocation tests

A drug provocation test is the controlled administration of a drug to a patient in supervised conditions to detect drug hypersensitivity reactions. They are considered as a gold standard test to detect ADRs. It is generally contraindicated in life-threatening drug reactions including drug-induced erythroderma and DRESS syndrome [65,66].

TREATMENT

Identifying the cause and management of erythroderma is important because of morbidity and mortality associated with the disease.

If not identified correctly, the causative drug can be life threatening if the patient is reexposed to the same drug. Also, wrong and overdiagnosis of a drug allergy can lead to the use of less-effective and costly drugs [7]. Determining the temporal relationship, epidemiological risk, and improvement on withdrawal of the drug, and excluding other differentials are important to identify the causative drug [7].

Erythroderma is a dermatological emergency. The patient should be hospitalized. Monitor the circulatory status, body temperature, renal function tests, serum electrolyte, and fluid balance of the patient. Prompt withdrawal of the culprit drug and avoiding all other nonessential drugs is important. A high-protein diet, emollients, topical steroids, and antihistamines are given [14]. Systemic steroids can be given in severe cases [34]. The patient is counseled to avoid the culprit drug in the future.

COMPLICATIONS

Complications can be the same as for other causes of erythroderma. These include fluid and electrolyte abnormalities, temperature dysregulation, cardiac failure, pneumonia, and septicemia [13]. Hair loss, nail dystrophy, and dyspigmentation in skin can be seen in long-standing cases [34]. Complications can arise secondary to systemic involvement in cases of erythroderma with DRESS syndrome.

PROGNOSIS

Prognosis is good in drug-induced erythroderma as after prompt withdrawal of the offending drug it recovers completely in a period of 2–6 weeks [14]. However, in DRESS syndrome prognosis is worse in cases of systemic involvement. Clinical features may take weeks to months to resolve after discontinuation of the culprit drug [49].

APPROACH TO PATIENT OF DRUG-INDUCED ERYTHRODERMA

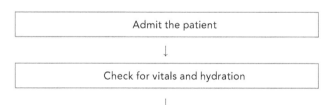

Admit the patient

↓

Check for vitals and hydration

↓

Detailed history
a. Duration and onset of rash
b. Site of onset and progression of rash
c. Type of lesions at onset, whether oozy, dry scaly, or fluid-filled lesions
d. History of any constitutional features
e. Any history of previous erythroderma
f. Any history of previous dermatoses
g. Any history of drug intake: new as well as chronic, indication for which the patient was using the drug, duration between drug intake and time of onset of rash, time of stopping the drug, past history of use of similar drug
h. Personal and family history of drug rash and atopy
i. Occupation of patient
j. Any comorbid condition
k. History of loss of weight, loss of appetite

↓

Detailed examination

a. General physical examination: check for vitals, facial edema, pedal edema, lymphadenopathy, icterus

b. Systemic examination for hepatosplenomegaly or any other systemic involvement

c. Mucocutaneous examination: predominant sites involved; involvement of palms, soles, scalp; type of scales; any oral lesions; also examine hair and nails

↓

Investigations: complete hemogram, liver function test, renal function test, random blood sugar, serum electrolytes, chest X-ray, urine routine microscopy, skin biopsy, fine needle aspiration cytology in case of lymphadenopathy

↓

Treatment: general measures—maintain ambient temperature, adequate nutrition, hydration, input/output charting, and vital monitoring

↓

Stop the culprit drug and other nonessential drugs in cases of drug-induced erythroderma

↓

Topical emollients, topical steroids, antihistamines, oral antibiotics in cases of focus of infection

↓

Oral steroids in severe cases

Counseling of patient: to avoid the culprit drug in the future

CONCLUSION

Drug-induced erythroderma is a common cause of erythroderma, especially in the very young and elderly. Allopurinol, antiepileptics, and antibiotics are common agents causing drug-induced erythroderma. If diagnosed early and the drug is stopped immediately, prognosis is good.

KEY POINTS

- Cutaneous drug reactions are one of the most common presentations of ADRs.
- DRESS syndrome is multifactorial, which includes genetic predisposition, environmental factors, immunogenic properties of the drug, and immune dysregulation.
- Causality assessment determines the causal relation between the drug administered and the occurrence of the adverse event.
- Peripheral eosinophilia is common in drug-induced erythroderma but is not specific.
- Drug-induced erythrodema has the best prognosis, with cessation of the culprit drug.

REFERENCES

1. Verma R, Vasudevan B, Pragasam V. Severe cutaneous adverse drug reactions. *Med J Armed Forces India* 2013;69(4):375–83.
2. Sigurdsson V et al. Expression of VCAM-1, ICAM-1, E-selectin, and P-selectin on endothelium in situ in patients with erythroderma, mycosis fungoides and atopic dermatitis. *J Cutan Pathol* 2000;27(9):436–40.
3. Hulmani M et al. Clinico-etiological study of 30 erythroderma cases from tertiary center in South India. *Indian Dermatol Online J* 2014;5(1):25–9.
4. Sarkar R, Sharma RC, Koranne RV, Sardana K. Erythroderma in children: A clinico-etiological study. *J Dermatol* 1999;26(8):507–11.
5. Botelho LF, Porro AM, Enokihara MM, Tomimori J. Adverse cutaneous drug reactions in a single quaternary referral hospital. *Int J Dermatol* 2016;55(4):198–203.
6. Huang HY, Luo XQ, Chan LS, Cao ZH, Sun XF, Xu JH. Cutaneous adverse drug reactions in a hospital-based Chinese population. *Clin Exp Dermatol* 2011;36(2):135–41.
7. Lee HY, Tay LK, Thirumoorthy T, Pang SM. Cutaneous adverse drug reactions in hospitalised patients. *Singapore Med J* 2010;51(10):767–74.
8. Patel RM, Marfatia YS. Clinical study of cutaneous drug eruptions in 200 patients. *Indian J Dermatol Venereol Leprol* 2008;74(4):430.
9. Yuan XY, Guo JY, Dang YP, Qiao L, Liu W. Erythroderma: A clinical-etiological study of 82 cases. *Eur J Dermatol* 2010;20(3):373–7.
10. Khaled A, Sellami A, Fazaa B, Kharfi M, Zeglaoui F, Kamoun MR. Acquired erythroderma in adults: A clinical and prognostic study. *J Eur Acad Dermatol Venereol* 2010;24(7):781–8.
11. Li J, Zheng HY. Erythroderma: A clinical and prognostic study. *Dermatology* 2012;225(2):154–62.
12. Hasan T, Jansen CT. Erythroderma: A follow-up of fifty cases. *J Am Acad Dermatol* 1983;8(6):836–40.
13. Karakayli G, Beckham G, Orengo I, Rosen T. Exfoliative dermatitis. *Am Fam Physician* 1999;59(3):625–30.
14. Sehgal VN, Srivastava G, Sardana K. Erythroderma/ exfoliative dermatitis: A synopsis. *Int J Dermatol* 2004;43(1):39–47.
15. Thakur BK, Verma S, Mishra J. Lichenoid drug reaction to isoniazid presenting as exfoliative dermatitis in a patient with acquired immunodeficiency syndrome. *Int J STD AIDS* 2015;26(7):512–5.
16. Bandyopadhyay D. Exfoliative dermatitis induced by leflunomide therapy. *J Dermatol* 2003;30(11):845–6.
17. Kuhnley EJ, Granoff AL. Exfoliative dermatitis during lithium treatment. *Am J Psychiatry* 1979;136(10):1340–1.

18. Ghura HS, Carmichael AJ, Bairstow D, Finney R. Fatal erythroderma associated with pentostatin. *BMJ* 1999;319(7209):549.

19. Oztas P et al. Imatinib-induced erythrodermia in a patient with chronic myeloid leukemia. *Acta Derm Venereol* 2006;86(2):174–5.

20. Kuznetsov AV, Weisenseel P, Flaig MJ, Ruzicka T, Prinz JC. Photoallergic erythroderma due to doxycycline therapy of erythema chronicum migrans. *Acta Derm Venereol* 2011;91(6):734–6.

21. Liu A, Giroux L. A suspected case of silodosin-induced erythrodermia. *Drug Saf Case Rep* 2015;2(1):1.

22. Rener-Primec Z, Balkovec V. Valproate-related erythrodermia with reversible encephalopathy: A rare but serious adverse reaction, case report. *Acta Dermatovenerol Alp Pannonica Adriat* 2014;23(2):35–8.

23. Arai S, Mukai H. Erythroderma induced by morphine sulfate. *J Dermatol* 2011;38(3):288–9.

24. Langtry JA, Harper JI, Staughton RC, Barrington P. Erythroderma resembling Sézary syndrome after treatment with Fansidar and chloroquine. *Br Med J (Clin Res Ed)* 1986;292(6528):1107–8.

25. Choi CU et al. Extensive exfoliative dermatitis induced by non-ionic contrast medium iodixanol (Visipaque) used during percutaneous coronary intervention. *Int J Cardiol* 2008;124(2):e25–7.

26. Danno K, Kume M, Ohta M, Utani A, Ohno S, Kobashi Y. Erythroderma with generalized lymphadenopathy induced by phenytoin. *J Dermatol* 1989;16(5):392–6.

27. Gallelli L, Ferraro M, Mauro GF, De Sarro G. Generalized exfoliative dermatitis induced by interferon alfa. *Ann Pharmacother* 2004;38(12):2173–4.

28. Igawa K, Konishi M, Moriyama Y, Fukuyama K, Yokozeki H. Erythroderma as drug eruption induced by intravesical mitomycin C therapy. *J Eur Acad Dermatol Venereol* 2015;29(3):613–4.

29. Sanghavi SA, Dongre AM, Khopkar US. Imatinib mesylate induced erythroderma. *Indian J Dermatol Venereol Leprol* 2012;78(3):408.

30. Sharma G, Govil DC. Allopurinol induced erythroderma. *Indian J Pharmacol* 2013;45(6):627–8.

31. Garg Y, Gore R, Jain S, Kumar A. A rare case of isoniazid-induced erythroderma. *Indian J Pharmacol* 2015;47(6):682–4.

32. Kumar S, Mahajan BB, Kaur S, Banipal RP, Singh A. Imatinib mesylate induced erythroderma: A rare case series. *J Cancer Res Ther* 2015;11(4):993–6.

33. Mahe E, Descamps V, Baikian B, Toulon A, Crickx B. Acitretin-induced erythroderma in a psoriatic patient. *J Eur Acad Dermatol Venereol* 2006;20(9):1133–4.

34. Marzano AV, Borghi A, Cugno M. Adverse drug reactions and organ damage: The skin. *Eur J Intern Med* 2016;28:17–24.

35. Ram-Wolf C, Mahe E, Saiag P. Escitalopram photo-induced erythroderma. *J Eur Acad Dermatol Venereol* 2008;22(8):1015–7.

36. Rowe CJ, Robertson I, James D, McMeniman E. Warfarin-induced erythroderma. *Australas J Dermatol* 2015;56(1):e15–7.

37. Sanchez-Borges M, Gonzalez-Aveledo L. Exfoliative erythrodermia induced by pantoprazole. *Allergol Immunopathol (Madr)* 2012;40(3):194–5.

38. Husain Z, Reddy BY, Schwartz RA. DRESS syndrome: Part I. Clinical perspectives. *J Am Acad Dermatol* 2013;68(5):693.

39. Kumari R, Timshina DK, Thappa DM. Drug hypersensitivity syndrome. *Indian J Dermatol Venereol Leprol* 2011;77(1):7–15.

40. Choudhary S, McLeod M, Torchia D, Romanelli P. Drug reaction with eosinophilia and systemic symptoms (DRESS) syndrome. *J Clin Aesthet Dermatol* 2013;6(6):31–7.

41. Aihara M. Pharmacogenetics of cutaneous adverse drug reactions. *J Dermatol* 2011;38(3):246–54.

42. Chantarangsu S et al. HLA-B*3505 allele is a strong predictor for nevirapine-induced skin adverse drug reactions in HIV-infected Thai patients. *Pharmacogenet Genomics* 2009;19(2):139–46.

43. Bharatiya PR, Joshi PB. Study of exfoliative dermatitis. *Indian J Dermatol Venereol Leprol* 1995;61(2):81–3.

44. Fiszenson-Albala F et al. A 6-month prospective survey of cutaneous drug reactions in a hospital setting. *Br J Dermatol* 2003;149(5):1018–22.

45. Banerjee S, Ghosh S, Mandal RK. A study of correlation between clinical and histopathological findings of erythroderma in North Bengal population. *Indian J Dermatol* 2015;60(6):549–55.

46. Shelley WB, Shelley ED. Shoreline nails: Sign of drug-induced erythroderma. *Cutis* 1985;35(3):220–2.

47. Jeung YJ, Lee JY, Oh MJ, Choi DC, Lee BJ. Comparison of the causes and clinical features of drug rash with eosinophilia and systemic symptoms and Stevens-Johnson syndrome. *Allergy Asthma Immunol Res* 2010;2(2):123–6.

48. Okoduwa C et al. Erythroderma: Review of a potentially life-threatening dermatosis. *Indian J Dermatol* 2009;54(1):1–6.

49. Kano Y, Ishida T, Hirahara K, Shiohara T. Visceral involvements and long-term sequelae in drug-induced hypersensitivity syndrome. *Med Clin North Am* 2010;94(4):743–59.

50. Das S, Sharma N. Erythroderma: How to know if it is drug induced? *Indian J Drugs Dermatol* 2017;3(2):98–9.

51. Belhekar MN, Taur SR, Munshi RP. A study of agreement between the Naranjo algorithm and WHO-UMC criteria for causality assessment of adverse drug reactions. *Indian J Pharmacol* 2014;46(1):117–20.

52. Naranjo CA et al. A method for estimating the probability of adverse drug reactions. *Clin Pharmacol Ther* 1981;30(2):239–45.

53. Doherty MJ. Algorithms for assessing the probability of an adverse drug reaction. *Respir Med CME* 2009;2:63–7.

54. Kim GK, Del Rosso JQ. Drug-provoked psoriasis: Is it drug induced or drug aggravated?: Understanding pathophysiology and clinical relevance. *J Clin Aesthet Dermatol* 2010;3(1):32–8.

55. Scott LA, Stone MS. Viral exanthems. *Dermatol Online J* 2003;9(3):4.

56. Mathew R, Sreedevan V. Erythroderma: A clinico-pathological study of 370 cases from a tertiary care center in Kerala. *Indian J Dermatol Venereol Leprol* 2017;83(5):625.

57. Jowkar F, Aslani FS, Shafiee M. Erythroderma: A clinicopathological study of 102 cases. *J Pak Assoc Dermatol* 2006; 16(3):129–33.

58. Patterson JW, Berry AD3rd, Darwin BS, Gottlieb A, Wilkerson MG. Lichenoid histopathologic changes in patients with clinical diagnoses of exfoliative dermatitis. *Am J Dermatopathol* 1991;13(4):358–64.

59. Ortonne N et al. Histopathology of drug rash with eosinophilia and systemic symptoms syndrome: A morphological and phenotypical study. *Br J Dermatol* 2015;173(1):50–8.

60. Walsh S et al. Drug reaction with eosinophilia and systemic symptoms: Is cutaneous phenotype a prognostic marker for outcome? A review of clini-copathological features of 27 cases. *Br J Dermatol* 2013;168(2):391–401.

61. Barbaud A, Gonçalo M, Bruynzeel D, Bircher A; European Society of Contact Dermatitis. Guidelines for performing skin tests with drugs in the investigation of cutaneous adverse drug reactions. *Contact Dermatitis* 2001;45(6):321–8.

62. Barbaud A et al. Toxidermies group of the French Society of Dermatology. A multicentre study to determine the value and safety of drug patch tests for the three main classes of severe cutaneous adverse drug reactions. *Br J Dermatol* 2013;168(3):555–62.

63. Pichler WJ, Tilch J. The lymphocyte transformation test in the diagnosis of drug hypersensitivity. *Allergy* 2004;59(8):809–20.

64. Rive CM, Bourke J, Phillips EJ. Testing for drug hypersensitivity syndromes. *Clin Biochem Rev* 2013;34(1):15–38.

65. Aberer W et al. European Network for Drug Allergy (ENDA); EAACI interest group on drug hypersensitivity. Drug provocation testing in the diagnosis of drug hypersensitivity reactions: General considerations. *Allergy* 2003;58(9):854–63.

66. Brockow K et al. Guideline for the diagnosis of drug hypersensitivity reactions: S2K-Guideline of the German Society for Allergology and Clinical Immunology (DGAKI) and the German Dermatological Society (DDG) in collaboration with the Association of German Allergologists (AeDA), the German Society for Pediatric Allergology and Environmental Medicine (GPA), the German Contact Dermatitis Research Group (DKG), the Swiss Society for Allergy and Immunology (SGAI), the Austrian Society for Allergology and Immunology (ÖGAI), the German Academy of Allergology and Environmental Medicine (DAAU), the German Center for Documentation of Severe Skin Reactions and the German Federal Institute for Drugs and Medical Products (BfArM). *Allergo J Int* 2015;24(3):94–105.

17

Pityriasis rubra pilaris induced erythroderma

RUBY VENUGOPAL AND D. V. LAKSHMI

INTRODUCTION

Pityriasis rubra pilaris (PRP) is a chronic papulosquamous disorder characterized by skin and nail involvement. It can be familial or acquired. The exact etiology of the disease is still debatable. Clinically it is characterized by reddish-orange plaques with follicular keratoses and pityriasiform scaling along with palmoplantar keratoderma. To begin with, the lesions are circumscribed but can progress to erythroderma, especially in adults. Erythroderma is a potentially fatal dermatological emergency that warrants intensive care. Hence, even though PRP is a self-limiting dermatological condition, its tendency to progress to erythroderma needs to be always kept in mind. A good understanding of the disease will help in early diagnosis and intervention, which are crucial and will directly affect the outcome of the patients.

EPIDEMIOLOGY

PRP is an uncommon dermatoses of juvenile or adult onset. Due to the rarity of the disease, there are limited epidemiological data available. PRP has been estimated to occur in about 1 in 50,000 new dermatological patients in India [1], as against 1 in 5,000 in the United Kingdom [2]. The reported incidence of PRP-induced erythroderma varies considerably. Dicken reported that PRP "almost always progress to a generalized Erythroderma" [3], and Albert and Mackool stated that PRP frequently turns erythrodermic [4]. In contrast, in a study conducted in 168 PRP cases of Thai origin, only 14 developed erythroderma [5]. Allison et al. [6], reported that 17% of 30 children with PRP developed erythroderma. PRP appears to affect both genders equally [7]. The age distribution is usually bimodal with familial

PRP usually occurring in the first decade and acquired PRP developing in the fifth or sixth decades of life.

ETIOPATHOGENESIS

The pathomechanism of PRP remains elusive. Certain possible mechanisms mentioned in the literature are abnormal vitamin A metabolism in the skin, association with internal malignancies, autoimmune diseases, or infections, particularly HIV. This has led to the speculation that it might be the result of abnormal immune response to some antigenic stimuli [4]. The disease is mostly acquired, although familial forms with both autosomal dominant and recessive inheritance are mentioned in the literature [8,9].

Mutations in the caspase recruitment domain family member 14 gene (CARD 14), an activator of NF-κB signaling, has been identified in the genetic forms of the disease and rarely in sporadic forms [10,11]. The role of the IL-23/Th 17 pathway has been identified in the pathogenesis, which explains the clinical and histopathological similarity of the disease with psoriasis [12].

PATHOLOGY

Histopathological changes in PRP, although not pathognomonic, can help in differentiating it from other causes of erythroderma, especially psoriasis. The histology changes with the evolution of the disease. There is psoriasiform dermatitis with irregular hyperkeratosis and alternating vertical and horizontal orthokeratosis and hyperkeratosis. This pattern has been referred to as the *checkerboard pattern* [13]. There is follicular plugging with foci of parakeratosis in the perifollicular shoulder. There can be patchy or confluent hypergranulosis. There is dilatation of dermal capillaries; however, they are not tortuous as seen in psoriasis. Acantholysis and focal acantholytic dyskeratosis in the epidermis have been described, and these features also help in distinguishing PRP from psoriasis [14]. However, it is unknown whether this finding is incidental or a rare but definite histologic change in PRP.

CLINICAL FEATURES

PRP has considerable clinical heterogeneity. Based on age of onset, course of the disease, morphologic features, and prognosis, Griffiths categorized PRP into five clinical subtypes: type 1, classic adult type; type 2, atypical adult type; type 3, classic juvenile type; type 4, circumscribed juvenile type; and type 5, atypical juvenile type [2]. Later, a sixth subtype, namely HIV-associated PRP, has been added [16].

The more recognizable and common clinical subtypes (type 1 and type 3) are generalized forms and can progress into erythroderma. Progression to erythroderma is more common in adults. HIV-associated PRP also frequently progresses to erythroderma. The atypical adult form has less of a tendency to become erythrodermic. The lesions tend to have an acute onset. The rash usually begins on the head near the scalp margins, neck, or upper trunk as erythematous slightly scaly macules that resemble seborrheic dermatitis clinically. Within days to weeks, the rash progresses with the appearance of erythematous follicular hyperkeratotic papules that gradually coalesce (Figures 17.1 through 17.3). Interfollicular erythema begins to appear, and the follicular lesions get gradually submerged in sheets of erythema progressing cephalocaudally. The face assumes a uniform red-orange hue with mild to moderate

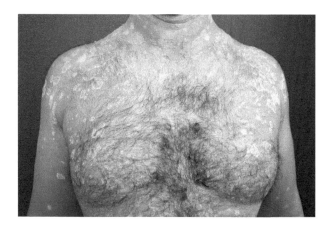

Figure 17.2 Erythroderma with pityriasiform scaling: extensive scaling on the chest.

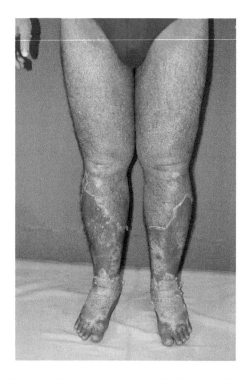

Figure 17.3 Erythroderma with pityriasiform scaling: extensive scaling and erythema on the lower limbs.

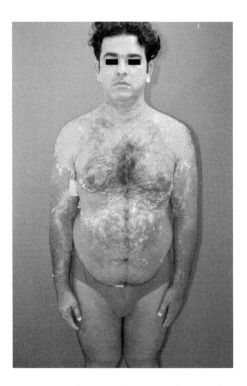

Figure 17.1 Erythroderma with pityriasiform scaling: extensive scaling and erythema visible on the trunk and upper limbs.

ectropion. Pruritus and irritation can be pronounced in later stages of the disease. Diffuse bran-like scales are present on the scalp. The rash may involve the oral mucosa in the form of white spots and lines, pale blue lines, and erythematous lesions covered with white streaks [17,18]. The lesions can affect buccal mucosa, gingivae, and the tongue and can mimic lichen planus.

The disease can progress from a limited form to erythroderma within 2–3 months of the course of the disease. Prolonged erythema can result in peripheral edema and may precipitate high-output cardiac failure in the elderly. Lymphadenopathy can be present. Those patients who present to a health-care facility for the first time after erythroderma sets in can be a diagnostic challenge. Certain distinctive clinical features can aid in diagnosis. "Islands of normal skin"

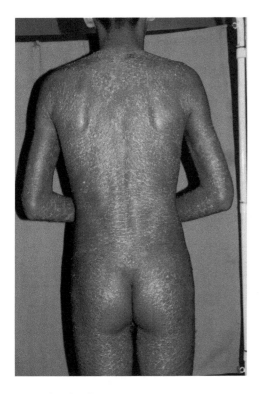

Figure 17.4 Islands of sparing.

(*nappes claires*), which are sharply demarcated areas of uninvolved skin present as islands in the sheets of erythema, are often present (Figure 17.4). These islands are considered as a diagnostic feature in PRP erythroderma; however, they have also been reported in other conditions such as cutaneous T-cell lymphoma, psoriasis, pemphigus foliaceus, and sarcoidosis [19]. Sometimes, circumscribed areas of deeper erythema are also seen. The palms and soles are involved in the form of yellowish hyperkeratosis, often referred to as the *PRP sandal* (Figure 17.5). Horny follicular papules are present on knees and elbows and on the proximal phalanges of fingers (nutmeg grater appearance) (Figure 17.6). Nail changes are nonspecific in the form of thickening and distal discoloration of nail plate and splinter hemorrhages. Unlike psoriasis, there

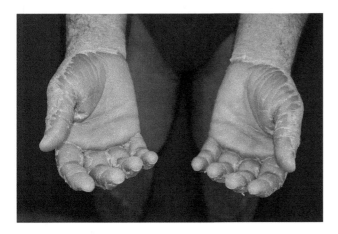

Figure 17.5 Palmar keratoderma.

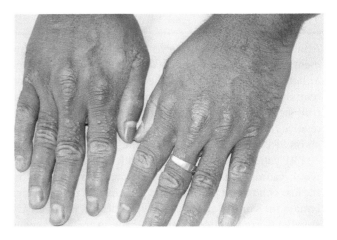

Figure 17.6 Grouped follicular papules on knuckles.

Table 17.1 Differentials in erythrodermic pityriasis rubra pilaris

Serial number	Differential diagnosis
1	Psoriasic erythroderma
2	Extensive seborrheic dermatitis
3	T-cell lymphoma
4	Erythroderma progressive symmetrica
5	Erythrokeratoderma variabilis
6	Follicular eczema
7	Follicular ichthyosis
8	Generalized hypersensitivity reaction

is minimal pitting in nails and no dystrophy of the nail plate. There can be an appearance of eruptive seborrheic keratoses along with the erythrodermic flare-up of PRP which later involute and fall off when the erythroderma resolves [20,21].

Dermoscopy is an important auxiliary tool in the differentiation of common types of erythroderma. Dermoscopy in PRP erythroderma has distinct patterns. Apart from diffuse whitish scaling and scattered dotted vessels over a reddish background, which can be found in erythrodermic psoriasis as well, PRP has unique findings in the form of several orange blotches, and islands of nonerythematous (spared) skin displaying reticular vessels [22].

The differentials to be considered in erythrodermic PRP are enumerated in Table 17.1.

DISEASE COURSE AND PROGNOSIS

The classical types of PRP can progress from limited disease to erythroderma within weeks, but in a majority of cases they resolve spontaneously [23].

INVESTIGATIONS

Diagnosis is usually based on clinical features. Histology can be used to confirm the diagnosis. No serological markers are available for PRP.

TREATMENT

Although PRP usually resolves within 1–3 years, treatment of the disease is generally difficult. It is often resistant to both topical and systemic therapies. Since spontaneous remission can occur in the disease course, evaluating the true merit of any therapeutic agent is difficult. Due to the relative rarity of the disease, no randomized controlled trials on PRP have been published in the literature.

PRP patients presenting acutely with erythroderma often require admission for intensive supportive care to cater to the loss of homeostasis. The basic principles of management remain the same in all types of erythroderma. Bland greasy emollients are the ideal topical therapy to treat cutaneous inflammation and restore barrier function. Some patients experience intense pruritus and often require systemic antihistamine therapy. Corticosteroid mouth rinses are useful in case of oral involvement.

Systemic retinoids remain the first line of therapy in most cases of erythrodermic PRP. Acitretin at a dose of up to 50 mg/day should be considered for a period of 3–6 months. In pediatric cases of erythrodermic PRP, oral retinoids can be considered, as short-term use of systemic retinoids in otherwise healthy children seems to be safe and well tolerated [24].

When retinoids fail or when they are contraindicated, methotrexate can be favored as second-line treatment. Methotrexate is given in doses of up to 20 mg/week. It can also be combined with acitretin [3].

Therapeutic approaches in PRP have been largely based on the resemblance of the disease to psoriasis. Therefore, TNF-α antagonists are being increasingly used in refractory and erythrodermic psoriasis. Infliximab at a dose of 5 mg/kg has been used to treat erythrodermic adult-onset PRP, both as an adjuvant to conventional therapy and as a rescue therapy where conventional agents have failed [25,26]. Etanercept also has been reported as a successful therapy in PRP [27–29]. Since this drug has been approved by the U.S. Food and Drug Administration for use in pediatric psoriasis, it can be a promising treatment option in juvenile PRP. Adalimumab has also been reported to be successful in type 1 PRP [30].

There are several case reports of successful use of ustekinumab, the anti-IL-12/IL-23 antibody in refractory cases of PRP [15,31–34]. The mechanism of action in PRP is by suppression of activation of the NF-κB pathway. Marked improvement has been reported in both familial and sporadic cases. Ustekinumab may be considered in preference to TNF-α inhibitors in severe or erythrodermic PRP when acitretin and methotrexate have been ineffective or are contraindicated.

In cases of HIV-associated PRP, antiretroviral therapy may result in complete response. However, relapses can be frequent. Acitretin can be added if indicated.

Several other therapies like azathioprine, cyclosporine, mycophenolate mofetil, fumaric acid, and extracorporeal phototherapy and their varying success have been reported in the literature. A therapeutic ladder for PRP is provided in Table 17.2.

Table 17.2 Therapeutic ladder in erythrodermic pityriasis rubra pilaris

Systemic drugs: Therapeutic ladder in erythrodermic pityriasis rubra pilaris

First line
 1. Acitretin
Second line
 1. Methotrexate
 2. Ustekinumab
Third line
 1. TNF-α antagonists
 2. Extracorporeal photochemotherapy

KEY POINTS

- PRP is a rare keratinization disorder with mostly unknown pathogenesis.
- PRP is clinically characteristic with diagnostic features of follicular plugging and palmoplantar keratoderma.
- Progress to erythroderma can occur and is difficult to treat.
- Retinoids are the first choice of treatment.

CONCLUSION

To date, no standardized therapeutic approach has been established in PRP. Basic supportive care is the most vital part in managing erythrodermic forms. Biologics have been a promising and significant addition to the therapeutic armamentarium in a difficult-to-treat case. Further studies are required to understand the pathophysiology and therapeutic interventions possible in the disease.

REFERENCES

1. Sehgal VN, Jain MK, Mathur RP. Pityriasis rubra pilaris in Indians (Letter). *Br J Dermatol* 1989;121:821–2.
2. Griffiths WA. Pityriasis rubra pilaris. *Clin Exp Dermatol* 1980;5:105–12.
3. Dicken CH. Treatment of classic pityriasis rubra pilaris. *J Am Acad Dermatol* 1994;31:997–9.
4. Albert MR, Mackool BT. Pityriasis rubra pilaris. *Int J Dermatol* 1999;38:1–11.
5. Piamphongsant T, Akaraphant R. Pityriasis rubra pilaris: A new proposed classification. *Clin Exp Dermatol* 1994;19:134–8.
6. Allison DS et al. Pityriasis rubra pilaris in children. *J Am Acad Dermatol* 2002;47:386–9.
7. Griffiths WA. Pityriasis rubra pilaris: A historical approach and clinical features. *Clin Exp Dermatol* 1976;1:37–50.
8. Vanderhooft SL, Francis J. Familial pityriasis rubra pilaris. *Arch Dermatol* 1995;131:448–53.

9. Sehgal VN, Srivastava G, Dogra S. Adult onset pityriasis rubra pilaris. *Indian J Dermatol Venereol Leprol* 2008;74:311–21.

10. Fuchs-Telem D et al. Familial pityriasis rubra pilaris is caused by mutations in CARD14. *Am J Hum Genet* 2012;91(1):163–70.

11. Li Q et al. Analysis of CARD14 polymorphisms in pityriasis rubra pilaris: Activation of NF-κB. *J Invest Dermatol* 2015;135(7):1905–8.

12. Feldmeyer L et al. Interleukin 23–helper T cell 17 axis as a treatment target for pityriasis rubra pilaris. *JAMA Dermatol* 2017;153(4):304–8.

13. Soeprono FF. Histologic criteria for the diagnosis of pityriasis rubra pilaris. *Am J Dermatopathol* 1986;8(4):277–83.

14. Magro CM, Crowson AN. The clinical and histomorphological features of pityriasis rubra pilaris: A comparative analysis with psoriasis. *J Cutan Pathol* 1997;24(7):416–24.

15. Eytan O, Sarig O, Sprecher E, van Steesel, MAM. Clinical response to ustekinumab in familial pityriasis rubra pilaris caused by a novel mutation in CARD14. *Br J Dermatol* 2014;171:420–1.

16. Misery I, Faure M, Claidy A. Pityriasis rubra pilaris and human immunodeficiency virus infection: Type 6 pityriasis rubra pilaris? *Br J Dermatol* 1996;135(6):1008–9.

17. Kurzydlo A-M, Gillespie R. Paraneoplastic pityriasis rubra pilaris in association with bronchogenic carcinoma. *Australas J Dermatol* 2004;45:130–2.

18. Martinez Calixto LE et al. Oral pityriasis rubra pilaris. *Oral Sur Oral Med Oral Pathol Oral Radiol Endod* 2006;101:604–7.

19. Pal S, Haroon TS. Erythroderma; A clinic-etiologic study of 90 cases. *Int J Dermatol* 1998;37:104–7.

20. Sahin MT et al. Transient eruptive seborrhoeic keratoses associated with erythrodermic pityriasis rubra pilaris. *Clin Exp Dermatol* 2004;29:554–5.

21. Gleeson CM et al. Eruptive seborrhoeic keratoses associated with erythrodermic pityriasis rubra pilaris. *J Eur Acad Dermatol Venereol* 2009;23:217–8.

22. Errichetti E, Piccirillo A, Stinco G. Dermoscopy as an auxiliary tool in the differentiation of the main types of erythroderma due to dermatological disorders. *Int J Dermatol* 2016;55:e616–8.

23. Griffiths WA. Pityriasis rubra pilaris: The problem of its classification. *J Am Acad Dermatol* 1992;26:140–2.

24. Brecher AR, Orlow SJ. Oral retinoid therapy for dermatologic conditions in children and adolescents. *J Am Acad Dermatol* 2003;49:171–82.

25. Liao WC, Mutasim DF. Infliximab for the treatment of adult-onset pityriasis rubra pilaris. *Arch Dermatol* 2005;141:423–5.

26. Manoharan S, White S, Gumparthy K. Successful treatment of type 1 adult onset pityriasis rubra pilaris with infliximab. *Australas J Dermatol* 2006;47:124–9.

27. Davis KF et al. Clinical improvement of pityriasis rubra pilaris with combination etanercept and acitretin therapy. *Arch Dermatol* 2007;143:1597–9.

28. Seckin D, Tula E, Ergun T. Successful use of etanercept in type I pityriasis rubra pilaris. *Br J Dermatol* 2007;158:642–3.

29. Cox V et al. Treatment of juvenile pityriasis rubra pilaris with etanercept. *J Am Acad Dermatol* 2009;59:S113–4.

30. Walling HW, Swick BL. Pityriasis rubra pilaris responding rapidly to adalimumab. *Arch Dermatol* 2009;145:99–101.

31. Foo SH, Rowe A, Maheshwari MB, Abdullah A. The challenge of managing pityriasis rubra pilaris: Success at last with ustekinumab? *Br J Dermatol* 2014;171(suppl S1):155.

32. Feldmeyer L, Hohl D, Gilliet M, Conrad C. Pityriasis rubra pilaris treated with ustekinumab. *J Invest Med* 2014;62:723.

33. Di Stefani A, Galluzzo M, Talamonti M, Chiricozzi A, Costanzo A, Chiment IS. Long term ustekinumab treatment for refractory type I pityriasis rubra pilaris. *J Dermatol Case Rep* 2013;7:5–9.

34. Wohlrab J, Kreft B. Treatment of pityriasis rubra pilaris with ustekinumab. *Br J Dermatol* 2010;163:655–6.

PART 5

Pediatric Emergencies–1 (Neonatal)

SAHANA M. SRINIVAS AND VISHAL SONDHI

18

Neonatal erythroderma

APARNA PALIT AND ARUN C. INAMADAR

INTRODUCTION

Neonatal erythroderma is a rare condition presenting at birth or during the first month of life. The causes of neonatal erythroderma are manifold; most of these disorders are unique to this age group, some others are commonly seen in older children and adults.

Erythroderma is defined as "any inflammatory condition involving more than 90% body surface area" [1]. In neonates widespread erythema is almost always present; in addition there may be scaling, vesiculation, and eczematization alone or in various combinations. This often leads to use of the term *red scaly baby* for erythrodermic neonates. It can be a manifestation of various primary cutaneous disorders or a cutaneous reaction pattern to systemic illnesses.

The common causes of neonatal erythroderma are infections, inflammatory disorders, and congenital ichthyoses [2]. Some disorders of immunodeficiency and inborn errors of metabolism may also present with erythroderma in this age group.

Neonatal erythroderma is a diagnostic and therapeutic challenge for clinicians. Disruption of the cutaneous barrier predisposes these children to infections, dehydration, and metabolic disturbances. Early accurate diagnosis is crucial for survival of the baby as some of the underlying causes are treatable. An integrated approach by neonatologists and dermatologists is imperative for the management of neonatal erythroderma.

EPIDEMIOLOGY

The true incidence of neonatal erythroderma in various populations is not known, indicating its rarity. In an Indian study the incidence of childhood erythroderma has been quoted as 0.11% ($n = 17$) of whom three (18%) were neonates [3]. In a French study including 51 cases of neonatal and infantile erythroderma, 16 (32%) had onset at birth; of them 15 neonates had congenital ichthyosis and one had Omenn syndrome [4].

CLASSIFICATION AND CLINICAL FEATURES

Various causes of erythroderma in the neonatal period are listed in Table 18.1 and presented schematically in Figure 18.1 [2,5–8]. Important clinical features of individual disorders have been highlighted subsequently.

Infections

STAPHYLOCOCCAL SCALDED SKIN SYNDROME

Staphylococcal scalded skin syndrome (SSSS) is caused by staphylococcal exotoxins A and B (ETA and ETB) that target epidermal cadherin desmoglein-1 at the granular cell layer [8]. This results in a split below the stratum granulosum causing widespread flaccid bulla formation, followed by erosions and scaling [8,9].

SSSS can occur in neonates either as a community or hospital-acquired infection. Though it is more common in older children, neonates are susceptible to this infection because of lack of immunity against the exotoxins and renal immaturity leading to poor clearance of the toxins [9].

Preterm neonates (born before 36 weeks of gestation), very low birth weight (VLBW, less than 1500 g at birth) and extremely low birth weight (ELBW, less than 1000 g at birth) babies may rarely get the infection [8,10–13]. These babies may develop recurrent episodes of SSSS even after full antibiotic therapy [12].

Unlike other severe neonatal infections where the source of organisms is the birth canal, *Staphylococcus aureus* is

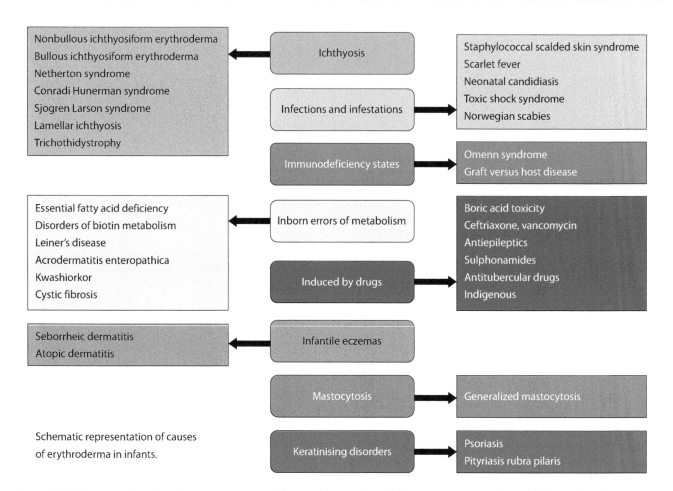

Figure 18.1 Causes of erythroderma in neonates (birth to 1 month) and infants (1 month to 1 year). (Remember the mnemonic: 6 I's in Mini Kids as the main causes of erythroderma in infants.)

Table 18.1 Causes of neonatal erythroderma

Infection	Staphylococcal scalded skin syndrome, neonatal toxic shock syndrome–like exanthematous disease, congenital cutaneous candidiasis
Nonsyndromic congenital ichthyosis	Bullous epidermolytic ichthyosis, nonbullous ichthyosiform erythroderma, lamellar ichthyosis, harlequin ichthyosis
Syndromic congenital ichthyosis	Netherton syndrome, Sjögren-Larsson syndrome, Conradi-Hünermann-Happle syndrome, Chanarin-Dorfman syndrome, keratitis-ichthyosis-deafness syndrome
Ectodermal dysplasia	Anhidrotic/hypohidrotic ectodermal dysplasia
Infiltrative disorder	Langerhans cell histiocytosis, diffuse cutaneous mastocytosis
Immunodeficiency disorders	Severe combined immunodeficiency, Omenn syndrome
Inborn errors of metabolism	Neutral lipid storage disease, multiple carboxylase deficiency, urea cycle defects, neonatal biotinidase deficiency
Cutaneous adverse drug reactions	Reported drugs: Ceftriaxone, vancomycin

Source: Dhar S et al. Indian J Dermatol 2012;57:475–8; Hoeger PH, Harper JI. Arch Dis Child 1998;79:186–91; Fraitag S, Bodemer C. Curr Opin Pediatr 2010;22:438–44; Bedocs LA et al. Neo Reviews 2011;12:e325–33; Davidson J et al. AJP Rep 2017;7(2):e134–7.

usually acquired from health-care givers [14]. The initial localization of the organism is at the umbilical stump or conjunctiva or at the genitalia following a very early ritual circumcision [14]. Approximately 30% of neonates acquire S. aureus infection by the first 6 days of life, and symptoms of SSSS may arise by the 3rd–16th days of life [15]. Usually the cases are sporadic, but outbreaks of SSSS have been reported in neonatal intensive care units due to handling of the babies by infected or asymptomatic carriers of S. aureus. SSSS occurring within 24 hours of birth (congenital SSSS) as part of maternal puerperal infection has been reported [14]. When caused by the methicillin-resistant strain of *S. aureus* (MRSA), it may be life threatening in neonates [9,16].

In neonates the initial focal infection may go unrecognized, and the baby develops diffuse, bright, blanchable erythema simulating acute sunburn [14]. It is followed by wrinkling of the skin on periorificial areas of the face and flaccid thin-walled, large, clear bullae and/or erosions appear all over the body. Nikolsky sign is positive. The erosions give rise to glistening, wet areas surrounded by rolled-up, thin scales [14].

NEONATAL TOXIC SHOCK SYNDROME–LIKE EXANTHEMATOUS DISEASE

Neonatal toxic shock syndrome–like exanthematous disease (NTED) is induced by toxic shock syndrome-1 toxin (TSST-1), mostly produced by MRSA [17]. TSST-1 acts as a bacterial superantigen and induces the immune response; the symptomatology is collectively designated as NTED [17].

Fever, chills, bright macular erythema that may desquamate later, and thrombocytopenia are the features of NTED [17]. It is a mild disease in neonates as compared to toxic shock syndrome in older children and adults. Rapid recovery is usual in this age group [17,18].

CONGENITAL CUTANEOUS CANDIDIASIS

This is a rare infective cause of neonatal erythroderma. Generalized cutaneous candidiasis may be present in newborns when there is chorioamnionitis due to ascending infection in the mother [19]. Babies of mothers with a foreign body in the uterus (specifically, a high cervical suture or an intrauterine device) are susceptible to developing congenital cutaneous candidiasis (CCC) [19].

Skin lesions are present in the initial 24 hours of life as widespread or patchy erythema (Figure 18.2) [19]. Thereafter, generalized erythematous papulopustular lesions develop; palms and soles are typically involved, and the oral cavity and diaper area are relatively spared. Subsequently, there are vesicles and bullae formation followed by erosions and desquamation. Paronychia and nail involvement may be present [19]. In term neonates, the condition is self-limiting and aggressive intervention is not indicated.

Preterm neonates (VLBW and ELBW) are prone to develop severe manifestations of CCC because of immature keratinization [5,19,20]. They may have the classical presentation as previously discussed. More commonly, there is diffuse erythema, erosions, and scaling or multiple erosions present at birth. There may be a stillborn baby. There is risk of candidemia, pneumonitis, and meningitis. Death is a common sequel in preterm babies with CCC.

Congenital ichthyosis

A baby born with collodion membrane is termed as a *collodion baby*. In natural course, the collodion membrane is shed, gradually giving rise to a glazed erythematous and scaly body surface resulting in neonatal erythroderma (Figure 18.3) [21]. Subsequently, these babies may develop a form of congenital ichthyosis, most commonly congenital ichthyosiform erythroderma (CIE), recessive X-linked ichthyosis (RXLI), or lamellar ichthyosis (LI) [21]. Hence, all of these variants of congenital ichthyosis may give rise to neonatal erythroderma. In 10%–20% of neonates born with collodion membrane there may be complete resolution by the third month of life, known as *self-healing collodion baby* [21].

Bullous epidermolytic ichthyosis (EI) or "bullous congenital ichthyosiform erythroderma" is an uncommon disorder where neonates are born with generalized flaccid bullae and erosions resulting from friction during passage through the birth canal [21]. Superficial EI or "ichthyosis bullosa of Siemens" is a milder variant starting at the neonatal period [21]. Lesions start as short-lasting bullae that rupture shortly with annular peeling and collarette-like border (mauserung) [21].

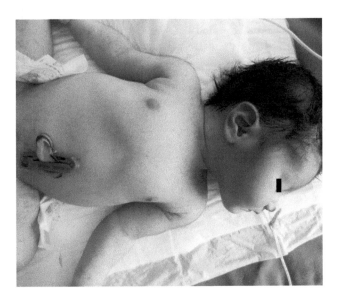

Figure 18.2 Patchy erythema in a case of congenital mucocutaneous candidiasis.

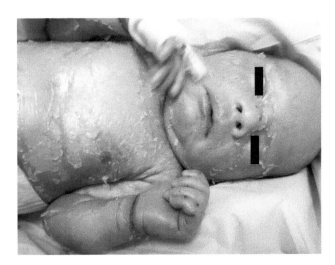

Figure 18.3 Shedding collodion membrane in a neonate. The baby developed clinical features of congenital ichthyosiform erythroderma afterward.

Some of the syndromic ichthyoses may present as collodion baby at birth. These include ichthyosis follicularis, alopecia, and photophobia (IFAP) syndrome; Netherton syndrome (NS); and Sjögren-Larsson syndrome (SLS) [21]. Gradually these children develop the classical features of individual syndrome.

NS and Conradi-Hünermann-Happle syndrome (CHHS) present as neonatal erythroderma [21]. In NS, the classical feature is bright orange-red scaly skin and sparse hair (scalp, eyebrow, eyelashes) at birth (Figures 18.4 and 18.5); during infancy the baby develops the classical double-edged polycyclic scales (ichthyosis linearis circumflexa). In CHHS, the scales are often aligned in swirls and whorls in Blaschkoid pattern [5–7,21].

Patients with keratitis ichthyosis deafness (KID) syndrome have transient erythroderma at or soon after birth [21]. Chanarin-Dorfman syndrome presents with erythroderma at birth due to generalized ichthyosis [21].

Ectodermal dysplasia

ANHIDROTIC/HYPOHIDROTIC ECTODERMAL DYSPLASIA

Patients with this type of ectodermal dysplasia are sometimes born with collodion membrane. It is shed by a few days after birth giving rise to transient erythroderma. The neonate may have the classical midfacial hypoplasia and periorbital wrinkling, which point to the diagnosis. Evolution of the classical manifestations of the disorder occurs through infancy and childhood.

Congenital psoriasis

Psoriasis at the neonatal age is usually localized involving the diaper area and flexures. However, congenital psoriasis, presenting as neonatal erythroderma, has rarely been reported (Figure 18.6) [2,5–7,22].

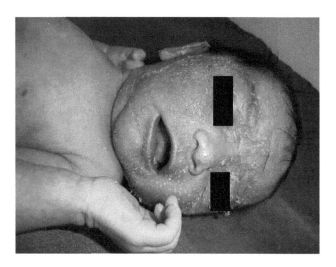

Figure 18.4 A baby with Netherton syndrome at birth. Note the orange-red erythema and double-edged polycyclic scales on the forehead.

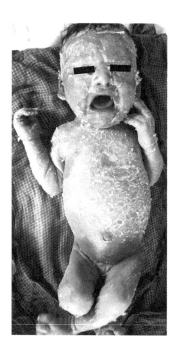

Figure 18.5 The neonate with Netherton syndrome on the seventh day of life with diffuse scaling.

Eczema

ATOPIC DERMATITIS

Atopic dermatitis (AD) may occasionally present as localized lesions in a typical facial distribution in neonates. AD presenting as neonatal erythroderma is extremely rare [2,5–7].

SEBORRHEIC DERMATITIS

The usual presentation of seborrheic dermatitis (SD) in neonates is localized on the scalp (cradle cap) and perineum (diaper dermatitis). Erythroderma resulting from SD may occur in early infancy. However, in a large series of patients with infantile SD, the disease onset was recorded even during the neonatal period [2,5–7,23]. The difference between atopic dermatitis and seborrheic dermatitis is presented in Table 18.2.

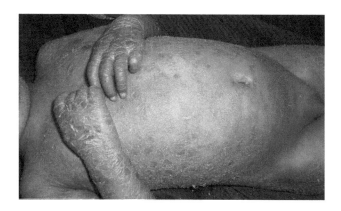

Figure 18.6 Extensive scaling on trunk and upper limbs in a case of congenital psoriasis.

Table 18.2 Differentiating features between atopic and seborrheic dermatitis

Atopic dermatitis	Seborrheic dermatitis
Erythroderma rare in neonatal period	Presents in first few months of life
Dermatitis characterized by vesicles and exudation	Inflammatory, yellowish scaling on the scalp
Itching only after 3 months of age	Erythematous patches are well demarcated and less pruritic
Sparing of napkin area and axilla	Diarrhea, failure to thrive
Positive family history of atopy	Involvement of neck, axilla, and groin

Proliferative disorders

LANGERHANS CELL HISTIOCYTOSIS

Langerhans cell histiocytosis (LCH) is a rare proliferative disorder that may present at birth or in the early neonatal period with diffuse involvement of the skin [24]. Cutaneous involvement may be part of single-system skin-only LCH (SS-LCH), also known as congenital self-healing reticulohistiocytosis (CSHRH) or Hashimoto-Pritzker disease [24]. Otherwise it may be part of multisystem LCH (MS-LCH), also known as Letterer-Siwe disease [24].

The neonate presents with a generalized polymorphic eruption composed of papules, vesicles, crusts, telangiectasias, petechiae, and ulcers (Figure 18.7). The classical feature is seborrheic dermatitis-like greasy, yellow, crusted papules accentuated over the scalp and diaper area observed in 75%–100% cases [24]. As the name suggests CSHRH is a self-regressive disorder, whereas Letterer-Siwe disease carries a poor prognosis requiring systemic therapy [24].

DIFFUSE CUTANEOUS MASTOCYTOSIS

Diffuse cutaneous mastocytosis (DCM) may present at birth. There is generalized involvement of skin with infiltrated papules giving rise to a doughy feel [5–7]. The skin may become erythematous due to handling or cuddling, and Darier's sign may be positive. Occasionally there may be vesicle or bulla formation (Figure 18.8).

Immunodeficiency disorders

Neonates with several congenital immunodeficiency disorders may present with erythroderma at birth or during the second to third week of life due to graft versus host disease (GVHD). The GVHD results from transplacental transfer and engraftment of maternal lymphocytes to the fetus (either self or from nonirradiated blood/blood product transfusion during pregnancy) [5,7]. This may also result due to postnatal exchange transfusion to the neonate [5]. In contrast to immunocompetent neonates where GVHD is mild and self-resolution is common, it is severe in immunodeficient babies [5].

SEVERE COMBINED IMMUNODEFICIENCY

Neonates with severe combined immunodeficiency (SCID) may present with exfoliative erythroderma due to GVHD resulting from severe T-cell immunodeficient state [7]. In severe cases there are extensive erosions simulating toxic epidermal necrolysis (TEN) [7].

OMENN SYNDROME

Omenn syndrome (OS) is considered as a variant of SCID. Neonates with OS present with erythrodermic eczematous eruptions at birth, and it is a constant feature of the disorder [25]. Often the skin has a pachydermatous appearance due to diffuse infiltration which is strongly suggestive of this

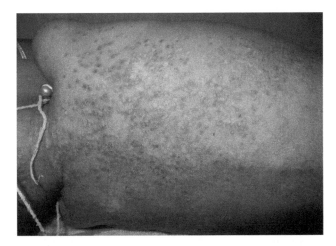

Figure 18.7 Extensive papular eruption in Langerhans cell histiocytosis.

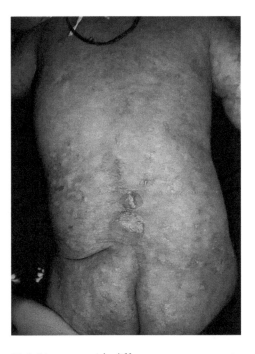

Figure 18.8 Neonate with diffuse cutaneous mastocytosis present since birth. Note the thick skin and erosions on the lower back.

condition [4,6]. There is near total lack of scalp and body hairs at birth [5,26]. Widespread, marked lymphadenopathy, hepatosplenomegaly, and ascites develop subsequently. Recurrent diarrhea, episodes of septicemia, and food intolerance are the causes of failure to thrive in neonates with OS. Life span is short, up to early infancy. The mother often gives the history of death of earlier children in the neonatal period [5].

OTHER IMMUNODEFICIENCY SYNDROMES

Widespread dermatitis is a feature of several primary immunodeficiency disorders like hyper-IgE syndrome, Wiskott-Aldrich syndrome, common variable immunodeficiency, selective IgA deficiency, and X-linked agammaglobulinemia [25]. Sometimes these patients may present with neonatal erythroderma.

Hereditary metabolic disorders

Some rare inborn errors of metabolism may present with erythroderma during early infancy and childhood and rarely during the neonatal period. These conditions are listed in Table 18.3 [27]. Severe metabolic abnormalities dominate the clinical picture in these children, manifesting as poor feeding, recurrent vomiting, dehydration, respiratory distress, lethargy, hepatosplenomegaly, severe ketoacidosis, hypotonia, seizures, and gradual deterioration of consciousness [27].

Rarely, these neonates may present with generalized eczematous rash with accentuation in acral, periorificial areas of the face, perineum, and genitalia simulating acrodermatitis enteropathica (acrodermatitis enteropathica-like eruptions) [27]. There may be erosions and scaling simulating SSSS. The skin lesions may be psoriasiform giving rise to erythroderma [27]. Thinning of hair and alopecia may be seen in these children.

These conditions are fatal with poor prognosis, and death is the eventuality in most of the cases.

Table 18.3 Inborn errors of metabolism that may present as neonatal erythroderma

Organic acidemia	Methylmalonic academia, propionic academia, maple syrup urine disease, glutaricacidemia type 1
Urea cycle defects	Carbamoyl phosphate synthetase deficiency, ornithine transcarbamoylase deficiency, citrullinemia
Neonatal biotin deficiency	Biotinidase deficiency

Source: Inamadar AC, Palit A. In: Inamadar AC, Palit A (Eds), *Advances in Pediatric Dermatology.* New Delhi: Jaypee Brothers Medical Publishers; 2011:234–48.

DIAGNOSIS

Clinical clues

Diagnosis of a case of neonatal erythroderma is mostly clinical. However, misdiagnosis of the underlying condition is frequent because of the common clinical presentation of erythroderma. Some conditions present initially with bullae and erosions (wet disorders), whereas scaling is the primary finding in others (dry disorders). Neonates with wet disorders like SSSS, CCC, and EI often become scaly following rupture of bullae and subsequent drying up of the erosions. Flowchart 18.1 presents the diagnostic clues to various underlying causes of neonatal erythroderma based on the cutaneous features at presentation [2,5–7].

Often systemic involvements may be associated with erythroderma and point to the diagnosis of underlying disorder. Flowchart 18.2 presents the systemic clues to the underlying causes of erythroderma [2,5–7].

Investigations

Laboratory investigations are supportive to clinical diagnosis in neonatal erythroderma.

BEDSIDE LABORATORY PROCEDURES

A few simple bedside laboratory procedures may be helpful in the diagnosis of some cases of neonatal erythroderma. These are presented in Table 18.4 [2,5–7].

SKIN BIOPSY AND HISTOPATHOLOGY

Histopathology of skin is not diagnostic in all cases of neonatal erythroderma. However, early skin biopsy and histopathological examination are imperative to detect suggestive findings if there are any [2,5–7].

BIOCHEMICAL AND HEMATOLOGICAL INVESTIGATIONS

Biochemical and hematological investigations have a supportive role in the diagnosis of neonatal erythroderma. Table 18.5 presents the list of these investigations helpful in etiological diagnosis [2,5–7]. Complete hemogram is imperative in all cases where systemic involvement is suspected as well as in neonatal infections. Serum electrolytes should be estimated when NS is a diagnostic possibility to detect hypernatremia at an early stage [2,5]. Estimation of the serum IgE level is helpful in conditions with eczematous skin lesions. If hereditary metabolic disorders are suspected, a panel of plasma amino acid level and urinary organic acid levels is to be estimated [6,7]. However, these tests may not be available in routine neonatal setup and can be performed at specialized centers.

Neonates with erythroderma due to conditions like nonsyndromic congenital ichthyosis and psoriasis do not require any biochemical and hematological investigation at the outset. However, the clinical course of a case of neonatal erythroderma may be complicated at any point of patient

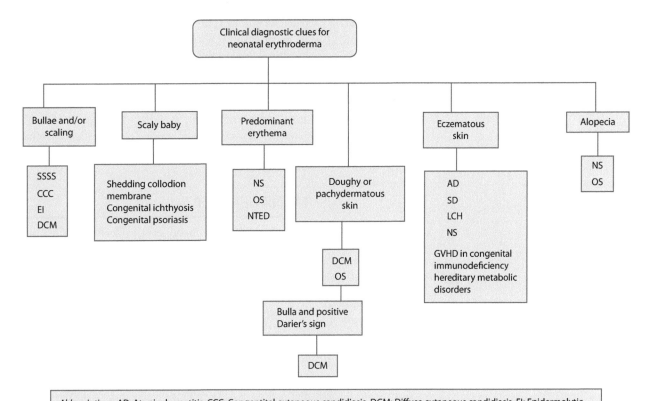

Flowchart 18.1 Clinical diagnostic clues in neonatal erythroderma. (From Dhar S et al. *Indian J Dermatol* 2012;57:475–8; Hoeger PH, Harper JI. *Arch Dis Child* 1998;79:186–91; Fraitag S, Bodemer C. *Curr Opin Pediatr* 2010;22:438–44; Bedocs LA et al. *Neo Reviews* 2011;12:e325–33.)

care due to gross cutaneous barrier dysfunction, infective complications, and metabolic disturbances. In such situations, serial monitoring of biochemical and hematological parameters is necessary. Increased total leukocyte count is indicative of sepsis.

MICROBIOLOGICAL INVESTIGATIONS

When the underlying cause of erythroderma is infection (SSSS, NTED, CCC), isolation of the organism by culture may be attempted if there is any primary focus. Umbilical stump, genitalia, maternal vaginal canal (high up), or

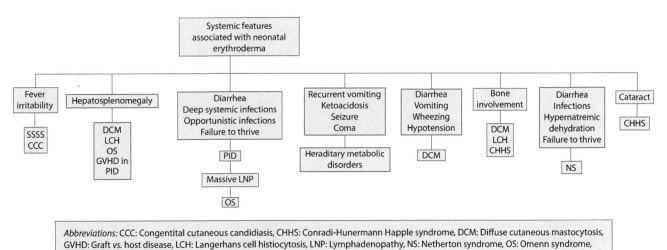

Flowchart 18.2 Systemic involvement in neonatal erythroderma. (From Dhar S et al. *Indian J Dermatol* 2012;57:475–8; Hoeger PH, Harper JI. *Arch Dis Child* 1998;79:186–91; Fraitag S, Bodemer C. *Curr Opin Pediatr* 2010;22:438–44; Bedocs LA et al. *Neo Reviews* 2011;12:e325–33.)

Table 18.4 Various bedside laboratory procedures helpful in the diagnosis of neonatal erythroderma

Procedure	Result	Underlying condition
Tzanck smear	Acantholytic cells	Staphylococcal scalded skin syndrome
Potassium hydroxide preparation from skin lesions, umbilical cord of newborn and placenta, and high vaginal swab of mother	Pseudohyphae and spores	Congenital cutaneous candidiasis
Light microscopy of hair (scalp/eyebrow/eyelashes)	Trichorrhexis invaginata	Netherton syndrome

Source: Dhar S et al. Indian J Dermatol 2012;57:475–8; Hoeger PH, Harper JI. Arch Dis Child 1998;79:186–91; Fraitag S, Bodemer C. Curr Opin Pediatr 2010;22:438–44; Bedocs LA et al. Neo Reviews 2011;12:e325–33.

Table 18.5 Biochemical and hematological tests helpful in the diagnosis of neonatal erythroderma

High serum IgE level and eosinophilia	Netherton syndrome, Omenn syndrome, atopic dermatitis
Neutrophilia	Staphylococcal scalded skin syndrome, neonatal toxic shock syndrome–like exanthematous disease, congenital cutaneous candidiasis
Thrombocytopenia	Langerhans cell histiocytosis, neonatal toxic shock syndrome–like exanthematous disease
Lymphopenia	Congenital immunodeficiency syndromes
Hypoproteinemia	Omenn syndrome
Low serum bicarbonate level: acidosis	Hereditary metabolic disorders
Serum electrolytes: hypernatremia	Netherton syndrome
Raised plasma amino acids, high urinary organic acids, urinary ketone bodies	Hereditary metabolic syndromes

Source: Dhar S et al. Indian J Dermatol 2012;57:475–8; Hoeger PH, Harper JI. Arch Dis Child 1998;79:186–91; Fraitag S, Bodemer C. Curr Opin Pediatr 2010;22:438–44; Bedocs LA et al. Neo Reviews 2011;12:e325–33.

placenta may bear the evidence of primary infection [14,19]. In premature neonates with CCC, blood, urine, and cerebrospinal fluid samples should be cultured to rule out invasive infection by Candida. In the presence of sepsis in an erythrodermic neonate, repeated culture sensitivity test from the fissures on skin or blood culture may be necessary as and when indicated.

Other disease-specific specialized investigations that can confirm the diagnosis of certain disorders are presented in Table 18.6 [2,5–7].

MANAGEMENT

Management of neonatal erythroderma is difficult and requires devoted care from dermatologists and neonatologists. The two challenges are the very young age of the patient and disruption of the cutaneous barrier.

General measures

Management in a neonatal intensive care unit is compulsory, and stringent maintenance of ambient temperature and humidity is essential. This minimizes transepidermal water loss in erythrodermic neonates, especially preterm babies. Close monitoring of fluid and electrolyte balance and maintenance of intake-output chart are necessary. Vital parameters to be monitored in an erythrodermic neonate are presented in Box 18.1 [5–7].

Collodion baby and erythroderma due to congenital ichthyoses present with eclabium, making breastfeeding and

Table 18.6 Confirmatory tests for diagnosis of certain disorders causing neonatal erythroderma

Disorder	Confirmatory test
Netherton syndrome	• LEKTI immunostaining of skin specimen • SPINK5 mutation analysis
Severe combined immunodeficiency	• RAG1 and 2 mutation analysis (null mutation)
Omenn syndrome	• Lymphocyte subset profile; lack of B cells and aberrant expansion of oligoclonal T cells (TH2 subtype) • RAG1 and 2 mutation analysis (hypomorphic mutation)
Bullous epidermolytic ichthyosis	• Keratin (K5 and K10) mutation analysis
Hereditary metabolic disorders	• Metabolic analysis of cultured fibroblasts

Source: Dhar S et al. Indian J Dermatol 2012;57:475–8; Hoeger PH, Harper JI. Arch Dis Child 1998;79:186–91; Fraitag S, Bodemer C. Curr Opin Pediatr 2010;22:438–44; Bedocs LA et al. Neo Reviews 2011;12:e325–33.

BOX 18.1: Monitoring a neonate with erythroderma

- Pulse, blood pressure, respiratory rate
- Body temperature
- Fluid input and level of hydration
- Urine output
- Level of consciousness (alert with good reflexes or lethargic)
- Evidence of cutaneous infection (skin fissures, umbilical stump, genitalia)
- Evidence of systemic infection (pulmonary, meningeal)

Source: Hoeger PH, Harper JI. *Arch Dis Child* 1998;79:186–91; Fraitag S, Bodemer C. *Curr Opin Pediatr* 2010;22:438–44; Bedocs LA et al. *Neo Reviews* 2011;12:e325–33.

assisted feeding difficult. Neonates with hereditary metabolic disorders are usually lethargic and refuse feeding. These babies require assisted feeding through nasogastric tubes.

Ectropion is a common association in erythrodermic neonates, especially in conditions associated with scaling. Frequent lubrication of the eyes with artificial tears and protective eye pads or shields are to be used to prevent exposure keratitis.

Flexion contracture of digits and limbs are common in these children, which can be prevented by frequent gentle passive movements. In neonates with adherent collodion membrane or severe erythroderma due to congenital ichthyosis, restriction in chest movement may occur; these babies should be observed for respiratory distress. Accumulated scales in the external nares and auditory canal may result in blockage and require periodical cleaning.

Daily cleansing is necessary, especially the flexures, genitalia, and perianal areas to minimize colonization by pathogenic organisms.

Use of long adhesive tapes for fixation of various gadgets (intravenous canula, nasogastric tube) to the skin of neonates with SSSS and EI should be avoided as these babies have fragile skin; either short strips of adhesive tapes or roller bandage can be used if the situation permits.

BOX 18.2: Indications of systemic retinoid therapy in neonatal erythroderma due to congenital ichthyoses

1. Severe ectropion and eclabium causing difficulty in feeding
2. Respiratory distress due to adherent, taut collodion membrane on thoracic region
3. Flexion contractures of digits and limbs

Excessive handling, rubbing, and cuddling should be avoided in neonates with DCM. Such stimulations may induce flushing episodes and bullae formation in these babies.

Specific treatment

TOPICAL

Bland emollients like white soft paraffin should be applied all over in neonates with ichthyotic and eczematous skin conditions several times a day. In the presence of large erosions resulting from rupture of bullae, the denuded areas can be covered with liquid paraffin embedded gauze dressings.

Psoriasis and eczematous conditions like atopic and seborrheic dermatitis are mostly treated with mild topical corticosteroids like hydrocortisone. Caution should be undertaken to prevent enhanced absorption of topical corticosteroids due to the damaged cutaneous barrier. Topical tacrolimus ointment (0.03%) can be used in addition in some cases with atopic dermatitis. The latter agent should never be used in erythrodermic neonates where NS is a diagnostic possibility; a very high serum concentration of tacrolimus may be attained in these babies due to the damaged skin barrier [5–7].

SYSTEMIC

Neonatal erythroderma due to infections are treatable and curable. SSSS and NTED are treated with an IV antistaphylococcal antibiotic such as cloxacillin [5–7]. If MRSA is isolated, vancomycin is the drug of choice [5–7]. CCC is treated with systemic antifungal agents such as oral fluconazole or in severe cases with IV amphotericin B. Topical clotrimazole cream can be added to a systemic regimen.

Disabling erythroderma due to congenital ichthyosis requires treatment with systemic retinoids, either isotretinoin or acitretin (0.5–1 mg/kg). Indications of starting systemic retinoids in these patients are presented in Box 18.2.

Neonates with erythroderma due to DCM are treated with a combination of histamine receptor (H1 and H2) blockers. Oral sodium chromoglycate can also be used [6]. Potential mast-cell degranulating drugs must be avoided in these patients [6].

Superficial and deep pyogenic infections in primary immunodeficiency disorders, OS, and NS are treated with appropriate antibiotics. If blood transfusion is required for the neonates with SCID and OS, irradiated blood must always be used to prevent a chance of occurrence of GVHD [5,6]. Bone marrow transplantation is the specific therapy for OS [5,6].

CONCLUSION

It is difficult to reach a definitive diagnosis of erythroderma in neonates. Persistent collodion membrane and congenital ichthyosis are the most common causes of erythroderma present at birth. Infective causes prevail within a few days to 2 weeks of life. Hereditary metabolic disorders

---

KEY POINTS

- Erythroderma due to staphylococcal scalded skin syndrome in premature neonates may be recurrent in spite of complete antibiotic therapy.
- Premature neonates with erythroderma due to congenital cutaneous candidiasis require blood, urine, and cerebrospinal fluid culture to rule out invasive infection.
- Erythroderma with predominant systemic features at presentation may be indicative of rare hereditary metabolic disorders or primary immunodeficiency disorders.
- A combination of consistent presence of erythroderma, pachydermatous skin, and near total lack of scalp and body hair are the clinical pointers to the diagnosis of Omenn syndrome.
- Generalized eczematous rash rather than scaling with periorificial accentuation is a clinical pointer to rare organic acidemias, and the neonate should be screened accordingly. In a neonate with erythroderma if Netherton syndrome is a diagnostic possibility, serum electrolytes are to be estimated to rule out hypernatremia.

---

and primary immunodeficiency disorders are distinct by predominant systemic features. A close look at the erythrodermic neonate may provide clinical clues to the diagnosis. Histopathological examinations of skin and laboratory tests are helpful in some cases. A collaborative approach is essential for effective management of the baby. Prognosis is better in infective conditions and nonsyndromic group of ichthyosis. Preterm baby and systemic involvement are the two poor prognostic factors irrespective of the underlying cause.

REFERENCES

1. Ingram JR. Eczematous disorders. In: Griffiths C, Barker J, Bleiker T, Chalmers R, Creamer D (Eds), *Rook's Textbook of Dermatology*. Volume 2. 9th ed. Oxford: Wiley Blackwell; 2016:39.1–35.
2. Dhar S, Banerjee R, Malakar R. Neonatal erythroderma: Diagnostic and therapeutic challenges. *Indian J Dermatol* 2012;57:475–8.
3. Sarkar R, Sharma RC, Koranne RV, Sardana K. Erythroderma in children: A clinico-etiological study. *J Dermatol* 1999;26:509–11.
4. Pruskowski A, Bodemer C, Fraitag S, Teillac-Hamel D, Amoric JC, deProst Y. Neonatal and infantile erythroderma: A retrospective study of 51 patients. *Arch Dermatol* 2000;136:875–80.
5. Hoeger PH, Harper JI. Neonatal erythroderma: Differential diagnosis and management of the "red baby." *Arch Dis Child* 1998;79:186–91.
6. Fraitag S, Bodemer C. Neonatal erythroderma. *Curr Opin Pediatr* 2010;22:438–44.
7. Bedocs LA, O'Regan GM, Bruckner AL. Red scaly babies: Neonatal erythroderma. *Neo Reviews* 2011;12:e325–33.
8. Davidson J, Polly S, Hayes PJ, Talati AJ, Patel T. Recurrent staphylococcal scalded skin syndrome in an extremely low-birth-weight neonate. *AJP Rep* 2017;7(2):e134–7.
9. De D, Dogra S. Erythroderma in children. In: Inamadar AC, Palit A, Ragunatha S (Eds), *Textbook of Pediatric Dermatology*. 2nd ed. New Delhi: Jaypee Brothers Medical Publishers; 2014:373–80.
10. Rieger-Fackeldey E, Plano L R, Kramer A, Schulze A. Staphylococcal scalded skin syndrome related to an exfoliative toxin A- and B-producing strain in preterm infants. *Eur J Pediatr* 2002;161(12):649–52.
11. Kapoor V, Travadi J, Braye S. Staphylococcal scalded skin syndrome in an extremely premature neonate: A case report with a brief review of literature. *J Paediatr Child Health* 2008;44(6):374–6.
12. Duijsters CE, Halbertsma FJ, Kornelisse RF, Arents NL, Andriessen P. Recurring staphylococcal scalded skin syndrome in a very low birth weight infant: A case report. *J Med Case Reports* 2009;3(1):7313.
13. Saida K et al. Exfoliative toxin A staphylococcal scalded skin syndrome in preterm infants. *Eur J Pediatr* 2015;174(4):551–5.
14. Loughead JL. Congenital staphylococcal scalded skin syndrome: Report of a case. *Pediatr Infect Dis J* 1992;11:413–4.
15. Dancer SJ, Simmons NA, Poston SM, Noble WC. Outbreak of staphylococcal scalded skin syndrome among neonates. *J Infect* 1988;16:87–103.
16. Hörner A et al. Staphylococcal scalded skin syndrome in a premature newborn caused by methicillin-resistant *Staphylococcus aureus*: Case report. *Sao Paulo Med J* 2015;133:450–3.
17. Kaga A, Watanabe H, Miyabayashi H, Metoki T, Kitaoka S, Kumaki S. A term infant of neonatal toxic shock syndrome-like exanthematous disease complicated with hemophagocytic syndrome. *Tohoku J Exp Med* 2016;240:167–70.
18. Paller AS, Mancini AJ. Bacterial, mycobacterial, and protozoal infections of the skin. In: Paller AS, Mancini AJ (Eds), *Hurwitz Clinical Pediatric Dermatology*. 4th ed. Edinburgh: Elsevier Saunders; 2011:321–47.
19. Darmstadt G, Dinulos J, Miller Z. Congenital cutaneous candidiasis: Clinical presentation, pathogenesis and management guidelines. *Pediatrics* 2000;105:438–44.
20. Smolinski K, Shah S, Honig P, Yan A. Neonatal cutaneous fungal infections. *Curr Opin Pediatr* 2005;17:486–93.

21. Oji V et al. Revised nomenclature and classification of inherited ichthyosis: Results of the first ichthyosis consensus conference in Soréze 2009. *J Am Acad Dermatol* 2010;63:607–41.

22. Salleras M, Sanche-Regana M, Umbert P. Congenital erythrodermic psoriasis: Case report and literature review. *Pediatr Dermatol* 1995;12:231–4.

23. Menni S, Piccinno R, Baietta S, CiuVreda A, Scotti L. Infantile seborrheic dermatitis: A seven year follow-up and some prognostic criteria. *Pediatr Dermatol* 1989;6:13–5.

24. Tran TH, Pope E, Weitzman S. Cutaneous histiocytoses. In: Griffiths C, Barker J, Bleiker T, Chalmers R, Creamer D (Eds), *Rook's Textbook of Dermatology*. Volume 4. 9th ed. Oxford: Wiley Blackwell; 2016:136.1–29.

25. Gniadecki R. The skin and disorders of the haemato-poietic and immune systems. In: Griffiths C, Barker J, Bleiker T, Chalmers R, Creamer D (Eds), *Rook's Textbook of Dermatology*. Volume 4. 9th ed. Oxford: Wiley Blackwell;2016:148.1–19.

26. Dyke MP, Marlow N, Berry PJ. Omenn's disease. *Arch Dis Child* 1991;66:1247–8.

27. Inamadar AC, Palit A. Acrodermatitis enteropath-ica-like eruptions: many faces, one expression. In: Inamadar AC, Palit A (Eds), *Advances in Pediatric Dermatology*. New Delhi: Jaypee Brothers Medical Publishers; 2011:234–48.

19

Collodion baby and harlequin ichthyosis

D. V. LAKSHMI AND SAHANA M. SRINIVAS

INTRODUCTION

Congenital ichthyosis (CI) is an inherited heterogenous group of cornification disorders characterized by excessive scaling and desquamation of the skin. It can be an isolated entity or syndromic, often posing a diagnostic challenge for clinicians. The collodion baby and harlequin fetus are phenotypic forms of CI, a mere outlook of underlying primary ichthyosiform disorder. Both collodion and harlequin fetus are high-risk newborns to be nursed in intensive care during the neonatal period due to a disrupted skin barrier that worsens the physiologically fragile skin of the newborn. Thus, a primary genodermatosis with skin barrier dysfunction manifesting at birth is a call for intensive care and intervention.

COLLODION BABY

Introduction

The term *collodion baby* (CB) refers to a phenotypic entity and not a specific disease per se. It is defined as a phenotypic presentation of a newborn encased by a membrane that is inelastic, translucent, and tight, and has a parchment-like sheet of skin on the entire body surface that eventually detaches to unveil underlying ichthyosiform genodermatosis. It is so named for its resemblance to a dried film of "collodion," a sticky brown nitrocellulose solution in ether and alcohol used previously as a wound sealant. *Collodion baby* as a term was coined by Hallopeau and Watelet in 1892 [1–3].

Etiopathogenesis

The collodion membrane occurs due to a genetic defect in epidermal cornification, keratinocyte protein, and lipid metabolism. Autosomal recessive congenital ichthyosis (ARCI) and nonbullous congenital ichthyosiform erythroderma are seen in the majority of infants due to a defect in the transglutaminase 1 gene (TGM1) mutation localized on chromosome 14q11 [4]. Moreover, five different gene localizations have been detected in ARCI. Lipoxygenases gene (ALOX 12B, ALOXE3), ATP-binding cassette transporter (ABCA12), and ichthyin receptor and a cytochrome p450 family member FLJ39501 are the newer genes detected. Approximately 80% of ARCI is due to involvement of these six genes [5–9].

TGM1 is an enzyme responsible for cross-linking proteins in the cornified cell envelope, and lipoxygenases are a group of dioxygenase enzymes involved in lipid metabolism of lamellar granules or intercellular lipid lamellae in epidermis. Different combinations of TGM1 mutations causing phenotypic variations with respect to severity have also been reported [5]. Ichthyin acts as a receptor for the hepoxilin pathway that leads to abnormalities of the granular layer of the epidermis and abnormal lamellar granules [8]. In a self-healing collodion membrane, compound heterozygous transglutaminase mutation ALOXE3 and ALOX12B genes have been found [10].

Causes of collodion baby

The causes are listed in Table 19.1.

Clinical features

Collodion babies are usually premature at birth. The membrane is a glistening, taut, inelastic sheet with obliteration of normal skin markings (Figures 19.1 and 19.2). It is also described as "sausage or plastic skin," "cling-film-like" or dipped in a wax appearance. It covers the entire skin surface

Table 19.1 Causes of collodion baby

- Autosomal recessive congenital ichthyoses (ARCI) (lamellar ichthyosis, congenital ichthyosiform erythroderma [nonbullous form])
- Epidermolytic hyperkeratosis (bullous congenital ichthyosiform erythroderma)
- Sjögren-Larsson syndrome
- Self-healing collodion baby
- Neutral lipid storage disease
- Trichothiodystrophy
- Annular epidermolytic erythema
- Loricrin keratoderma
- X-linked hypohydrotic ectodermal dysplasia
- Type 2 Gaucher disease [11]
- Neu-Laxova syndrome [12]
- Conradi-Hünermann-Happle syndrome
- Netherton syndrome [13]
- Hay-Wells syndrome
- Holocarboxylase deficiency [14]

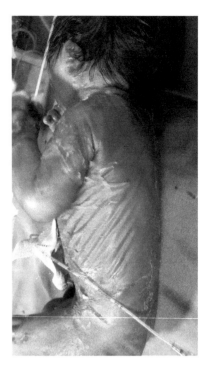

Figure 19.2 Collodion membrane and deformed ears. (Photo courtesy of Dr. Rachana Shekar.)

fissuring postnatally. The fissuring is more at the flexures and around the joints. It peels off completely by 2–4 weeks, but the epidermal barrier dysfunction will be present (Figures 19.3 and 19.4). It may be persistent for up to 3 months in a few neonates. The residual skin gradually becomes dry and

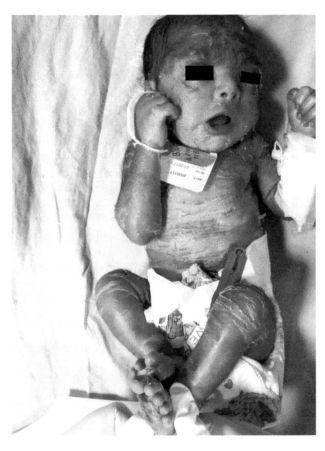

Figure 19.1 Collodion baby: Parchment-like membrane-encased neonate. Also note the ectropion. (Photo courtesy of Dr. Rachana Shekar.)

minimally limiting the respiration, body movements, and sucking function of the neonate; otherwise the general condition of the neonate is usually normal. But, the membrane is inelastic, so respiration and body movements provoke

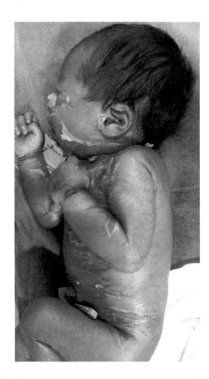

Figure 19.3 Peeling of collodion membrane of the baby in Figure 19.1. Also note the normalcy of the ear in due course. (Photo courtesy of Dr. Rachana Shekar.)

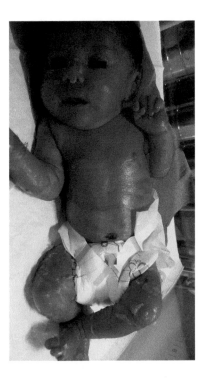

Figure 19.4 Resolution of collodion membrane of baby in Figure 19.1. The ectropion is improving. (Photo courtesy of Dr. Rachana Shekar.)

tough, but the tight membrane on the limbs may lead to constriction bands, pseudocontractures, and loss of function. Sausage-shaped swelling of the digits is also not uncommon.

The eyelids and the lips may be everted and tethered leading to ectropion and eclabion, respectively (Figure 19.5). The chronic ectropion state leads to exposure keratitis due to xerophthalmia and eventually blindness. There may be obliteration of nasal passages. The pinnae may be flattened due to the deforming action of the membrane on the soft auricular cartilage. As the child grows up, the primary diseases that have caused the collodion baby begin to manifest.

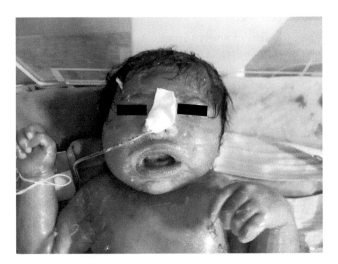

Figure 19.5 Collodion baby: Fish mouth appearance and ectropion.

Variations in collodion membrane

The collodion membrane at the time of presentation can vary in form from the conventional, generalized form. Varied forms include the following:

1. Collodion babies may not develop any ichthyosiform dermatosis, and this is then termed a *self-healing collodion baby/lamellar ichthyosis of the newborn*. Because many of these patients, when reexamined later in childhood or as adults, have a variable degree of anhidrosis, heat intolerance, and mild signs of ichthyosis such as xerosis and fine desquamation, particularly in the axillary and neck regions, the term *self-improving collodion ichthyosis* may be more appropriate.
2. An acral self-healing collodion membrane is confined to the extremities.
3. Segmental collodion membranes are seen in Conradi-Hunermann syndrome.
4. A collodion membrane may be followed by isolated palmoplantar keratoderma.
5. An incomplete or localized collodion membrane may peel away and reform with the same pattern over a period of weeks.

Complications and prognosis

The collodion membrane, though it clears in a few weeks, can cause neonatal complications in 45% of cases, leading to mortality in up to 11% in the first few weeks of life [15]. The skin of a collodion baby is prone to transepidermal water loss (TEWL), six times more than TEWL in normal skin [16]. This leads to fluid and electrolyte imbalances. Newborn collodion babies are at a higher risk of hypernatremic dehydration and hypothermia. The metabolic complications can also lead to renal failure and neurological damage.

Difficulties with sucking and breathing lead to hypoxia with risk for aspiration pneumonia from amniotic debris. Constrictive bands form around the extremities and digits, which impairs blood circulation. The cutaneous fissures and erosions can get secondarily infected and lead to sepsis. Due to a barrier defect, increased use of topical medications may result in drug toxicity.

Differentials

1. *Chrysalis babies*: These babies have intermediate features of collodion and harlequin ichthyosis.
2. *Harlequin ichthyosis*: The neonate will have armor-like plate adherent scales with grotesque appearance. It is a lethal autosomal recessive condition.
3. *Restrictive dermopathy or stiff baby syndrome*: This presents as thick, taut, tethered skin that does not dessicate in the neonatal period. The prognosis is poor, and the child succumbs early due to respiratory failure.

Table 19.2 Sample format for evaluation of a collodion baby

1. Day of life: Sex:	Informant:..		
	Maternal history:............	Obstetric index:......................	
	Chronic maternal illness if any:		Consanguinity:............
Antenatal history:	Birth history:	Method of delivery:	Pedigree charting:
Antenatal ultrasonography Findings if available:	If Preterm:	Postnatal events: Feeding:	Family history of ichthyosis:
	Current presenting dermatological complaints:		
	Examination findings:		
Look for syndromic associations:			
Sample collected for examination: (e.g., hair for microscopy, blood samples of parents and neonate, skin biopsy for gene testing)			
Provisional diagnosis:			

Evaluation of collodion baby

HISTORY TAKING

The chart provided in Table 19.2 is a sample format that can be useful prior to a walk into the intensive care unit. Clinical clues that help in early diagnosis are a positive history of ichthyosiform disorder in other sibling(s), consanguinity between parents, and another keratotic cutaneous disorder in other children. Consanguineous families may have a higher incidence of an affected newborn "higher hit rate" than anticipated in autosomal recessive inheritance.

Laboratory investigations

BASELINE COMPLETE HEMOGRAM AND ESTIMATION OF SERUM ELECTROLYTES

Baseline investigations should be done in all neonates, as they help to treat underlying electrolyte disturbances accordingly and prevent overcorrection and fluid overload.

Estimation of renal functions: Blood urea nitrogen, creatinine, and urine output.
Estimation of liver functions and serum lipid levels: It is particularly of importance if retinoid therapy is to be instituted.
Total protein, albumin
Skin surface cultures
Vitamin D level estimation
Skin biopsy for histopathology

Light microscopy and special stains

Light microscopic examination of the skin specimens of a neonate with a collodion membrane in the early phase shows an eosinophilic, periodic acid schiff (PAS)-positive stratum corneum with hyperkeratosis. The granular layer is reduced causing attenuation of the epidermis. The rest of the dermal components are unremarkable.

Electron microscopy

Electron microscopy reveals dense intracytoplasmic granules and convoluted corneocytes with prominent nuclear debris in the upper portion of the stratum corneum. The thinned granular layer is structurally normal. Lamellar bodies are numerous in the intercellular space with well-preserved desmosomes. Frenk et al. found that evaluation of ultrastructural changes at day 1 and intermittently at day 15 can help in determining the prognosis [17]. This can help to distinguish the self-healing variant from ichthyotic outcomes. The self-healing form shows normal ultrastructural changes, whereas the ichthyotic form may show changes in the stratum corneum, keratohyaline granules, and tonofilaments.

GENE TESTING

The diagnosis of nonsyndromic ARCI is difficult to establish by skin findings at birth in the collodion baby. A multigene panel that includes 12 known genes associated with ARCI is ideal [18]. It is found that 15% of affected families may not have these known genes. If unavailable, single-gene testing can be considered starting with *ABCA12* in individuals with harlequin ichthyosis, *TGM1* in individuals with ARCI without harlequin presentation at birth, and *SLC27A4* in those presenting with ichthyosis-prematurity syndrome.

HARLEQUIN ICHTHYOSIS

Harlequin ichthyosis (HI) is the most devastating form of ARCI. HI presents at birth with severely thickened, plate-like scales and grooved skin over the entire body, significantly distorting surface features and causing movement restriction. The disease incidence is estimated to be 1 in 300,000 births [19]. In 1750, the first case who suffered from thickened and cracked skin over the whole body was reported by Reverend Oliver Hart in his diary that was published in 1932 [20]. Harlequin refers to the resemblance of facial features and diamond-shaped scales to the comic servant character costume [21].

Pathogenesis

The pathogenesis of the disease is attributed to structural and functional default of keratin, filaggrin, and the lamellar body. These are the main elements of the stratum corneum. Abnormal localization of epidermal lipids, abnormalities of keratinocyte nuclei, and distorted ultrastructure of lamellar granules lead to hyperkeratosis with hypergranulosis and parakeratosis of the epidermis, suggesting that the process of terminal differentiation is incomplete [22]. Alterations in protein phosphatase activity and calcium-mediated signaling are also implicated [23,24]. The causative genes were filaggrin, claudins, PP2A, and calpain 1 for the array of cellular phenotypes in HI. Also, in another study, the occurrence of serine-threonine protein phosphatase enzyme deficiency related to protein phosphatase gene mutations localized on the 11th chromosome were noted as another possible cause of this disease [24].

ROLE OF ABCA12 IN HARLEQUIN ICHTHYOSIS

In 2005, a Japanese dermatologist identified ABCA12 on chromosome 2q35 as the causative gene in HI on the basis of the principle of homozygosity. ABCA12 is a lipid transporter from the Golgi apparatus to the lamellar granule in differentiated keratinocyte, and the lack of ABCA12 leads to a marked reduction of lipid content in the horny layer, premature keratinocyte differentiation, and defective secretion of lipids from the lamellar granules into the extracellular space. In HI epidermis, the expression of kallikrein 5 and cathepsin D proteases was also found to be reduced [25,26].

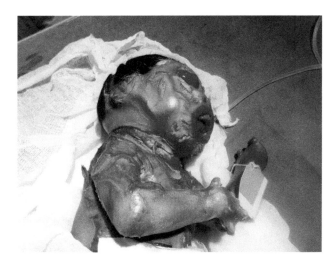

Figure 19.7 Armor-like scales and deep fissures.

Clinical features

The neonate is usually premature and encased in a hyperkeratotic coat of armor, which is a thick, yellow-brown, firmly adherent, plaque covering the entire body surface (Figure 19.6). The armor is taut and inflexible. It splits causing deeper fissures into the dermis (Figure 19.7). The facial appearance is distorted with nasal hypoplasia, ectropion, eclabium, and lack of external ears (Figure 19.8). The skull may be microcephalic. The ears are flattened because of the loss of skin elasticity and thus appear rudimentary (Figure 19.9). The scalp feels boggy. The hands and feet may be encased within hyperkeratotic casts like a mitten or a membrane (Figure 19.10). This may lead to digital necrosis. Other signs are hypoplastic digits including absence of nails, pseudo-contractures, and restricted joint mobility.

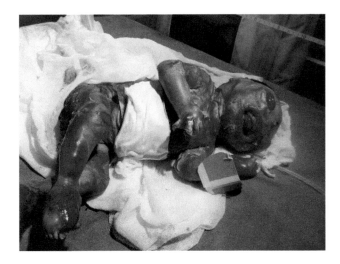

Figure 19.6 Harlequin fetus.

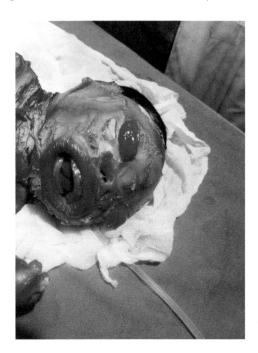

Figure 19.8 Fish mouth appearance.

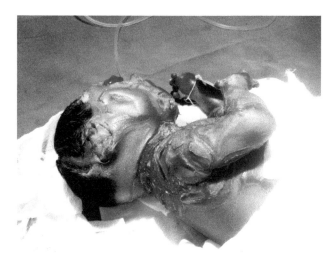

Figure 19.9 Deformed ears.

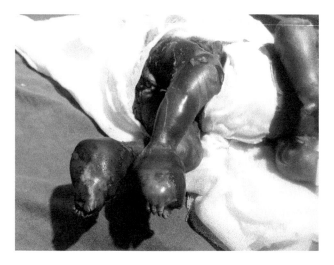

Figure 19.10 Mitten extremities and contractures at the lower leg causing foot edema.

The cast may shed to leave erythrodermic skin, and NBIE may develop.

Investigations

HISTOPATHOLOGY

The epidermis shows compact hyperkeratosis, hypergranulosis with parakeratosis. The hyperkeratosis extends to involve the follicular epithelium and pilosebaceous units. The stratum basale and spinosum appear normal, though vacuolization can be seen. Papillomatosis and dermal infiltration may be present but rare.

ELECTRON MICROSCOPY

Ultrastructurally, HI epidermis showed lamellar granule abnormalities. Reported morphological abnormalities include abnormal lamellar granules in the granular layer keratinocytes and lack of extracellular lipid lamellae in the stratum corneum, which leads to defective lipid transport by lamellar granules and disruption of intercellular lipid layers.

It shows vacuoles, lipid droplets, and cellular remnants in corneocytes. The spinous and granular layer shows the absence or reduction of lamellar bodies. The intercellular lipid lamellae are also not well formed at the junction of granulosum and corneum.

Complications

These babies have serious complications including hypothermia and hyperthermia, dehydration, absence of effective sucking, respiratory difficulty, hypoventilation, poor feeding, hypernatremia, seizures, and skin infection.

Prognosis of harlequin fetus

The outcome is poor in these infants owing to stillbirth and early neonatal death. There have been reports of few favorable outcomes. Thus, with every right to survival, if an intensive support system is available, a care plan should be drawn in every case.

A survival rate of 56% has been reported and is expected to further increase with improved neonatal intensive care and treatment options, such as early topical and/or systemic retinoids [27]. Surviving children eventually shed this armor and develop generalized scaling and intense redness of the skin (erythroderma, severe chronic idiopathic erythroderma–like phenotype). Harlequin ichthyosis remains a serious and chronic skin disorder, and severe ectropion, eclabium, alopecia, palmoplantar keratoderma with painful fissures and digital contractures, and growth delay are common.

TREATMENT OF COLLODION AND HARLEQUIN BABIES

Intensive care is largely supportive in these neonates and involves a multidisciplinary team of neonatologist, dermatologist, genetics, ophthalmologist, otolaryngologist, orthopedic specialist and nursing team. It is indeed extremely important to counsel the parents that the striking physical appearance is transient. Because of significant mortality, especially in HI, it is essential to discuss the treatment protocol (e.g., ventilatory support, retinoids, potential risk of demise) with parents.

The main principles in management include

1. Treatment of manifestations
2. Prevention of secondary complications
3. Avoidance of irritants
4. Surveillance and follow-up
5. Genetic counseling

Treatment of manifestations and secondary complications

1. *Fluid and electrolytes*: In collodion babies fluid and electrolyte balance and temperature are to be monitored

periodically; monitor serum electrolytes, urine output, and daily weight gain/loss. Serum albumin, creatinine, and blood urea nitrogen levels should be periodically estimated. Monitoring of daily weight is needed.

2. *Humid environment*: Humidified incubators help in providing a temperature-controlled, humidified environment that decreases the degree of TEWL. The humidity in incubator settings often ranges from 40% to 60%, though 90% to 100% is also advocated. Gradually taper incubator humidity to an ambient humidity of the neonatal intensive care unit, so it can be well tolerated. The newborn should be maintained in an incubator for at least 4 weeks or until the membrane sheds. However, if the neonate is stable, it can be shifted to an open crib earlier [28–30]. If there is respiratory failure, ventilatory support may be needed. In HI, transfer to a nonhumidified environment can be instituted early as humidity can increase skin colonization with pseudomonas.

3. *Emollients*: Bland emollients need to be applied frequently and liberally. They should be applied postfeed and after a diaper change. Frequent emollient application can help in débridement of scales. Application of keratolytic-containing emollients should be avoided due to percutaneous absorption and toxicity. Topical ceramide containing emollients has not shown to improve barrier function, though ceramides can stimulate ABCA12 expression through PPARδ receptors [31].

Avoid first bath, avoid manual débridement of scales, and encourage aseptic handling of the neonate to reduce risk of infection. Daily buffered dilute hypochlorite baths have been suggested. This is done by dampening roll gauze with 0.125% warmed sodium hypochlorite mixed in 1:10 proportion with warmed sterile water. Gauze is applied as a wet wrap for 10–20 minutes [32,33].

Securing IV Lines: Infants have fragile skin, but securing an IV line is essential for hydration, parenteral nutrition, and laboratory sampling. It can be secured through a central venous umbilical line, peripheral scalp vein, or central catheter line.

4. *Ophthalmologic evaluation* is essential. Suitable eye care should be carried out for the collodion babies with ectropion. Lubricant ophthalmic ointment should be applied to margins of lids every 6–12 hours. They need to be followed up regularly at an eye outpatient unit. As retinoids (topical tazarotene and oral retinoids) promote desquamation of stratum corneum, it may be effective in reducing ectropion [34,35].

5. *Systemic antibacterials, antifungals, and analgesia*: The collodion and HI babies with extensive skin erosions are always at risk of infections and sepsis; therefore, suitable local and systemic antibacterial agents must be cautiously determined and initiated. Candidal infections are frequent in the fissures in the inguinal folds with high humidity as a risk factor. In cases of epidermolytic hyperkeratosis (bullous congenital ichthyosiform erythroderma) that show generalized erythema, bullae, and erosions, an antibacterial will be needed along with the standard therapy.

Serial surveillance swabs for bacterial and fungal cultures from sites (skin folds, nares, ear canals, perianal area) are to be sent daily for the first week of life and once weekly for the rest of the neonatal intensive care unit stay [36].

In HI, the fissuring is deep and often painful. This may require parenteral analgesia.

6. *Nutrition and feeding*: Increased TEWL and skin turnover increase the caloric demands. Eclabium further interferes with sucking. If sucking reflex is sufficient, oral/breast feeding should be encouraged. If poor, nasogastric tube feeding may be needed. Parenteral alimentation and enteral feed may be needed for proper calorie intake.

Vitamin D deficiency and rickets have been well established in neonates with ichthyosis. Monitoring vitamin D levels and supplementation may be necessary.

Avoidance of irritants

The drugs such as salicylic acid, lactic acid, and propylene glycol may be applied in order to remove the hyperkeratotic sheets from the skin. But in such cases with generalized lesions, particularly in newborns, it must not be forgotten that the application of salicylic acid locally in extreme doses may cause salicylic acid toxemia. Therefore, local remedy in these cases should be cautiously monitored and carried out in this way. However, in the collodion babies with localized lesions, local retinoic acid and calcipotriol treatments have been reported to be successful.

Role of retinoids

Systemic retinoids are the currently preferred oral drugs giving impressive results in cases with generalized lesions. Acitretin has been successfully used at the dose of 0.5–0.75 mg/kg/day in collodion babies. In HI, Rajpopat et al. reported 83% survival among 25 treated infants, and 92% survival among 12 infants treated with retinoids was reported by Shibata et al. In cases of lamellar ichthyosis, systemic retinoids have been begun at doses of 0.5 mg/kg/day and later the doses have been increased to 2 mg/kg/day [37].

Although harlequin fetus is rare among all the ichthyosiform diseases, without any dispute it is the most severe form. Hence, high mortality rates have been observed. Nonetheless, these rates have also declined because of systemic retinoids.

Treatment initiation within the first 7 days of life is highly recommended. Acitretin is the retinoid most often administered, though lack of commercially available liquid formulation is a major setback. Capsular acitretin is compounded, and liquid formulation is to be prepared. The acitretin dose administered is 0.5–1 mg/kg/day. It should be titrated to the lowest dose based on clinical improvement and monitoring of side effects. Retinoids not only hasten desquamation, they also improve digital, thoracic constrictions and aid in functional movement and breathing [34].

When oral retinoids cannot be tolerated, topical retinoids have been found to be beneficial. Also found useful is 0.1% tazarotene cream. It can be used successfully in older infants as oral retinoids are tapered [38].

Surveillance and monitoring for sequelae

More than 60% of infants born with a collodion membrane eventually develop ichthyosis [39]. Differentiation of ichthyosis subtypes in the neonatal period is difficult. Skin histology in the first few weeks of life is not specific and therefore not helpful. The final diagnosis emerges after weeks or months of follow-up and depends on the genetic analysis. In 2009, the first ichthyosis consensus conference was held and established an international nomenclature and classification of inherited ichthyoses: syndromic versus nonsyndromic forms. Based on this classification, once the clinical subtype is suspected, the results of genetic analyses will help to provide proper treatment and genetic counseling. In severe congenital ichthyosis, DNA-based prenatal diagnosis is possible.

More than 60% of affected CBs will develop one of the following two subtypes later in life: lamellar ichthyosis or NBIE. In 10%–20%, the membrane resolves leaving a normal appearing skin [40,41].

Genetic counseling

Genetic counseling is the process of providing individuals and families with information on the nature, inheritance, and implications of genetic disorders to help them make informed medical and personal decisions. The families need to be advised about the course and outcome. Prenatal diagnosis in future pregnancies and gene testing are recommended.

PRENATAL DIAGNOSIS

The need for prenatal diagnosis is important in congenital ichthyosis as the quality of life of patients is seriously affected in some cases. Recent advances in DNA-based prenatal diagnoses for congenital ichthyosis families by sampling chorionic villus or amniotic fluid in the earlier stages of pregnancy have been promising. These are superior to prenatal diagnoses by fetal skin biopsy [42].

Earlier, fetal skin biopsy and electron microscopy at 19–23 weeks were performed for diagnosis, but any interruption for termination at this late stage of pregnancy posed a serious threat to the fetus. After the identification of *ABCA12* as the causative gene for HI, DNA-based prenatal diagnoses by chorionic villus or amniotic fluid sampling in the first trimester are promising and also have significantly lowered iatrogenic fetal risk and reduced the burden on mothers [43]. Amniocentesis at 17 and 19 weeks is also diagnostic [44,45]. Biopsy of fetal skin can confirm the diagnosis at 20–23 weeks of gestation.

By sonography, detecting the characteristic mouth shape at 17 weeks of gestation can help in early diagnosis [46]. Other features include echogenic amniotic fluid, joint contractures, short limbs, and intrauterine growth restriction. Dense floating particles in amniotic fluid may be seen in HI and are known as the "snowflake sign" [47].

GENE TESTING

As mentioned earlier, gene testing is the newer advancement in ichthyosis identification [18]. The diagnosis of ARCI is to be first established in proband (infant). A multigene panel is the diagnostic test of choice as it helps also in evaluating syndromic forms. In harlequin ichthyosis, analysis of *ABCA12* should be performed first; in individuals with ARCI without harlequin presentation at birth, analysis of *TGM1* should be performed first.

CONCLUSION

The clinical features in a collodion baby do not predict the final diagnosis or prognosis of the underlying ichthyosis phenotype. In addition, histopathologic features of skin biopsy specimens in the first few weeks will not be useful in differentiating the different types of ichthyosis. Thus, to determine the underlying cause for the collodion membrane, a protocol must be established following the shedding of the collodion membrane for management and follow-up. It is important to note though that accurately diagnosing a collodion baby can be a difficult and long process, especially since patients may change from predominantly scaly skin to predominantly erythematous skin as they get older in age.

KEY POINTS

- Collodion baby is a phenotypic prodromal state that precedes the onset of an underlying disease condition.
- The collodion membrane is an evanescent state of the neonatal skin, yet neonatal complications can occur in 45%, with a mortality rate of ~11% in the first few weeks of life. Harlequin ichthyosis is a devastating form with significant mortality.
- Autosomal recessive congenital ichthyosis typically presents with collodion membrane or ichthyosiform erythroderma at birth.
- The severity of the ichthyosiform condition develops gradually; it cannot be predicted in the state of collodion membrane.
- The outcome of each case forms a key component for genetic counseling of the family; the scope of prenatal diagnosis is vital in future pregnancies.
- Intensive care is vital in stabilizing the neonates and requires a multidisciplinary approach.

REFERENCES

1. Hallopeau H, Watelet R. Sur une forme attenuee de la maladie dite ichthyose foetale. *Ann Derm Syph* 1892;3:149–52.

2. Cockayne EA. *Inherited abnormalities of the skin and its appendages.* London: Oxford University Press; 1933.

3. Fox GH. The alligator boy: A case of ichthyosis. *J Cutan Venereol Dis* 1884;2:97–9.

4. Rusell LJ et al. Mutations in gene for transglutaminase 1 in autosomal recessive lamellar ichthyosis. *Nat Genet* 1995;9:279–83.

5. Fischer J. Autosomal recessive congenital ichthyosis. *J Invest Dermatol* 2009;129:1319–21.

6. Jobard F et al. Lipoxygenase 3 and 12R lipoxygenase are mutated in nonbullous congenital ichthyosiform erythroderma linked to chromosome 17p13.1. *Hum Mol Genet* 2002;11:107–13.

7. Lefevre C et al. Mutations in the transporter ABCA12 are associated with lamellar ichthyosis type 2. *Hum Mol Genet* 2003;12:2369–78.

8. Lefevre C et al. Mutations in ichthyin, a new gene on chromosome 5q33 in a new form of autosomal recessive congenital ichthyosis. *Hum Mol Genet* 2004;13:2473–82.

9. Lefevre C et al. Mutation in new cytochrome p450 gene in lamellar ichthyosis type 3. *Hum Mol Genet* 2006;15:767–76.

10. Vahlquist A et al. Genotypic and clinical spectrum of self-improving collodion ichthyosis: ALOX12B, ALOXE3, and TGM1 mutation in Scandinavian patients. *J Invest Dermatol* 2010;130:438–43.

11. Ince Z et al. Gaucher disease associated with congenital ichthyosis. *Eur J Pediatr* 1995;63:854–6.

12. Hickey P et al. Neu-Laxova syndrome: A case report. *Pediatr Dermatol* 2003;20:25–7.

13. Chavanas S et al. Localization of the Netherton syndrome gene to chromosome 5q32, by linkage analysis and homozygosity mapping. *Am J Hum Genet* 2000;66:914–21.

14. Arbuckle HA, Morelli J. Holocarboxylase synthetase deficiency presenting as ichthyosis. *Pediatr Dermatol* 2006;23:142–4.

15. Chiaverini C. Congenital ichthyosis. *Ann Dermatol Venereal* 2009;136:923–34.

16. Buyse L, Graves C, Marks R, Wijeyesekera K, Alfaham M, Finlay AY. Collodion baby dehydration: The danger of high transepidermal water loss. *Br J Dermatol* 1993;129:86–8.

17. Frenk E. A spontaneously healing collodion baby: A light and electron microscopical study. *Acta Derm Venereol* 1981;61:168–71.

18. Richard G. Autosomal recessive congenital ichthyosis. 2001 January 10 [Updated 2017 May 18]. In: Adam MP et al. (Eds) *GeneReviews® [Internet].* Seattle: University of Washington; 1993–2018. https://www.ncbi.nlm.nih.gov/books/NBK1420/

19. Ahmed H, O'Toole EA. Recent advances in the genetics and management of harlequin ichthyosis. *Pediatr Dermatol* 2014;31:539–46.

20. Kouskoukis C, Minas A, Tousimis D. Ichthyosis congenital fetalis. *Int J Dermatol* 1982;21:347–8.

21. Multani AS et al. Three siblings with Harlequin ichthyosis in an Indian family. *Early Hum Dev* 1996;45:229–33.

22. Buxmann MM et al. Harlequin ichthyosis with an epidermal lipid abnormality. *Arch Dermatol* 1979;115:189–93.

23. Kam E et al. Protein phosphatase activity in human keratinocytes cultured from normal epidermis and epidermis from patients with harlequin ichthyosis. *Br J Dermatol* 1997;137:874–82.

24. Judge MR. Collodion baby and Harlequin ichthyosis. In: Harper J, Oranje A, Prose N. *Textbook of Pediatric Dermatology.* 2nd ed. Malden, MA: Blackwell; 2006:118–25.

25. Kensell DP et al. Mutations in ABCA12 underlie the severe congenital skin disease harlequin ichthyosis. *Am J Hum Genet* 2005;76:794–803.

26. Sakai K et al. Localization of ABCA12 from Golgi apparatus to lamellar granules in human upper epidermal keratinocytes. *Exp Dermatol* 2007;16:920–6.

27. O'Toole EA, Kelsell DP. Harlequin ichthyosis. In: Irvine A, Hoeger P, Yan A (Eds), *Harper Textbook of Pediatric Dermatology.* 3rd ed. Oxford: Wiley Blackwell; 2011:175.

28. Elias S, Mazur M, Sabbagha R, Esterly NB, Simpson JL. Prenatal diagnosis of harlequin ichthyosis. *Clin Genet* 1980;17:275–80.

29. Prado R, Ellis LZ, Gamble R, Funk T, Arbuckle HA, Bruckner AL. Collodion baby: An update with a focus on practical management. *J Am Acad Dermatol* 2012;67:1362–74.

30. Nguyen MA, Gelman A, Norton SA. Practical events in management of a collodion baby. *JAMA Dermatol* 2015;151:1031–2.

31. Haller JF et al. Endogenous β glucocerebrosidase activity in ABCA12 epidermis elevates ceramide levels after topical lipid application but does not restore barrier function. *J Lipid Res* 2014;55:493–503.

32. Koochek A, Choate KA, Milstone LM. Harlequin ichthyosis: Neonatal management and identification of new ABCA12 mutation. *Pediatr Dermatol* 2014;31:e63–4.

33. Milstone LM. Scaly skin and bath pH: Rediscovering baking soda. *J Am Acad Dermatol* 2010;62:885–6.

34. Digiovanna JJ, Mauro T, Milstone LM, Schmuth M, Toro JR. Systemic retinoids in the management of ichthyosis and related skin types. *Dermatol Ther (Heidelb)* 2013;26:26–38.

35. Craiglow BG, Choate KA, Milstone LM. Topical Tazarotene for the treatment of ectropion in ichthyosis. *JAMA Dermatol* 2013;149:598–600.

36. Glick JB, et al. Improved management of Harlequin ichthyosis with advances in neonatal intensive care. *Pediatrics* 2017;139(1):e20161003.

37. Tuzun Y, Iscimen A, Pehlivan O. Collodion baby. *J Turk Acad Dermatol* 2008;2:82201r.

38. Harvey HB, Shaw MG, Morell DS. Perinatal management of Harlequin ichthyosis: A case report and literature. *J Perinatol* 2010;30:66–72.

39. Aradhya SS, Srinivas SM, Hiremagalore R, Shanmukappa AG. Clinical outcome of collodion baby: A retrospective review. *Indian J Dermatol Venereol Leprol* 2013;79:553.

40. Vahlquist A et al. Genotypic and clinical spectrum of self-improving collodion ichthyosis: ALOX12B, ALOXE3, and TGM1 mutations in Scandinavian patients. *J Invest Dermatol* 2010;130:438–43.

41. Larrègue M et al. Collodion baby: 32 new case reports. *Ann Dermatol Venereol* 1986;113:773–85.

42. Akiyama M, Shimizu H. An update on molecular aspects of the non-syndromic ichthyoses. *Exp Dermatol* 2008;17:373–82.

43. Akiyama M. Updated molecular genetics and pathogenesis of ichthyoses. *Nagoya J Med Sci* 2011;73:79–90.

44. Akiyama M et al. Characteristic morphologic abnormality of harlequin ichthyosis detected in amniotic fluid cells. *J Invest Dermatol* 1994;102:210–13.

45. Akiyama M, Suzumori K, Shimizu H. Prenatal diagnosis of harlequin ichthyosis by the examination of keratinized hair canals and amniotic fluid cells at 19 weeks estimated gestation age. *Prenat Diagn* 1999;19:167–71.

46. Bongain A et al. Harlequin fetus: Three-dimensional sonographic findings and new diagnostic approach. *Ultrasound Obstet Gynecol* 2002;20:82–5.

47. Rajpopat S et al. Harlequin ichthyosis: A review of clinical and molecular findings in 45 cases. *Arch Dermatol* 2011;147:681–6.

20

Sclerema neonatorum

SWETHA MUKHERJEE AND SHEKHAR NEEMA

INTRODUCTION

Sclerema neonatorum (SN) is a rare condition with grave prognosis seen in premature neonates. It generally occurs in the first week of life and is associated with sepsis and hypothermia. The neonate presents with generalized hardening of the skin. SN was first described by Underwood in the eighteenth century [1]. Histopathological features were described by Ballyntyne [2].

EPIDEMIOLOGY

SN occurs more commonly in the premature neonate. It is predominantly seen in males.

PATHOGENESIS

The exact pathogenesis of SN is not known. Various theories have been proposed. The most widely accepted theory is of differential composition of neonatal fat from adult fat. Neonatal fat contains more saturated fat, such as stearic acid and palmitic acid, and less unsaturated fatty acid, such as oleic acid. It has a high melting point and a low solidification point and so can harden with falling body temperature, which may occur in conditions such as circulatory shock [3].

The second theory states that SN occurs due to a defect in the lipid transport mechanism. The level of free fatty acid in serum at birth is low and starts rising after birth due to mobilization from adipose tissue. These fatty acids are incorporated in triglycerides by the liver and used for metabolic requirements and for maintaining body temperature. Defective mobilization of fatty acids due to a defect in the adipose lipolytic enzyme may result in this thickening [4].

There are other theories that suggest that SN is a sign of severe toxicity and can result from various underlying disease processes. There is still another theory that suggests that SN is a form of edema affecting connective tissue septa [5].

CLINICAL FEATURES

SN generally occurs in severely ill premature neonates in the first week of life. The patient presents with rigid skin involving the whole body but sparing the palms, soles, and genitalia. The skin is cool, waxy, and has mottled discoloration (Figure 20.1). It may be associated with sepsis, hypothermia, hypocalcemia, and congenital anomalies. Other systemic features are respiratory distress due to bound down skin, congestive heart failure, intestinal obstruction, and diarrhea. Death usually occurs due to septicemia in the majority of cases. Maternal complications such as premature rupture of membranes, preeclampsia, eclampsia, and placenta previa may be associated [6].

Subcutaneous fat necrosis of the newborn (SCFN) and scleredema are other differential diagnoses of SN. Clinical features to differentiate these diseases from SN are presented in Table 20.1.

TREATMENT

The treatment of SN is unsatisfactory, and it carries a bad prognosis. In a majority of patients, the outcome is fatal, and death results from sepsis. Early diagnosis of SN is of paramount importance, as early treatment of sepsis can reverse features of SN. Treatment strategies that can be followed in the case of SN are as follows [6,9,10]:

- Early institution of broad-spectrum antibiotics.
- Correction of fluid and electrolyte imbalance.
- Prevention of hypothermia.

Table 20.1 Differential diagnosis of sclerema neonatorum

Disease	Onset	Clinical feature	Associated disease/ precipitating disease	Histopathology	Treatment	Outcome
Sclerema neonatorum	Premature neonate, first week of life	Diffuse hardening of skin, sparing palms, soles, and genitalia; skin is cool, waxy, and mottled	Sepsis, hypothermia, congenital anomalies, respiratory distress, congestive heart failure, diarrhea, intestinal obstruction	Septal thickening; sparse to absent inflammation; needle-shaped clefts in lipocytes	Treatment of underlying sepsis, supportive care	Poor; fatal in majority of cases
Subcutaneous fat necrosis [7]	Post mature neonate, first 4 weeks of life	Circumscribed, erythematous subcutaneous nodules especially over cheeks, buttocks, shoulder, thigh (Figure 20.2)	Precipitated by asphyxia, mechanical trauma, hypothermia; hypercalcemia occurs during resolution phase	Granulomatous lobular panniculitis with needle-shaped cleft in lipocytes and giant cells	Supportive therapy	Good
Scleredema [8]	Premature neonate, first week of life	Generalized firm, pitting edema starting in lower extremities	Cold injury, infection, diarrhea	Skin and subcutaneous tissue edema with inflammatory cell infiltrate	Supportive therapy	Good

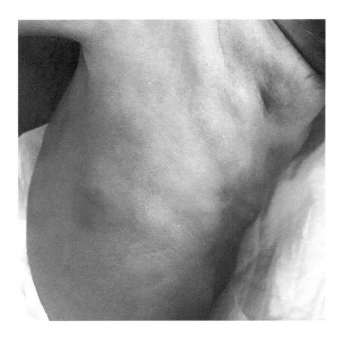

Figure 20.1 Sclerema neonatorum.

- Steroids, adrenocorticotrophic hormone (ACTH), and IV immunoglobulins have been used successfully by various authors. These treatments can be tried if supportive treatment fails.

CONCLUSION

SN is a neonatal emergency. The diagnosis of this disease requires immense clinical acumen as the diagnosis is largely based on clinical features. The dermatologist needs to identify the disease accurately and rule out other differential diagnoses promptly. Rapid institution of therapy is of paramount importance as the disease has a very poor prognosis. Counseling the parents about the prognosis is important.

KEY POINTS

- Sclerema neonatorum is a medical emergency occurring in preterm infants.
- Occurs in the first week of life.
- Manifests as thickening of skin with systemic abnormalities.
- Spares palms, soles and genitalia.
- Respiratory distress, congestive heart failure and septicemia are most important complications.

REFERENCES

1. Djojodiguno ST. Sclerema neonatorum (literature review). *Paediatrica Indonesiana* 1965;5:28–34.

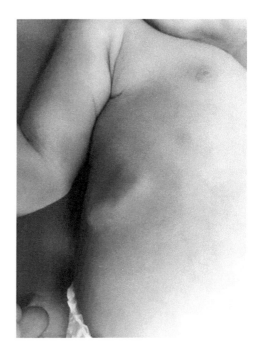

Figure 20.2 Subcutaneous fat necrosis.

2. Gray AM. On the identity of adiponecrosis subcutanea neonatorum with sclerema neonatorum. *Br J Dermatol* 1933;45:498–506.
3. Hughes WE, Hammond ML. Sclerema neonatorum. *J Pediatr* 1948;32:676–92.
4. Kellum RE, Ray TL, Brown GR. Sclerema neonatorum. Report of a case and analysis of subcutaneous and epidermal–dermal lipids by chromatographic methods. *Arch Dermatol* 1968;97:372–80.
5. Elliott RI. Sclerema. *Proc R Soc Med* 1959;52:1018–21.
6. Shrestha S, Chaudhary N, Koirala S, Gupta R. Sclerema neonatorum treated successfully with parenteral steroids: An experience from a resource poor country. *Case Rep Pediatrics* 2017;2017:4836142.
7. Burden AD, Krafchik BR. Subcutaneous fat necrosis of the newborn: A review of 11 cases. *Pediatr Dermatol* 1999;16:384–7.
8. Kumar R, Agarwal PK, Wakhlu AK, Wakhlu I. Scleredema in a 6-week-old baby. *Indian Pediatr* 1991;28:1195–7.
9. Zeb A, Darmstadt GL. Sclerema neonatorum: A review of nomenclature, clinical presentation, histological features, differential diagnoses and management. *J Perinatol* 2008;28:453.
10. Buster KJ, Burford HN, Stewart FA, Sellheyer K, Hughey LC. Sclerema neonatorum treated with intravenous immunoglobulin: A case report and review of treatments. *Cutis* 2013;92:83–7.

PART 6

Pediatric Emergencies–2 (Childhood)

SAHANA M. SRINIVAS AND VISHAL SONDHI

21

Epidermolysis bullosa

SAHANA M. SRINIVAS

INTRODUCTION

The term *epidermolysis bullosa* (EB) refers to a heterogeneous group of inherited mechanobullous disorders characterized by blistering of the skin and the mucous membrane in response to minor frictional trauma or no apparent trauma. The hallmarks of the disease are mechanical fragile skin and easily inducible blisters and erosions from birth or early infancy. Inherited EB encompasses over 30 phenotypically or genetically distinct entities [1]. Many subtypes of EB affect various organs including the cardiovascular system, gastrointestinal tract, eyes, bones, and joints, making it a neonatal dermatological emergency. There are four major types of EB: simplex, junctional, dystrophic, and mixed based on the level of cleavage at the dermoepidermal basement membrane zone (BMZ).

EPIDEMIOLOGY

The most accurate epidemiological data are derived from the National EB Registry project from the United States and also from Scotland. According to the EB Registry, the incidence and prevalence are 1 in 50,000 live births, and the prevalence is 1:20,000–1:10,0000 population in the United States and Europe [2]. Among the types of EB, EB simplex (EBS) is more common than junctional EB (JEB) and dystrophic EB (DEB). There are no epidemiological data from India. EB can occur anytime from birth to infancy. Worldwide data suggest that there is no gender, racial, or geographical predilection of EB.

It is known that many variants of inherited EB cause premature death, and most of the deaths occur during childhood. Complications and death are more common in JEB than in other types. In a cross-sectional study of risk of childhood deaths in EB from the National EB Registry, risk of death during infancy and childhood was shown to be greatest in JEB, with cumulative and conditional risk of EB of 40%–44.7% by age 1 year, rising to 61.8% in children with generalized subtype JEB and 48.2% in those with intermediate-type JEB. The cumulative risk of death by age of 1 year of 2.8% was seen in some children with EBS, generalized type [3].

CLASSIFICATION OF EPIDERMOLYSIS BULLOSA

The types and subtypes of EB have been classified based on the mode of inheritance, phenotype, ultrastructural, immunohistochemical, and molecular findings. Since the last international consensus meeting on diagnosis and classification was published in 2008, many new phenotypes and causative genes have been identified, and a new classification was proposed (onion skin approach) in 2014. Based on the level of blisters, EB can be classified into EBS, intraepidermal; within the dermoepidermal junction, JEB; beneath the basement membrane, DEB; and mixed pattern, Kindler syndrome (KS) (Figure 21.1) [3]. Subtypes of EB are classified based on phenotypic features, distribution (localized/generalized), severity, and some additional features like exuberant granulation tissue, mottled pigmentation, and pseudosyndactyly (Table 21.1) [3].

PATHOPHYSIOLOGY

Inherited EB results from mutations in any of several structural proteins present within the keratinocyte or the skin BMZ. Severity of skin and extracutaneous diseases is a reflection of the type of mutation that is present, as well as the ultrastructural location of the targeted protein. In EBS, blister cleavage occurs in basal or spinous layers of the epidermis, and keratinocytes have abnormal density and

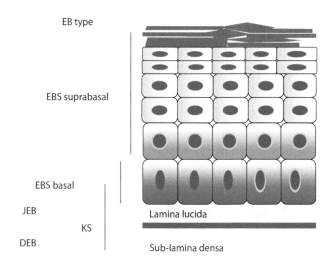

Figure 21.1 Classification of epidermolysis bullosa.

organization of keratin filaments. In JEB, blisters form in lamina lucida, where hemidesmosome structure and density are frequently diminished. In DEB, a blister cavity is formed beneath the lamina densa, and anchoring fibrils appear abnormal, reduced, or altogether absent. In Kindler syndrome, multiple cleavage planes may be seen with the same sample of skin [4–6]. The localized, generalized, and Dowling-Meara variants of EBS are caused by missense mutations in keratin-5 and keratin-14 genes (KRT5, KRT14). JEB-generalized is associated with premature termination codons in both alleles of any one of the three genes, LAMA3, LAMB3, and LAMC2, encoding the three constituent polypeptide chains of the laminin-332 gene. In JEB localized, there is a premature termination codon in one allele and another less disruptive mutation in the paired allele. DEB is caused by mutations in the collagen VII gene [3].

Table 21.1 Recent classification of epidermolysis bullosa

Type	Major types	Subtypes	Targeted proteins
Epidermolysis bullosa simplex (EBS)	Suprabasal	Acral peeling skin syndrome	Transglutaminase 5
		EBS superficialis (EBSS)	Unknown
		Acantholytic EBS (EBS-acanth)	Desmoplakin, plakoglobin
		Skin fragility syndromes	Desmoplakin, plakoglobin, plakophilin
	Basal	EBS, localized (EBS-loc)	K5, K14
		EBS, generalized severe (EBS-gen sev)	K5, K14
		EBS, generalized intermediate (EBS-gen intermed)	K5, K14
		EBS with mottled pigmentation (EBS-MP)	K5
		EBS, migratory circinate (EBS-migr)	K5
		EBS, autosomal recessive K14 (EBS-AR K14)	K14
		EBS with muscular dystrophy (EBS-MD)	Plectin
		EBS with pyloric atresia (EBS-PA)	Plectin, $\alpha6\beta4$ integrin
		EBS-Ogna (EBS-og)	Plectin
		EBS, autosomal recessive-BP230 deficiency	Bullous pemphigoid antigen-1
		EBS, autosomal recessive-exophilin 5 deficiency	Exophilin 5
Junctional epidermolysis bullosa	JEB, generalized	JEB, severe generalized	Laminin-332
		JEB, generalized intermediate	Laminin-332
		JEB, with pyloric atresia	Collagen XVII
		JEB, late onset	Collagen XVII
		JEB, with respiratory and renal involvement	Integrin $\alpha3$ subunit

(Continued)

Table 21.1 (*Continued*) Recent classification of epidermolysis bullosa

Type	Major types	Subtypes	Targeted proteins
	JEB, localized	JEB, localized (JEB-loc)	Collagen XVII, α6β4 integrin, laminin-332
		JEB, inversa	Laminin-332
		JEB-LOC syndrome	Laminin-332 Isoform α3 chain
Dystrophic epidermolysis bullosa (DEB)	Dominant dystrophic epidermolysis bullosa (DDEB)	DDEB, generalized (DDEB-gen)	Collagen VII
		DDEB, acral (DDEB-ac)	Collagen VII
		DDEB, pretibial (DDEB-pt)	Collagen VII
		DDEB, pruriginosa (DDEB-pr)	Collagen VII
		DDEB, nails only (DDEB-na)	Collagen VII
		DDEB, bullous dermolysis of newborn (DDEB-BDN)	Collagen VII
	Recessive dystrophic epidermolysis bullosa (RDEB)	RDEB, generalized severe	Collagen VII
		RDEB, generalized intermediate	Collagen VII
		RDEB, inversa	Collagen VII
		RDEB, localized	Collagen VII
		RDEB, pretibial	Collagen VII
		RDEB, pruriginosa	Collagen VII
		RDEB, centripetalis	Collagen VII
		RDEB, bullous dermolysis of newborn	Collagen VII
Kindler syndrome			Kindlin-1 (Fermitin family homolog 1)

CLINICAL FEATURES

Epidermolysis bullosa simplex

Most of the subtypes of EBS are not very severe, except the EB severe generalized variant that can be fatal. EBS presents at birth or infancy. Localized or generalized blisters are present, healing with postinflammatory hypopigmentation. Rarely, milia and scarring can be seen. Nails are dystrophic. The scalp is usually normal. The localized form presents in early childhood with blistering more commonly on the hands and feet that rarely scars (Figure 21.2). In the generalized variant of EBS, blistering is present in a herpetiform or clustered pattern (Figure 21.3). There is a risk of death in two-thirds of children with generalized EBS due to sepsis, and occasionally due to tracheolaryngeal strictures or stenoses; this is well documented in the EB Registry study population [3]. The majority of EBS subtypes have a good prognosis, except lethal acantholytic and plakoglobin deficiency that can lead to early death [7]. Death usually occurs in acantholytic EB in the neonatal period, with possible causes including anemia and heart failure. Plakoglobin deficiency EB suprabasal type leads to progressive cardiomyopathy and eventually death, but most reported cases are still children [3].

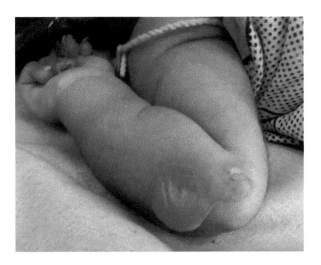

Figure 21.2 Epidermolysis bullosa simplex showing flaccid bulla on right forearm with dystrophic nails.

Clinical features of major subtypes of EBS are summarized in Tables 21.2 and 21.3 [3,5]. EBS with mottled pigmentation is a rare variant with induced blisters leaving mottled pigmentation. Muscular dystrophy may be congenital or can occur in the fourth decade. Risk of mortality

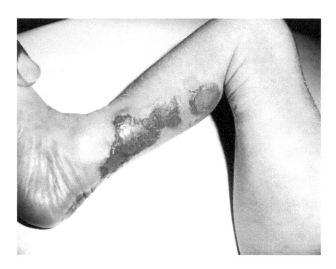

Figure 21.3 Erosions with vesicle in a herpetiform pattern on right lower leg in generalized epidermolysis bullosa simplex.

increases in EBS with muscular dystrophy and pyloric atresia due to anemia, growth retardation, and tracheolaryngeal strictures [3]. The Ogna variant of EBS can present with seasonal blistering, hemorrhagic blisters, generalized bruising tendency, and onychogryphosis of great toenails.

Junctional epidermolysis bullosa

Clinical features of subtypes of JEB are summarized in Table 21.4 [3,5]. Severe generalized JEB presents with large erosions, granulation tissue around the periorificial region, alopecia, nail dystrophy, dental enamel hypoplasia, hoarseness of voice, and gastrointestinal and genitourinary tract involvement (Figure 21.4). JEB generalized intermediate presents with similar features but with less granulation tissue (Figure 21.5) [8]. Death occurs in about half of those with generalized severe JEB and generalized intermediate

EB within the first 2 years of life with a further increase in the cumulative risk of death in the former JEB subtype. With increasing age, the most common complications include sepsis, upper airway occlusion, pneumonia, renal failure, and failure to thrive eventually leading to death. Risk of squamous cell carcinoma (SCC) in JEB occurs after 15 years and is estimated at 18% in generalized severe JEB according to the National EB Registry. Renal failure is more common in generalized intermediate JEB [3,5].

JEB with pyloric atresia is lethal in the neonatal period and has poor prognosis with death within a few months of life. There is generalized blistering with variable anemia and growth retardation. Laryngoonychocutaneous (LOC) syndrome is a rare variant of JEB. It is seen in individuals of Punjabi Muslim origin. There are short-lived blisters with erosions, exuberant granulation tissue, dystrophy of nails, and laryngeal involvement (hoarseness) [9]. Complications in LOC syndrome include anemia and growth failure. JEB with respiratory and renal involvement is a rare autosomal recessive type of JEB presenting with generalized blisters and renal and respiratory involvement present at birth or later. Mortality occurs during the neonatal period due to severe respiratory distress and interstitial pneumopathy. Rarely, patients can present with congenital nephritic syndrome [3].

Dystrophic epidermolysis bullosa

Dominant DEB (DDEB) is the most common subtype of DEB. Clinical features of major subtypes of DEB are summarized in Table 21.5 [5]. Recessive DEB (RDEB) generalized severe presents at birth with widespread blistering, scarring, and deformity. Loss of fluid, blood, and protein leads to malnutrition, hypoalbuminemia, and severe anemia. There is increased risk of glomerulonephritis, renal amyloidosis, and IgA nephropathy in RDEB and rarely in

Table 21.2 Clinical features of suprabasal types of epidermolysis bullosa simplex (EBS)

Clinical features	EBS superficialis	Lethal acantholytic EBS	Plakophilin deficiency
Mode of transmission	Autosomal dominant	Autosomal recessive	Autosomal recessive
Onset	Birth/early infancy	Birth	Birth
Skin distribution	Generalized, acral	Generalized	Generalized
Skin findings	• Superficial erosions • Intact blisters rarely noted • Milia, scarring present	• Mimics pemphigus • Oozing erosions, not blisters • Milia, scarring absent	• Erosions, erythema, bullae, desquamation • With age localized to flexures • Milia, scarring absent • Perioral erythema, circinate scaly erosions
Other features	Dystrophic nails	Dystrophic nails, alopecia, neonatal teeth	Dystrophic nails, woolly hair, alopecia, fissuring of palms and soles, tongue erosions
Extracutaneous features	None	None	Constipation, esophageal stricture
Ocular findings	Absent	Absent	Blepharitis, absent/sparse eyelashes, astigmatism

Table 21.3 Clinical features of basal types of epidermolysis bullosa simplex (EBS)

Clinical features	EBS, localized	EBS, generalized	EBS, other generalized
Mode of transmission	Autosomal dominant	Autosomal dominant/sporadic	Autosomal dominant/sporadic
Onset	Birth to early adulthood	Birth/within first week	Birth/infancy
Skin distribution	Hands, feet	Generalized	Generalized, infancy on occiput, back, legs
Skin features	Nonscarring bullae, worse during summer, increases with trauma	Grouped herpetiform blisters on trunk, proximal limbs, tendency of blistering decreases with age • Milia, scarring present	Nonscarring bullae, tense, serous, blister worse in summer, improvement with puberty • Milia, scarring present
Other features	Dystrophic nails, palmoplantar keratoderma	Nail shedding, flexion deformities of digits	Associated with congenital absence of skin, focal palmoplantar keratoderma
Extracutaneous features	Intraoral, palatal erosions	Intraoral blistering, hoarse cry due to laryngeal involvement, constipation, gastroesophageal reflex	Soft tissue abnormalities are variable
Improvement with age	Persistent, learn to modify lifestyle	Reduces, can be troublesome	Improves

Table 21.4 Clinical features of subtypes of junctional epidermolysis bullosa (JEB)

Clinical features	JEB, generalized severe	JEB, generalized intermediate	JEB, localized
Mode of transmission	Autosomal recessive	Autosomal recessive	Autosomal recessive
Onset	Birth	Birth	Birth
Skin distribution	Generalized	Generalized	Localized
Skin features	Blisters, milia, atrophic scarring, granulation tissue	Blisters, milia, scarring, granulation tissue absent or rarely present	Blisters, milia, no scarring, no granulation tissue
Other features	Scalp erosions, palmoplantar keratoderma absent	Diffuse nonscarring to scarring alopecia, focal palmoplantar keratoderma, EB nevi	Nail dystrophy
Extracutaneous features	Anemia, growth retardation, soft tissue abnormalities, enamel hypoplasia, caries, gastrointestinal tract involvement, genitourinary tract, ocular abnormalities, pseudosyndactyly, delayed puberty	Anemia, growth retardation, soft tissue abnormalities, enamel hypoplasia, caries, gastrointestinal tract and ocular not involved	Soft tissue abnormalities, excessive caries
Death	Common	Uncommon	None

DDEB. Death usually occurs in generalized severe RDEB during infancy and childhood as a result of septicemia, pneumonia, or renal failure. Dilated cardiomyopathy is an uncommon complication seen in 4.5% of patients by the age of 20 years, but it may be fatal if it occurs along with chronic renal failure. Other complications include anal scarring leading to constipation, urethral stenosis, urinary retention, hypertrophy of the bladder, and hydronephrosis [3,5]. RDEB generalized intermediate presents with more esophageal issues with advancing age. Risk of SCC in RDEB is 7.5%, 68%, 80%, and 90% by the age of 20, 35, 45, and 55 years of age. Regular inspection of a nonhealing wound is necessary, and if any suspicion is present, biopsy is mandatory. Children with RDEB generally survive in the neonatal and infantile periods but may develop infections later in childhood or cutaneous carcinomas in adulthood [3].

Pretibial DDEB/RDEB occurs at birth or infancy. Clinically it presents with pruritus, bullae, papular, plaque-like lesions, atrophic scarring, and milia on shins. EB pruriginosa presents in childhood with generalized or localized blisters, healing with atrophy, and milia (Figures 21.6 through 21.8). Nails are dystrophic. Constipation is present. Intractable pruritus is characteristic of EB pruriginosa. Bullous dermolysis of newborn is a rare subtype, onset is at birth or infancy and presents as generalized neonatal skin blistering that improves during childhood and remits completely. Blister heals with atrophic scarring, milia, and mild hypopigmentation [10,11].

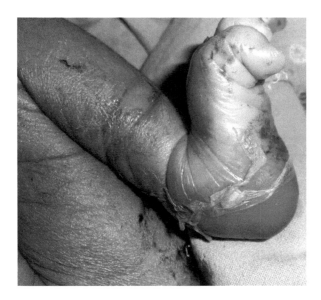

Figure 21.4 Large erosion in junctional epidermolysis bullosa on left lower leg extending onto soles.

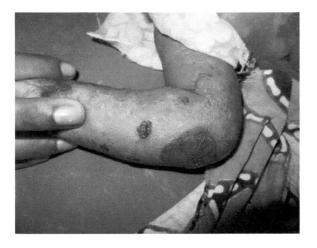

Figure 21.5 Erosions, milia, scarring in junctional epidermolysis bullosa.

KINDLER SYNDROME

Kindler syndrome is autosomal recessively inherited. It presents with blistering at birth or infancy. Blisters are generalized, usually subsiding in late childhood, giving rise to poikiloderma. Other features include photosensitivity, dystrophic nails, webbing of toes, gingival hyperplasia, periodontal disease, and rarely presents with complications such as esophagitis, esophageal strictures, colitis, urethral stricture, and ectropion requiring emergency management [5]. SCC can develop after the age of 30 years; hence, early and regular surveillance is important.

LABORATORY APPROACH

Although diagnosis of EB is clinical, laboratory tests are necessary to determine the type of EB, whether it is epidermolysis bullosa simplex, junctional, or dystrophic variant. Routine blood counts, liver and renal function tests, serum electrolytes, bone profile, and vitamins A and B12 assay should be done every 6 months to recognize early complications. Skin biopsy must be sent for ultrastructural examination or for antigen mapping to confirm the subtype of EB. Biopsy is usually taken from unaffected skin. A microblister is induced by rubbing the skin with a fingertip or pencil eraser. Skin should be stroked 30–40 times to induce the blister. Incision and punch biopsy are usually avoided due to skin fragility. A shave biopsy would be ideal in EB [3].

Monoclonal antibodies are used in antigen mapping to find the likely mutated protein, thus determining the subtype of EB. This test is simple and available in India and is less expensive than other tests. Collagen IV, keratin 14, laminin-332, and collagen VII are four antibodies used to determine the level of blistering. Antibodies to type XVII collagen, plectin, α6β4 integrin, are used to categorize the subtype of EB [12].

Transmission electron microscopy (TEM) visualizes the level of tissue separation or blister formation and various components of the dermoepidermal junction. In EBS the split is seen in the lower part of the epidermis. In EBS, generalized severe apart from the intraepidermal cleavage, there are abnormal clumps of tonofilaments. In JEB there is a split at the level of lamina lucida. In severe generalized JEB there is diminutive hemidesmosomes, attenuated subbasal dense plates, and reduced anchoring filaments. The cleavage plane is below the lamina densa in DEB [13]. This test is very expensive and requires expert opinion. TEM is now used mainly in a reference laboratory and is less applicable as a primary diagnostic procedure.

Although molecular testing is available at a few centers in India, it is very expensive; but this test helps to determine the mode of genetic transmission, determine the prenatal or preimplantation diagnosis, and confirm the few rare variants of EB. Molecular testing helps to identify the genes responsible for the different types of EB and determines the location and type of mutations in disease causation. Molecular testing requires DNA samples of the proband, siblings, and parents. Next-generation sequencing testing is done on the affected child. Once the mutation is confirmed, it is validated by Sanger sequencing for the affected child, siblings, and parents. Mutational screening techniques are based on polymerase chain reaction amplification of target DNA or RNA sequences. Prenatal testing along with counseling is an important part in the management of families at risk of developing EB. Prenatal techniques include analysis of fetal skin biopsy in the second trimester or examination of DNA from the first trimester by chorionic villous sampling.

MANAGEMENT OF EPIDERMOLYSIS BULLOSA

There is no cure for EB. Management of EB is mainly supportive. Management of a child with EB is focused on

Table 21.5 Clinical features of subtypes of dystrophic epidermolysis bullosa (DEB)

Clinical features	Dominant DEB (DDEB), generalized	Recessive DEB (RDEB), severe generalized	RDEB, generalized intermediate
Mode of transmission	Autosomal dominant	Autosomal recessive	Autosomal recessive
Onset	Birth	Birth	Birth
Skin distribution	Generalized, trunk, limbs, bony prominences	Generalized, frictional areas	Generalized
Skin findings			
Blisters	Follow sharp knocks rather than mild friction	Mildest trauma produces blister, erosions, crusting	Milder, localized
Milia	Present	Constant feature	Present, not significant
Atrophic scarring	Present	Present	Present
Granulation tissue	Absent	Rare	Absent
Nail involvement	Dystrophy, scarring of nail bed, flexion contractures of fingers	Dystrophic	Dystrophic
Scalp abnormalities	Telogen effluvium	Scarring alopecia, decreased body hair	Scarring alopecia, less pronounced
Palms and soles (keratoderma)	Absent	None	None
Other features	Albopapuloid lesions, congenital absence of skin	Pruritus present, flexion contractures at axillae, knees, elbows by adulthood, delayed puberty, dilated cardiomyopathy, decreased bone mineralization, bone pain, fracture of calcanei, vertebral bodies	None
Extracutaneous involvement			
Anemia	25%	Present	Less common
Growth retardation	Rare	Present, thin, short stature	Less common
Oral cavity			
Soft tissue abnormalities	Mild	Ankyloglossia, microstomia, gums fragile, tongue atrophic	Oral blisters
Enamel hypoplasia	Absent	Absent	Absent
Caries	Normal frequency	Excessive	Normal frequency
Gastrointestinal tract	Dysphagia, microstomia, constipation, anal fissures	Constipation, dysphagia, fibrosis, stricture, poor nutrition	Dysphagia, anal fissures
Genitourinary tract	Rare	Urethral stenosis, urinary retention, postinfectious glomerulonephritis, hydronephrosis, renal amyloid, IgA nephropathy, renal failure	Rare
Ocular findings	Absent	Symblepharon, limbal broadening, ectropion, pannus, corneal opacities	Present, less common
Pseuodosyndactly	Rare	Present, mitten-like appearance of hands, feet in 90%–100%	Rare
Respiratory tract	Absent		Absent
Malignancy			
Squamous cell carcinoma (SCC)	Present in older patients	Multiple SCC by 35 years (67.8%), 90.1% by 55 years	SCC less common
Death	None	Die by third to fourth decade	Death less common

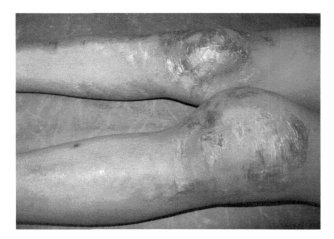

Figure 21.6 Dystrophic epidermolysis bullosa showing atrophic scarring.

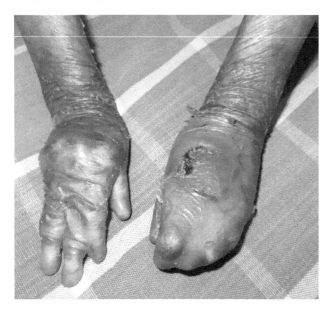

Figure 21.7 Pseudosyndactyly with mitten hands in dystrophic epidermolysis bullosa.

minimizing new blisters, preventing infection, controlling pain, providing nutritional support, caring for any wounds, managing potential complications, and providing psychological support to patients and family members [14].

General care in epidermolysis bullosa

- Counseling should be provided to all family members about the disorder and importance of regular follow-up.
- Caregivers must be taught to handle the child gently to prevent new blisters. Roll the baby away from you and gently roll back onto hands while lifting. Alternatively, lift the baby on the mattress the baby is lying on.
- Multiple handlers for the child are to be avoided.
- The environment should not be too warm. Nursing the child in a cot or bassinette is better, unless indicated for reasons such as prematurity when the child can be put in a soft incubator mattress.

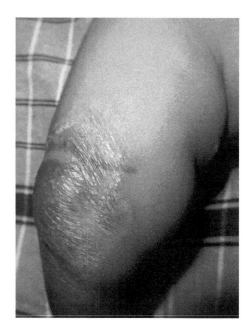

Figure 21.8 Dystrophic epidermolysis bullosa showing atrophic scarring and milia formation.

- Clamping the umbilical cord should be replaced by ligature tying.
- Parents should be taught to pop the blisters by using a lancet or sterile needle. The needle should pierce from one end of the blister to the other end without deroofing, allowing slow drainage. Gentle pressure with a gauze swab can be used to encourage the fluid to drain.
- The child should be bathed daily with mild cleansers.
- Diapers with no elastic or soft cotton diapers must be used. Clothing should be loose soft cotton, with seams covered.
- Hanging skin must be trimmed. Nails should be cut regularly.
- Moisturizers such as liquid paraffin are to be used all over the body except on raw wounds to prevent itching and for lubrication.
- Prevent trauma in elderly children.
- Palms and soles must be kept dry in the summer season. Cotton mittens can be used to prevent itching. Wear two pairs of cotton socks to minimize friction. Cornstarch can be sprinkled into shoes or socks to reduce friction.
- Good nutrition should be maintained. A soft teat or latex teat can be used for bottle feeding. Teething gel may be used if the mouth is sore. In severe cases, a nasogastric tube may be indicated.
- A soft-bristled toothbrush should be used. Short blisters may be needed for microstomia.

Wound care in epidermolysis bullosa

- Adequate analgesic can be given half an hour prior to dressing (Syrup Paracetamol most commonly used) [15,16].
- Wound dressing should start from legs upward, trunk, face, and then scalp.

- There are two types of wound care; they are different for a raw wound and a healing wound.
- Moisturizers should be applied for dry and healing wounds (petroleum jelly or bland emollients).
- Dressings are mainly three layers:
  - *First layer/primary layer*: Nonsticky, silicone nonadherent woven mesh-like dressing/Mepitel/ Vaseline-impregnated gauze/burns mesh/collagen dressings.
  - *Second layer/secondary*: Absorptive dressings, foam-based dressings used. Mepilex if available/dressing pad can be used.
  - *Third layer*: To hold the dressing in place. Mepitac or roller gauze can be used.

- Other dressing substitutes include dermal allograft, Apligraf, Dermagraft (a fibroblast-derived skin substitute harvested from neonatal foreskin), or amniotic membrane.

Prevention and treatment of infections

Inspection of wounds regularly for purulent exudates is necessary. Regular swabbing for culture and sensitivity should be done. The choice of antibiotic is based on culture sensitivity and may be needed for long periods. Topical measures such as regular bathing, emollient lotions containing antimicrobials, or bleach baths can be routinely used to keep the colonization count at a low level so that wound healing

Table 21.6 Management of complications

Complications	Clinical features	Management
Gastrointestinal tract	• Painful and ulcerated mouth	Analgesics, Haberman Feeder with lubrication, nonstinging mouthwashes
	• Difficulty in swallowing with narrowing/pharyngoesophageal strictures	Fluoroscopically guided balloon esophageal dilatation
	• Feeding problems	Supplements, special feeds (recommended by dietician), gastrostomy feeding
	• Reflux	Proton pump inhibitors
	• Constipation	Increased fiber diet, increased fluid intake, regular laxative
	• Anemia	Nutritional supplement, IV iron, blood transfusions, treatment of underlying cause
Genitourinary tract	• Decreased urine flow	Treatment of infections
	• Pain on voiding	Enough fluids
	• Recurrent infections	Avoid unnecessary procedures and surgery (catheterization/urethral dilatation, electroresection)
	• Urethral meatal stenosis or strictures	Monitor blood pressure, blood and urine test regularly
	• Bladder distension	
	• Hydroureter	
	• Hydronephrosis	
	• Chronic renal failure	
Respiratory tract	• Tracheolaryngeal strictures	Tracheostomy
	• Pneumonia	Antibiotics
Cardiovascular system	• Dilated cardiomyopathy	Avoid potential medicines in epidermolysis bullosa that can damage the heart
		Echo from the age of 2 years
		Early treatment of symptoms
Ear, nose, throat	• Hoarse cry	Nebulizations, nebulized steroids
	• Noisy breathing	Oral steroids
		Tracheostomy
Eyes	• Corneal dryness	Lubricants
	• Corneal abrasions	Surgery
	• Scarring	Amniotic membrane transplant
Bones	• Osteopenia	Biphosphonates
	• Osteoporosis	
	• Vertebral fractures	
Hand	• Pseudosyndactyly	Hand occupational therapist
		Surgery (releasing all contractures)
Carcinomas	• Squamous cell carcinoma (SCC)/basal cell carcinoma	Excision/surgical debulking
		Radiation therapy
		Amputation (SCC of hands and feet)

is not impaired. Prophylactic antibiotics are not indicated, and umbilical and IV lines should not be placed routinely.

Management of complications in epidermolysis bullosa

A multidisciplinary approach is necessary to manage complications. An EB team consists of trained nurses, dermatologist, pediatrician, gastroenterologist, dentist, ophthalmologist, plastic surgeon, dietician, occupational therapist, and geneticist. Management of complications is summarized in Table 21.6.

Novel therapies in epidermolysis bullosa

Understanding the molecular basis of EB has led to the development of novel genetic and cellular therapies. Hematopoietic cell transplantation, gene therapy, protein replacement therapy, and cell-based therapies have been researched for the treatment of EB [17]. Gene and cell therapies hold great promise, especially for recessive forms of EB. The first skin gene therapy trial was done in JEB. Intradermal injection of allogeneic fibroblasts temporarily stimulates increased expression of type VII collagen in patient fibroblasts in the less severe form of RDEB. Mesenchymal stem cell transplant has been shown to produce collagen VII to the basement membrane and improvement in RDEB [17].

Care of child who has epidermolysis bullosa in intensive care unit

- Name band should be taped to child's clothes, rather than worn around wrist or ankle, which may rub and cause blistering [18].
- For skin preparation do not rub the skin, gently swipe with an alcohol swab.
- No finger or heel pricks. Long-line IV access is needed for more than 48 hours.
- Place padding around the arm before application of blood pressure cuff.
- Pulse oximetry should be done using nonadhesive sensor or an adhesive sensor over plastic wrap or Mepitel.
- Electrocardiogram electrodes can be applied over Mepitel dressing.
- Avoid sticking adhesive tapes directly to the skin.
- Transfer the patient on a draw sheet ideally in conjunction with a slide sheet to avoid shearing.

CONCLUSION

EB is a rare group of inherited skin disorders with variable prognosis. The prognosis depends on the subtype, type of inheritance, and association with systemic complications. There is high mortality associated with severe recessive forms of EB. Early recognition of these complications associated with EB and appropriate management may increase

KEY POINTS

- Epidermolysis bullosa is an inherited group of mechanobullous disorders affecting multiorgans.
- Severe autosomal recessive forms of EB are associated with systemic complications and bad prognosis.
- Complications include anemia, failure to thrive, sepsis, oesophageal and tracheolaryngeal strictures, pneumonia, renal failure and eventually death.
- Risk of moratlity increases in neonatal period in JEB generalized severe and RDEB due to sepsis, respiratory distress and interstitial pneumonia.
- Death usually occurs during infancy and childhood in RDEB and JEB generalized severe.
- Carcinoma are late complications seen after the age of 15 years in severe forms.
- Management includes early recognition of complications, multidisciplinary approach, counselling and regular follow up.

life expectancy and improve quality of life. Counseling parents about the conditions and associated complications is an important aspect of management. A multidisciplinary approach with regular follow-up is necessary.

REFERENCES

1. Maldonado-Colin G, Hernandez-Zepeda C, Duran-McKinster C, Garcia-Romero MT. Inherited epidermolysis bullosa: A multisystem disease of skin and mucosae fragility. *Indian J Paediatr Dermatol* 2017;18:267–73.
2. Pfendner E, Uitto J, Fine JD. Epidermolysis bullosa carrier frequencies in the US population. *J Invest Dermatol* 2001;116:483–4.
3. Fine JD et al. Inherited epidermolysis bullosa: Updated recommendations on diagnosis and classification. *J Am Acad Dermatol* 2014;70:1103–26.
4. Horn HM, Tidman MJ. The clinical spectrum of epidermolysis bullosa simplex. *Br J Dermatol* 2000;142:468–72.
5. Fine JD et al. The classification of inherited epidermolysis bullosa (EB): Report of the Third International Consensus Meeting on Diagnosis and Classification of EB. *J Am Acad Dermatol* 2008;58:931–50.
6. Intong LR, Murrell DF. Inherited epidermolysis bullosa: New diagnostic criteria and classification. *Clin Dermatol* 2012;30:70–7.
7. Antherton DJ, Denyer J. *Epidermolysis Bullosa: An Outline for Professionals*. Berkshire, UK: DebRA; 2003:1–48.
8. Hore I et al. The management of disease specific ENT problems in children with epidermolysis bullosa: A retrospective case note review. *Int J Pediatr Otorhinolaryngol* 2007;71:385–91.

9. Philips RJ, Atherton DJ, Gibbs ML, Stobel S, Lake BD. Laryngo-onycho-cutaneous syndrome: An inherited epithelial defect. *Arch Dis Chils* 1994;70:319–26.

10. Lee JY, Chen HC, Lin SJ. Pretibial epidermolysis bullosa: A clinicopathological study. *J Am Acad Dermatol* 1993;29:974–81.

11. McGrath JA, Schofield OM, Eady RA. Epidermolysis bullous pruriginosa: Dystrophic epidermolysis bullosa with distinctive clinicopathological features. *Br J Dermatol* 1994;130:617–25.

12. Hiremagalore R, Kubba A, Bansel S, Jerajani H. Immunofluorescence mapping (IFM) in inherited epidermolysis bullosa: A study of eighty-six cases from India. *Br J Dermatol* 2015;172:384–91.

13. Eady RA, Dopping-Hepenstal PJ. Transmission electron microscopy for the diagnosis of epidermolysis bullosa. *Dermatol Clinic* 2010;28:211–2.

14. Gonzalez ME. Evaluation and treatment of the newborn with epidermolysis bullosa. *Semin Pernatol* 2013;37:32–9.

15. Lara-Corrales I, Arbuckle A, Zarinehbaf S, Pope E. Principles of wound care in patients with epidermolysis bullosa. *Pediatr Dermatol* 2010;27:229–37.

16. Denyer JE. Wound management for children with epidermolysis bullosa. *Dermatol Clin* 2010;28:257–64.

17. Wong T et al. Potential of fibroblast cell therapy for recessive dystrophic epidermolysis bullosa. *J Invest Dermatol* 2008;128:2179–89.

18. Atherton DJ, Denyer J. *Epidermolysis Bullosa: An Outline for Professionals.* Berkshire, UK: DebRA; 1997.

22

Ichthyotic disorders

SAHANA M. SRINIVAS

INTRODUCTION

Many ichthyotic disorders can present as neonatal erythroderma and thus present as an emergency dermatological condition. Ichthyotic disorders presenting as erythroderma can be congenital in onset or can present in less than 1 month or greater than 1 month of life. Congenital ichthyosis is a group of hereditary disorders characterized by variable degrees of generalized, persistent scaling, with a chronic, lifelong course. Ichthyosis can be part of clinical syndromes with various systemic involvement. Nonsyndromic and syndromic ichthyosis can cause erythroderma in infants and children [1]. In a retrospective study of neonatal erythroderma conducted by Pruszkowski et al., ichthyosis was the cause in 24% of cases [2]. Sarkar et al. found ichthyosiform erythroderma to be the etiological diagnosis in 25% of neonatal erythroderma cases [3]. Different ichthyoses that can present as dermatological emergencies are denoted in Table 22.1.

NONSYNDROMIC ICHTHYOSIS

Nonbullous congenital ichthyosiform erythroderma

Nonbullous ichthyosiform erythroderma (NBIE), also called congenital ichthyosiform erythroderma (CIE), is an autosomal recessive congenital ichthyosis. NBIE is caused by mutations in adenosine triphosphate (ATP) binding cassette protein A12 (ABCA12), arachidonate lipoxygenases, ceramide synthetase 3, lipase N, and transglutaminase (TGM1) [4]. Affected children are usually born with collodion membrane (Figure 22.1). After shedding of the collodion membrane, there is erythroderma and scaling. Erythroderma may persist throughout in severe cases.

Scales are fine on the face and trunk and are lamellar type on the extremities (Figure 22.2). There is hyperkeratosis of palms and soles. Other features include dystrophic nails, moderate to severe hypohidrosis, and sometimes scarring alopecia [5]. The disease course is mild to severe. Extracutaneous involvement includes failure to thrive and short stature. Histology shows hyperkeratosis, normal or moderately thickened granular layer, parakeratosis, and acanthosis [6].

Bullous congenital ichthyosiform erythroderma

Bullous congenital ichthyosiform erythroderma (BCIE) is a rare type of keratinopathic ichthyotic phenotype with blister formation. It is inherited as an autosomal dominant pattern, but due to the heterogeneity of this disorder, it can be inherited as an autosomal recessive disorder or sporadic form. BCIE is caused by mutations in epidermal keratin 1 (KRT 1) and keratin 10 (KRT 10). Palmoplantar keratoderma (PPK) with BCIE is more often associated with the KRT 1 gene mutation than the KRT 10 gene. Clinically it presents as generalized blister formation with multiple erosions and erythroderma. BCIE does not present as collodion membrane at birth. At birth there is generalized erythema with tender erosions which decreases with age and progresses to epidermolytic hyperkeratosis in adulthood [7]. Thick hyperkeratosis at the flexures is very characteristic of this disorder. Hyperkeratosis may be seen on elbows, wrists, and ankles. Flaccid bullae rupture to leave tender raw areas. Molting is present (periodic shedding of scales). There may be PPK. Rarely extracutaneous features like mental retardation, ventricular septal defect, breast hypoplasia, and congenital club foot have been reported [8]. Histology shows hyperkeratosis and acanthosis with granular degeneration.

Table 22.1 Classification of ichthyotic disorders manifesting as dermatological emergencies

Nonsyndromic
Bullous congenital ichthyosiform erythroderma
  (epidermolytic ichthyosis)
Nonbullous congenital ichthyosiform erythroderma
Lamellar ichthyosis (congenital ichthyosiform
  erythroderma)
Syndromic ichthyosis
Netherton syndrome
Sjögren-Larsson syndrome
Keratitis-ichthyosis-deafness syndrome
Chanarin-Dorfman syndrome
Conradi-Hünermann syndrome
Congenital hemidysplasia with ichthyosiform
  erythroderma and limb defects (CHILD) syndrome
Ichthyosis prematurity syndrome
Trichothiodystrophy

Lamellar ichthyosis

Lamellar ichthyosis (LI) is a severe form of autosomal recessive congenital ichthyosis (ARCI). In the Asian population, LI is mainly caused by mutation in the TGM1 and ABCA12 genes. Clinically children present with collodion membrane at birth. After shedding of the collodion membrane, the skin is covered by large, thickened, quadrilateral, adherent

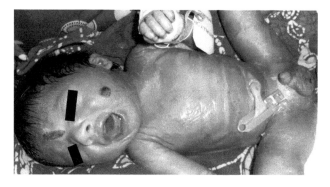

Figure 22.1 Newborn with collodion membrane.

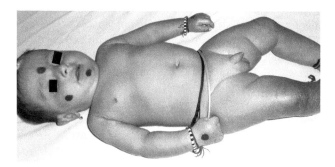

Figure 22.2 Child showing mild erythema with fine scales on trunk and lamellar scales on extremities after shedding of collodion membrane.

lamellar scales all over the body, including the face, palms, and soles (Figure 22.3) [5]. There is diffuse hyperkeratosis with maceration and fissuring at flexural sites. Erythema is usually mild or absent. PPK is present in all cases of Lamellar ichthyosis (Figure 22.4) [9]. Ectropion is usually seen leading to dryness of the cornea and conjunctiva with exposure keratitis (Figure 22.5). Nails are thickened with subungual hyperkeratosis. Histology shows marked hyperkeratosis, hypergranulosis and moderate acanthosis, and few parakeratotic cells.

SYNDROMIC ICHTHYOSIS

Netherton syndrome

Netherton syndrome (NS) is a rare autosomal recessive disorder characterized by erythroderma, ichthyosis, hair

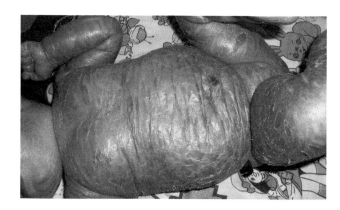

Figure 22.3 Lamellar ichthyosis with lamellar scaling all over the body.

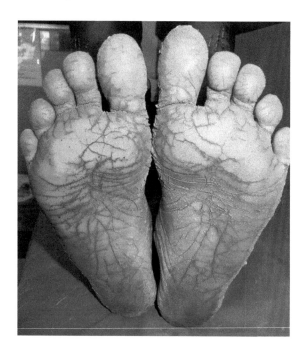

Figure 22.4 Diffuse palmoplantar keratoderma in lamellar ichthyosis.

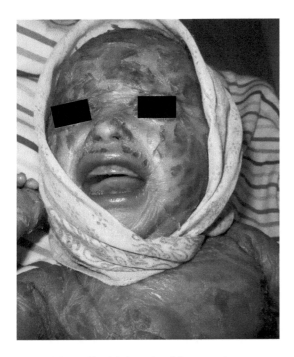

Figure 22.5 Lamellar ichthyosis with ectropion.

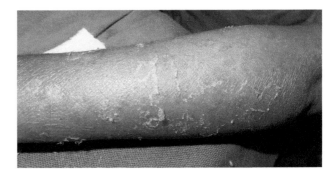

Figure 22.7 Child showing ichthyosis linearis circumflexa on forearm after 2 years of age.

shaft defects, and atopy. NS is caused by mutations in the SPINK 5 gene which encodes lymphoepithelial Kazal-type-related inhibitor (LETK1). NS manifests at birth as generalized scaling and erythroderma at birth or during the early infantile period but not with collodion baby phenotype (Figure 22.6) [10]. After 2 years, they develop characteristic ichthyosis called *ichthyosis linearis circumflexa* (ILC). ILC presents as migratory, polycyclic scaly lesions with a peripheral double-edged scale (Figure 22.7). Associated features include failure to thrive, hypernatremic dehydration secondary to excess fluid loss from the defective skin barrier, delayed growth, short stature, and recurrent infections. Approximately 75% of those with NS develop atopic manifestations with increased serum IgE levels. The pathognomic feature of NS is the hair shaft defect called *trichorrhexis invaginata* (TI) or a ball-and-socket defect (Figure 22.8). Trichorrhexis nodosa and pili torti can also be seen in NS [11]. Examining eyebrow hairs is more informative for diagnosing hair shaft defects. Histology shows psoriasiform dermatitis. Any child presenting with neonatal erythroderma should be investigated for hair shaft defects to rule out NS.

Sjögren-Larsson syndrome

Sjögren-Larsson syndrome (SLS) is an autosomal recessive disorder characterized by clinical symptoms of congenital ichthyosis, spastic paresis, and mental retardation. SLS is caused by mutation in the gene fatty aldehyde dehydrogenase. SLS presents at birth or in the neonatal period with varying degrees of erythema and ichthyosis. The collodion phenotype is rarely seen. Erythema is seen at birth but may not be evident after 1 year of age. Ichthyosis is usually fine to lamellar type and predominantly affects the lower abdomen, sides, and nape of neck and flexures (Figure 22.9) [12]. PPK is seen in 50% of cases. Neurological features include speech and motor delay, spastic paresis, and seizures. One-third of patients present with foveal and perifoveal glistening dots that appear after several years of age. Bilateral glistening yellow white dots involving the foveal and parafoveal regions are present from the age of 1–2 years. The number of dots increases with age, although the extent of maculae involvement does not correlate with systemic severity. Diagnosis is confirmed by the measurement of enzyme activity in cultured skin fibroblasts or leucocytes.

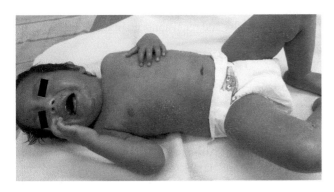

Figure 22.6 Generalized scaling erythroderma in Netherton syndrome.

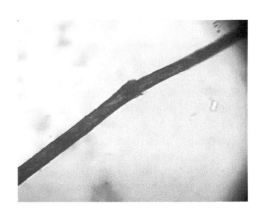

Figure 22.8 Trichorrhexis invaginata in Netherton syndrome.

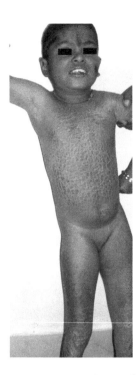

Figure 22.9 Sjögren-Larsson syndrome showing lamellar scaling with spastic paresis.

Keratitis-ichthyosis-deafness syndrome

Keratitis-ichthyosis-deafness (KID) syndrome is a rare hereditary cornification disorder due to mutation in connexin 26, a protein necessary for intercellular communication. It is a clinical triad of keratitis, congenital ichthyosis, and bilateral sensorineural deafness. At birth there is erythematous skin that progresses and becomes thickened and leathery at the first month of life. A characteristic feature of KID syndrome is the presence of generalized stippled papules and well-defined verrucous plaques on the face and limbs. Ichthyosis is generalized and severe [13]. Alopecia is seen in 25% of patients. Nails are dystrophic with the stippled pattern of PPK. Extracutaneous features include hypotrichosis, anhidrosis, and recurrent infections, especially candidiasis.

Chanarin-Dorfman syndrome

Chanarian-Dorfman syndrome, also called *neutral lipid storage disease with ichthyosis*, is a rare autosomal recessive disorder where there is accumulation of triglycerides in all tissues. There is a mutation in the comparative gene identification (CGI) 58 gene located on chromosome 3p21. Ichthyosis is of the CIE phenotype. They usually present with collodion membrane at birth with ectropion and eclabium. Other clinical features include liver steatosis, hepatomegaly, muscle weakness, myopathy, ataxia, neurosensory deafness, subcapsular cataract, nystagmus, and mental retardation [14]. Diagnosis is confirmed by the presence of lipid droplets in granulocytes and monocytes in peripheral smear (Jordan anomaly).

Conradi-Hünermann-Happle syndrome

Conradi-Hünermann-Happle (CHH) syndrome is a rare X-linked dominant multisystem disorder. It occurs due to postzygotic mutation in the EBP (emopamil binding protein) gene on chromosome Xp11.23. It is characterized by linear ichthyosis, chondrodysplasia punctata, cataract, and short stature. The child is born with severe ichthyosiform erythroderma, and the scales are arranged in swirls and whorls along the lines of Blaschko. With age, ichthyosis improves and mild ichthyosis presents on the extremities along with follicular atrophoderma along the lines of Blaschko with hypopigmented and hyperpigmented streaks on the trunk. There may be persistent psoriasiform lesions in intertriginous areas (ptychotrophism) [15]. Localized scarring alopecia may be seen. Other features include asymmetrical skeletal involvement with stippled calcification of the epiphyseal region resulting in shortening of long bones, severe kyphoscoliosis, congenital dislocation of the hip, facial dysplasia, congenital heart defects, sensorineural deafness, renal anomalies, and ophthalmological changes like cataract, microphthalmia, and microcornea.

Congenital hemidysplasia with ichthyosiform erythroderma and limb defects syndrome

Congenital hemidysplasia with ichthyosiform erythroderma and limb defects (CHILD) syndrome, also called *unilateral CIE*, manifests with features of congenital hemidysplasia, ichthyosiform erythroderma, and limb defects. The characteristic feature is the presence of unilateral ichthyosiform erythroderma with sharp midline demarcation with ipsilateral hypoplasia of the bony structures. It is an X-linked-dominant condition seen in females and lethal in hemizygous males. It is caused by mutation in the encoding NADPH steroid dehydrogenase-like protein (NSDHL) at Xq28 [16]. Ichthyosiform erythroderma presents at birth or after a few months of life. Yellow to waxy scaling and streaks of inflammation may follow Blaschko lines, and streaks of normal skin may be present within the area of CHILD syndrome. Other features include unilateral alopecia and severe nail dystrophy. Lesions improve with age or clear spontaneously. Extracutaneous features include ipsilateral skeletal hypoplasia, lobster claw deformity, and cardiovascular and renal abnormalities.

Ichthyosis prematurity syndrome

Ichthyosis prematurity syndrome (IPS) is an autosomal recessive disorder with neonates born more than 6 weeks prematurely. It is caused by mutation in the solute carrier family 27 member 4 SLC27A4 gene/fatty acid transport protein 4 (FATP4). At birth there is thick, spongy desquamating skin that resembles vernix caseosa, which is accentuated more on the scalp and eyebrows. Later in the neonatal period, there is moderate erythroderma with scaling resembling a cobblestone appearance. Associated features include

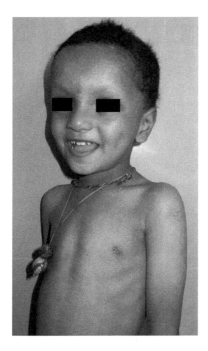

Figure 22.10 Fine scaling on face and trunk with brittle hair in trichothiodystrophy.

polyhydramnios, neonatal respiratory distress, peripheral eosinophilia, atopic dermatitis, dermographism, food allergy, and asthma.

Trichothiodystrophy

Trichothiodystrophy (TTD) is an autosomal recessive disorder with dry, brittle, cysteine-deficient hair with multisystem involvement. Patients usually present with collodion baby phenotype with CIE at birth. There is erythema with fine to lamellar scaling all over the body (Figure 22.10).

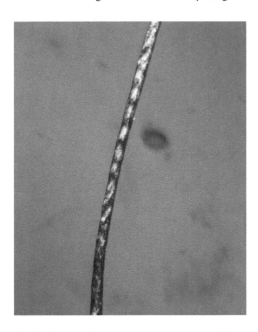

Figure 22.11 Tiger tail appearance in polarized light microscopy in trichothiodystrophy.

With age, ichthyosis improves, leaving the mild lamellar type of ichthyosis. Palmoplantar keratoderma is present. Syndromes associated with TTD include IBIDS (ichthyosis, brittle hair, impairment of intelligence, decreased fertility, and short stature) and PIBIDS (photosensitivity, ichthyosis, brittle hair, impairment of intelligence, decreased fertility, and short stature) syndromes [16]. Diagnosis of TTD can be confirmed by hair shaft examination under polarized light microscopy, which shows alternate light and dark bands (tiger-tail appearance) (Figure 22.11).

CONCLUSION

Ichthyotic disorders presenting as dermatological emergencies can have varied manifestations. Many ichthyotic disorders present as collodion baby phenotype, which gives a clue to recognize possible underlying ichthyotic disorders. A systematic approach is necessary to recognize these conditions to prevent life-threatening complications. Early evaluation of these disorders and management prevent mortality. Long-term follow-up and counseling are important.

KEY POINTS

- Ichthyotic disorders can present as an emergency condition in the form of erythroderma.
- Approximately 25% cases of neonatal erythroderma are due to an ichthyotic disorder.
- Both nonsyndromic and syndromic ichthyosis can present as dermatological emergencies.
- Many of the congenital ichthyosis disorders present at birth as collodion baby phenotype. Recently due to improved care in the intensive care unit, mortality due to collodion baby is reduced.
- Early recognition of the complications associated with ichthyotic disorders can prevent mortality.
- Genetic counseling and long-term follow-up form the mainstay of management in ichthyotic disorders.

REFERENCES

1. Kumar S, Sehgal VN, Sharma RC. Common genodermatoses. *Int J Dermatol* 1996;35:685–94.
2. Pruszkowski A, Bodemer C, Fraitag S, Teillac-Hamel D, Amoric JC, de Prost Y. Neonatal and infantile erythroderma: A retrospective study of 51 patients. *Arch Dermatol* 2000;136:875–80.
3. Sarkar R. Neonatal and infantile erythroderma. "The red baby." *Indian J Dermatol* 2006;51:178–81.
4. Sugiura K, Akiyama M. Update on autosomal recessive congenital ichthyosis: mRNA analysis using hair samples is a powerful tool for genetic diagnosis. *J Dermatol Sci* 2015;79:4–9.

5. Akiyam M, Sawamura D, Shimizu H. The clinical spectrum of non bullous ichthyosiform erythroderma and lamellar ichthyosis and lamellar ichthyosis. *Clin Exp Dermatol* 2003;28:235–40.

6. Akiyama M. Severe congenital ichthyosis of the neonate. *Int J Dermatol* 1998;37:722–8.

7. Judge MR, Mclean WH, Munro CS. Disorder of keratinization. In: Burns T, Breathnach S, Cox N, Griffiths C (Eds), *Rook's Textbook of Dermatology*. 8th ed. Oxford, London: Blackwell Science; 2010:19.29–33.

8. Math A et al. Identification of a *de novo* keratin 1 mutation in epidermolytic hyperkeratosis with palmoplantar involvement. *Eur J Dermatol* 2006;16:507–10.

9. Takeichi T, Akiyama M. Inherited ichthyosis: Non-syndromic forms. *J Dermatol* 2016;43:242–51.

10. Aradhya SS, Srinivas SM, Hiremagalore R, Shanmukappa AG. Netherton syndrome masquerading as psoriatic erythroderma. *Indian J Paediatr Dermatol* 2014;15:89–91.

11. Srinivas SM, Hiremagalore R, Suryanarayan S, Budamakuntala L. Netherton syndrome with pili torti. *Int J Trichology* 2013;5:225–6.

12. Srinivas SM, Raju KV, Hiremagalore R. Sjögren-Larsson syndrome. A study of clinical symptoms in six children. *Indian Dermatol Online J* 2014;5:185–8.

13. Inamdar AC, Raghunatha S. Inherited ichthyosis and other disorders of keratinization. In: Inamdar AC, Palit A, Raghunatha S (Eds), *Textbook of Pediatric Dermatology*. 2nd ed. New Delhi: Jaypee; 2014:89–111.

14. Mi XB, Luo MX, Guo LL, Zhang TD, Qiu XW. CHILD syndrome: Case report of a Chinese patient and literature review of the NAD [P]H steroid dehydrogenase-like protein gene mutation. *Pediatr Dermatol* 2015;32:e277–82.

15. Kiely C, Devaney D, Fischer J, Lenane P, Irvine AD. Ichthyosis prematurity syndrome: A case report and review of known mutations. *Pediatr Dermatol* 2014;31:517–8.

16. Lambert WC, Gagna CE, Lambert MW. Trichothiodystrophy: Photosensitive, TTD-P, TTD, Tay syndrome. *Adv Exp Med Biol* 2010;685:106–10.

23

Kasabach-Meritt phenomenon

SANJAY SINGH AND NEETU BHARI

INTRODUCTION

In 1940, Kasabach and Merritt described a case of extensive capillary hemangioma with the presence of thrombocytopenic purpura and coagulopathy in a male child [1,2]. Kasabach-Merritt phenomenon (KMP) is a life-threatening situation characterized by thrombocytopenic consumptive coagulopathy (severe thrombocytopenia, elevated fibrin degradation products, and hypofibrinogenemia). The risk of mortality is as high as 10%–37% even if treated [3,4]. Many pharmacological agents (steroids, vincristine, propranolol, interferons, etc.) have been used to treat the condition, but the therapeutic response is variable. Sirolimus has shown good results, but evidence is limited to a few case series. Since surgical excision cannot be done in all cases, the need for an effective pharmacological agent is crucial. KMP is almost exclusively associated with two rare tumors, i.e., kaposiform hemangioendotheliomas (KHEs) and tufted angiomas (TAs), and is occasionally seen in association with angiosarcoma [5–7].

CLINICAL PRESENTATION OF KAPOSIFORM HEMANGIOENDOTHELIOMA AND TUFTED ANGIOMA

KHE and TA are both vascular tumors, and just like infantile hemangioma, they also present during infancy.

Mixed KHEs are commonly seen over the extremities, head, neck, and trunk with deeper infiltration, while deep KHEs are noncutaneous lesions limited to deeper tissues such as joints, retroperitoneum, and mediastinum [8]. It presents as an erythematous to violaceous or purpuric, ill-defined, indurated plaque with pebbly texture and deeper infiltration [9]. A large referral center observed the incidence of KHE to be approximately 0.07/100,000 children per year [9]. Histopathology shows infiltrating nodules composed of poorly canalized slit-like/crescentic vessels lined by spindle-shaped endothelial cells [2]. The risk of KMP increases if the lesion is of large size, has deeper involvement, or has a retroperitoneal location [8]. KHE is characterized by progressive fibrosis and deeper infiltration that may result in encasement and compression of surrounding vital structures; thus, the long-term risk of morbidity and mortality is significant [10].

TA, also known as *angioblastoma of Nagakawa*, presents as a firm, dusky, solitary, erythematous nodule (Figure 23.1) [5]. The usual age of onset is around 1–5 years, but it may even present at the time of birth. Compared to KHEs, TAs have a benign course with only a few reports of local invasion or an aggressive nature. Lesions may partially involute with time but rarely disappear completely [11]. Proximal extremities, neck, and upper trunk are the most common sites involved. Histopathology shows densely packed capillaries (vascular tufts) scattered in the dermis surrounded by crescentic spaces within tumor stroma (Figure 23.2). This classical presentation is called a "cannonball" configuration [11].

Both KHE and TA are CD31 and CD34 positive immunohistochemically with focal lymphatic marker positivity (LYVE1, PROX1, and D2-40). Both of them have intermediate malignancy potential. They are locally aggressive, and distant metastasis has not been described [2]. If untreated, both show the tendency to progress or may show partial spontaneous resolution but never disappear completely.

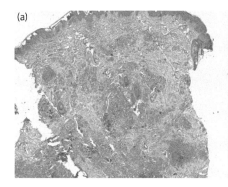

Figure 23.1 Dusky erythematous plaque over the right mandibular area, extending to the right side of the neck and chest. Sudden increase in the size, erythema, and firmness of the plaque is suggestive of Kasabach-Merritt phenomenon.

ASSOCIATION OF KAPOSIFORM HEMANGIOENDOTHELIOMA AND TUFTED ANGIOMA WITH KASABACH-MERRITT PHENOMENON

Croteau et al. studied 107 patients of KHE of which 71% of the cases developed KMP. The risk was significantly higher, i.e., 18-fold in the case of retroperitoneal or intrathoracic involvement. Lesions present at retroperitoneal and intrathoracic sites developed KMP in 85% and 100% cases, respectively. Also, those with KHE infiltrating into muscle or deeper were at 6.3-fold higher risk of KMP [9]. Another review of 19 patients of KMP had 18 (94.7%) patients of KHE and just one (5.3%) case of TA as components [5,12].

PATHOGENESIS

KMP is characterized by abnormal platelet function in an abnormal vasculature. These structurally abnormal vessels trap the platelets leading to platelet activation. Activated

platelets activate two main mechanisms in these vascular lesions:

1. Consumption as well as degradation of fibrinogen and other coagulation factors.
2. Release of adenosine diphosphate (ADPs) leading to further activation of platelets.

This cascade of events leads to an increase in prothrombin time (PT), activated partial thromboplastin time (aPTT), fibrin degradation products (FDPs), D-dimer, and low fibrinogen levels. These parameters are similar to disseminated intravascular coagulation (DIC), but DIC is a systemic phenomenon while KMP is localized to the lesion only [2]. Also, endothelial cells of KHE and platelets release vascular endothelial growth factors (VEGFs), which further leads to stimulation of angiogenesis and increase in the size of the lesion [2].

CLINICAL FEATURES AND EVALUATION

KMP is clinically characterized by a rapid increase in the size of the preexisting vascular plaque. In addition, the plaque becomes dusky erythematous, firm, and tender (Figure 23.1).

Patients may have bleeding from the lesions, hepatomegaly, jaundice, painful petechiae, signs of high-output cardiac failure in the form of tachycardia, feeding difficulty, and pallor due to anemia. The features resemble sepsis. As the size of the lesion increases and the child grows, symptoms can become more severe.

The bleeding can occur at distant sites as well. If there are no cutaneous lesions, suspect internal bleeding. Aggressive infiltration presenting as ulceration can also occur rarely, and it can become secondarily infected.

On hematological investigations, features of consumptive coagulopathy, i.e., derangement of blood coagulation parameters in the form of thrombocytopenia, microangiopathic hemolytic anemia, reduced fibrinogen, elevated fibrin degradation products, elevated D-dimer, and prolonged PT and aPTT are seen. Blood counts, blood culture, and genetic tests to identify the causative gene are ancillary.

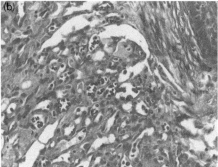

Figure 23.2 (a) Hematoxylin and eosin stain (10×) of a punch biopsy showed nodular aggregates in the upper, mid, and lower dermis giving a cannonball appearance. (b) Hematoxylin and eosin stain (40×) of a punch biopsy showed these nodular aggregates are composed of proliferating endothelial cells, capillaries, and lymphatics.

Radiological imaging helps to determine the extent of the lesion. Computed tomography scan, magnetic resonance imaging, Doppler, and radionuclide scanning help to delineate lesions better. Histological evaluation can be done for the confirmation of the diagnosis of primary lesion (Figure 23.2).

TREATMENT

There are no well-established, strong, evidence-based management strategies for KMP in the literature so far because of the rare incidence of this phenomenon. Currently available treatment options come from case reports and small case series only, as there are no randomized controlled trials and prospective studies available that evaluate their efficacy and safety (Table 23.1).

Surgical modalities

EMBOLIZATION

A number of agents have been tried for embolization in KMP, such as cellulose porous beads, platinum thrombogenic microcoils, polyvinyl alcohol particles, and drugs like bleomycin or iodinated oil [2,13,14]. In the case of rapid progression, embolization can be a life-saving procedure. However, if there are multiple feeding vessels, the embolization is not an ideal choice of treatment. The risk of tissue necrosis persists, and other rare reported complications are limb loss and stroke [2].

Ryan et al. found a partial response in KMP in 10/15 (66.6%) patients, and Wang et al. found good response in 9/14 (64%) patients with embolization [15,16]. Embolization has been used successfully in combination with vincristine [15].

SURGICAL EXCISION

Surgical excision of the primary lesion is the most definitive mode of treatment, if feasible. In 2011, a multidisciplinary expert panel proposed urgent surgical intervention in patients who are hemodynamically unstable or those with threatened limb loss. However, only in a limited number of cases, surgical intervention is amenable because of infiltration of the lesion into adjacent structures [17]. Furthermore, surgical and anesthetic complications with deranged coagulation profile in infants and younger children are significantly high.

Medical treatment

HEMOSTASIS SUPPORT

A patient presenting with KMP should always be assessed for hemodynamic instability. Platelet counts in KMP can be alarmingly low, but clinicians should not be apprehensive as despite the profound thrombocytopenia, life-threatening hemorrhages are uncommonly seen. Cryoprecipitate or fresh frozen plasma (10–15 mL/kg) should be given in settings of deranged coagulation profile, hypofibrinogenemia (fibrinogen <1 g/dL), platelet counts <10,000/μL, active bleeding, or prior to planned surgery [15]. In case of active bleeding, recombinant human factor VIIa can also be used. Despite deranged coagulation parameters including abnormal PT, aPTT, and international normalized ratio, use of heparin and low molecular weight heparin is not recommended in the management of KMP [18].

STEROIDS

Steroids continued to be the mainstay of treatment of KMP in spite of low efficacy and high relapse rates. There is a rapid and quick onset of response, but long-term efficacy is less than 30% [2]. The standard dose used is 2–5 mg/kg but can be as high as 30 mg/kg, and even pulse steroids have been used in life-threatening situations. A North American expert panel suggested that a uniform approach of systemic steroids with weekly vincristine should be accepted for all patients of KHE with KMP [6,18].

VINCRISTINE

Vincristine is a chemotherapeutic agent used as an anticancer drug in lymphoproliferative disorders. It is a natural vinca alkaloid and binds to tubulin, thereby interfering with mitotic spindle microtubules and inhibiting mitosis [1,2]. It also induces apoptosis of the endothelial cells and tumor

Table 23.1 Various drugs used in the management of Kasabach-Merritt phenomenon

Drug used	Dose	Mechanism of action	Level of evidence
Steroids	2–5 mg/kg or pulse dose	Increases vasoconstriction, inhibits fibrinolysis, disrupts angiogenesis	1
Vincristine	1–1.5 mg/m^2 or 0.05–0.065 mg/kg/week	Interferes with mitotic spindle activity and inhibits mitosis	1
Interferon-α	1 × 10^6 U/m^2/day in first week then 3 × 10^6 U/m^2/day for 3–9 months	Inhibits angiogenesis by suppressing basic fibroblast growth factor	2
Sirolimus	0.8 mg/m^2 twice daily then monthly (trough to 10–15 ng/mL)	Inhibits lymphangiogenesis	1/2
Propanolol	1–2 mg/kg/day	Nonselective ß-blocker; inhibits angiogenesis	3

cells and stops angiogenesis. Vincristine may cause mild bone marrow suppression, but the use is limited because of its neurotoxicity [1,2]. Vincristine has been used in combination with oral steroids, aspirin, ticlopidine, embolization, and radiotherapy [19–21]. A meta-analysis compared the efficacy of vincristine and steroids and concluded that it was better in KHE/TA in terms of efficacy and complication rates [19]. The standard dose used is 1–1.5 mg/m² or 0.05–0.065 mg/kg at weekly intervals via central access [1].

SIROLIMUS

Sirolimus causes decrease in size of the vascular tumor and improvement in hematological parameters. It also inhibits lymphangiogenesis [22,23]. In a multicenter retrospective cohort study of 52 patients with KHE, patients were treated with sirolimus alone or in combination with a short course of steroids in the presence of severe symptoms of KMP. Of these, 96% and 98% of the patients showed significant improvement in both groups, respectively, at 6 and 12 months [24]. Another retrospective study with eight patients of vincristine-resistant KMP found 100% response in hematologic parameters with sirolimus [25]. Sirolimus has been used for renal transplant in children with good safety margin; however, a risk related to angiogenesis inhibition in the developing infant has been claimed [2]. A study evaluating the response of sirolimus in refractory KHE found rapid response with average time for clinical response of 5.3 days and stabilization of platelet count >100 × 10⁹/L at 15.1 days with fewer and mild side effects in the form of mucositis, grade 1 elevation of transaminases, thrombocytosis, etc. [26]. Besides its antiangiogenesis property, sirolimus has shown antifibrotic activity in animal models [27]. Although efficacy of sirolimus is well established in KMP, there are occasional reports of therapeutic failure [28].

INTERFERON-ALPHA (IFN-α)

Interferon-α (IFN-α) has been used in KMP when other primary drugs have failed. Equal efficacy is seen with both IFN-α2a and 2b [2,29]. The dosage used is 3 million IU units/m²/day. However, the use is limited because of serious side effects including irreversible spastic diplegia in infants [2,6]. Other reported side effects are flu-like symptoms, fatigue, deranged liver enzymes, and cytopenia [2].

In a meta-analysis by Michaud et al., 11 (0.025%) of 441 children developed irreversible spastic diplegia when given IFN-α for vascular lesions, while 16 (0.036%) children developed reversible motor developmental disturbances [29]. In another study of 12 patients of KHE treated with subcutaneous IFN-α (1 × 10⁶U/m²/day in first week then 3 × 10⁶U/m²/day for 3–9 months), 11 patients showed a greater than 50% reduction in tumor size [30].

PROPRANOLOL

Propranolol is a β-adrenergic receptor (nonselective) blocker that has gained fair acceptance in the treatment of infantile hemangiomas. Isolated case reports have shown good response of KMP with propranolol (mono or combined therapy) [31–33], but in larger case series, propranolol

has failed to show promising results [2]. Currently it is considered as a third-line drug for the management of KMP.

ANTIPLATELET DRUGS

Aspirin, dipyridamole, ticlopidine, and pentoxifylline have all been used for KMP either as monotherapy or in combination as dual antiplatelet therapy. Antiplatelet drugs are safe in KMP, and there is no increased risk of bleeding complications in these patients. An aspirin and ticlopidine combination has been most commonly used in clinical practice, and dual therapy is more efficacious than monotherapy. Aspirin irreversibly inhibits cyclooxygenase activity leading to inhibition of platelet aggregation, while ticlopidine selectively blocks ADP-induced platelet aggregation. Although combination therapy has been found to be effective in many case reports and series [34], a few reports have shown unsuccessful results [35].

Physical modalities

RADIATION THERAPY

Response rates as high as 75% have been described using radiotherapy in combination with steroids without any radiation injury even up to a follow-up of 6 years [2,36]. But, there is risk of secondary malignancies and growth disturbances with the use of radiotherapy, so the use is limited to life-threatening situations only or if other safer modalities have failed in the past [37].

COMPRESSION THERAPY

Compression causes decreased blood flow to the involved limb, and this effect might decrease the risk of impending high cardiac output failure. Compression cannot be the definitive mode of treatment but is only effective as an adjuvant to other mainstay treatment options.

MISCELLANEOUS DRUGS AND TREATMENT OPTIONS

Shen et al. used intralesional absolute ethanol every 3 days in eight pediatric patients with KMP at a dose of 0.5–1 mL/kg body weight. All patients had shown blood coagulation profile improvements after being treated for 2 weeks. After 2 weeks, weekly doses were given. In the 1-year to 3-year follow-up periods, there was no recurrence. Minor complications such as pain, transient bruises, flush on face, local scars, and small areas of local necrosis were noted in this study [38]. Similarly, Yuan et al. described good results with intralesional absolute ethanol [12]. Isolated reports of everolimus, an mTOR inhibitor, leading to complete remission of KMP exist in literature [39,40]. Tranexamic acid and aminocaproic acid have been used extensively in KMP, usually in combination therapy [41–43]. Combination chemotherapy has been used successfully in cases resistant to conventional therapies [44,45]. Fuchimoto et al. treated a child with KHE accompanied by KMP with four cycles of combined vincristine, actinomycin D, and cyclophosphamide (VAC). Interestingly, multimodal treatments including steroids, interferon-α, radiation, embolization therapy, and vincristine as monotherapy failed in this case [44]. Rarely, drugs such as carboplatin, tetrahydro-pyranyl, adriamycin, gemcitabine, and vinorelbine have been used in difficult to treat cases [46,47].

CONCLUSION

KMP is a life-threatening emergency, most commonly seen with preexisting atypical vascular lesions as kaposiform hemangioendothelioma and tufted angioma. Early recognition and treatment are of crucial importance. There are no well-established, strong, evidence-based management strategies for KMP in the literature so far because of the rare incidence of this phenomenon. In a child presenting with KMP, hemodynamic stability should be achieved as soon as possible with the use of fresh frozen plasma infusions. Surgical excision and embolization, when feasible, are the first line of treatment. Oral prednisolone with or without vincristine can be used in the cases where surgical excision is not feasible. Oral sirolimus has shown its efficacy and safety in recent reports and case series. Other drugs and combination therapies are used in nonresponsive recalcitrant cases.

KEY POINTS

- Kasabach Merritt phenomenon is a consumptive coagulopathy.
- It is usually found in Kaposiform hemangioendothelioma and Tufted angioma.
- Rapid increase in size of lesion, bleeding and systemic complications are characteristic findings.
- Surgical modalities like excision and embolization and medications like steroids, vincristine and sirolimus are good treatment options.

REFERENCES

1. Yadav D, Maheshwari A, Aneja S, Seth A, Chandra J. Neonatal Kasabach-Merritt phenomenon. *Indian J Med Paediatr Oncol Off J Indian Soc Med Paediatr Oncol* 2011;32:238–41.
2. O'Rafferty C, O'Regan GM, Irvine AD, Smith OP. Recent advances in the pathobiology and management of Kasabach-Merritt phenomenon. *Br J Haematol* 2015;171:38–51.
3. Arunachalam P, Kumar VRR, Swathi D. Kasabach-Merritt syndrome with large cutaneous vascular tumors. *J Indian Assoc Pediatr Surg* 2012;17:33–6.
4. Kwok-Williams M, Perez Z, Squire R, Glaser A, Bew S, Taylor R. Radiotherapy for life-threatening mediastinal hemangioma with Kasabach-Merritt syndrome. *Pediatr Blood Cancer* 2007;49:739–44.
5. Bhari N et al. Tufted angioma with recurrent Kasabach-Merritt phenomenon. *Indian J Dermatol Venereol Leprol* 2018;84:121.
6. Mahajan P, Margolin J, Iacobas I. Kasabach-Merritt phenomenon: Classic presentation and management options. *Clin Med Insights Blood Disord* 2017;10:1179545X17699849.
7. Wadhwa S, Kim TH, Lin L, Kanel G, Saito T. Hepatic angiosarcoma with clinical and histological features of Kasabach-Merritt syndrome. *World J Gastroenterol* 2017;23:2443–7.
8. Alaqeel AM, Alfurayh NA, Alhedyani AA, Alajlan SM. Sirolimus for treatment of kaposiform hemangioendothelioma associated with Kasabach-Merritt phenomenon. *JAAD Case Rep* 2016;2:457–61.
9. Croteau SE et al. Kaposiform hemangioendothelioma: Atypical features and risks of Kasabach-Merritt phenomenon in 107 referrals. *J Pediatr* 2013;162:142.
10. Schaefer BA, Wang D, Merrow AC, Dickie BH, Adams DM. Long-term outcome for kaposiform hemangioendothelioma: A report of two cases. *Pediatr Blood Amp Cancer* 2017;64:284–6.
11. Rambhia KD, Khopkar US. Tufted angioma. *Indian Dermatol Online J* 2016;7:62.
12. Yuan SM, Shen WM, Chen HN, Hong ZJ, Jiang HQ. Kasabach-Merritt phenomenon in Chinese children: Report of 19 cases and brief review of literature. *Int J Clin Exp Med* 2015;8:10006–10.
13. Zhou S, Li H, Mao Y, Liu P, Zhang J. Successful treatment of Kasabach-Merritt syndrome with transarterial embolization and corticosteroids. *J Pediatr Surg* 2013;48:673–6.
14. Khant ZA et al. Successful transarterial embolization with cellulose porous beads for occipital haemangioma in an infant with Kasabach-Merritt syndrome. *BJRcase Rep* 2017;2:20170004.
15. Ryan C et al. Kasabach-Merritt phenomenon: A single centre experience. *Eur J Haematol* 2010;84:97–104.
16. Wang P, Zhou W, Tao L, Zhao N, Chen X-W. Clinical analysis of Kasabach-Merritt syndrome in 17 neonates. *BMC Pediatr* 2014;14:146.
17. Sasson M, Flippin JA, Birken G, Alkhoury F. Surgical intervention for Kasabach-Merritt syndrome: A case report. *J Pediatr Surg Case Rep* 2015;3:462–5.
18. Drolet BA et al. Consensus-derived practice standards plan for complicated kaposiform hemangioendothelioma. *J Pediatr* 2013;163:285–91.
19. Liu X et al. Clinical outcomes for systemic corticosteroids versus vincristine in treating kaposiform hemangioendothelioma and tufted angioma. *Medicine (Baltimore)* 2016;95:e3431.
20. Wang Z, Li K, Yao W, Dong K, Xiao X, Zheng S. Steroid-resistant kaposiform hemangioendothelioma: A retrospective study of 37 patients treated with vincristine and long-term follow-up. *Pediatr Blood Cancer* 2015;62:577–80.

21. Garcia-Monaco R et al. Kaposiform hemangioendothelioma with Kasabach-Merritt phenomenon: Successful treatment with embolization and vincristine in two newborns. *J Vasc Interv Radiol* 2012;23:417–22.

22. Huber S et al. Inhibition of the mammalian target of rapamycin impedes lymphangiogenesis. *Kidney Int* 2007;71:771–7.

23. Ando K et al. The efficacy and safety of low-dose sirolimus for treatment of lymphangioleiomyomatosis. *Respir Investig* 2013;51:175–83.

24. Ji Y et al. Sirolimus for the treatment of progressive kaposiform hemangioendothelioma: A multicenter retrospective study. *Int J Cancer* 2017;141:848–55.

25. Wang H, Duan Y, Gao Y, Guo X. Sirolimus for vincristine-resistant Kasabach-Merritt phenomenon: Report of eight patients. *Pediatr Dermatol* 2017;34:261–5.

26. Kai L, Wang Z, Yao W, Dong K, Xiao X. Sirolimus, a promising treatment for refractory kaposiform hemangioendothelioma. *J Cancer Res Clin Oncol* 2014;140(3):471–6.

27. Oza VS, Mamlouk MD, Hess CP, Mathes EF, Frieden IJ. Role of sirolimus in advanced kaposiform hemangioendothelioma. *Pediatr Dermatol* 2016;33:e88–92.

28. Triana PJ et al. Pancreatic kaposiform hemangioendothelioma not responding to sirolimus. *Eur J Pediatr Surg Rep* 2017;05:e32–5.

29. Michaud A-P, Bauman NM, Burke DK, Manaligod JM, Smith RJH. Spastic diplegia and other motor disturbances in infants receiving interferon-alpha. *Laryngoscope* 2004;114:1231–6.

30. Wu HW et al. Interferon-alpha therapy for refractory kaposiform hemangioendothelioma: A single-center experience. *Sci Rep* 2016;6:36261.

31. Oksiuta M, Matuszczak E, Dębek W, Dzienis-Koronkiewicz E, Hermanowicz A. Successful exclusive propranolol therapy in an infant with life-threatening Kasabach-Merritt syndrome. *J Pediatr Surg Case Rep* 2013;1:200–2.

32. Mizutani K et al. Successful combination therapy of propranolol and prednisolone for a case with congenital Kasabach-Merritt syndrome. *J Dermatol* 2017; 44:1389–91.

33. Jiang RS, Zhao ZY. Multimodal treatment of Kasabach-Merritt syndrome arising from tufted angioma: A case report. *Oncol Lett* 2017;13:4887–91.

34. Fernandez-Pineda I, Lopez-Gutierrez JC, Chocarro G, Bernabeu-Wittel J, Ramirez-Villar GL. Long-term outcome of vincristine-aspirin-ticlopidine (VAT) therapy for vascular tumors associated with Kasabach-Merritt phenomenon. *Pediatr Blood Cancer* 2013;60:1478–81.

35. Enjolras O et al. [Kasabach-Merritt syndrome on a congenital tufted angioma]. *Ann Dermatol Venereol* 1998;125:257–60.

36. Shin HY, Ryu KH, Ahn HS. Stepwise multimodal approach in the treatment of Kasabach-Merritt syndrome. *Pediatr Int Off J Jpn Pediatr Soc* 2000;42:620–4.

37. Atahan IL, Cengiz M, Ozyar E, Gürkaynak M. Radiotherapy in the management of Kasabach-Merritt syndrome: A case report. *Pediatr Hematol Oncol* 2001;18:471–6.

38. Shen W, Cui J, Chen J, Zou J, Xiaoying Z. Treating kaposiform hemangioendothelioma with Kasabach-Merritt phenomenon by intralesional injection of absolute ethanol. *J Craniofac Surg* 2014;25:2188–91.

39. Matsumoto H et al. Successful Everolimus treatment of kaposiform hemangioendothelioma with Kasabach-Merritt phenomenon: Clinical efficacy and adverse effects of mTOR inhibitor therapy. *J Pediatr Hematol Oncol* 2016;38:e322–5.

40. Uno T, Ito S, Nakazawa A, Miyazaki O, Mori T, Terashima K. Successful treatment of kaposiform hemangioendothelioma with everolimus. *Pediatr Blood Cancer* 2015;62:536–8.

41. Warrell RP, Kempin SJ. Treatment of severe coagulopathy in the Kasabach-Merritt syndrome with aminocaproic acid and cryoprecipitate. *N Engl J Med* 1985;313:309–12.

42. Ortel TL, Onorato JJ, Bedrosian CL, Kaufman RE. Antifibrinolytic therapy in the management of the Kasabach-Merritt syndrome. *Am J Hematol* 1988;29:44–8.

43. Dresse MF et al. Successful treatment of Kasabach-Merritt syndrome with prednisone and epsilon-aminocaproic acid. *Pediatr Hematol Oncol* 1991;8:329–34.

44. Fuchimoto Y et al. Vincristine, actinomycin D, cyclophosphamide chemotherapy resolves Kasabach-Merritt syndrome resistant to conventional therapies. *Pediatr Int* 2012;54:285–7.

45. Hu B, Lachman R, Phillips J, Peng SK, Sieger L. Kasabach-Merritt syndrome-associated kaposiform hemangioendothelioma successfully treated with cyclophosphamide, vincristine, and actinomycin D. *J Pediatr Hematol Oncol* 1998;20:567–9.

46. Yasui N et al. Kasabach-Merritt phenomenon: A report of 11 cases from a single institution. *J Pediatr Hematol Oncol* 1998;20:567–9.

47. Read WL, Williams F. Metastatic angiosarcoma with Kasabach-Merritt syndrome responsive to gemcitabine and vinorelbine after failure of liposomal doxorubicin and paclitaxel: A case report. *Case Rep Oncol* 2016;9:177–81.

PART 7

Infections and Infestations

K. P. ANEESH

24

Staphylococcal scalded skin syndrome

RESHAM VASANI

INTRODUCTION

Staphylococcal scalded skin syndrome (SSSS) describes a spectrum of superficial blistering disorders caused by the exfoliative toxin of *Staphylococcus aureus*. Generally, SSSS is regarded as a mild disease, but in neonates and in immunocompromised adults, it is considered serious and occasionally fatal. It also shares a resemblance to toxic epidermal necrolysis from which it is essential to differentiate and hence qualifies as a dermatological emergency.

The first description of the disease was by Baron Von Rittershain, a German physician in 1878 [1]. The condition is hence also called *Ritter disease* or *Ritter Von Ritterschein disease* [2].

ETIOLOGY

Approximately 35% of the general population are commensal carriers of *S. aureus* [3,4]. Patients of contact dermatitis, psoriasis, and atopic dermatitis are pronounced carriers of *S. aureus*. Nursing homes and hospitals are common sources of this bacterium because of insufficient infection control practices (like regular handwashing and cleaning stethoscopes). Newborns are at high risk because bacteria are colonized within 6 days of birth. In neonates, *S. aureus* can be isolated from skin, eyes, umbilicus, perineum, and wound sites [5].

Initial studies revealed that phage lytic group II staphylococci were mainly responsible for exfoliative toxin and cause SSSS, but now it is known that all phage groups are able to produce exfoliative toxin [6,7]. Approximately 5% of *S. aureus* produce exfoliative toxin [3,8,9] and have two different serotypes affecting humans (ETA and ETB) [10].

Childhood cases of SSSS are primarily associated solely with ETA production, but the frequencies of different toxins in adult cases are unclear.

PATHOGENESIS

S. aureus enters the skin through a break in the barrier (such as erosions, atopic dermatitis, and varicella lesions), but hematogenous spread is usually limited by the presence of antitoxin antibodies [10,11]. This results in the clinical presentation of localized forms like bullous impetigo (Figure 24.1). In the generalized form, toxin is produced at distant sites like nares, eyes, umbilicus, groin, wound site, or an infected systemic site (in conditions such as pneumonia, osteomyelitis, or endocarditis). Lack of protective antibodies allows the toxin to spread through the bloodstream to reach the mid-epidermis via dermal capillaries to produce generalized exfoliation [12].

Desmoglein-1 (Dsg1) is a desmosomal cadherin involved in intercellular adhesion and is found only in the superficial dermis. It plays an important role in maintaining epidermal integrity. Disruption of this structure would result in the loss of cell-to-cell adhesion and separation at the level of the zona granulosa. ETA acts like an atypical glutamate-specific serine protease that binds and cleaves Dsg1 in the region of amino acid number 10, where there are several glutamic acid residues.

Recent work suggests that exfoliative toxins may possess unique and specific superantigenic activity though it is unlikely to play a major role in the pathogenesis. It may be important in other diseases where superantigens are thought to be involved, such as acute exacerbations of atopic dermatitis, Kawasaki disease, staphylococcal

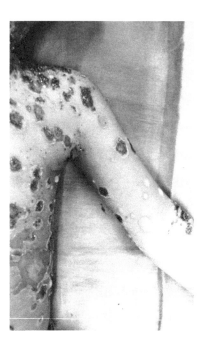

Figure 24.1 Bullous impetigo.

nephritis, rheumatoid arthritis, and other autoimmune diseases [11].

CLINICAL FEATURES

Localized staphylococcal scalded skin syndrome

Like bullous impetigo, localized SSSS presents with few localized fragile superficial blisters filled with colorless or purulent fluid [13]. The surrounding skin appears normal. There are no systemic symptoms. In neonates, the lesions are more common around the umbilicus and perineum. In older children, lesions are more common on the extremities (Figure 24.1) [14].

Generalized staphylococcal scalded skin syndrome

AGE AT PRESENTATION

Generalized SSSS usually can occur at any age but is commonly evident in childen younger than 5 years of age. The possible reasons for this age predilection are lack of protective antibodies against staphylococcal toxins and immature kidneys that are unable to excrete the toxin.

Though uncommon in adults, the greatest risk factor is underlying illness, especially renal disease that accounts for a mortality rate of >60%. Specific risk factors for SSSS include a suppressed immune system as seen in conditions such as diabetes, malignancy, chronic alcohol abuse, and HIV, where patients cannot produce antibodies to exfoliative toxins, and conditions such as renal failure and treatments such as hemodialysis where patients cannot excrete toxins.

Outbreaks of SSSS have been reported in the neonatal intensive care unit (NICU) due to handling of babies by infected or asymptomatic carriers of *Staphylococci*. Breastfeeding may confer protection against SSSS.

CLINICAL FEATURES

The prodromal phase includes irritability, malaise, and fever. There is initially a localized infection of the conjunctiva, throat, nares, perineum, or umbilicus (Figure 24.2). In most cases, no focus of infection is found or the infection is not apparent before the SSSS rash appears [15].

A scarlatiniform eruption is followed by a scalded appearance of skin (Figure 24.3). This is further followed by formation of flaccid bullae (Figure 24.4). Nikolsky sign is positive [14,17]. Superficial blisters quickly rupture, especially at the sites of friction, leaving raw, red, moist skin with appearance similar to a hot water scald (Figure 24.5) [15]. The eruption

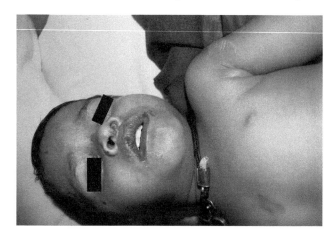

Figure 24.2 Initial lesions around the nares and perioral area.

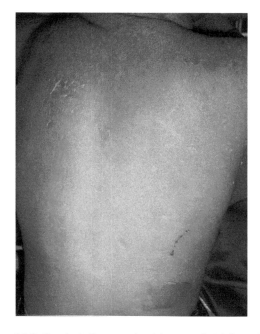

Figure 24.3 Scarlatiniform rash with superficial flaccid blistering and peeling.

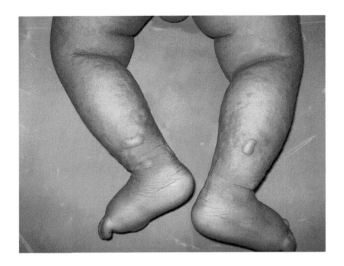

Figure 24.4 Bullae over an erythematous base.

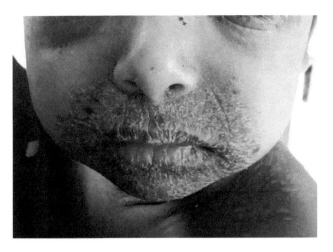

Figure 24.7 Perioral crusting.

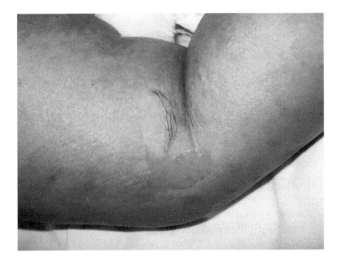

Figure 24.5 Blisters rupture to show raw red moist skin.

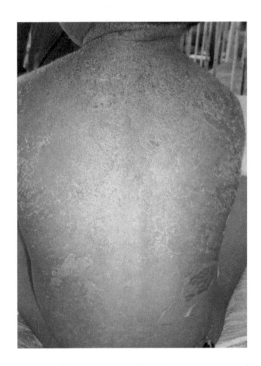

Figure 24.8 Exfoliation seen after the acute episode.

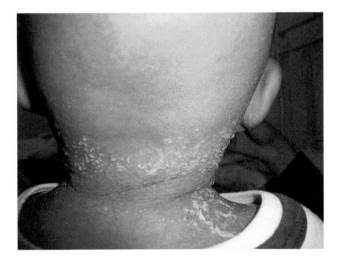

Figure 24.6 Pustules on neck.

is more prominent over the flexures like axillae and neck (Figure 24.6) and the facial appearance is characteristic with separation of perioral crusts, leaving behind radial fissures around the mouth (Figure 24.7).

Though most patients do not appear severely ill, in advanced erythrodermic cases, generalized malaise, fever, irritability, skin tenderness, and poor feeding are seen. Generalized denudation carries a risk of fluid loss, dehydration, and altered thermoregulation. Premature infants are particularly at risk of secondary gram-negative infection with *Pseudomonas aeruginosa* and also septicemia [18,19]. Generalized tissue paper–like wrinkling of the epidermis appears around the 10th day (Figure 24.8). Since the condition is toxin mediated, exfoliation usually continues 24–48 hours after starting appropriate antibiotic treatment [16]. The skin heals rapidly within 7–14 days without scarring, because of the high level of split in the epidermis.

Clinical features in adults are essentially similar to those found in children except that the majority grow *S. aureus* in blood culture. Fever is associated with edematous erythema of

Table 24.1 Differences in presentation of staphylococcal scalded skin syndrome (SSSS) in children and adults

Criterion	SSSS in children	SSSS in adults
Age at presentation	<5 years	Immunocompromised and those with renal failure
Cause	Absence of antibodies against the exfoliative toxins and immature renal function	Due to inability to produce antibodies against exfoliative toxins on account of immunosuppression and inability to excrete toxins on account of renal failure
Site of primary infection	Difficult to identify the site of primary infection in most cases	Pneumonia, osteomyelitis, septic arthritis
Blood culture	Negative	Positive
Associated diseases	Child is otherwise in good health	Immunocompromised-chronic renal disease, HIV, malignancy, chemotherapy, IV drug abuse, diabetes mellitus
Mortality	<5%	40%–63%

the eyelids and nostrils, and the condition is associated with a significantly high mortality rate. The clinical features in adults versus those in children are summarized in Table 24.1.

DIAGNOSIS

The investigations are directed toward a thorough examination to identify the potential focus of staphylococcal infection, fluid status of the patient, and any evidence of secondary infection.

- *Tzanck smear*: Shows the presence of acantholytic cells without the presence of inflammatory cells.
- *Culture specimen*: Can be obtained from the eye, nose, throat, or pyogenic foci on skin for isolation of *S. aureus*. Exfoliated skin and intact blisters do not yield any organisms since it is caused by hematogenous spread of the exfoliative toxin.
- *Antibiotic sensitivity profile*: The antibiotic sensitivity profile of *S. aureus* isolated may be useful where empiric treatment is not successful because of antibiotic resistance [20].
- *Blood culture*: This is positive in less than 5% of the cases [21].
- *X-Ray chest*: This may rule out pneumonia as the original focus of infection.
- *Erythrocyte sedimentation rate (ESR)*: ESR is elevated in most cases.
- *Electrolytes/renal function tests*: The results are closely followed in severe cases where fluid loss via dehydration is a concern.
- *Skin biopsy*: Though not practical in children, skin biopsy is the most useful test in case of a diagnostic confusion. In SSSS, biopsy shows a midepidermal splitting at the level of zona granulosa without cytolysis, cell necrosis, or inflammatory reaction [22].
- *Polymerase chain reaction, reverse passive latex agglutination, enzyme-linked immunosorbent assay, and radioimmunoassay*: These methods can identify toxin production by *S. aureus* [23] but rely on isolation of *S. aureus*, which is neither sensitive nor specific. The time taken to isolate the organism from peripheral and

blood specimens would help only to make a retrospective diagnosis [24]. Gene sequence detection by DNA hybridization is a recently developed system for exfoliative toxins of SSSS. The major drawback of these techniques is that they are meant for laboratory-based research rather than clinical applications, and techniques are too costly and time consuming for routine analysis [25].
- The detection of phage group II will strongly support the diagnosis of SSSS even though other phage types show identical clinical features [26].

DIFFERENTIAL DIAGNOSIS

The closest differential diagnosis is toxic epidermal necrolysis, since both the conditions exhibit positive Nikolsky sign, skin tenderness, and scalded skin appearance [27].

Table 24.2 summarizes the differential diagnosis of SSSS.

MANAGEMENT

Localized lesions of bullous impetigo

In localized lesions of bullous impetigo, the organisms are present in the lesion. Because of this, oral antibiotics with topical antibiotics such as topical mupirocin and fusidic acid are used.

Generalized lesions

For generalized lesions, treatment is preferable and best accomplished in an intensive care or burn unit. Start antibiotics as soon as possible though SSSS will continue to progress for another 24–48 hours after onset until the circulating antitoxin is neutralized by antibodies or excreted by the kidneys [28]. Central venous access is preferable for blood sampling of urea, electrolytes, and blood gases every 8–12 hours. Urinary catheterization to measure urine output is helpful.

As most strains of *S. aureus* causing SSSS are methicillin sensitive, penicillinase-resistant ß-lactam agents such

Table 24.2 Differential diagnosis of staphylococcal scalded skin syndrome (SSSS)

Entity	Similarity to SSSS	Difference from SSSS
Toxic epidermal necrolysis	• Scalded appearance • Skin tenderness • Positive Nikolsky sign	• Seen in adults • Usually secondary to drug intake • Can cause extensive erosions in mouth, conjunctiva, trachea, bronchi, esophagus, and genitalia • Carries a high mortality rate [25] • On histopathology, separation is at the level of dermoepidermal junction versus the split in granular layer in SSSS; inflammatory infiltrate is present unlike SSSS
Infections caused by human enterovirus, echovirus, coxsackie virus, enterovirus 71	Superficial blistering that does not involve the oral cavity	Epidermal necrosis with keratinocyte dyskeratosis
Drug-related rash, eosinophilia, and systemic symptoms	Fever followed by appearance of erythematous eruption on face, trunk, and extremities and can be followed by bulla formation	• Follows intake of anticonvulsants and sulfonamides • Appears weeks after the intake of drug • Elevated serum IgG to HHV6 • Histopathology shows a perivascular lymphocytic infiltrate with eosinophils
Staphylococcal toxic syndrome	Mild forms can be associated with exfoliation	Have associated petechiae and desquamation of palms and soles predominantly, while in SSSS there are bullae with a positive Nikolsky sign that desquamates; facial and skin fold involvement is more commonly seen in SSSS

as cloxacillin, dicloxacillin, oxacillin, flucloxacillin, and nafcillin are the first-line antibiotics [15]. In case of penicillin allergic patients, clarithromycin or cefuroxime are the possible options. If the patient is not responding to these agents, then methicillin-resistant strains of *S. aureus* (MRSA) should be suspected, for which vancomycin is the drug of choice [30]. For secondary gram-negative infection, amikacin or gentamicin injections can be administered. Table 24.3 summarizes the dosages of antibiotics used in the treatment of SSSS.

Ninety-one percent of adults have antibodies against ETA. Systemically unwell children can hence be administered fresh frozen plasma (10 mg/kg) to neutralize exotoxin antibodies, and if no response, can be administered a 5-day course of IV immunoglobulin (0.4 g/kg/d).This approach should be successful in both children and adults but has only been reported to work in children. Double-blinded randomized placebo trials have not been performed [31,32].

Rapid sensitive and specific tests are being developed using Desmoglein as an antigen for quantification of toxin in plasma or other biological fluids taken from suspected cases of SSSS. Synthesis of analogues of toxin binding regions of desmoglein to inhibit toxins and therefore prevent exfoliation in a similar pattern as has been shown with L-monocytogenes would be of benefit. Their ability to invade epithelial cells and inhibition by N-terminal fragments and recombinant proteins of E cadherin (CDH-1 gene) makes them theoretically useful in high-risk cases

such as adults with underlying disease and children with extensive disease.

Fluids

In pediatric patients, fresh frozen plasma can be given as a bolus (10% of a child's circulating volume [70 mL/kg])

Table 24.3 Dosages of drugs that can be administered in a case of staphylococcal scalded skin syndrome (SSSS)

Drug	Dosage
Flucloxacillin	50–100 mg/kg/day
Cloxacillin	25 mg/kg/day in divided doses every 6 hours
Nafcillin	100 mg/kg/day IV in four divided doses
Penicillin G Procaine	300 KU/day intramuscularly (IM) for <30 kg, 600 K to 1 million U/day IM for >30 kg
Cefazolin	100 mg/kg/day IV in four divided doses
Cephalexin	40 mg/kg/day in four divided doses × 7–10 days
Clindamycin	40 mg/kg/day IV in four divided doses
Bactrim	10 mg/kg/day in two doses × 7–10 days
Vancomycin	10–15 mg/kg/day in two divided doses up to 1 gm q12hr

followed by maintenance fluid of dextrose 4% in saline 0.18% at a weight-dependent rate using the 4-2-1 rule [33].

Despite a significant risk of hypovolemia from fluid loss, the risk of hyponatremia exists because of inappropriate release of vasopressin with the excess of IV fluids given. Hence, 0.45% saline + 5% dextrose should be given as maintenance fluid [28].

Dressings

For denuded areas, soft silicone primary dressings covered by saline-soaked gauze are preferred. Povidone iodine and silver sulfadiazine dressings are avoided due to the risk of systemic absorption of iodine and silver, respectively. If skin loss is small, sterile dressings of silver sulfadiazine cream and paraffin-impregnated gauze covered by gauze and cotton tissue can be used for the trunk. As areas heal, hydrocolloid dressings can be applied [29].

Analgesia

Paracetamol is the analgesic of choice in SSSS. Avoiding nonsteroidal anti-inflammatory drugs that are excreted by the kidneys and cause an increased risk of bleeding is important. Opiates like fentanyl can be administered as needed [29].

Other measures

Midazolam 50–100 μg/kg/h may be of benefit for sedation. For pruritus in children, medication may be used as required. Bedding must be comfortable. Forced-air warming blankets are better replacements for heavy blankets as they provide a core temperature of 37°C –38°C. Physiotherapy is to be done to ensure mobility of joints [28]. Nasogastric/nasojejunal tube should be used to provide enteral nutrition.

PROGNOSIS

If treatment including nasogastric feeding, IV fluids, and IV antibiotics are begun early, denuded skin will reepithelialize in 12 days without scarring. Mortality is low with appropriate care in children (up to 5%) [14,15,18]. It can reach almost 60% in adults who have an underlying illness even with initiation of appropriate antibiotics. More extensive involvement in a younger patient is associated with a worse outcome.

PREVENTION

Asymptomatic nasal carriage is an important source of infection in neonates; hence, strict control measures should be taken, such as isolation of the infected patients, barrier nursing, and antiseptic handwashing by staff and visitors to the unit. Screening of staff and patients is necessary.

Exfoliative toxin may serve as a target for development of vaccines in the future.

KEY POINTS

- Staphylococcal scalded skin syndrome is a spectrum of superficial blistering disorders caused by exfoliative toxin of *Staphylococcus aureus*.
- In the generalized variant, following a prodrome there is a scarlatiniform eruption that eventuates into formation of flaccid bullae leading to erosions and exfoliation that are more prominent over the flexures.
- Due to the superficial level of split in the epidermis, there is rapid healing with appropriate treatment usually within 10 days.
- Investigations are directed toward identifying a potential focus of staphylococcal infection, fluid status of the patient, and any evidence of secondary infection.
- The primary focus of infection is obscure in children but is detectable in adults in most cases.
- Hospitalization of the patient with administration of fluids to maintain electrolyte and fluid balance, infection control with antibiotics, and pain management are the mainstay of treatment.
- Mortality is low in children but is higher in adults on account of an associated immunocompromised state.

REFERENCES

1. Von Rittershain GR. Die exfolitive dermatitis jungener senglinge. *Z Kinderheilkd* 1878;2:3–23.
2. Melish ME, Glasgow LA. The staphylococcal scalded skin syndrome: Development of an experimental model. *N Engl J Med* 1970;282:1114–9.
3. Dancer SJ, Noble WC. Nasal, axillary and perineal carriage of *Staphylococcus aureus* among pregnant women: Identification of strains producing epidermolytic toxin. *J Clin Pathol* 1991;44:681–4.
4. Noble WC. *The Micrococci*. London: Lloyd-Luke; 1981:152–81.
5. Dancer SJ, Simmons NA, Poston SM, Noble WC. Outbreak of staphylococcal scalded skin syndrome among neonates. *J Infect* 1988;16:87–103.
6. Dajani AS. The scalded skin syndrome: Relation to phage group II staphylococci. *J Infect Dis* 1972; 125:548.
7. Kondo I, Sakurai S, Sarai Y. New type of exfoliatin obtained from staphylococcal strains belonging to phage group other than group II, isolated from patients with impetigo and Ritter's disease. *Infect Immun* 1974;10:851–61.

8. Adesiyun AA, Lenz W, Schaal KP. Exfoliative toxin production by *Staphylococcus aureus* strains isolated from animals and human beings in Nigeria. *Microbiologica* 1991;14:357–62.

9. Elsner P, Hartman AA. Epidemiology of ETA- and ETB-producing staphylococci in dermatological patients. *Zentbl Bacterial Mikrobiol Hyg Series A* 1988;268:534.

10. Papageorgiou AC, Plano LR, Collins CM, Acharya KR. Structural similarities and differences in *Staphylococcus aureus* exfoliative toxins A and B as revealed by their crystal structure. *Protein Sci* 2000;9:610–8.

11. Ladhani S, Joannou CL, Lochrie DP, Evans RW, Poston SM. Clinical, microbial and biochemical aspects of the exfoliative toxins causing staphylococcal scalded skin syndrome. *Clin Microbiol Rev* 1999;12:224–42.

12. Melish ME, Chen FS, Sprouse S, Stuckey M, Murata MS. Epidermolytic toxin staphylococcal infection: Toxin levels and host response. In: Jeljaszewicz J (Ed), *Staphylococci and Staphylococcal Infections*. Stuttgart: Gustav Fischer-Verlag; 1981:287–98.

13. Lyell A. Toxic epidermal necrolysis (the scalded skin syndrome): A reappraisal. *Br J Dermatol* 1979;100:69–86.

14. Melish ME. Staphylococci, streptococci and the skin: Review of impetigo and staphylococcal scalded skin syndrome. *Semin Dermatol* 1982;1:101–9.

15. Cribier B, Piemont Y, Grosshans E. Staphylococcal scalded skin syndrome in adults: A clinical review illustrated with a new case. *J Am Acad Dermatol* 1984;30:319–24.

16. Ladhani S, Newson TA. Familial outbreak of staphylococcal scalded skin syndrome. *Pediatr Infect Dis J* 2000;19:578–9.

17. Moss C, Gupta E. The Nikolsky sign in staphylococcal scalded skin syndrome. *Arch Dis Child* 1998;79:290.

18. Gemmell CG. Staphylococcal scalded skin syndrome. *J Med Microbiol* 1997;43:318–27.

19. Hoffmann RR, Lohner M, Bohm N, Schaefer HE, Letitis J. Staphylococcal scalded skin syndrome and consecutive septicaemia in a preterm infant. *Pathol Res Pract* 1994;190:77–81.

20. Yokota S, Imagawa T, Kataakura S, Mitsuda T, Arai TS. Staphylococcal scalded skin syndrome caused by exfoliative toxin B-producing methicillin-resistant *Staphylococcus aureus*. *Eur J Pediatr* 1996;155:722.

21. Goldberg NS, Ahmed T, Robinson B, Ascensao H, Horwitz H. Staphylococcal scalded skin syndrome mimicking acute graft-versus-host disease in a bone marrow transplant recipient. *Arch Dermatol* 1989;15:385–9.

22. Gentilhomme E, Faure M, Piemont Y, Binder P, Thivolet J. Action of staphylococcal exfoliative toxins on epidermal cell cultures and organotypic skin. *J Dermatol* 1990;17:526–32.

23. Ladhani S et al. Development and evaluation of detection systems for staphylococcal exfoliative toxin A responsible for the scalded skin syndrome. *J Clin Microbiol* 2001;39:2050–4.

24. Ladhani S, Joannou CL. Difficulties in the diagnosis and management of staphylococcal scalded skin syndrome. *Pediatr Infect Dis J* 2000;142:1251–5.

25. Ladhani S, Evans RW. Staphylococcal scalded skin syndrome. *Arch Dis Child* 1998;78(1):85–8.

26. Curran JP, Al-Salihi FL. Neonatal staphylococcal scalded skin syndrome: Massive outbreak due to an unusual phage type. *Pediatrics* 1980;66(2):285–90.

27. Revuz J et al. Toxic epidermal necrolysis: Clinical findings and prognostic factors in 87 patients. *Arch Dermatol* 1987;123:1166–70.

28. Blyth M, Estela C, Young AE. Severe staphylococcal scalded skin syndrome in children. *Burns* 2008;34:98–103.

29. Greenwood JE, Dunn KW, Davenport PJ. Experience with severe extensive blistering skin disease in a paediatric burn unit. *Burns* 2000;26:82–7.

30. Ladhani S, Joannou CL. Difficulties in diagnosis and management of the staphylococcal scalded skin syndrome. *Pediatr Infect Dis J* 2000;19:819–21.

31. Schmidt H, Lissner R, Struff W, Thamm O, Karch H. Antibody reactivity of a standardized human serum protein solution against a spectrum of microbial pathogens and toxins: Comparison with fresh frozen plasma. *Ther Apher* 2002;6:145–53.

32. Tenendbaum T et al. Exchange transfusion in a preterm infant with hyperbilirubinemia, staphylococcal scalded skin syndrome (SSSS) and sepsis. *Eur J Pediatr* 2007;166:733–5.

33. Strauss RG. Blood and blood component transfusions. In: Kliegman RM et al. (Eds), *Nelson Textbook of Pediatrics*, Vol. 1. 18th ed. Philadelphia, PA: Elsevier Saunders; 2011:1955–8.

25

Toxic shock syndrome

ASEEM SHARMA AND MADHULIKA MHATRE

INTRODUCTION

The origins of this lethal disease date back to 1978, when pediatric case reports started flowing into the Centers for Disease Control and Prevention regarding this novel entity. Toxic shock syndrome (TSS) was first described as a febrile, bacterial toxin-mediated, hyperacute, multiorgan system disease with mucocutaneous manifestations. The next few years saw a surge in the cases of toxic shock syndrome among menstruating women, ascribed to the usage of superabsorbent tampons. In recent times, with the advent of cotton and rayon-based tampons, the incidence of menstrual TSS has gone down drastically. However, TSS continues to be reported across all age groups and sexes, owing to cutaneous and aural infections, gynecological and surgical procedures, and as a sequelae to burns [1,2].

The incriminated gram-positive bacteria are *Staphylococcus aureus* and *Streptococcus pyogenes* (group A *Streptococcus* spp. [GAS], Lancefield) capable of producing a multitude of toxic proteins, including exotoxins and superantigens (SAgs). On interaction with antigen-presenting cells (APCs), SAgs induce a massive cytokine cascade via T-cell proliferation, culminating in the classic quartet of TSS: fever, capillary leak, rash, and subsequent hypotension [3]. Needless to say, early recognition of symptomatology and causation is of paramount importance, to prevent morbidity and mortality.

EPIDEMIOLOGY

Hereinafter, for simplicity, this chapter deals with TSS under two separate headings, based on the etiological bacterial agents.

Staphylococcal toxic shock syndrome

Synonyms: Toxic staphylococcal syndrome

The early 1980s marked a rise in this entity, especially in Caucasian women in the reproductive age group, and came to be known as "tampon-TSS" or "menstrual-TSS." Rarer in this millennium, a Minnesota study reported 61 cases between 2004 and 2006, 33 being tampon induced [4]. The age distribution was younger than standard. The clinical presentation is difficult to distinguish from staphylococcal TSS stemming from other etiologies. Menstrual TSS, overall, is extremely rare in this millennium, following discontinuation of absorbent tampons. The global incidence now stands between 20 and 25/100,000. Nonmenstrual TSS is accounted for by nearly half occurring in the age group below 2 years, and 62% have cutaneous lesions.

Streptococcal toxic shock syndrome

Synonyms: Toxic streptococcal syndrome, streptococcal toxic shock–like syndrome

Invasive GAS infections show a fairly consistent global incidence of 2–4 per 100,000 [5]. An Ontario-based prospective study in the early 1990s identified 323 patients with soft tissue infection (48%), hematological bacteremia (14%), and pyogenic pneumonia (11%), in decreasing order of incidence. Thirteen percent of subjects developed streptococcal toxic shock syndrome (STSS), 6% contracted necrotizing fasciitis, and 2% showed pyomyonecrosis. STSS invariably has milder dermatological symptoms vis-à-vis staphylococcal TSS, albeit with severe systemic involvement, morbid complications, and a higher fatal outcome. The age and sex distribution is more uniform, with significantly fewer cases of menstrual TSS.

ETIOPATHOGENESIS

Staphylococcal toxic shock syndrome

TSS falls under the purview of bacterial toxin-mediated disorders, amid the following: staphylococcal scalded skin syndrome (SSSS), bullous impetigo, recurrent perineal erythema and desquamative disease, scarlet fever, Kawasaki disease, guttate psoriasis, infective endocarditis, and rheumatic fever.

The toxins producing the aforementioned comprise the following:

1. Exfoliative toxins
2. Endotoxins

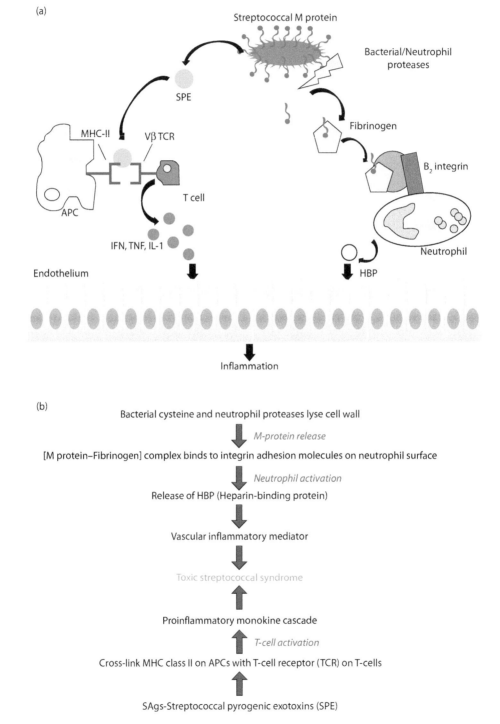

Figure 25.1 Etiopathogenesis of streptococcal toxic shock syndrome.

3. Exotoxins (enterotoxins, cytotoxins, neurotoxins, and vasculotoxins)
4. Specialized toxins: staphylokinase and Panton-Valentine leukocidin
5. SAgs: Staphylococcal TSS toxin-1 (TSST-1), streptococcal superantigen (SSA)

TSS is principally Sag mediated. Staphylococcal strains produce TSST-1 and enterotoxins A, B, C, D, E, and I. Individual susceptibility to this disease also depends on the presence of antibodies against TSST-1, coded by the *tstH* gene [6]. The potency of SAgs is that they can stimulate over 20% of host T cells, thereby causing polyclonal activation. These host cells are activated via interaction of the T-cell receptor (TCR) with major histocompatibility complex (MHC-II) on antigen-presenting cells (APCs), and the CD28 protein that acts as a costimulator. The resultant activation releases a massive cytokine storm with interleukins 1,6 and tumor necrosis factor-α (TNF-α), which induces vascular toxicity and shock.

MENSTRUAL TOXIC SHOCK SYNDROME

The human vagina has a physiological anaerobic habitus. However, with tampon usage, oxygen is introduced which modifies the milieu and allows aerobic bacteria to thrive. The high absorbency of older tampons acts as a culture medium for the same. Menstrual TSS is almost exclusively caused by *Staphylococcus*, mediated by TSST-1, which has a very high propensity to penetrate mucosal surfaces, among all SAgs. It may occur within 2–3 days of menstruation. It is ascribed to a paucity of antibodies to TSST-1 in susceptible patients.

NONMENSTRUAL TSS

Nonmenstrual TSS comprises nearly half of modern-day TSS. It is the effect of an existing nidus of infection, viz.,

- Postsurgical
- Postpartum wound infections
- Gynecological procedures
- Mastitis
- Postseptorhinoplasty
- Rhinosinusitis
- Osteomyelitis
- Arthritis
- Post-burns
- Perianal abscesses
- Aural infections
- Respiratory infections—influenza, pneumonitis
- Insulin sites, infusion pumps
- Nasal packing

Streptococcal toxic shock syndrome

Please refer to Figure 25.1(a and b). Group A *Streptococcus* spp. primarily produce pyrogenic and mitogenic exotoxins, and M proteins leading to the pathology.

CLINICAL MANIFESTATIONS

A typical case of TSS presents to the emergency unit with a fever and rash. There is a strong history of precession by myalgia, sore throat, nausea, vomiting, and/or watery diarrhea. Fever may vary in intensity and frequency, depending on the etiology. The patient presents with orthostatic hypotension or in frank shock; a reduced capillary refill time or decreased urine output may be the presenting complaints in cases of covert shock.

Cutaneous manifestations

STAPHYLOCOCCAL TOXIC SHOCK SYNDROME

The most common manifestation is a truncal, macular erythroderma similar to the classic "scarlatina" of scarlet fever, albeit reduced in intensity and sans the gritty, sandpaper-like feel (Figure 25.2). It is nontender and does not progress to purpuric lesions. Bullous lesions, akin to those in SSSS, have been reported, fragile and showing negativity on Nikolsky sign (Figure 25.3a and b). Conjunctival, mucosal, and pharyngeal hyperemia with a red or white strawberry/raspberry tongue may be seen (Figures 25.4 and 25.5). Patients who survive present with classical desquamation, initially over the tips of digits, progressing to involve the palms and soles, after 2–4 weeks. It differs from the periungual peeling seen post-Kawasaki disease. Clinical features are appended as per the Centers for Disease Control and Prevention (CDC) case definition (Table 25.1).

STREPTOCOCCAL TOXIC SHOCK SYNDROME

An infective focus, surgical procedure, or trauma is a prerequisite for development of STSS. In cases where no definitive nidus is localized, transient oropharyngeal bacteremia has been suggested, after ruling out the previously mentioned conditions. Signs of systemic toxicity, sepsis, a hyperacute and progressive clinical outcome, and a case fatality rate exceeding 50% distinguish it from toxic staphylococcal syndrome. The difference between STSS and toxic staphylococcal syndrome are appended (Table 25.2).

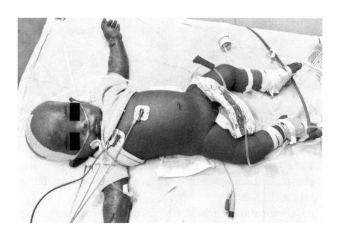

Figure 25.2 Macular erythroderma in staphylococcal toxic shock syndrome.

(a)

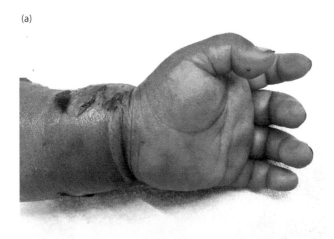

(b)

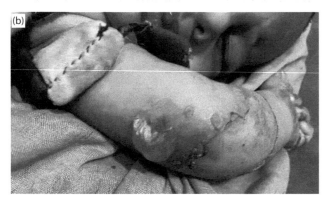

Figure 25.3 (a, b) Bullous lesions in staphylococcal toxic shock syndrome.

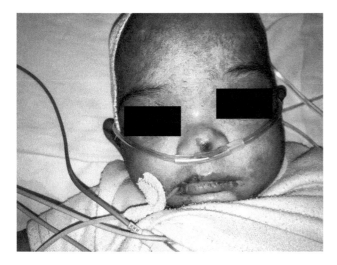

Figure 25.4 Facial and mucosal involvement in toxic shock syndrome.

In the last decade, severely invasive GAS infections have been reported frequently, with multiorgan system failure and shock [6–9].

Complications include streptococcal myonecrosis, bacteremia, adult respiratory distress syndrome (ARDS), septic shock, and acute renal failure; death occurs despite modern therapeutic regimens [10–12].

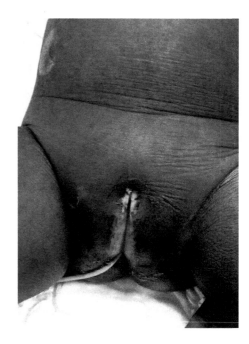

Figure 25.5 Genital mucosal involvement in staphylococcal toxic shock syndrome.

Symptoms

1. *Pain*: Pain is the most common symptom. Severe and abrupt in onset, and confirmed as tenderness on palpation. Extremity pain is the most frequent, but it may also mimic other conditions like pelvic inflammatory disease, serositis (pleural, pericardial, peritoneal), pneumonitis, or an acute coronary event. Approximately 20% have an influenza-like syndrome with fever, myalgia, chills and rigor, nausea, diarrhea, and vomiting [13].
2. *Fever*: Fever is the earliest sign, but patients in shock may present with hypothermia [14,15].
3. *Disorientation, mental confusion, or disrupted higher mental functions*: This may be seen in 55% of patients [16].
4. *Skin*: Eighty percent of patients show signs of soft tissue infection, viz., localized erythema and swelling, of which 70% of patients progress to necrotizing fasciitis or pyomyositis or muscle necrosis and often require fasciotomy, surgical débridement, or even amputation [17]. Progression of the swelling to vesicles leading to formation of bullae with a bluish hue is an ominous sign, suggesting necrotizing fasciitis (Figures 25.6 and 25.7). Only 10% of STSS patients show a diffuse, scarlatiniform rash. The case definitions of streptococcal TSS and necrotizing fasciitis by the CDC are given in Table 25.3.

Necrotizing fasciitis (STSS-NF)

Necrotizing fasciitis is defined as a deep-seated infection of the hypodermic tissue, progressing to destroy fascia, and sparing muscle tissue (Figures 25.8 through 25.12). The most common causal agent is GAS. A history of superficial, blunt trauma precedes the infection. Early distinction from simple cellulitis is often difficult, distinguished by "out-of-proportion" pain. Late markers comprise tense edema, stark erythema, and bullae

Table 25.1 Case definition of staphylococcal toxic shock syndrome (Centers for Disease Control and Prevention case definition 2011)

Major criteria	Minor criteria (≥3)

Fever >38.8°C (102°F)
  • Erythematous rash, macular erythroderma
  • Skin desquamation, 7–14 days after onset of illness
Hypotension (systolic <90 mm Hg or less than fifth percentile by age)
Negative serology, Rocky Mountain spotted fever, measles, leptospirosis, dengue (*revised*)
	Gastrointestinal (vomiting, diarrhea)
	Central nervous system (altered sensorium in absence of fever and hypotension)
	Mucosal hyperemia (conjunctival, oropharyngeal, genital) (Figures 25.4 and 25.5)
	Muscular (severe myalgia or raised creatine kinase, aldolase levels by twofold)
	Hepatic (raised transaminases/bilirubin by twofold)
	Hematologic: thrombocytopenia, platelets <100,000/mm^3
	Renal impairment (urea or creatinine deranged by twofold, pyuria or ≥5 leukocytes per high-power field in the absence of urinary tract infection)

impending rupture, which turn bluish over time. NF is associated with a multitude of systemic symptoms and high morbidity, in spite of usage of antibiotics, dialysis, ventilators, IV fluids, and improved surgical techniques. It is postulated that newer strains of GAS are highly virulent, and thereby somewhat resistant to conventional therapy [17].

Clinical features of streptococcal toxic shock syndrome-necrotizing fasciitis

For the CDC case definition, refer to Table 25.4.

- Skin pain—continuous, severe
- Vesiculobullous formation

Table 25.2 Differences between staphylococcal and streptococcal toxic shock syndrome

Variables	Toxic staphylococcal syndrome	Toxic streptococcal syndrome
Microbial isolation		
Nonsterile site		+
Sterile site		+
Fever	+	
Hypotension	+	+
Rash	++	+
Desquamation	+	
Multisystem		
involvement		+
≥2 of the following		
Gastrointestinal	++	+
Muscular	+	
Mucous membrane	++	
Renal	+	+
Hepatic	+	+
Hematologic	+	+
Neurological	+	
Respiratory		+
Soft tissue necrosis		++

- Cutaneous necrosis
- Ecchymosis (bruising), preceding cutaneous necrosis
- Edema extending beyond the erythematous margin
- Systemic toxicity [18–20]
- Rapid progression

LABORATORY DIAGNOSIS

Hematological and biochemical

Investigations are done as per the protocol for acute skin failure. Leukocytosis is a common finding, with occasional neutrophilia. Thrombocytopenia may be seen, which mandates further investigation to establish disseminated intravascular coagulation. Liver function tests show derangement, both with regard to raised bilirubin and transaminases. Serum creatinine phosphokinase levels are elevated, consistent with myalgia and myositis. Renal functions are deranged, representing a prerenal effect, signifying

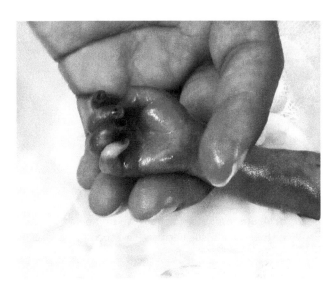

Figure 25.6 Necrosis and digital gangrene in streptococcal toxic shock syndrome.

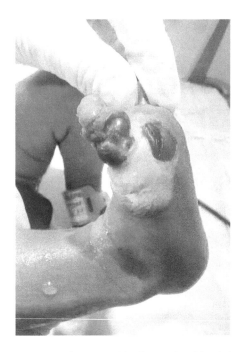

Figure 25.7 Vesiculation and bullae with a bluish hue suggesting impending necrotizing fasciitis in streptococcal toxic shock syndrome.

hypotension and dehydration. Renal tubular necrosis may ensue if blood pressure correction is not done with alacrity. Dyselectrolytemia is common, with serum calcium levels showing significant reduction [14].

Specific laboratory anomalies in STSS patients are as follows:

1. Hypoalbuminemia (85%)
2. Hypocalcemia (79%)
3. Elevated liver transaminase levels (63%)

Table 25.3 Case definition of streptococcal toxic shock syndrome and necrotizing fasciitis (Centers for Disease Control and Prevention case definition 2010)

Streptococcal toxic shock syndrome
 A. Isolation of group A *Streptococcus* spp.
  1. Sterile site
  2. Nonsterile body site
 B. Signs and symptoms
  1. Hypotension
  2. Clinical and laboratory abnormalities (≥2)
   a. Renal impairment
   b. Coagulopathy
   c. Liver abnormalities
   d. Acute respiratory distress syndrome
   e. Extensive tissue necrosis, i.e., necrotizing fasciitis
   f. Erythematous rash

Definite = A1 + B (1 + 2)
Probable = A2 + B (1 + 2)

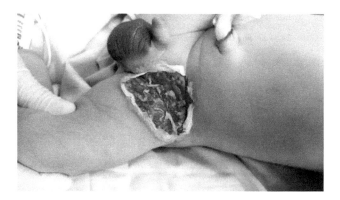

Figure 25.8 Necrotizing fasciitis in streptococcal toxic shock syndrome.

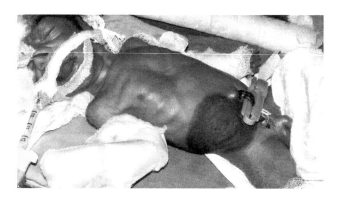

Figure 25.9 Necrotizing fasciitis over the inguinal region in streptococcal toxic shock syndrome.

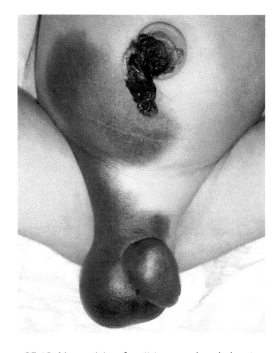

Figure 25.10 Necrotizing fasciitis over the abdomino-scrotal region in streptococcal toxic shock syndrome.

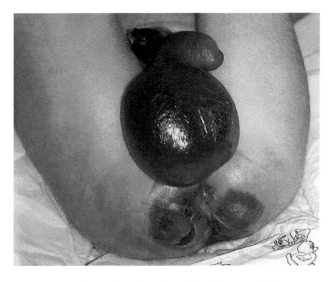

Figure 25.11 Scrotal and perineal fasciitis mimicking Fournier gangrene.

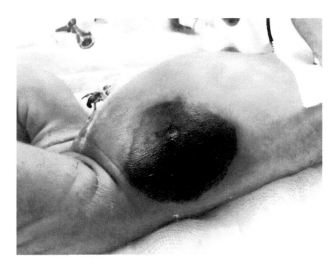

Figure 25.12 Streptococcal toxic shock syndrome-necrotizing fasciitis over the flank.

4. Prolonged prothrombin time and/or activated partial thromboplastin time (60%–71%)
5. Elevated creatinine level (40%–89%)

Microbiology

Gram stain and cultures are done to elicit the following:

1. *Staphylococcus aureus, Streptococcus pyogenes*: Isolated from a well-defined focus of infection (e.g., abscess, wound infection).
2. *Menstrual TSS*: 90% of patients demonstrate the organism in cervical and vaginal fluid cultures, even in subclinical infection.

Imaging studies

These are done specifically to rule out ARDS in cases of STSS, or for confirming clinical evidence of serosal involvement

Table 25.4 Case definition of streptococcal necrotizing fasciitis (Centers for Disease Control and Prevention case definition)

Necrotizing fasciitis
A. Definite
   1. Soft tissue + fascial involvement
PLUS
   2. Serious systemic disease ($\geq$1)
      a. Death
      b. Shock (systolic <90 mm Hg)
      c. Disseminated intravascular coagulopathy
      d. Failure of organ systems
        i. Respiratory failure
        ii. Liver failure
        iii. Renal failure
   3. Isolation of group A streptococcus from a normally sterile body site
B. Suspected case
   1. 1 + 2 and serologic confirmation of group A streptococcal infection by a fourfold rise against
      a. Streptolysin-O
      b. DNase B
   2. 1 + 2 and histologic confirmation
      Gram-positive cocci in a necrotic soft tissue infection

in STSS-NF. A chest skiagram usually suffices for the same. Also, muscle sonography and magnetic resonance imaging may need to be done for pyomyonecrosis.

Histology

Skin biopsies are often inconclusive and nonspecific. They may show spongiosis, necrotic keratinocytes in the epidermis, and moderate dermal perivascular polymorphonuclear and lymphocytic infiltrate. Clefting is seen at the subepidermal level, in case of bullae.

Renal biopsies are indicated to diagnose tubular necrosis, as a sequel to STSS-NF, with profound and prolonged hypotension.

PROGNOSIS

Early recognition, treatment in a tertiary care center by arresting the progression of septic shock, prompt circulatory shock, and hemodynamic support help recovery in patients in over 3–4 weeks. Having said that, the overall global mortality still rests between 7% and 12% in toxic staphylococcal syndrome. The mortality rates for STSS are fivefold higher.

DIFFERENTIAL DIAGNOSES

The authors propose a diagnostic approach similar to any case with fever, rash, and hypotension. Approaching TSS starts with early establishment of the diagnosis by ruling out other differentials such as the following:

- SSSS (fewer complications, better prognosis)
- Streptococcal scarlet fever ("scarlatina" rash)
- Kawasaki disease
- Leptospirosis (early petechial rash)
- Measles
- Rocky Mountain spotted fever
- Stevens-Johnson syndrome/toxic epidermal necrolysis
- Drug reaction with eosinophilia and systemic symptoms (DRESS) syndrome/drug hypersensitivity syndrome
- Pediatric peeling skin syndromes

MANAGEMENT

TSS is a dramatic, fulminant syndrome, where early recognition is imperative for initiating management and preventing mortality. General measures for managing septic shock and acute skin failure must be followed irrespective of the etiological type. They include the following:

- Hospitalization
- Strict barrier nursing (single, double barrier with septic precautions, control of moisture, odor, temperature)
- Early and adequate antibiotic therapy to combat septic shock
- Vasopressin, fluid replacement
- Early hemodynamic resuscitation and continued circulatory support
- Corticosteroids (refractory vasopressor-dependent shock, and progressive macular erythroderma)
- Control of vital clinical and laboratory parameters
- Dialysis
- Ventilator (in case of ARDS)

Staphylococcal toxic shock syndrome (specific)

- Removal of the tampon in menstrual TSS
- Other nidi of infection to be searched for—blood, urine, stool cultures
- Antibiotics—for the focus of infection and antitoxin anti-inflammatory action (refer to Table 25.5 for details)
- Corticosteroid therapy for its anti-inflammatory action against leukocyte accumulation and T-cell homing [21].
- Intravenous immunoglobulin (IVIg)—transfers antibodies against TSST-1, helps neutralize circulating toxin

Streptococcal toxic shock syndrome (specific)

ß-Lactam antibiotics were the mainstay of treatment for many years, highly effective against the susceptible streptococcal microbe, and numerous studies have corroborated the same. However, studies have found the efficacy of clindamycin to be superior in fulminant streptococcal infections, gaining U.S. Food and Drug Administration approval status for the same [22,23].

Table 25.5 Antistaphylococcal therapies for streptococcal toxic shock syndrome

Classification	Antimicrobial agents
β-Lactams	Methicillin, oxacillin, cephalosporins
Glycoproteins	Vancomycin
Lipopeptides	Daptomycin
Macrolides	Erythromycin, clarithromycin, and azithromycin
Lincosamides	Clindamycin
Oxazolidinones	Linezolid, tedizolid
Streptogramins	Quinupristin/dalfopristin
Aminoglycosides	Gentamicin, streptomycin, kanamycin, and amikacin
Tetracyclines	Tetracycline, minocycline, doxycycline, and tigecycline
Sulfonamides	Trimethoprim sulfamethoxazole

Source: Lin Y-C, Peterson ML. *Expert Rev Clin Pharmacol* 2010;3(6):753–67.

Clindamycin: The heightened efficacy of this lincosamide antibiotic lies in its multipronged action. It is immune to the inoculum stage [24,25] and acts as a superpotent suppressor of bacterial toxinogenesis. It inhibits M-protein synthesis and causes bacterial phagocytosis [26]. Clindamycin has a longer postantibiotic effect than its contemporaries. Last, it inhibits lipopolysaccharide-induced monocyte synthesis of TNF. All in all, it acts as a potent immunomodulator in addition to its antibacterial action. The dosage used is (parenteral) 30–45 mg/kg/day, given in three divided doses. Vancomycin at the dose of 50 mg/kg/day, in two divided doses, is added to increase the spectrum against virulent strains, as well.

Intravenous immunoglobulin (IVIg)

1. Considered second-line in the management of TSS, its mechanism of action includes
   a. Anti-inflammatory effect
      i. Decreased production of proinflammatory cytokines—tumor necrosis factor (TNF)-α, interleukin (IL)-1,6
   b. Downregulation of adhesion molecules and chemokine-receptor expression
   c. Neutralization of SAgs
2. IgM-fortified IVIg has shown a significantly higher efficacy.
3. A standard dosage of 2 g/kg initially, followed by 0.4 g/kg/day for 4 days is the most effective schedule.

Surgical intervention

The dictum that is followed for the management of STSS-NF is that once suspected, surgical débridement is warranted. However, various studies have debated this issue as to when débridement should be performed. It has been postulated that early débridement helps limit the sepsis, removes dead necrotic tissue, and also curbs the spread of infection. But a few studies are of the opinion that delaying surgery may decrease morbidity by allowing the development of a line of demarcation, separating necrotic from vital tissue, and thereby limiting the extent of tissue resection. It may also decrease mortality by allowing the patient to stabilize hemodynamically before surgery. Initiating an immunomodulator early that neutralizes the toxin, such as IVIg, may help the patient stabilize faster and delay surgical intervention [3].

An observational study by Norrby-Teglund suggested that an initial conservative surgical approach combined with the use of immunomodulators may reduce morbidity in hemodynamically unstable patients without increasing mortality [27].

RECENT TRENDS

- Monoclonal antibodies under development against (staphylococcal) enterotoxin-B (SEB) include pagabaximab, Aurograb, and Aurexis.
- Molecular studies on the *tstH* gene are under way to understand the pathogenesis of TSST-1 in detail.

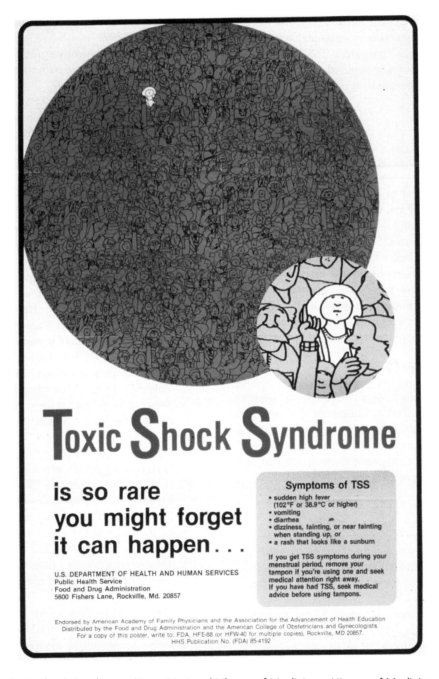

Figure 25.13 Poster: Toxic Shock Syndrome. (From National Library of Medicine—History of Medicine via WikiCommons. https://commons.wikimedia.org/wiki/File:Toxic_shock_syndrome_is_so_rare_you_might_forget_it_can_happen_-_ (6946668685).jpg.)

- Experimental targeted agents, include:
  - Glycerol monolaurate (GML), which inhibits the growth of *Staphylococcus aureus* and delays toxin production.
  - Hemoglobin subunit targets that inhibit exoprotein induction.
  - V-b peptides compete with the TCR binding site to prevent T-cell activation (via staphylococcal enterotoxin-B).
- The latest FDA-approved antibacterials for gram-positive cutaneous infections, oritavancin, dalbavancin, and tedizolid are effective, against the staphylococcal superfamily. Their anti-inflammatory role though has not been delineated.
- Vaccination—Anti-staphylococcal vaccines have not garnered enough attention with regard to TSST modulation, and lack efficacy in hitherto completed clinical trials. The list, for academic purposes, at present is as follows:
  - StaphVAX
  - Altastaph V710
  - STEBVax [28]

CONCLUSION

TSS, be it staphylococcal or streptococcal, is associated with significant mortality and morbidity. Interplay between M-protein-induced neutrophil activation and the cytokine storm brought about by the SAg family punctuates this disease that has spanned well over three decades. It is a fitting example of how skin can serve as an early marker to prevent near-certain organ system failure and subsequent death. However, this would require a high index of clinical suspicion, prompt hemodynamic replacement and compensation, and a multidisciplinary approach (Figure 25.13).

ACKNOWLEDGMENT

We would like to acknowledge and extend our heartfelt gratitude to Dr. Samir Sheikh, Consultant Neonatologist, Wockhardt Hospitals, Mumbai, and Dr. Rachita Dhurat, Professor and H.O.D, Department of Dermatology, Lokmanya Tilak Municipal Medical College and General Hospital, Sion Mumbai, for the clinical photographs.

KEY POINTS

- Toxic shock syndrome is a toxin mediated multi-system disease with high mortality.
- Its incidence has reduced due to the decreased use of tampons.
- Staphylococcal and streptococcal TSS are the two variants.
- Complications include septic shock, ARDS, myonecrosis, renal failure and coagulopathy.
- Antibiotics, IVIg and supportive care are cornerstones of therapy.

REFERENCES

1. National Organization for Rare Disorders. Toxic shock syndrome (accessed on September 10, 2017).
2. Womenshealth.gov. Menstruation and the menstrual fact sheet (accessed on September 10, 2017).
3. Low DE. Toxic shock syndrome. *Crit Care Clin* 2013;29(3):651–75.
4. Centers for Disease Control and Prevention (CDC). Update: Toxic-shock syndrome–United States. *MMWR Morb Mortal Wkly Rep* 1983;32:398–400.
5. DeVries AS et al. Staphylococcal toxic shock syndrome 2000–2006: Epidemiology, clinical features, and molecular characteristics. *PLOS ONE* 2011;6:e22997.
6. Steer AC et al. Invasive group a streptococcal disease: Epidemiology, pathogenesis and management. *Drugs* 2012;72:1213–27.
7. Brosnahan AJ, Schlievert PM. Gram-positive bacterial superantigen outside-in signaling causes toxic shock syndrome. *FEBS J* 2011;278:4649–67.
8. Wharton M et al. Case definitions for public health surveillance. *MMWR Recomm Rep* 1990;39:1–43.
9. Kohler W, Gerlach D, Knoll H. Streptococcal outbreaks and erythrogenic toxin type A. *ZblBaktHyg* 1987;266:104–15.
10. Martin PR, Hoiby EA. Streptococcal serogroup A epidemic in Norway 1987–1988. *Scand J Infect Dis* 1990;22:421–9.
11. Holm S. Fatal group A streptococcal infections. *Presented at the 89th Conference of the American Society for Microbiology*, New Orleans, LA, 1989.
12. Wheeler MC, Roe MH, Kaplan EL, Schlievert PM, Todd JK. Outbreak of group A streptococcus septicemia in children: Clinical, epidemiologic, and microbiological correlates. *JAMA* 1991;266:533–7.
13. Holm SE, Norrby A, Bergholm AM, Norgren M. Aspects of pathogenesis of serious group A streptococcal infections in Sweden, 1988–1989. *J Infect Dis* 1992;166:31–7.
14. Stegmayr B, Bjorck S, Holm S, Nisell J, Rydvall A, Settergren B. Septic shock induced by group A streptococcal infections: Clinical and therapeutic aspects. *Scand J Infect Dis* 1992;24:589–97.
15. Demers B et al. Severe invasive group A streptococcal infections in Ontario, Canada: 1987–1991. *Clin Infect Dis* 1993;16:792–800.
16. Stevens DL. Invasive group A streptococcal infections: The past, present and future. *Pediatr Infect Dis J* 1994;13:561–6.
17. Stevens DL. Invasive group A streptococcus infections. *Clin Infect Dis* 1992;14:2–13.
18. Svane S. Peracute spontaneous streptococcal myositis: A report on 2 fatal cases with review of literature. *ActaChirScand* 1971;137:155–63.
19. Yoder EL, Mendez J, Khatib R. Spontaneous gangrenous myositis induced by *Streptococcus pyogenes*:

Case report and review of the literature. *Rev Infect Dis* 1987;9:382–5.

20. Todd JK. Toxic shock syndrome. *Clin Microbiol Rev* 1988;1:432–40.

21. Todd JK, Ressman M, Caston SA, Todd BH, Wiesenthal AM. Corticosteroid therapy for patients with toxic shock syndrome. *JAMA.* 1984;252(24):3399–402.

22. Stevens DL, Gibbons AE, Bergstrom R, Winn V. The eagle effect revisited: Efficacy of clindamycin, erythromycin, and penicillin in the treatment of streptococcal myositis. *J Infect Dis* 1988;158:23–8.

23. Stevens DL, Bryant AE, Yan S. Invasive group A streptococcal infection: New concepts in antibiotic treatment. *Int J Antimicrob Agents* 1994;4:297–301.

24. Stevens DL, Yan S, Bryant AE. Penicillin-binding protein expression at different growth stages determines penicillin efficacy *in vitro* and *in vivo*: An explanation for the inoculum effect. *J Infect Dis* 1993;167:1401–5.

25. Yan S, Bohach GA, Stevens DL. Persistent acylation of high-molecular weight penicillin-binding proteins by penicillin induces the post-antibiotic effect in *Streptococcus pyogenes. J Infect Dis* 1994;170:609–14.

26. Gemmell CG et al. Potentiation of opsonization and phagocytosis of *Streptococcus pyogenes* following growth in the presence of clindamycin. *J Clin Invest* 1981;67:1249–56.

27. Norrby-Teglund A, Muller MP, McGeer A, Gan BS, Guru V, Bohnen J, Thulin P, Low DE. Successful management of severe group A streptococcal soft tissue infections using an aggressive medical regimen including intravenous polyspecific immunoglobulin together with a conservative surgical approach. *Scand J Infect Dis* 2005 Mar 1;37(3):166–72.

28. Lin Y-C, Peterson ML. New insights into the prevention of staphylococcal infections and toxic shock syndrome. *Expert Rev Clin Pharmacol* 2010;3(6):753–67.

26

Cellulitis and necrotizing fasciitis

VIKAS PATHANIA

INTRODUCTION

Skin and soft tissue bacterial infections often present as a dermatological emergency whether in an outpatient department or more commonly in an inpatient setting. Cellulitis and erysipelas are essentially acute infection and inflammation of the dermis and the subcutaneous connective tissue. While both are considered under an umbrella term of nonnecrotizing skin and soft tissue infections (SSTIs), they differ in their clinical presentation and prognosis [1]. Erysipelas is confined to the upper dermis and subcutaneous tissue with predominant involvement of lymphatics and with sharp demarcation from surrounding skin. Cellulitis is a more deep-seated inflammation of the lower dermis and subcutis with ill-defined margins [2]. Necrotizing skin and soft tissue infections (NSTIs) include necrotizing fasciitis, gangrenous cellulitis, and myonecrosis and are characterized by being locally destructive and spreading via tissue planes. They are often associated with serious systemic complications [3]. Group Aβ hemolytic streptococci and *Staphylococcus aureus* are the two bacteria most commonly implicated in causation; however, other groups of streptococci, coagulase-negative *Staphylococcus aureus*, as well as *Haemophilus influenzae*, *Vibrio vulnificus*, and *Enterococcus* with other gram-negative organisms have been isolated in a subset of cases and in special situations and age groups. The rise of methicillin-resistant *Staphylococcus aureus* has further contributed to incidence as well as morbidity and mortality arising from these infections [2,4]. Early clinical diagnosis and systemic antibiotics remain the cornerstone of treatment of these dermatological emergencies.

EPIDEMIOLOGY

Cellulitis is the most common dermatological condition requiring admission, almost accounting for as high as 56%

in one recent study [5]. It affects mostly adults in the age group between the fourth and sixth decades, and males are more commonly affected than females [2,6]. However, certain subsets such as facial cellulitis and perianal cellulitis are seen more commonly in children, while the polymicrobial variant of necrotizing fasciitis is seen more commonly in the elderly, diabetics, those infected with HIV, and other immunocompromised patients [4].

ETIOPATHOGENESIS

Cellulitis and erysipelas are most commonly caused by group Aβ hemolytic streptococci (GAS) in immunocompetent hosts [2]. However, community-acquired methicillin-resistant *Staphylococcus aureus* (CA-MRSA) has become an important etiologic agent in recent times, superseding GAS in certain studies [7,8]. Childhood periorbital cellulitis and erysipelas, once a complication of sinusitis due to *Haemophilus influenzae* type b, is now rare to find in the postvaccination era [2,9,10].

Cellulitis in the setting of venous insufficiency and following lymphatic stasis post–breast surgery is caused predominantly by non–group A streptococci [1,11,12]. *Aeromonas hydrophila*, *Vibrio vulnificus*, and *Vibrio alginolyticus* have been implicated in cellulitis following injuries with water and soil exposure [13,14]. Other uncommon causes include group B, C, and G *Streptococcus*, *Streptococcus pneumoniae*, *Pseudomonas*, and other gram-negative bacteria, especially in the setting of postoperative surgical site infection following abdominal and genitourinary surgery [2,15]. Necrotizing fasciitis has two spectra of flora, a type 1 polymicrobial variant caused by anaerobes like *Peptostreptococcus*, *Bacteroides* spp., and facultative species like non–group A streptococci and Enterobacteriaceae and the monomicrobial type II caused by group Aβ hemolytic streptococci [3,16]. Factors that initiate infection usually cause breaches in the skin, thereby providing a portal of entry (whether it be trauma, surgical procedures, bites, or stings). They can also commonly complicate dermatoses such as stasis eczema, web intertrigo, psoriasis, and chronic ulcers. Extremes of age, diabetes mellitus, nephrotic syndrome, lymphoedema (congenital and acquired), cancer, neutropenia, and acquired immunodeficiency syndrome are some of the important predisposing factors usually present in the background [1,3,17].

CLINICAL FEATURES

Classically, cellulitis presents as diffuse erythematous induration with local tenderness, pain, and raised local temperature. Erysipelas is similar in appearance but with better definition of its margins (Figure 26.1) and overlying *peau d'orange* appearance [1]. The overlying skin may undergo blistering sometimes with hemorrhagic fluid. There may be associated lymphangitis and tender regional lymphadenopathy [2]. Systemic constitutional upset is often present with erysipelas, but it is a constant feature with cellulitis in the form of fever, chills, malaise, and tachycardia [7]. Lower extremities are the most common sites to be affected in a setting of stasis eczema, nonhealing ulcer, or a toe web intertrigo in a diabetic. These are the usual portals of entry for infective pathogens (Figure 26.2). Less commonly, facial involvement, which may be bilateral and often without an identifiable source of infection, is usually the case in erysipelas [2]. Cellulitis occurring in a postoperative wound would, in addition to inflammation and tenderness of wound margins, also have purulent discharge and often yield the causative organism in cultures. Cellulitis complicating bedsores and pressure ulcers in the elderly and nonambulatory patients is characterized by polymicrobial etiology and invasion of underlying structures. These patients are at high risk for bacteremia [1,7,15]. Facial cellulitis in children, once commonly caused by *Haemophilus influenzae B* with meningitis as a feared complication, has now dramatically decreased in

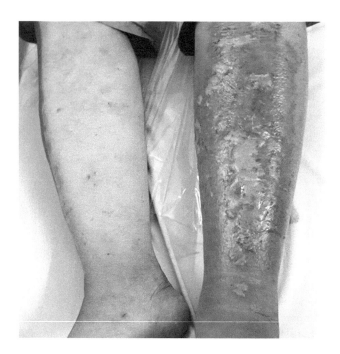

Figure 26.2 Cellulitis of lower limb with overlying blistering.

incidence following the advent of *H. influenza* vaccination. Perianal cellulitis in children, caused by *Streptococcus pyogenes*, presents as perianal erythema, painful defecation, and blood-tinged stools [4,9,10]. Rarely, genitalia can also be affected (Figure 26.3).

Necrotizing fasciitis initially presents with local erythema, edema, and tenderness. This is soon followed by bluish gangrenous discoloration of overlying skin due to the occlusion of small blood vessels and tenderness replaced by anesthesia due to the destruction of subcutaneous nerves, signifying rapid extension of fasciitis by "flesh-eating bacteria" beyond the margin of cutaneous necrosis. There may be overlying bulla formation and even frank necrosis of the overlying skin. Constitutional symptoms with high-grade fever and toxicity accompany early progression. Type 1 necrotizing fasciitis, the more common variant, is polymicrobial

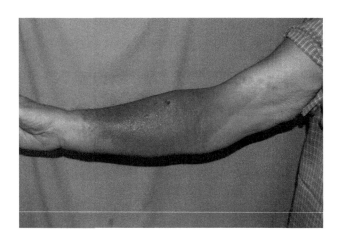

Figure 26.1 Erysipelas of the forearm.

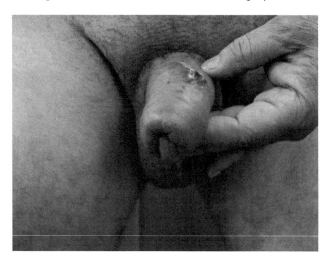

Figure 26.3 Cellulitis of the penis.

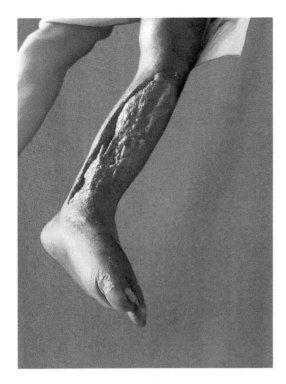

Figure 26.4 Necrotizing fasciitis of lower limb showing necrotic tendon sheaths and fascia following breakdown of overlying skin.

in origin with anaerobes and facultative aerobes delivered in susceptible debilitated patients undergoing surgery, bowel perforation, and penetrating trauma. Common sites include the extremities, abdominal wall, perineum, and postoperative wounds. Type II necrotizing fasciitis is monomicrobial in origin with group A streptococci being the predominant microorganism, although incidence of MRSA has been rising. The clinical presentation is similar to type I necrotizing fasciitis, but progression is faster with early and rapid necrosis of overlying skin, thus revealing underlying structures like muscles and tendon sheaths (Figure 26.4) [3,4,18].

Certain anatomic variants have also been described. Synergistic necrotizing cellulitis is similar to type 1 necrotizing fasciitis and presents as multiple perineal sinuses draining pale "dishwater" exudate containing fragments of necrotic fat [19]. Meleney gangrene is another variant of type I necrotizing fasciitis presenting as necrotic ulcer at postoperative sites, fistulous tracts, or wire-stay sutures [3,20]. Cervical necrotizing fasciitis is another anatomical variant of type 1 necrotizing fasciitis originating from dental or pharyngeal infection, while craniofacial necrotizing fasciitis is caused by group A streptococci following trauma [21]. Fournier gangrene is another genital form of type 1 necrotizing fasciitis involving skin and subcutaneous tissue of genitals, but characteristically sparing the testes, glans penis, and spermatic chord, which have a different blood supply [22,23]. Necrotizing fasciitis when associated with clostridium gangrenous cellulitis may also demonstrate crepitus [3,15].

DIAGNOSIS

Considering the emergent nature of these conditions, diagnosis remains clinical. Differential diagnoses to be considered in cases of erysipelas and cellulitis are similar presentations of other infections such as necrotizing fasciitis, early herpes zoster, deep fungal infections, erysipeloid, cutaneous anthrax, and atypical mycobacterial infections. Noninfective conditions such as chronic lymphoedema, stasis dermatitis, deep vein thrombosis, panniculitis, sweet syndrome, scleroderma, scleredema, lupus erythematosus, sarcoidosis, eosinophilic cellulitis, bites and stings, and drug hypersensitivity may often mimic these entities [1,2,24–26]. In case of necrotizing fasciitis, infective differentials include cellulitis, osteomyelitis, herpes zoster, deep fungal infections, atypical mycobacterial infections, and septic emboli. While among noninfective conditions, cutaneous vasculitis, warfarin necrosis, panniculitis with liquefactive necrosis, hidradenitis suppurativa, pyoderma gangrenosum, and metastatic Crohn disease should be kept in mind [3,27,28].

Treatment is generally not deferred by investigations; however, attempts should be made to isolate the causative microorganism with its antibiotic sensitivity pattern and to rule out other conditions. In case of erysipelas and cellulitis, surface swabs are generally not helpful as they grow contaminants rather than the implicated organism [1]. Similarly, blood cultures are also not very useful with only 2%–5% yield [29,30]. However, needle aspiration following infusion of nonbacteriostatic saline in the advancing edge of the lesion may yield growth in 4%–42% cases [31]. Punch biopsies for Gram stain and culture can yield organisms in up to 20%–30% of cases. Histopathologically, the dermis shows intense edema with vascular and lymphatic dilatation and overlying epidermal spongiosis. Direct immunofluorescence can demonstrate streptococcal organisms with sensitivity up to 70% [1].

Necrotizing fasciitis is often diagnosed at the operating table with the appearance of dead and devitalized structures on blunt dissection, which are demonstrated as grayish, foul smelling, and do not bleed with lack of adherence to surrounding tissues [18,28]. Wong et al. in 2004 developed a laboratory risk indicator for necrotizing fasciitis (LRINEC) with parameters for scoring, such as elevated C-reactive protein, leukocytosis, anemia, hyponatremia, renal failure, and hyperglycemia with a positive predictive value of 92% and a negative predictive value of 96% [32,33]. Tissue from surgical specimen or biopsy is more likely to demonstrate the organism as opposed to that in the case of cellulitis. Histopathology is likely to demonstrate prominent angiitis with focal dermal necrosis and spread along tissue planes. There is fibrinoid necrosis of the media of vessels with fibrin thrombi and coagulative necrosis. Cellular infiltrate of polymorphonuclear and mononuclear leukocytes with gram-positive cocci is usually present [3].

Table 26.1 Antibiotic treatment of cellulitis and necrotizing fasciitis

Disease	Antibiotic of choice	Alternative antibiotics
Erysipelas	Penicillin, amoxycillin, vancomycin	Cephalexin, cefoxitin, dicloxacillin, amoxycillin/ clavulanate, clindamycin, azithromycin
Cellulitis	Dicloxacillin, cephalexin, ampicillin/ sulbactam, ticarcillin/clavulanate, piperacillin/tazobactam, imipenem/ cilastatin, meropenum	Vancomycin, clindamycin, linezolid (if methicillin-resistant Staphylococcus aureus [MRSA] suspected)
Type 1 necrotizing fasciitis	Ampicillin/sulbactam, imipenem/ cilastatin, meropenem, ticarcillin/ clavulanate, vancomycin (if MRSA suspected)	Cefoxitin, clindamycin, metronidazole + aminoglycoside
Type II necrotizing fasciitis	Penicillin G + clindamycin	Ceftriaxone + clindamycin, vancomycin, linezolid, quinupristin/dalfopristin, daptomycin

Imaging in the form of ultrasound, computed tomography, and magnetic resonance imaging are helpful especially in demonstrating soft tissue swelling, involvement of fascial planes, and entrapped air [34–36].

TREATMENT

Both erysipelas and cellulitis may be treated on an outpatient basis. More severe cases of cellulitis merit inpatient care with parenteral antibiotics. It is prudent to start antibiotics empirically without waiting for culture and sensitivity, following which the same may be changed accordingly. Traditionally in an uncomplicated cellulitis, a penicillinase-resistant penicillin such as dicloxacillin or an oral cephalosporin such as cephalexin should be effective. β-Lactam antibiotics such as clarithromycin or clindamycin can be considered where hypersensitivity to penicillin is documented. Where MRSA is suspected, linezolid and vancomycin can be considered. Supportive adjunctive therapies include rest and elevation of the part, sterile saline dressings, and moist heat [1,2,37].

The management of necrotizing fasciitis includes a combination of urgent surgical débridement, parenteral antibiotics, and adjunct therapy. Surgical exploration and débridement of all necrotic tissue as also amputation of the limb, if required, can be lifesaving measures. Specimens thus obtained can be submitted for staining, culture, and histopathological examination. Pending cultures, a broad-spectrum parenteral antibiotic should be empirically exhibited to cover the polymicrobial spectrum of microorganisms as provided in (Table 26.1) [3,15,18,38]. Adjunctive therapies such as hyperbaric oxygen and IV immunoglobulin have been tried with some success [39]. The role of nonsteroidal anti-inflammatory drugs remains controversial, as they may contribute to progression of the disease by masking the signs and symptoms for early detection of sepsis [40].

DISEASE COURSE AND PROGNOSIS

Cellulitis and erysipelas follow an acute course but generally respond favorably to conservative treatment. Rarely they may progress to necrotizing fasciitis and sepsis, if left untreated. Recurrent episodes are common with lymphatic compromise such as that following mastectomy and immunocompromised states such as diabetes and AIDS [1]. Necrotizing fasciitis follows a more hyperacute course with progression to sepsis and multiorgan failure when surgical intervention is delayed. Mortality and limb loss in such cases range from 17% to 49% in such cases with predictors for amputation being diabetes mellitus, soft tissue swelling, skin necrosis, gangrene, and serum creatinine values $\geq$1.6 mg/dL on admission [3,41], and hence lies the importance of a high index of suspicion and early diagnosis in such cases. An approach to cellulitis and necrotising fasciitis is provided in Chart 1.

> ## KEY POINTS
>
> - Cellulitis and erysipelas are forms of nonnecrotizing skin and soft tissue infections (SSTIs).
> - Necrotizing skin and soft tissue infections include necrotizing fasciitis, gangrenous cellulitis, and myonecrosis (NSSTI).
> - Necrotizing fasciitis may be polymicrobial (type I) or monomicrobial (type II).
> - Incidence of both SSTIs and NSSTIs is increasing with emergence of methicillin-resistant Staphylococcus aureus.
> - While cellulitis is managed conservatively with antibiotics with favorable outcome, necrotizing fasciitis requires in addition urgent surgical exploration and débridement.
> - Early clinical diagnosis and institution of empirical antibiotics with surgical intervention is the cornerstone of management of these pyodermas.

Chart 1: Approach to cellulitis and necrotizing fasciitis

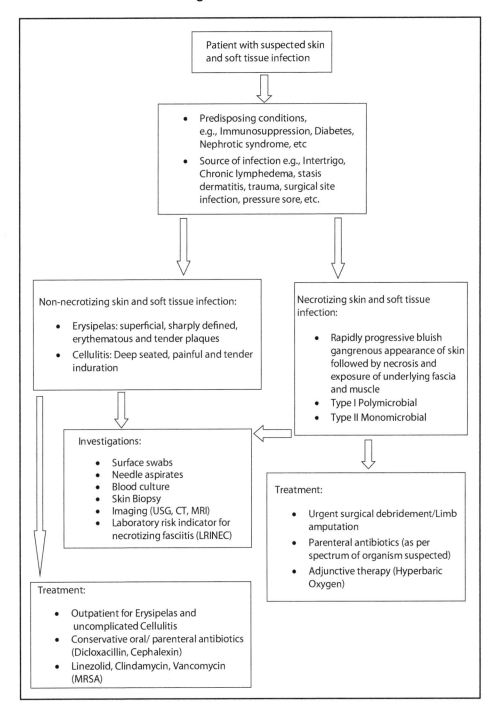

REFERENCES

1. Lipworth AD, Saavedra AP, Weinberg AN, Johnson RA. Chapter 178: Non-necrotizing infections of the dermis and subcutaneous fat: Cellulitis and erysipelas. In: Goldsmith LA, Katz SI, Gilchrest BA, Paller AS, Leffell D, Wolff K (Eds), *Fitzpatrick's Dermatology in General Medicine*. 8th ed. New York: McGraw-Hill; 2012:2160–8.

2. Hay RJ JR. Cellulitis and erysipelas. In: Griffiths C, Barker J, Bleiker T, Chalmers R, Creamer D (Eds), *Rook's Textbook of Dermatology*. 9th ed. West Sussex, UK: Blackwell; 2016:26.17–21.

3. Lipworth AD, Saavedra AP, Weinberg AN, Johnson RA. Chapter 179: Necrotizing soft tissue infections: Necrotizing fasciitis, gangrenous cellulitis, and myonecrosis. In: Goldsmith LA, Katz SI, Gilchrest BA, Paller AS, Leffell D Wolff K (Eds), *Fitzpatrick's Dermatology in General Medicine*. 8th ed. New York: McGraw-Hill; 2012:2169–77.

4. Bhat MR. Bacterial infections. In: Sacchinanad S, Oberai C, Inamadar AC (Eds), *IADVL Textbook of Dermatology*. 4th ed. Mumbai, India: Bhalani Publishing; 2015:440–1.

5. Lai-Kwon JE, Weiland TJ, Jelinek GA, Chong AH. Which patients with dermatological conditions are admitted via the emergency department? *Australas J Dermatol* 2014;55:255–9.

6. Hadzovic-Cengic M et al. Cellulitis—Epidemiological and clinical characteristics. *Med Arch (Sarajevo, Bosnia Herzegovina)* 2012;66(3 Suppl 1):51–3.

7. Gunderson CG. Cellulitis: Definition, etiology, and clinical features. *Am J Med* 2011;124:1113–22.

8. Chira S, Miller LG. *Staphylococcus aureus* is the most common identified cause of cellulitis: A systematic review. *Epidemiol Infect* 2010;138:313.

9. Rath E, Skrede S, Mylvaganam H, Bruun T. Aetiology and clinical features of facial cellulitis: A prospective study. *Infect Dis (Lond)* 2018;50(1):27–34.

10. Barone SR, Aiuto LT. Periorbital and orbital cellulitis in the *Haemophilus influenzae* vaccine era. *J Pediatr Ophthalmol Strabismus* 2017;34:293–6.

11. Woo PC, Lum PN, Wong SS, Cheng VC, Yuen KY. Cellulitis complicating lymphoedema. *Eur J Clin Microbiol Infect Dis* 2000;19:294–7.

12. Teerachaisakul M, Ekataksin W, Durongwatana S, Taneepanichskul S. Risk factors for cellulitis in patients with lymphedema: A case-controlled study. *Lymphology* 2013;46:150–6.

13. Bateman JL, Tu RP, Strampfer MJ, Cunha BA. *Aeromonas hydrophila* cellulitis and wound infections caused by waterborne organisms. *Heart Lung* 1988;17:99–102.

14. Howard RJ, Lieb S. Soft-tissue infections caused by halophilic marine vibrios. *Arch Surg* 1988;123:245–9.

15. Brook I. Microbiology and management of soft tissue and muscle infections. *Int J Surg* 2008;6:328–38.

16. Paramythiotis D, Koukoutsis H, Harlaftis N. Necrotizing soft tissue infections. *Surg Pract* 2007;11:17–28.

17. Iacopi E, Coppelli A, Goretti C, Piaggesi A. Necrotizing fasciitis and the diabetic foot. [Internet] 2015;14(4):316–27. http://dx.doi.org/101177/1534734615606534

18. Carter PS, Banwell PE. Necrotising fasciitis: A new management algorithm based on clinical classification. *Int Wound J* 2004;1:189–98.

19. Stone HH, Martin JD, Jr. Synergistic necrotizing cellulitis. *Ann Surg* 1972;175:702.

20. Puyo Villafane E. [Hemolytic streptococcal gangrene (Meleney)]. *Prensa Med Argent [Internet]* 1954 [cited 2017 November 19];41(39):2791–5.

21. Antunes AA, Avelar RL, de Melo WM, Pereira-Santos D, Frota R. Extensive cervical necrotizing fasciitis of odontogenic origin. *J Craniofac Surg* 2013;24:e594–7.

22. Mallikarjuna MN, Vijayakumar A, Patil VS, Shivswamy BS. Fournier's gangrene: Current practices. *ISRN Surg* 2012;2012:942437.

23. Parry N. Fournier gangrene. *Clin Case Reports* 2015;3:198.

24. Keller EC, Tomecki KJ, Alraies MC. Distinguishing cellulitis from its mimics. *Cleve Clin J Med* 2012;79:547–52.

25. Hirschmann JV, Raugi GJ. Lower limb cellulitis and its mimics: Part II. Conditions that simulate lower limb cellulitis. *J Am Acad Dermatol* 2012;67:177.e1–9; quiz:185–6.

26. Falagas ME, Vergidis PI. Narrative review: Diseases that masquerade as infectious cellulitis. *Ann Intern Med* 2005;142:47.

27. Sharma P, Dhungel S. All that is red is not cellulitis. Pyoderma gangrenosum. *Eur J Intern Med* 2014;25:e17–8.

28. Bonne SL, Kadri SS. Evaluation and management of necrotizing soft tissue infections. *Infect Dis Clin North Am* 2017;31(3):497–511.

29. Trenchs V, Hernandez-Bou S, Bianchi C, Arnan M, Gene A, Luaces C. Blood cultures are not useful in the evaluation of children with uncomplicated superficial skin and soft tissue infections. *Pediatr Infect Dis J* 2015;34:924–7.

30. Malone JR, Durica SR, Thompson DM, Bogie A, Naifeh M. Blood cultures in the evaluation of uncomplicated skin and soft tissue infections. *Pediatrics* 2013;132(3).

31. Liles DK, Dall LH. Needle aspiration for diagnosis of cellulitis. *Cutis* 1985;36(1):63–4.

32. Wong C, Khin L, Heng K, Tan K, Low C. The LRINEC (laboratory risk indicator for necrotizing fasciitis) score: A tool for distinguishing necrotizing fasciitis from other soft tissue infections. *Crit Care Med* 2004;32:1535–41.

33. Swain R, Hatcher J, Azadian B, Soni N, De Souza B. A five-year review of necrotising fasciitis in a tertiary referral unit. *Ann R Coll Surg Engl* 2013;95:57.

34. Parenti GC, Marri C, Calandra G, Morisi C, Zabberoni W. [Necrotizing fasciitis of soft tissues: Role of diagnostic imaging and review of the literature]. *Radiol Med* 2000;99:334–9.

35. Kehrl T. Point-of-care ultrasound diagnosis of necrotizing fasciitis missed by computed tomography and magnetic resonance imaging. *J Emerg Med* 2014;47:172–5.

36. Carbonetti F et al. The role of contrast enhanced computed tomography in the diagnosis of necrotizing fasciitis and comparison with the laboratory risk indicator for necrotizing fasciitis (LRINEC). *Radiol Med* 2016;121:106–21.

37. Griffith ME, Ellis MW. Antimicrobial activity against CA-MRSA and treatment of uncomplicated non-purulent cellulitis. *Expert Rev Anti Infect Ther* 2013;11:777–80.

38. Ali A, Botha J, Tiruvoipati R. Fatal skin and soft tissue infection of multidrug resistant *Acinetobacter baumannii*: A case report. *Int J Surg Case Rep* 2014;5:532–6.

39. Korhonen K. Hyperbaric oxygen therapy in acute necrotizing infections with a special reference to the effects on tissue gas tensions. *Ann Chir Gynaecol Suppl* 2000;214:7–36.

40. Holder EP, Moore PT, Browne BA. Nonsteroidal anti-inflammatory drugs and necrotising fasciitis. *An update. Drug Saf* 1997;17:369–73.

41. Khamnuan P, Chongruksut W, Jearwattanakanok K, Patumanond J, Tantraworasin A. Necrotizing fasciitis: Epidemiology and clinical predictors for amputation. *Int J Gen Med* 2015;8:195–202.

27

Cutaneous manifestations of sepsis

K. P. ANEESH AND MAHASHWETA DAS

INTRODUCTION

Sepsis is defined as systemic inflammatory response syndrome (SIRS) secondary to a documented infection. The host response to infection leading to sepsis is a continuum that ranges from sepsis to severe sepsis to septic shock and multiple organ dysfunction syndrome (MODS) [1]. The symptoms of sepsis are often nonspecific and include fever with chills, confusion, anxiety, breathlessness, nausea, vomiting, malaise, and fatigue. But these symptoms are not universal or pathognomonic. Even though fever is a common symptom, some cases may have hypothermia in the presence of tachycardia and tachypnea. Like the other clinical features of sepsis, cutaneous manifestations are also not pathognomonic, but the presence of them may be extremely useful for the clinician to arrive at a diagnosis as well as to assess the severity of the condition.

DIAGNOSIS OF SEPSIS

Infection is typically identified by signs and symptoms along with laboratory investigations (Figure 27.1). However, the classical signs and symptoms may not always be present. For example, immunosuppressed patients may not develop fever and the presence of hypothermia in such patients and in the elderly indicates a grave prognosis [2]. It is often impossible to identify a source of infection, but proven microbiological invasion of a sterile environment (e.g., a positive peritoneal tap in a cirrhotic patient), points toward infection. Patients receiving antibiotics may also fail to yield positive test results for possible infections. Therefore, in such cases, unexplained organ dysfunction in the presence of other signs, including cutaneous findings, may be the only clue (Figure 27.2) [3–6].

PATHOPHYSIOLOGY OF SEPSIS

The primary event in pathogenesis of sepsis is presumed to be uncontrolled activation of the inflammatory response to a pathogen. The resultant inflammation leads to uncontrolled coagulation, which in turn leads to release of a battery of inflammatory cytokines. The initial burst of inflammatory activation is often mediated by TNF-α, which acts through pattern recognition receptors (PRRs), like toll-like receptors (TLRs), and leads to NF$\kappa\beta$ activation and secretion of a cascade of inflammatory mediators. The dysregulated immune response ultimately leads to organ failure. The organ failure in sepsis is functional and is largely due to cytokine-induced cellular hibernation rather than cellular death.

The cutaneous features of sepsis can point toward the underlying infection, the injury caused by the inflammatory response (such as vasculitis), or the resultant organ failure. A simplified representation of the pathogenesis and associated cutaneous features are given in Figure 27.3.

CUTANEOUS SIGNS OF INFECTIONS LEADING TO SEPSIS

Erythroderma

Erythroderma in a patient with sepsis suggests staphylococcal or streptococcal toxic shock syndrome (TSS). The patients of staphylococcal TSS are more likely to present with erythroderma, but they seldom yield positive results in blood culture. The patients may initially have a maculopapular rash that typically spares the areas compressed by occlusive clothing [7]. The rash progresses to diffuse erythroderma and desquamation in 5 days to 2 weeks of the onset of the illness. The condition may progress

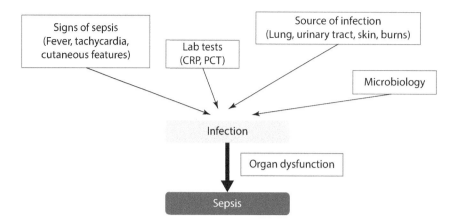

Figure 27.1 Diagnosis of Sepsis from Infection: An infection is diagnosed from clinical signs including cutaneous features, lab tests and/or microbiological positivity. When organ dysfunction is also identified, a diagnosis of sepsis is made. Note: CRP, C reactive Protein; PCT, Procalcitonin.

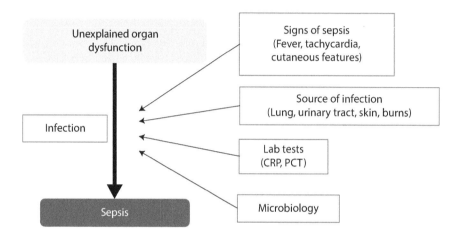

Figure 27.2 Diagnosis of Sepsis from Organ Dysfunction: Infection can be difficult to identify in critically ill patients, especially in patients on long-term antibiotic therapy. Unexplained organ dysfunction should raise the suspicion of sepsis and a thorough investigations needs to be done to identify the underlying infection. Note: CRP, C reactive Protein; PCT, Procalcitonin.

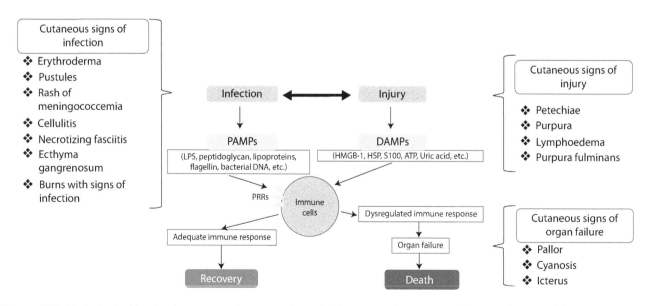

Figure 27.3 Pathological basis of cutaneous features of sepsis: Cutaneous features can be an indicator of the underlying infection. Alternatively they can be the consequence of cellular injury or the resultant organ failure.

into septic shock with development of hypotension, cold extremities, peripheral cyanosis, and oliguria. Myalgia is a common symptom and may mimic acute abdomen when there is guarding on palpation. Mucous membrane examination reveals conjunctival and oropharyngeal hyperemia with a red beefy tongue and punctate nonpurulent buccal ulcerations. There may be transient patchy alopecia and loss of one or more fingernails. Hyperemic and tender genitalia with malodorous vaginal discharge may also be present. Streptococcal TSS is commonly seen with a soft tissue infection, and blood culture for bacteria often yields positive results [8].

Pustules

The presence of generalized or localized pustules in a patient in sepsis, especially in neonates and immunocompromised patients, may suggest a fungal infection, particularly with *Candida* species. Even though congenital candidiasis seen in infants born to mothers with vaginal candidiasis is a skin-limited disease, in the setting of an immunocompromised state or evidence of sepsis, candidemia has to be considered [9,10]. A smear for fungi and potassium hydroxide mount will help confirm the diagnosis.

Pustules due to disseminated gonococcemia are acrally located and tender. They have a typical gun metal gray color or may be hemorrhagic or black. Intracellular gram-negative diplococci in Gram-stained smears are diagnostic [11,12].

Meningococcemia rash

Meningococcemia typically presents with a group of cutaneous findings. The initial rash may be a transient macular or papular rash that resembles a viral exanthem. The rash soon progresses to form the typical small and irregular petechiae with a smudged appearance. Most often the lesions are distributed on the extremities and trunk. Extensive hemorrhagic lesions with central necrosis may develop.

Cellulitis and erysipelas

Cellulitis and erysipelas are described in Chapter 26 [13–19].

Ecthyma gangrenosum

Ecthyma gangrenosum is a relatively rare disorder. Even though *Pseudomonas aeruginosa* was proposed as the etiological agent of ecthyma gangrenosum, various other bacteria like *Escherichia coli*, *Citrobacter freundii*, *Klebsiella pneumonia*, various other *Pseudomonas* species, and *Morganella morganii* may also be responsible [20–22]. The skin lesions begin as an erythematous nodule or hemorrhagic vesicle, usually macule first and then papule, which evolves into a necrotic ulcer with eschar. The lesions may be localized or widespread all over the body [23–25].

Table 27.1 Hard clinical signs suggestive of necrotizing soft tissue infections

Highly specific	Presence of bullae
	Skin ecchymosis that precedes skin necrosis
	Presence of gas in the tissues by examination or radiographic evaluation
	Cutaneous anesthesia
Less specific	Pain out of proportion to examination
	Edema that extends beyond the erythema
	Systemic toxicity
	Progression of infection despite antibiotic therapy

Source: Hakkarainen et al. *Curr Probl Surg* 2014;51(8):344–62.

Necrotizing fasciitis

Sepsis is a common sequelae of necrotizing soft tissue infections (NSTIs), which is described in Chapter 26. Some "hard" clinical signs that are more suggestive of NSTIs are listed in Table 27.1 [26–31].

CUTANEOUS SIGNS OF SEPSIS DUE TO ENDOTHELIAL INJURY

Acute vascular endothelial injury and dysfunction is a central event in the pathogenesis of sepsis, increasing vascular permeability, promoting activation of the coagulation cascade, leading to tissue edema, and compromising the perfusion of vital organs. Sepsis induces a proadhesive, procoagulant, and antifibrinolytic state in endothelial cells, altering hemostasis, leukocyte trafficking, inflammation, barrier function, and microcirculation. The appearance of skin lesions such as petechiae, purpura, and lymphoedema are primarily due to acute injury to the endothelial cells and their dysfunction.

Purpura fulminans

Purpura fulminans (PF) is described in detail in Chapter 34 [32–37].

Petechiae and purpura

The vasculitis and coagulopathy that can occur in sepsis may cause purpura, sometimes prominent in the nail folds and small capillaries. Patients with infections causing thrombocytopenia are more likely to develop such lesions.

CUTANEOUS SIGNS OF ORGAN FAILURE

The final result of dysregulated immune response in sepsis is organ failure, which may involve multiple organ systems. Even though acute involvement of these organ systems fails to produce striking cutaneous changes, subtle signs may point toward possible compromise of the concerned organ system. Peripheral cyanosis in the presence of other features of sepsis, such as hyper- or hypothermia, tachycardia, and tachypnea, points toward pulmonary failure. Peripheral pitting edema may also induce acute cardiorespiratory failure. Cutaneous signs relevant to involvement of other organ systems include icterus, pruritus, and pallor [38,39].

CONCLUSION

Sepsis is a major clinical challenge to clinicians working in emergency and critical care medical units. The clinical signs of sepsis are largely variable and may indicate a spectrum based on the severity. Cutaneous signs are an important pointer toward the possible etiology, severity, and prognosis of sepsis and help in early diagnosis of the condition.

KEY POINTS

- Cutaneous manifestations of sepsis are early clues to their diagnosis.
- Erythroderma, pustules, necrotising fasciitis, purpura and echthyma gangrenosum are some cutaneous morphological manifestations of sepsis.
- Early identification of cutaneous features leads to early diagnosis of sepsis and thus prevents morbidity and mortality.

REFERENCES

1. Singer M et al. The Third International Consensus Definitions for Sepsis and Septic Shock (Sepsis-3). *JAMA* 2016;315(8):801–10.
2. Kushimoto S et al. The impact of body temperature abnormalities on the disease severity and outcome in patients with severe sepsis: An analysis from a multicenter, prospective survey of severe sepsis. *Crit Care* 2013;17:R271.
3. Vincent JL et al. International study of the prevalence and outcomes of infection in intensive care units. *JAMA* 2009;302:2323–9.
4. Heenen S, Jacobs F, Vincent JL. Antibiotic strategies in severe nosocomial sepsis: Why do we not deescalate more often? *Crit Care Med* 2012;40:1404–9.
5. Vincent JL et al. Rapid Diagnosis of Infection in the Critically Ill (RADICAL), a multicenter study of molecular detection in bloodstream infections, pneumonia and sterile site infections. *Crit Care Med* 2015;43:2283–91.
6. Phua J et al. Characteristics and outcomes of culture-negative versus culture-positive severe sepsis. *Crit Care* 2013;17:R202.
7. Tofte RW, Williams DN. Clinical and laboratory manifestations of toxic shock syndrome. *Ann Intern Med* 1982;96:843–7.
8. Tofte RW, Williams DN. Toxic shock syndrome: Clinical and laboratory features in 15 patients. *Ann Intern Med* 1981;94(Part 2):149–55.
9. Guery BP et al. Management of invasive candidiasis and candidemia in adult non-neutropenic intensive care unit patients: Part I. Epidemiology and diagnosis. *Intensive Care Med* 2009;35(1):55–62.
10. Picazo JJ, González-Romo F, Candel FJ. Candidemia in the critically ill patient. *Int J Antimicrob Agents* 2008;32:S83–5.
11. Brown TJ, Yen-Moore A, Tyring SK. An overview of sexually transmitted diseases. Part I. *J Am Acad Dermatol* 1999;41:511.
12. O'Brien JP, Goldenberg DL, Rice PA. Disseminated gonococcal infection: A prospective analysis of 49 patients and a review of pathophysiology and immune mechanisms. *Medicine (Baltim)* 1983;62:395.
13. Stevens DL et al. Practice guidelines for the diagnosis and management of skin and soft tissue infections: 2014 update by the Infectious Diseases Society of America. *Clin Infect Dis* 2014;59(2):e10–52.
14. Gunderson CG, Martinello RA. A systematic review of bacteremias in cellulitis and erysipelas. *J Infect* 2012;64(2):148–55.
15. Dupuy A et al. Risk factors for erysipelas of the leg (cellulitis): Case-control study. *BMJ* 1999;318(7198):1591–4.
16. Ginsberg MB. Cellulitis: Analysis of 101 cases and review of the literature. *South Med J* 1981;74(5):530–3.
17. Koutkia P, Mylonakis E, Boyce J. Cellulitis: Evaluation of possible predisposing factors in hospitalized patients. *Diagn Microbiol Infect Dis* 1999;34(4):325–7.
18. Kulthanan K et al. Clinical and microbiologic findings in cellulitis in Thai patients. *J Med Assoc Thai* 1999;82(6):587–92.
19. Chira S, Miller LG. *Staphylococcus aureus* is the most common identified cause of cellulitis: A systematic review. *Epidemiol Infect* 2010;138(3):313–7.
20. Edelstein H, Cutting HO. *Escherichia coli* as cause of ecthyma gangrenosum. *Postgrad Med* 1986;79(2):44–5.
21. Rodot S, Lacour JP, van Elslande L, Castanet J, Desruelles F, Ortonne JP. Ecthyma gangrenosum caused by *Klebsiella pneumoniae*. *Int J Dermatol* 1995;34(3):216–7.
22. Soria A, Francès C, Guihot A, Varnous S, Bricaire F, Caumes E. Etiology of ecthyma gangrenosum: Four cases. *Ann Dermatol Venereol* 2010;137(6-7):472–6.
23. Pandit AM, Siddaramappa B, Choudhary SV, Manjunathswamy BS. Ecthyma gangrenosum in a newborn child. *Indian J Dermatol Venereol Leprol* 2003;69(1):52–3.
24. Agarwal S, Sharma M, Mehndirata V. Solitary ecthyma gangrenosum (EG)-like lesion consequent to *Candida albicans* in a neonate. *Indian J Pediatr* 2007;74(6):582–4.

25. Varghese GM, Eapen P, Abraham S. Ecthyma gangrenosum of a single limb. *Indian J Crit Care Med* 2011;15(3):188–9.
26. Shiroff A, Herlitz G, Gracias V. Necrotizing soft tissue infections. *J Intensive Care Med* 2014;29(3):138–44.
27. Umbert I, Oliver G, Winkelmann R, Peters M. Necrotizing fasciitis: A clinical, microbiological and histopathologic study of 14 patients. *J Am Acad Dermatol* 1989;20(5):774–81.
28. Howard R, Pessa M, Brennaman B, Ramphal R. Necrotizing soft-tissue infections caused by marine vibrios. *Surgery* 1985;98(1):126–30.
29. Goodell K, Jordan M, Graham R, Cassidy C, Nasraway S. Rapidly advancing necrotizing fasciitis caused by *Photobacterium (Vibrio) damsela*: A hyperaggressive variant. *Crit Care Med* 2004;32(1):278–81.
30. Wall D, Kleain S, Black S, de Virgilio C. A simple model to help distinguish necrotizing from nonnecrotizing soft-tissue infections. *J Am Coll Surg* 2000;191(3):227–31.
31. Hakkarainen TW, Kopari NM, Pham TN, Evans HL. Necrotizing soft tissue infections: Review and current concepts in treatment, systems of care, and outcomes. *Curr Probl Surg* 2014;51(8):344–62.
32. Darmstadt GL. Acute infectious purpura fulminans: Pathogenesis and medical management. *Pediatr Dermatol* 1998;15:169–83.
33. Talwar A, Kumar S, Gopal M, Nandini A. Spectrum of purpura fulminans: Report of three classical prototypes and review of management strategies. *Indian J Dermatol Venereol Leprol* 2012;78(2):228.
34. Brown DL, Greenhalgh DG, Warden GD. Purpura fulminans and transient protein C and S deficiency. *Arch Dermatol* 1998;124:119–23.
35. Madden RM, Gill JC, Marlar RA. Protein C and protein S levels in two patients with acquired purpura fulminans. *Br J Haematol* 1990;75:112–7.
36. Hautekeete ML et al. Purpura fulminans in pneumococcal sepsis. *Arch Intern Med* 1986;146:497–9.
37. Francis RB. Acquired purpura fulminans. *Semin Thromb Haemostat* 1990;16:310–25.
38. Canet E et al. Acute respiratory failure in kidney transplant recipients: A multicenter study. *Crit Care* 2011;15(2):R91.
39. Hazin R, Abu-Rajab Tamimi TI, Abuzetun JY, Zein NN. Recognizing and treating cutaneous signs of liver disease. *Cleve Clin J Med* 2009;76(10):599–606.

Viral infections

K. B. ANURADHA

INTRODUCTION

Most viral infections with cutaneous manifestations are self-limiting, but there are a few conditions that may be life threatening and can lead to emergencies. A prompt diagnosis and rapid initiation of treatment are paramount in the management of such conditions. The etiology, clinical features, diagnosis, and treatment of such viral infections are discussed in this chapter.

HERPES SIMPLEX VIRUS INFECTIONS

Herpes simplex virus (HSV) infections are generally self-limiting. However, HSV infection in neonates and immuno-compromised individuals, and eczema herpeticum should be considered as emergencies.

Neonatal herpes

HSV may be transmitted to the neonate during the intra-uterine (5%), intrapartum (85%), or postpartum (10%) periods [1]. The risk of transmission is highest (30%–50%) for women who acquire a genital HSV infection near the time of delivery. The risk of transmission is low (<1%–3%) for women with recurrent genital herpes. Seventy percent of neonatal HSV infections are caused by HSV-2. Neonatal HSV-1 infections are usually acquired through contact with a person with orolabial disease but can also occur intrapartum if the mother is genitally infected with HSV-1.

The clinical spectrum of perinatally acquired neonatal infections can be divided into the following three forms:

1. Localized infection of the skin, eyes, and/or mouth (SEM), which is characterized by vesicular eruptions, erosions, or peeling
2. Central nervous system (CNS) disease characterized by encephalitis that may present as lethargy, irritability, poor feeding, temperature instability, seizures, and a bulging fontanelle
3. Disseminated disease with encephalitis, hepatitis, pneumonia, and coagulopathy

In 68% of infected babies, skin vesicles are the presenting sign. However, 39% of neonates with disseminated disease, 32% with CNS disease, and 17% with SEM disease never develop vesicular skin lesions. The incubation period may be as long as 3 weeks and averages about 1 week.

The pattern of involvement at presentation is important prognostically. With treatment, localized skin disease is rarely fatal, whereas CNS or disseminated disease is fatal in 15%–50% of neonates so affected. More than 50% of patients with CNS or disseminated neonatal herpes have neurological disability.

Intrauterine HSV infection is rare and usually fatal. Very few children survive to present with characteristic wide-spread reticulate scarring of the whole body.

The diagnosis of neonatal herpes is confirmed by viral culture or preferably immediate direct fluorescent antibody (DFA) staining of material from skin or ocular lesions. CNS involvement is detected by polymerase chain reaction (PCR) of the cerebrospinal fluid (CSF). PCR of the CSF is negative in 24% of neonatal CNS herpes infections, so pending other testing, empiric therapy may be required.

Neonatal herpes infections are treated with IV acyclovir 10–20 mg/kg every 8 hours for 14 days in SEM disease and 21 days for CNS and disseminated disease.

The appropriate management of pregnancies complicated with genital herpes is still complex. The current recommendation is to perform cesarean section in the mother with active genital lesions or prodromal symptoms. Because the risk of neonatal herpes is much greater in mothers who experience their initial episode during pregnancy, antiviral treatment of all initial episodes of genital HSV infection in pregnancy is recommended. Standard acyclovir doses for initial episodes, 400 mg three times daily for 10 days, are recommended. Chronic suppressive therapy with acyclovir has been used from 36 weeks' gestation to delivery in women with an initial episode of genital HSV during pregnancy, to reduce outbreaks and prevent the need for cesarean section.

Herpes simplex virus infection in immunocompromised patients

Immunosuppressed patients are at risk of developing fulminant herpes infections. In such patients primary and recurrent cases of herpes simplex infections are more severe, persistent, and more resistant to therapy. Vesicles enlarge to form hemorrhagic blisters and deep ulcers [2]. Extension of oral HSV infection into the esophagus or trachea and ocular involvement from direct inoculation or from periorbital lesions are grave complications that require early diagnosis and treatment. As ocular HSV infection can lead to corneal ulceration, scarring, globe rupture, and blindness: it should certainly be treated as an emergency.

Death is often secondary to visceral involvement, the most common being herpes encephalitis. Herpes labialis is a coincidental finding in many cases of herpes encephalitis. Mortality is more than 70% in untreated cases, and residual neurologic defects are seen in most of the survivors.

Viral cultures from ulcer margins, DFA testing, and skin biopsy are the diagnostic aids.

In severe cutaneous herpes infections in the immunosuppressed, IV acyclovir 5–10 mg/kg every 8 hours can be given to control the disease. In patients with AIDS and those with persistent immunosuppression, consideration should be given to chronic suppressive therapy with oral acyclovir 400–800 mg two to three times daily, or oral valacyclovir 500 mg twice daily, or oral famciclovir 500 mg twice daily. Acyclovir resistance is a complication of such long-term therapy. The standard treatment of acyclovir-resistant herpes simplex infection is IV foscarnet.

Despite early treatment with IV acyclovir 10 mg/kg every 8 hours for 7–14 days, herpes encephalitis carries significant mortality and morbidity [3].

Eczema herpeticum (Kaposi varicelliform eruption)

Eczema herpeticum (EH) is a herpetic superinfection, usually due to HSV-1, presenting most often in children, especially in association with atopic dermatitis. The use of topical calcineurin inhibitors, hot tub exposures, and mutations in gene-encoding filaggrin are considered as risk factors. It can also occur in patients with impaired skin barrier due to other conditions such as burns, pemphigus, Darier disease, Hailey-Hailey disease, mycosis fungoides, Sézary syndrome, severe seborrheic dermatitis, allergic contact dermatitis, scabies, and ichthyoses.

In EH, herpetic lesions bypass the nerve endings and ganglions and directly spread to a diseased cutaneous region [4].

EH is clinically characterized by acute onset of widespread umbilicated vesicles leading to punched out erosions and hemorrhagic crusts. Patients may have associated fever, malaise, and lymphadenopathy. EH may be complicated by bacterial superinfection with *Staphylococcus aureus*. EH can be fatal, usually from *Staphylococcus aureus* septicemia, but also from visceral dissemination of herpes simplex.

Viral culture, skin biopsy, or DFA testing may be done to confirm the diagnosis.

Rapid initiation of IV acyclovir 5–10 mg/kg body weight every 8 hours for 5–7 days is crucial as HSV may completely disseminate and possibly lead to death [5].

A summary of the treatment of herpes simplex infection in neonates, the immunocompromised, and in eczema herpeticum is provided in Table 28.1.

VARICELLA ZOSTER VIRUS INFECTION

Varicella zoster virus (VZV) presents as varicella (chicken pox) as a primary infection and herpes zoster (shingles) when the virus is reactivated. Both varicella and herpes zoster are self-limiting diseases, but there are specific circumstances where VZV infections can lead to emergencies.

Varicella (chicken pox)

Varicella is characterized by outbreaks of vesicles (Figure 28.1), preceded by an incubation period of 2 weeks with or without prodromal symptoms. Airborne droplets are the usual route of transmission of varicella, although direct contact with vesicular fluid is another mode of spread. Mucosae can be affected with multiple aphthous-like ulcers.

Risk factors for severe varicella include age (the first month of life is a susceptible period, especially if the mother is seronegative), neonates with delivery before 28 weeks of gestation (because of the failed transplacental transfer of immunoglobulin G antibodies), doses of corticosteroid equivalent to 1–2 mg/kg/day of prednisolone, and malignancy (especially leukemia). Almost 30% of patients with leukemia have visceral dissemination of varicella, and 7% may die.

Neonatal varicella, which should be considered as an emergency, is seen in two clinical settings: primary VZV infection during pregnancy that is transmitted across the placenta or primary VZV infection during the perinatal period. The former can occur at any point during gestation and results in either congenital varicella syndrome and/or fetal death.

Table 28.1 Treatment of herpes simplex virus infections in neonates and immunocompromised individuals, and eczema herpeticum

Disease	Drug and dosage
Neonatal	Acyclovir: 20 mg/kg IV 8 hourly for 14–21 days
Immunocompromised	*Recommended use until all mucocutaneous lesions are healed*
	Acyclovir: 400 mg oral five times daily or 5 mg/kg (if age >12 years) to 10 mg/kg (if age <12 years) IV 8 hourly
	Famciclovir: 500 mg oral twice daily
	Valacyclovir: 1 g oral twice daily
Eczema herpeticum	*Recommended use for 10–14 days or until all mucocutaneous lesions healed*
	Acyclovir: 15 mg/kg (400 mg maximum) oral three to five times daily or, if severe, 5 mg/kg (if age >12 years) to 10 mg/kg (if age <12 years) IV 8 hourly
	Famciclovir: 500 mg oral twice daily
	Valacyclovir: 1 g oral twice daily
Chronic suppression in the setting of HIV infection	Acyclovir: 400–800 mg oral three times daily
	Famciclovir: 500 mg oral twice daily
	Valacyclovir: 500 mg oral twice daily
Acyclovir-resistant HSV in immunocompromised patients	Foscarnet: 40 mg/kg IV 8–12 hourly for 2–3 weeks (or until all lesions are healed)
	Cidofovir: 1% cream or gel four times daily for 2–3 weeks (for severe disease), 5 mg/kg IV weekly for 2 weeks then every other week (together with probenecid)

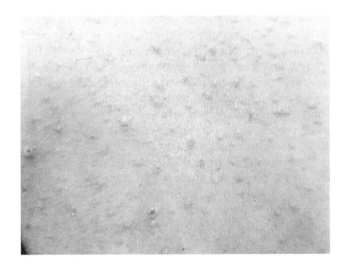

Figure 28.1 Papulovesicles, vesicles, and crusting on an erythematous base in varicella.

Congenital varicella syndrome occurs in 2% of children born to women who develop varicella during the first or second trimester of pregnancy and manifests as intrauterine growth retardation, microcephaly, cortical atrophy, limb hypoplasia, microphthalmia, cataracts, chorioretinitis, and cutaneous scarring [6]. Prognosis is poor, and death during infancy results from gastroesophageal reflux, aspiration pneumonia, or respiratory failure [7].

The second form of neonatal varicella is *perinatal varicella*, which occurs when there is maternal disease 5 days before delivery to 2 days after delivery. Infants develop the classic skin vesicles on an erythematous base. Dissemination may result in pneumonia, hepatitis, encephalitis, and severe coagulopathy [7]. Infants exposed to maternal infection should be given varicella zoster immunoglobulin (VZIG) if available or IV immunoglobulin (IVIG) at birth or as soon as maternal symptoms develop [8].

Varicella infections can be life-threatening in a few other circumstances. Immunocompromised individuals with varicella have an increased risk for systemic complications including pneumonitis, CNS involvement, pneumonia, thrombocytopenia, and liver function impairment.

Although less than 5% of varicella cases occur in immunocompetent adults, 55% of deaths due to varicella occur in adults. Adults with varicella infection are at increased risk of pneumonitis, and the most common cause of mortality is pneumonia with respiratory failure [9].

Hemorrhagic varicella is a malignant variant of chicken pox that may be associated with disseminated intravascular coagulation. Manifestations may be extremely severe and include macroscopic hematuria, necrotic purpura, and cerebrovascular thrombosis [10].

A clinical diagnosis can usually be made upon the history and physical examination. A Tzanck smear and/or DFA can rapidly help to confirm the diagnosis. Viral culture is specific, and PCR is highly sensitive. Serology is only useful in retrospect.

Varicella in immunocompromised individuals should be treated with acyclovir 10 mg/kg intravenously every 8 hours for 7–10 days or until crops of new lesions have ceased.

Herpes zoster

Herpes zoster, the latent reactivation of previous VZV, is rarely life-threatening, though disseminated disease can be associated with increased morbidity and mortality. Fluid from herpes zoster vesicles can transmit VZV to seronegative individuals leading to varicella.

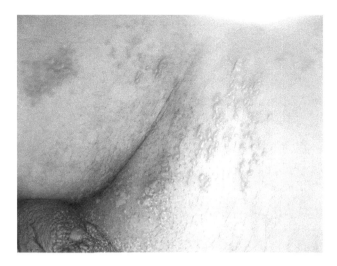

Figure 28.2 Grouped vesicles in a dermatomal distribution in herpes zoster.

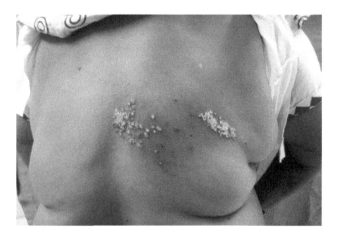

Figure 28.3 Pustular lesions in herpes zoster.

Herpes zoster usually manifests as an eruption of grouped vesicles in a dermatomal distribution (Figure 28.2). Lesions can become pustular (Figure 28.3) or hemorrhagic. In immunosuppressed patients, disseminated disease may occur, defined as more than 20 vesicles outside the area of the primary or adjacent dermatome. Common complications of disseminated disease include pneumonia, encephalitis, and hepatitis. VZV encephalitis may occur months after an episode of herpes zoster. Patients have a subacute clinical presentation with headache, fever, mental status changes, seizures, and focal neurologic defects. Cerebrospinal fluid analysis reveals VZV DNA by PCR. Death often results, although case reports have shown that high-dose IV acyclovir therapy may be efficacious [11].

Ramsay Hunt syndrome, also known as herpes zoster oticus, is a herpetic infection of the inner, middle, and external ear. It is a reactivation of latent VZV virus in the geniculate ganglion, the sensory ganglion of the facial nerve; however, reactivation affects both the facial nerve (cranial nerve VII) and the vestibulocochlear nerve (cranial nerve VIII) due to their close proximity. Patients present with severe ear pain, small vesicles on the pinna or oral mucosa, and facial palsy. Prompt diagnosis is paramount as initiation of antiviral therapy within 72 hours of the onset of symptoms leads to resolution of the facial palsy in as many as 75% of cases [12].

Herpes zoster ophthalmicus involves the ophthalmic division of the trigeminal nerve and occurs in up to 20% of patients with herpes zoster. Hutchinson sign is the appearance of a herpes zoster lesion on the tip or side of the nose and serves as a useful prognostic factor in the ensuing ocular inflammation. Clinically, patients develop lesions on the margin of the eyelid. Early complications include periorbital edema, residual ptosis, lid scarring, deep scalp pitting, entropion, ectropion, pigmentary changes, and lid necrosis [13]. Glaucoma, optic neuritis, encephalitis, hemiplegia, and acute retinal necrosis are more severe long-term complications, the risk of which may be reduced by half with prompt initiation of antiviral therapy. Chronic disease due to neurologic damage occurs in up to 30% of patients with this form of herpes zoster.

Uncomplicated zoster may be adequately treated with oral antivirals, such as valacyclovir 1 gm or famciclovir 500 mg every 8 hours for 7 days. Disseminated and severe infections require IV acyclovir 10 mg/kg every 8 hours for 7–14 days. Although corticosteroids may be added as an adjuvant therapy in herpes zoster infections due to their anti-inflammatory properties, studies have failed to show a beneficial effect on acute pain, and in some instances adverse effects including gastrointestinal symptoms, edema, and granulocytosis have been reported. However, in Ramsay Hunt syndrome, steroids may be added to antiviral therapy if there are no contraindications [14].

Zostavax is a live attenuated vaccine that is recommended in all persons 60 years or older for the prevention of herpes zoster and postherpetic neuralgia. The vaccine has been shown to reduce the incidence of herpes zoster by 51%, reduce the incidence of postherpetic neuralgia by 67%, and reduce the herpes zoster-related burden of illness by 61% [15]. Gabapentin has been approved since 2002 by the U.S. Food and Drug Administration (FDA) for the treatment of postherpetic neuralgia [16].

A summary of treatment of VZV infections is provided in Table 28.2.

CYTOMEGALOVIRUS INFECTION

Cytomegalovirus (CMV), or human herpesvirus-5 (HHV-5), is acquired by exposure to infected children, sexual transmission, and transfusion of CMV-infected blood products. CMV causes a mild form of infectious mononucleosis in most affected immunocompetent individuals. Fatal massive hepatic necrosis can occur in rare cases. Immunocompromised individuals, including those with HIV, malignancy, or postorgan transplant patients, may have severe, complicated CMV infections.

Congenital infection occurs in 0.5%–2% of newborns, often as a result of transplacental transmission of the

Table 28.2 Treatment of varicella zoster virus infections

Disease	Drug and dosage
Varicella	Acyclovir: 20 mg/kg (800 mg maximum) oral four times daily for 5 days Valacyclovir 20 mg/kg (1 g maximum) oral three times daily for 5 days
Herpes zoster	Acyclovir: 800 mg oral five times daily for 7–10 days Famciclovir: 500 mg oral three times daily for 7 days Valacyclovir: 1 g oral three times daily for 7 days
Immunocompromised	Acyclovir: 10 mg/kg (500 mg/m²) IV 8 hourly for 7–10 days or until cropping has ceased (depending on the setting, consider continuing until lesions are healed)

virus. Clinical manifestations are more severe in offspring whose mothers are primarily infected during pregnancy than in those whose mothers undergo reactivation; the earlier the gestational infection, the more severe the disease. Cutaneous manifestations of congenital CMV include jaundice, petechiae and purpura, referred to as "blueberry muffin" lesions, and complications include hearing loss and mental retardation [1].

Complications such as the Landry-Guillain-Barré syndrome, and involvement of the CNS with encephalitis and meningitis, have been reported to have a high risk of mortality. Postperfusion syndrome occurs after a blood transfusion and is practically a mononucleosis syndrome in which the involvement of the liver is usually prominent. The mortality rate is very high (80%–90%) in organ recipients and in those with HIV infection who frequently develop viremia with bouts of fever and variable liver, lung, gastrointestinal, and retinal involvement. Most often, CMV infection coexists with other opportunistic infections, and death is most often due to *Pneumocystis carinii* pneumonia.

Culture of CMV is the traditional diagnostic gold standard, but this takes weeks to days. In histology, an "owl's eye appearance" of the infected endothelial cell is diagnostic. Detection of CMV in tissue cultures within 24–48 hours is possible with the shell vial assay, in which monoclonal antibodies specific for early CMV antigens are employed.

The first-line agents for treatment (as well as prophylaxis) of CMV in immunocompromised patients are ganciclovir and valganciclovir. High-titer CMV immunoglobulins are also occasionally used [17]. Treatment of CMV-induced mononucleosis in immunocompetent individuals, however, is only supportive.

MEASLES (RUBEOLA)

Measles, due to the morbillivirus of Paramyxoviridae family, has markedly decreased in incidence since the development of vaccination against the virus. Generally, affected individuals are unvaccinated children less than 5 years of age or vaccinated school-age children who failed to develop immunity to the vaccine.

The virus is transmitted via respiratory secretions. After an asymptomatic incubation period of 10–11 days, high fever develops followed by rapid defervescence. Other symptoms include severe coryza, conjunctivitis, and a barking cough. The eruption consists of erythematous macules and papules appearing behind the ears and at the anterior hairline, coalescing and spreading slowly to the neck and trunk, and finally to the extremities (Figure 28.4), including the hands and feet. The eruption fades in the order of appearance, becoming brownish-yellow because of capillary hemorrhage. The typical enanthem is diagnostically characterized by bluish-gray areas on the tonsils (Herman spots) and punctate blue-white lesions surrounded by an erythematous ring (grains of sand on a red background) on the buccal mucosa, opposite the second molars (Koplik spots) that appear 1–2 days before the exanthem and remain for 2–3 days.

Complications are more common in the very young and in the malnourished. Encephalitis occurs unpredictably in 1 in 800 cases and results in death and brain damage only in a small minority of cases. Subacute sclerosing panencephalitis may develop later in 1 of 100,000 cases, resulting in mental and motor deterioration, personality changes, myoclonic seizures, coma, and death. Infection in pregnant patients has been associated with fetal death [18].

Laboratory diagnosis of measles can be accomplished by virus isolation or detection via PCR in nasopharyngeal secretions or urine as well as serological assays for measles-specific antibodies (IgM or IgG).

There is no specific antiviral therapy for measles. Vaccination is the gold standard for preventing infection. The measles, mumps, rubella (MMR) vaccine is a live attenuated vaccine and as a result cannot be used in immunocompromised patients. Although no antivirals have been effective in

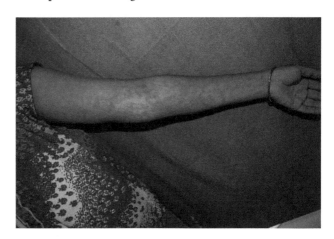

Figure 28.4 Maculopapular rash in measles.

treating measles infection, vitamin A supplementation may reduce deaths from measles by 50% as vitamin A deficiency has been shown to increase morbidity and mortality [19].

GERMAN MEASLES (RUBELLA)

Rubella is a viral infection caused by the rubella virus of the *Togaviridae* family. The disease is spread by respiratory droplets. After a 2-week incubation period where mild constitutional symptoms may be present (more severe in adults), an eruption develops. It starts on the face and spreads from head to foot, lasting about 3 days (3-day measles). In contrast with measles, erythema is paler and does not coalesce. Erythematous petechial macules may also be present on the soft palate (Forchheimer spots). Lymphadenopathy (postauricular, posterior cervical, and suboccipital) may precede the eruption and lasts longer.

Complications are uncommon but tend to occur more often in adults than in children. Arthritis or arthralgia is almost exclusive of women. More alarming is encephalitis that occurs in 1 in 6,000 cases [20]. This again is more often in women than in children and is fatal in up to 50% of cases. In children, hemorrhagic manifestations (1 per 3,000 cases) secondary to thrombocytopenia and vasculitis are more frequent. They may affect the gastrointestinal tract, brain, and kidneys. Most patients recover. Additional complications include orchitis, neuritis, hepatitis, pericarditis, and a rare late syndrome of progressive panencephalitis.

Infection with rubella virus in early gestation (first trimester) may cause a number of congenital defects, fetal death, spontaneous abortion, or premature delivery. Congenital rubella syndrome is characterized by cataracts, deafness, congenital cardiac defects (patent ductus arteriosus, ventricular septal defects) and CNS abnormalities (microcephaly, developmental delay). A "blueberry muffin baby" presentation due to dermal hematopoiesis is occasionally observed.

Rubella can be diagnosed by detection of antirubella IgM antibodies or a fourfold increase in specific IgG antibodies, virus isolation, or detection via reverse transcriptase polymerase chain reaction (RT-PCR).

Treatment of rubella is supportive. The current recommended immunization schedule for rubella vaccine (given in conjunction with measles and mumps vaccines) is for an initial dose at 9 months, second dose at 15 months, and a third dose at 4–6 years. If rubella-specific IgM antibodies or a diagnostic rise in IgG antirubella antibodies are detected in early pregnancy, the patient should be offered prenatal counseling.

PARVOVIRUS B19 INFECTION

Parvovirus B19 is a small, single-stranded DNA-containing virus causing a wide range of diseases varying from asymptomatic infections to fetal demise.

The most common form of infection is erythema infectiosum, or "fifth disease." In general, regardless of the clinical presentation, the virus is self-limited with the exception of a few circumstances [2]. It is transmitted through respiratory secretions, blood products, or vertically during pregnancy. Although parvovirus B19 is more common in children, infection does occur in adults.

Erythema infectiosum occurs after a 4–14-day incubation period. Individuals develop the classic "slapped-cheek" facial erythema that spares the nasal bridge and circumoral regions. One to four days later, erythematous macules and papules appear which progress to form a lacy, reticulate pattern most commonly observed on the extremities, lasting 1–3 weeks. Once cutaneous signs appear, the individual is no longer contagious [2]. Arthralgia or arthritis, seen in up to 10% of patients with erythema infectiosum, is more common in female adults and may occur in up to 60% of those infected [21].

Both children and adults may develop a distinct syndrome known as papular purpuric glove and socks syndrome, which is also secondary to parvovirus B19. Clinically, patients have edema and erythema of the palms and soles with petechiae and purpura associated with burning and pruritus.

Parvovirus B19 can cause complications in three situations: immunosuppression, pregnancy, and underlying hematologic disease. Patients with hematologic disease, such as sickle cell anemia or hereditary spherocytosis, who become infected with parvovirus B19 are at risk of developing severe transient aplastic anemia. Recovery is usually spontaneous, but heart failure and death may occur. Thrombocytopenia is another less common complication. Fetal infection with parvovirus B19 can result in miscarriage or nonimmune hydrops fetalis [2]. The greatest risk to the fetus is when infection is acquired before 20 weeks' gestation.

Diagnosis in the acute aplastic phase can be made by the detection of virus in the serum by electron microscopy or PCR amplification of viral DNA. By the time the rash appears, the virus is rapidly disappearing from the blood, and the diagnosis is made by finding specific IgM antibody to human parvovirus.

The mainstay of treatment is supportive. High-dose IV immunoglobulin has been shown to eliminate parvovirus B19 from the bone marrow. Intrauterine transfusions can reverse fetal anemia and reduce fetal demise. Prevention and measures to avoid susceptible people are often difficult, as once the rash appears and is recognized as parvovirus B19, patients are no longer contagious.

ENTEROVIRUS INFECTIONS

The enteroviruses, a subgroup of the picornavirus family, cause a wide array of illnesses associated with exanthems. The nonpolio enteroviruses include echoviruses and coxsackievirus types A and B. Enteroviral infections are usually transmitted via fecal-oral or respiratory routes, and they can also be spread from mother to infant in the peripartum period. The usual incubation period is 3–6 days.

Epidemics of hand-foot-and-mouth disease (HFMD) (Figure 28.5) are usually caused by coxsackievirus A16 or enterovirus 71. In addition, cases with coxsackievirus types A4–7, A9, A10, B1–3, and B5 have been reported. The infection

(a)

(b)

(c)

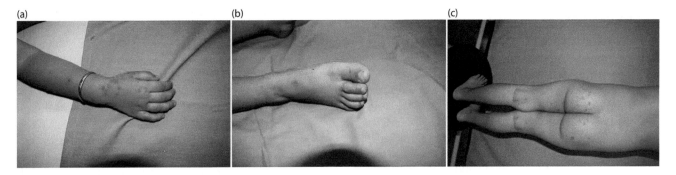

Figure 28.5 Vesicles in hand-foot-and-mouth disease on (a) hands, (b) feet, and (c) buttocks.

is more severe in infants and children than in adults, but generally, the disease has a mild course. Symptoms such as malaise, low-grade fever, and anorexia are often present, and occasionally, patients have high fever, marked malaise, diarrhea, and arthralgias. Myocarditis, pneumonia, meningoencephalitis, and even death have been reported. A large outbreak of HFMD in Taiwan caused by enterovirus 71 had a high mortality rate of 19.3% in the severe cases [2]. Deaths were due to pulmonary hemorrhage. Infection in the first trimester may lead to spontaneous abortion or intrauterine growth retardation.

Specific confirmation of enteroviral infection may be accomplished via the use of viral culture or PCR-based assays from throat or stool swab, cerebrospinal fluids, or fluid from cutaneous vesicles.

Supportive care suffices in most of the enteroviral infections as it is self-limiting. However, in certain patient populations, including immunosuppressed individuals or neonates, an enteroviral infection may be associated with potentially life-threatening complications. Pleconaril, a drug that interferes with enterovirus attachment and uncoating by binding to the protein capsid, has been demonstrated to be useful in clinical studies, and it holds promise as a specific antiviral therapy for serious enteroviral infections [22].

DENGUE FEVER

The hemorrhagic fevers are a group of zoonotic viral infections that range in severity from a mild, self-limited febrile illness to a severe, life-threatening disease. The most important disease with dermatological involvement is dengue fever. Dengue, also called breakbone fever, is an acute illness with fever and two or more of the following symptoms: headache, retro-orbital pain, myalgia, arthralgia, rash, and hemorrhagic manifestations. Fever and other symptoms may subside after 3–4 days, and the patient may recover completely, or the fever may return with an eruption within 1–3 days. Skin eruptions appear in 80% of patients during the remission period of the fever. This timely appearance is diagnostically important because differentiating from malaria, yellow fever, or influenza is difficult by just looking at the skin lesions. The eruption consists of a centrifugal macular, maculopapular, scarlatiniform, or petechial eruption, characteristically starting from the dorsum of the

hands and feet and spreading to the arms, legs, and torso. The face is rarely involved. Lesions may become confluent, with small round islands of sparing, the "white islands in a sea of red" [23], and last 2 hours to several days. Laboratory tests usually reveal a characteristic thrombocytopenia and leukopenia with pathological values of transaminases.

Life-threatening complications that are becoming increasingly frequent are hemorrhagic fever and shock syndrome [24]. Hemorrhagic fever begins with a sudden elevation in temperature that persists for 2–7 days and is followed by bleeding from sites of trauma and from the gastrointestinal and urinary tracts. Abdominal pain, vomiting, febrile seizures (in children), and a decreased level of consciousness are also observed. The average case fatality rate is about 5%. Shock syndrome can occur after the hemorrhagic fever, with symptoms of circulatory and respiratory failure that may result in death in about 2% of cases.

The diagnosis can be confirmed by recovery of the virus in culture, serological assays, or PCR analysis. No specific therapy exists for dengue, but with intensive supportive care the mortality rate can be decreased.

CONCLUSION

Viral infections with cutaneous manifestations are mostly self-limiting. However, in some instances, irreversible damage or death may ensue. Immunosuppressed patients are at a greater risk of developing such complications. Such cases should be promptly diagnosed and treated.

KEY POINTS

- Some viral infections with predominant cutaneous features can manifest as emergencies.
- These become more pronounced in immunocompromised states.
- Disseminated herpes simplex and zoster infections, neonatal varicella and herpes require emergent treatment.
- Measles, rubella, hand foot, and mouth disease can all have rare complications which can present as emergencies.

REFERENCES

1. Wolf R, Davidovici BB, Parish JL, Parish LC. *Emergency Dermatology.* New York: Cambridge University Press; 2010.

2. Rebora A. Life-threatening cutaneous viral diseases. *ClinDermatol* 2005;23(2):157–63.

3. Kusuhara T, Nakajima M, Inoue H, Takahashi M, Yamada T. Parainfectious encephalomyeloradiculitis associated with herpes simplex virus 1 DNA in cerebrospinal fluid. *Clin Infect Dis* 2002;34(9):1199–205.

4. Marcus B, Lipozencic J, Matz H, Orion E, Wolf R. Herpes simplex: Autoinoculation versus dissemination. *Acta Dermatovenerol Croat* 2005;13(4):237–41.

5. Sanderson IR, Brueton LA, Savage MO, Harper JI. Eczema herpeticum: A potentially fatal disease. *Br Med J (Clin Res Ed)* 1987;294(6573):693–4.

6. Pastuszak AL et al. Outcome after maternal varicella infection in the first 20 weeks of pregnancy. *N Engl J Med* 1994;330:901–5.

7. Smith CK, Arvin AM. Varicella in the fetus and newborn. *Semin Fetal Neonatal Med* 2009;14(4):209–17.

8. Chapman SJ. Varicella in pregnancy. *Semin Perinatol* 1998;22(4):339–46.

9. Selleger C. Fatal varicella pneumonia in adults. Report of two cases and review of literature (author's transl). *Rev Fr Mal Respir* 1979;7(1):9–18.

10. Olasode OA, Olasode BJ. Haemorrhagic varicella: A malignant variant of chicken pox. *Cent Afr J Med* 1998;44:205–6.

11. Gnann Jr JW. Varicella-zoster virus: A typical presentations and unusual complications. *J Infect Dis* 2002;186(Suppl 1):S91–8.

12. Murakami S, Hato N, Horiuchi J, Honda N, Gyo K, Yanagihara N. Treatment of Ramsay Hunt syndrome with acyclovir-prednisone: Significance of early diagnosis and treatment. *Ann Neurol* 1997;41(3):353–7.

13. Liesegang TJ. Herpes zoster ophthalmicus natural history, risk factors, clinical presentation, and morbidity. *Ophthalmology* 2008;115(2 Suppl):S3–12.

14. Dworkin RH et al. Recommendations for the management of herpes zoster. *Clin Infect Dis* 2007;44(Suppl 1):S1–26.

15. Sanford M, Keating GM. Zoster vaccine (Zostavax): A review of its use in preventing herpes zoster and postherpetic neuralgia in older adults. *Drugs Aging* 2010;27(2):159–76.

16. Thomas B, Farquhar-Smith P. Extended-release gabapentin in post-herpetic neuralgia. *Expert Opin Pharmacother* 2011;12(16):2565–71.

17. Meyers JD. Prevention and treatment of cytomegalovirus infection. *Ann Rev Med* 1991;42:179–87.

18. Scott LA, Seabury Stone M. Viral exanthems. *Dermatol Online J* 2003;9:4.

19. Hussey GD, Klein M. A randomized, controlled trial of vitamin A in children with severe measles. *N Engl J Med* 1990;323(3):160–4.

20. Rosa C. Rubella and rubeola. *Semin Perinatol* 1998;22:318–22.

21. Balkhy HH, Sabella C, Goldfarb J. Parvovirus: A review. *Bull Rheum Dis* 1998;47(3):4–9.

22. Rotbart HA, Webster AD. Treatment of potentially life-threatening enterovirus infections with pleconaril. *Clin Infect Dis* 2001;32:228–35.

23. Radakovic-Fijan S et al. Dengue hemorrhagic fever in a British travel guide. *J Am Acad Dermatol* 2002;46:430–3.

24. Anderson RC et al. Punctate exanthema of West Nile virus infection: Report of 3 cases. *J Am Acad Dermatol* 2004;51:820–3.

29

Fungal infections causing emergencies

R. MADHU, PRADEESH ARUMUGAM, AND V. HARI PANKAJ

INTRODUCTION

Many systemic fungal infections can manifest as emergencies, and dermatological findings can help in early diagnosis of such cases. Clinical manifestations of such mycoses depend on the virulence of the pathogen, host response, transmission route, and geographic factors. We discuss a few systemic fungal infections that can present as emergencies.

EPIDEMIOLOGY

Incidence and prevalence

There are limited numbers of epidemiologic studies on systemic fungal infections worldwide. Risk factors for these mycoses are given in Table 29.1. Marcoux et al. reported that systemic mycoses frequently occurred within the first 2 months of diagnosis of the underlying diseases, such as hematological malignancies and solid organ transplantation [1]. Tessari et al. showed that the peak incidence of systemic fungal infection was in the first 2 years after transplantation [2].

Gender

In the pediatric age group, boys outnumbered girls, reflecting the higher male prevalence of systemic fungal infections among patients with acute lymphoblastic leukemia (ALL) (almost 50% of the primary underlying diagnoses). The mean age of 8 years was also influenced by the average age of ALL onset [1]. Among the patients affected with zygomycosis, males are affected more than females, probably due to the protective role of estrogen in females (as seen in paracoccidioidomycosis).

ETIOPATHOGENESIS

Endemic infections (pathogenic fungal infections): Fungi that can cause systemic infection in people with normal immune function as well as those who are immune compromised include *Histoplasma capsulatum*, *Coccidioides immitis*, *Blastomyces dermatitidis*, *Paracoccidioides brasiliensis*, and *Talaromyces marneffei*, earlier known as *Penicillium marneffei*. These fungi are found in soil and wood debris.

Opportunistic fungal infections: Fungi that only result in systemic infection in immunocompromised or sick people include *Candida* species, *Aspergillus* species, *Cryptococcus* spp, *Zygomycetes*, etc. These fungi are found in or on normal skin as commensals, decaying vegetable matter, and bird droppings, respectively, but not exclusively. They are present throughout the world.

Solid organ transplantation, AIDS, systemic lupus erythematosus, systemic corticosteroid use, diabetes mellitus, and leukopenia are well-known risk factors for systemic fungal infections [3]. Other predisposing factors include the use of chemotherapeutic agents, malignancies, extensive surgery, trauma, and the use of broad-spectrum antimicrobial therapy [4].

Yeast infections appear to be much more frequent than mold infections. *Candida* infections are the most common, followed by *Aspergillus*, *Alternaria*, *Fusarium*, and others. Although *Candida albicans* is still the most common cause of invasive candidiasis, nonalbicans *Candida* species account for a growing proportion of cases nowadays. Aspergillosis occurs more frequently in medical patients, whereas candidiasis is more in surgical patients [5]. Patients with defective barrier function are more frequently infected by *Candida* than by *Aspergillus* species. In contrast, patients with hematologic disorders are infected more frequently

Table 29.1 Risk factors for development of systemic mycoses in immunocompromised hosts

Broad-spectrum antibiotics	90%
Hematological abnormalities	70%
Neutropenia	50%
Loss of barrier function	20%
Contamination	12%

by molds than by candidal yeasts [1]. The two major fungal pathogens in immunocompetent intensive care unit (ICU) patients are *Candida* spp. and *Aspergillus* spp. [6,7].

Source of pathogens

Candida species are frequent commensals of the human gastrointestinal, respiratory, and reproductive tracts, and the skin [4]. *Candida* colonization, whether endogenous or environmentally acquired, is a prerequisite for invasive candidiasis. Filamentous fungi, including *Aspergillus* and the *Mucorales*, are ubiquitous in the environment and are frequently inhaled. When the natural environment of such pathogenic molds is disrupted, the level of airborne spores is increased, thereby placing patients at elevated risk of exposure, colonization, and possible infection. Risk factors for colonization with filamentous fungi are as given in Table 29.2.

Host-pathogen interaction

Innate immunity is the dominant protective mechanism against disseminated candidiasis, zygomycosis, and aspergillosis [10–12]. Patients with quantitative and qualitative abnormalities of neutrophils and monocytes are at increased risk for development of these infections. Elevated serum glucose and renal failure may lead to impaired neutrophil and monocyte adherence, chemotaxis, phagocytosis, pathogen killing, and respiratory burst and has been associated with development of these infections [13,14].

Table 29.2 Risk factors for mucormycosis

• Uncontrolled diabetes mellitus	• Prolonged use of corticosteroids
• Diabetic ketoacidosis	• Graft-versus-host disease
• Hematologic malignancies	• Voriconazole prophylaxis in high-risk patients
• Solid organ or bone marrow transplants	• Premature neonates
• Severe neutropenia	• IV drug abuse
• Iron overload	*Nosocomial mucormycosis:*
• Deferoxamine iron chelation therapy	Construction work/contaminated air filters/wound dressings/wooden splints/IV catheters/tongue depressors, nonsterile tapes
• Burns/other wounds	
• Trauma, major surgery	

Source: Reiss E et al. (Eds). In: *Fundamentals of Medical Mycology.* New York: Wiley-Blackwell; 2012:431–55; Petrikkos G et al. *Clin Infect Dis* 2012;54(S1):S23–34.

Sporangiospores of *Mucorales* gain entry into the host through inhalation, direct inoculation into the abraded skin, or ingestion. In case of intact immunity, the macrophages are able to prevent the germination of spores into hyphae, while in immunosuppressed patients, this action is defective. Defective host immunity creates a contusive atmosphere for the spores to grow into sparsely septate hyphae that invade the small and large arteries by virtue of their predilection for the elastic lamina of the vessels producing thrombosis, hemorrhage, infarction, and necrosis [8,15].

CLINICAL FEATURES

Diagnosis of systemic mycoses is often very challenging because of the highly polymorphic nature of the skin lesions [16]. The clinical features of the illness depend on the specific infection and which organs have been affected. Infections in people with normal immune function may result in very minor symptoms or none at all (called *subclinical infection*). Cutaneous lesions are rare in these infections and may occur due to direct inoculation on an abraded skin (Table 29.3).

The common systemic fungal infections are as follows.

Candidiasis

Invasive candidiasis (IC) is a spectrum of syndromes, including (a) bloodstream infection (BSI) or candidemia,

Table 29.3 Cutaneous manifestation of systemic mycoses

Mycoses	Skin manifestation
Candidiasis	Single lesions, disseminated
	Erythematous papules, nodules
	Purpuric lesions
Aspergillosis	Few lesions, widespread
	Erythematous patches with necrotic centers
	Ulcers similar to pyoderma gangrenosum
Zygomycosis	Plaques, pustules, nodules, abscess, ulcers
Cryptococcosis	Umbilicated papules
	Papules, plaques, blisters, nodules, ulcers, sinuses, abscess, cellulitis, purpura (variety of lesions)
	Usually first sign of infection
Histoplasmosis	Papules, blisters, nodules, ulcers, abscess, sinuses
	Erythema multiforme
	Erythema nodosum
	Oral ulcers
Penicilliosis	Umbilicated papules
	Ulcers
Blastomycosis	Warty lesions
	Papules, nodules, abscesses, sinuses
	Oral lesions

(b) deep-seated *Candida* infections in the presence of BSI, and (c) deep-seated infections without BSI. Each contributes to almost a third of intensive care unit invasive candidiasis. The main species of *Candida* that are found to cause IC are *Candida albicans, Candida glabrata, Candida parapsilosis, Candida krusei,* and *Candida tropicalis. Candida parapsilosis* has the tendency to cause device and central catheter infections. Bronchial *Candida* isolates are generally considered nonpathogenic and reflect colonization.

Risk factors that could predict IC infection include the following:

- Antibiotics use combined with
- Central venous catheter placement within the last 3 days, in addition to two of the following risk factors:
  - Surgery
  - Immunosuppression
  - Steroid use
  - Pancreatitis, within the last 7 days
  - Total parenteral nutrition and/or dialysis within last 3 days.

By implementing this rule, clinicians can safely rule out patients who are not at high risk of IC (negative predictive value of 97%) [7].

Deep *Candida* infections can present differently as follows:

Candidemia: Immunocompromised patients, after complicated abdominal surgery, after prolonged intensive care treatment, severe burn patients, pancreatitis, broad-spectrum antibiotic use, and central venous catheter use
Deep Candida *abscess*: After abdominal or esophageal surgery
Candida esophagitis or deep mouth infections: Cancer treatment, AIDS patients
Candida endophthalmitis: After candidemia, intravenous drug abuse
Candida endocarditis: IV drug abuse, valvular surgery
Candida osteomyelitis: After candidemia, operation, IV drug abuse

TYPE OF *CANDIDA* SKIN LESIONS

- Multiple, erythematous papules with central pale vesicular, pustular, or necrotic lesions [17]
- Purpuric (most common)
- Maculopapules, nodules, or plaques—from 2 mm to 10 cm
- Generalized rash

The management of IC is time sensitive, because delaying diagnosis and delay in initiation of right antifungal therapy carries a high mortality risk.

Aspergillosis

Invasive aspergillosis (IA) is recognized as one of the invasive fungal infections that can affect nonneutropenic critically ill patients. *Aspergillus fumigatus* is the main pathogen to consider, followed by *A. niger* and *A. flavus* [18].

Risk factors for ICU patients include chronic obstructive pulmonary disease, malnutrition, diabetes mellitus, liver cirrhosis, abdominal surgical intervention, and those on peritoneal dialysis. Nonneutropenic patients who develop invasive aspergillosis respond better to treatment than the others [6].

SKIN MANIFESTATIONS OF ASPERGILLOSIS

Primary cutaneous aspergillosis usually involves sites of skin injury, namely, at or near IV access catheter sites (adhesive tapes), at sites of traumatic inoculation, and at sites associated with occlusive dressings, burns, or surgery [19]. Secondary cutaneous lesions result either from contiguous extension to the skin from infected underlying structures such as the paranasal sinuses, nasal cavity, or orbit, or from widespread blood-borne seeding of the skin. They are classified as follows:

- *HIV-related cutaneous aspergillosis*: The use of adhesive tape dressings was the most consistent risk factor associated. The range of clinical findings of primary cutaneous aspergillosis includes nodules, molluscum-like papules, plaques, and ulcers.
- *Non-HIV-infected immunocompromised patients*: High-risk individuals include burn victims, neonates, cancer patients, after stem cell transplantation, and after solid organ transplantation.
- *Otherwise healthy individuals*: Following surgical wounds, traumatic inoculation, or by exposure to high spore counts such as farming.

A. fumigatus is the most common species in HIV patients, while in non-HIV, nonburn patients, *A. flavus* is the most common followed by *A. fumigatus* and other species.

Cutaneous aspergillosis is polymorphic—erythematous plaques often with pustules, hemorrhagic bulla, large papules, umbilicated papules, centrally necrotic ulcers, deep abscesses, nodules, or pseudoepithelial hyperplasia or vegetative papules, eventually evolving into an eschar [1,18,20–22].

Mucormycosis (zygomycoses)

Mucormycosis is a rapidly progressing angioinvasive opportunistic fungal infection in which hematogenous dissemination can occur in 70% of cases even after aggressive surgical and systemic antifungal treatment. Mucorales are present ubiquitously in the environment, dead and decaying organic matter. Most common etiological agents causing mucormycosis belong to *Rhizopus, Mucor,* and *Lichtheimia* genera (Table 29.4). Mortality can be as high as 31% in such cases [23].

Mucorales infect a broader and more heterogeneous population and are unique among the filamentous fungi because of their disproportionately high capacity to cause devastating disease in persons with no underlying condition. Various types of mucormycosis are mucocutaneous (Figure 29.1), rhino-orbitocerebral (Figures 29.2 and 29.3), and disseminated mucormycosis (pulmonary, cardiac,

Table 29.4 Etiological agents of mucormycosis

Mucorales

Rhizopus arrhizus (formerly R. oryzae)
R. microsporus
Mucor racemosus
Lichtheimia corymbifera (formerly Absidia corymbifera)
Rhizomucor pusillus
Apophysomyces elegans
Cunninghamella bertholletiae
Saksenaea spp.
Syncephalastrum racemosum

gastrointestinal tract, and bones). Primary mucormycosis occurs in patients with severe burns, superficial ulcers in diabetes, contaminated wound dressings, and post-traumatic gangrenous cellulitis. Mucorales have a predilection

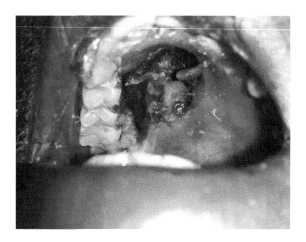

Figure 29.1 Mucormycosis—black eschar in the palate.

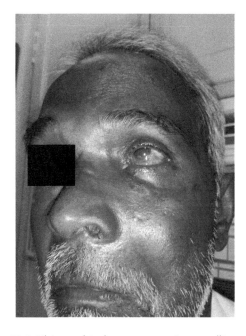

Figure 29.2 Rhino-orbital mucormycosis—swelling of the left cheek, discharge from left nostril, and chemosis of left eye seen.

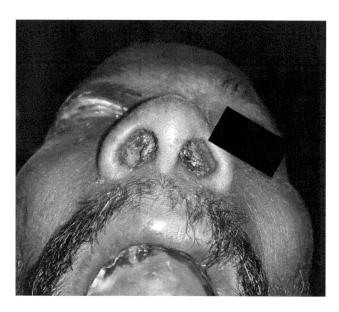

Figure 29.3 Rhino-orbito-cerebral mucormycosis—crusting in the right eye and both nostrils and eschar in the palate seen.

for angioinvasion and result in thrombus formation followed by ischemia and necrosis.

Cerebral infection through hematogenous spread is the most common presentation of zygomycosis. Symptoms range from unilateral headache, fever, numbness, nasal hypoesthesia, periorbital or retro-orbital pain, diplopia, blurred vision, amaurosis (unilateral or bilateral), rapid progression to blindness, swelling of the cheek, purulent discharge from the nostril, altered mental status, and convulsions.

Dermatological examination reveals the presence of crusted plaques, black eschars, or ulcers. Ocular signs are nystagmus, fixed pupil, orbital apex syndrome, or blindness. Visual loss may occur due to direct fungal invasion or retinal artery thrombosis. Neurological signs include cranial nerve palsies of second to seventh nerves. Cerebral edema and sometimes stroke may also occur.

Fusariosis

Fusariosis is the second most common mold infection in immunocompromised patients, next to aspergillosis [24,25]. The most common *Fusarium* sp. is *F. solani* followed by *F. oxysporum* and *F. moniliforme*. Skin involvement is common and usually precedes fungemia by about 5 days. In immunocompromised patients, skin lesions are disseminated in about 88% of fusariosis, while it is localized in 93% of immunocompetent patients.

TYPES OF SKIN LESIONS
- Disseminated papules and nodules
- Necrotic
- Ecthyma gangrenosum
- Surrounding erythema (target)
- Cellulitis

Fusarium species have a propensity for invading two sites (blood and skin) that can be easily sampled for diagnostic purposes.

Fungal infections in special situations: HIV

Invasive fungal infections in AIDS patients are mainly caused by conditional pathogenic fungi. *Candida* species is the most common followed by *Cryptococcus neoformans. Candida albicans* is the most common conditional pathogenic fungi isolated from AIDS patients [26]. Nonalbicans *Candida* species are of special concern, as some are highly virulent and are associated with treatment failure because of reduced susceptibility to antifungal agents. *Cryptococcus neoformans* is the most common cause of fungal meningitis worldwide and the fourth most common life-threatening opportunistic infection in individuals with AIDS. A timely lumbar puncture is recommended to determine whether cryptococcal meningitis exists when a patient with AIDS presents with symptoms and signs of meningitis or meningoencephalitis.

Oropharyngeal candidiasis is characterized by painless, creamy white, plaque-like lesions of the buccal or oropharyngeal mucosa, or tongue surface. Lesions can be easily scraped off with a tongue depressor or other instrument. Esophageal candidiasis is occasionally asymptomatic but often presents with fever, retrosternal burning pain or discomfort, and odynophagia. Candidal pneumonia presenting with fever, cough, chest pain, dyspnea, rales, or rhonchi and other signs of consolidation may occur.

Cryptococcosis: Cryptococcosis among patients with AIDS most commonly occurs as a subacute meningitis with fever, malaise, and headache. Classical meningitis symptoms and signs are neck stiffness or photophobia. Primary cutaneous cryptococcosis due to traumatic inoculation is rare. Lesions tend to be solitary and on the exposed sites. Secondary lesions are due to hematogenous dissemination and may range from molluscum contagiosum–like umbilicated papules, nodules, pustules, and plaques to abscess, ulcer, grouped vesicles, and cellulitis (Figure 29.4). Scalp, face, and neck are the most common sites to be involved. Differential diagnosis of molluscum contagiosum–like lesions includes histoid Hansen, penicilliosis, histoplasmosis, and other deep mycoses.

Penicilliosis: Penicilliosis, now known as talaromycosis, is an AIDS-defining illness. Persons with AIDS with CD4 <200/μL, solid organ transplant, hematological malignancy, and connective tissue diseases on immunosuppression are the high-risk groups.

The manifestations of penicilliosis marneffei include fever, lymphadenopathy, skin lesions, and weight loss. The skin lesions appear on the face, ears, trunk, and extremities. Lesions are polymorphic and occur as papules, nodules, or pustules. Some of the papules may have central umbilication resembling molluscum contagiosum.

Histoplasmosis: Pulmonary and CNS manifestations predominate. Cutaneous manifestations can be in the form of papules, plaques, nodules (even ulcerated), crusted lesions, and erythema multiforme-like lesions.

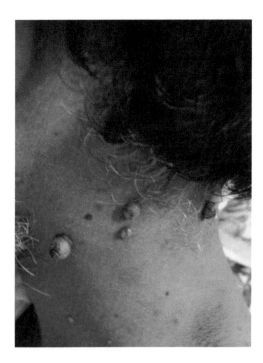

Figure 29.4 Cryptococcosis—molluscum contagiosum–like lesions seen on the left cheek.

INVESTIGATIONS

Direct microscopic examination of the specimens in 10% potassium hydroxide (KOH) wet mount is a very valuable tool that would aid an early diagnosis of systemic mycoses and prompt initiation of treatment which would significantly reduce the morbidity and mortality of these infections.

Mucorales appear as hyaline, coenocytic or sparsely septate, broad, ribbon-like hyphae with wide-angle or right-angle branching (Figure 29.5). In aspergillosis, hyphae are seen as thin, septate with acute-angle branching. In the case

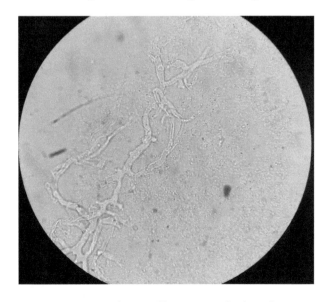

Figure 29.5 Mucorales—10% potassium hydroxide wet mount showing the hyaline, sparsely septate, broad ribbon-shaped hyphae with wide-angle branching.

of penicilliosis, intracellular or extracellular basophilic, spherical, or oval yeast-like organisms with a central septum can be seen in Wright/Giemsa stain. Cryptococci are seen as budding yeast cells with the refractile capsule seen as a distinct clear halo in Indian ink preparation. *Candida* appear as budding yeast cells and pseudo-hyphae in 10% KOH/Gram or Wright stains. Calcofluor examination has the advantage of rapid diagnosis but is available only in tertiary centers.

On histopathology, in neutropenic patients the inflammatory response can be minimal, and careful search of fungal elements has to be carried out. Angioinvasion with subsequent tissue infarction and necrosis can be evident. Mucorales and aspergillus can be identified by the characteristic features. In cryptococcosis, histopathology depends on the fungal load in the host. Periodic acid-Schiff and Grocott methenamine silver stains are special fungal stains that help to confirm the diagnosis when there is a diagnostic dilemma with hematoxylin and eosin section.

Fungal culture results can be obtained 1 week after seeding in the case of molds, although cultures are kept for a total of 28 days before reporting the culture findings as negative (Figures 29.6 through 29.8). *Candida* exhibits rapid growth, usually within 48–72 hours (Figure 29.9).

ß-D-Glucan is an important component of the fungal cell wall that has been targeted for detection of invasive fungal infections (IFIs). It has a high sensitivity and low specificity. It is also helpful in assessing the patient's response to therapy [27,28]. In disseminated fusariosis, blood culture is positive in greater than 50%.

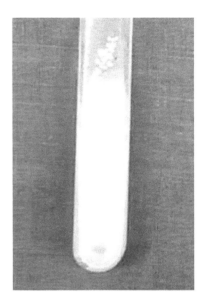

Figure 29.7 Culture of mucormycosis.

TREATMENT

Antifungal therapeutic strategies include prophylaxis of high-risk patients and preemptive, empirical, and targeted therapies. The armamentarium of currently available agents includes fluconazole, the echinocandins (caspofungin, micafungin, and anidulafungin), voriconazole, deoxycholate amphotericin B (AmB) and its lipid formulations, AmB lipid complex (ABLC), and liposomal AmB (L-AmB). Other agents including

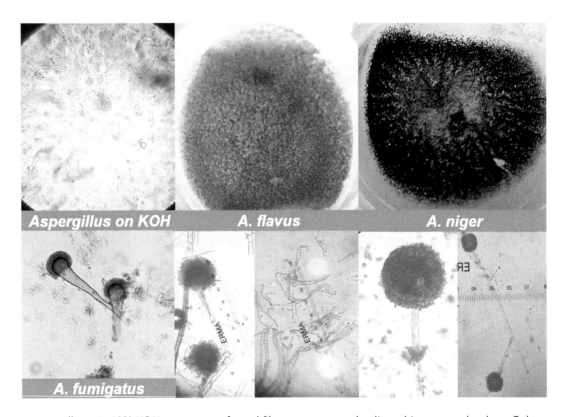

Figure 29.6 Aspergillus—in 10% KOH wet mount, fungal filaments seen as hyaline, thin septate hyphae. Culture and lactophenol cotton blue mount of *Aspergillus fumigatus*, *A. flavus*, and *A. niger* seen.

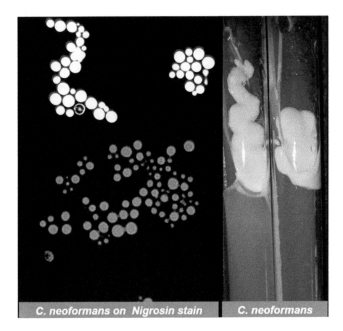

Figure 29.8 Cryptococcosis—yeast cells with refractile capsules in nigrosin stain and the culture in Sabouraud's dextrose agar (SDA).

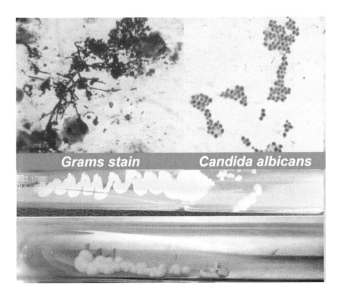

Figure 29.9 *Candida*—budding yeast cells and pseudo-hyphae seen in Gram stain and the yeasty colony of *Candida* species.

itraconazole, posaconazole, AmB colloidal dispersion (ABCD), and 5-fluorocytosine have limited use in the ICU and are generally not used as first-line therapy in this setting [4].

Invasive candidiasis: The recommended drug of choice in almost all invasive candidiasis cases is an echinocandin. The therapy has to be continued for at least 2 weeks from the first negative blood cultures. Therapy is usually extended to 4–6 weeks when dissemination and end-organ infection have occurred [29].

Aspergillosis: There are no current recommendations for invasive aspergillosis prophylaxis in nonneutropenic ICU patients. Itraconazole has activity against *Aspergillus* spp.; however, its limited oral bioavailability in ICU patients limits its usefulness in that population. Voriconazole, currently the gold standard, has been shown to be more efficacious than amphotericin B deoxycholate. Amphotericin B is active against all *Aspergillus* species except *Aspergillus terreus*. It is currently not recommended to use caspofungin monotherapy for treatment of invasive aspergillosis unless there are contraindications to the use of other agents.

Mucormycosis: Liposomal amphotericin B is the cornerstone for treatment of mucormycosis. Posaconazole is an emerging therapeutic option for mucormycosis, especially in patients with renal failure in whom amphotericin B cannot be used. Isavuconazole, a newer triazole antifungal agent, has been approved by the U.S. Food and Drug Administration for the treatment of invasive mucormycosis and aspergillosis [30].

Fusariosis: Given the poor outcome of fusariosis in hematopoietic stem cell transplantation (HSCT) recipients and the relative resistance of these fungi to antifungal agents, preventive nonchemotherapeutic measures are of paramount importance. Such measures include a thorough evaluation and treatment of skin lesions and tissue breakdown (particularly onychomycoses that serve as a portal of entry for *Fusarium* species) before and after receipt of HSCTs and adequate air and water infection control practices to avoid environmental exposure to this fungus [24,31].

Systemic mycoses in HIV/AIDS: Amphotericin B, fluconazole, and itraconazole are cornerstones of treatment in these cases. Amphotericin B is a polyene with a very broad spectrum of activity, but side effects are common, occurring in 50%–90% of cases, and hence it may not be appropriate for patients with marginal renal function or those at high risk for hepatotoxicity, in whom the use of lipid-associated products has been employed to overcome side effects, but the use of lipid-associated formulations is often restricted because of the high cost. Fluconazole is available in oral or IV formulations and is well tolerated, with fewer drug interactions than other azoles. It is inactive against filamentous fungi. Itraconazole has a wider spectrum than fluconazole. It is active against yeasts and molds, with the exception of *Fusarium* spp., *Scedosporium* spp., and the Mucorales. Use of fluconazole for prophylaxis has led to increased fungal resistance and to the emergence of intrinsically resistant or less-susceptible *Candida* species such as *C. krusei* and *C. glabrata*.

Immune reconstitution through HAART is the most important measure for preventing IFIs in patients with AIDS. Table 29.5 describes antifungals and their specific roles in management.

PROGNOSIS

Prognosis is poor in immunocompromised patients. Mortality from HIV-associated cryptococcal meningitis remains high (10%–30%), even in developed countries, because of the inadequacy of current antifungal drugs and combinations and the complication of raised intracranial

Table 29.5 Antifungal treatment in fungal infections

Antifungal	Acts against these fungal species
Fluconazole	Invasive candidiasis
	Cryptococcosis maintenance therapy
Voriconazole	Invasive candidiasis
	Aspergillosis
	Rare filamentous fungi
Amphotericin B	Invasive candidiasis
	Cryptococcosis
	Histoplasmosis
	Zygomycosis
	Empirical antifungal therapy
Echinocandins	Invasive candidiasis
	Aspergillus
	Empirical therapy
Others	Posaconazole, flucytosine

pressure [10–12]. A study conducted by Ecevit et al. [13] shows that increased recognition and timely diagnosis of cryptococcal meningitis may improve outcomes. Mucormycosis has been reported to have an overall mortality rate of 44%.

CONCLUSION

In view of the rising trend of invasive fungal infections in this era of increased immunosuppressive states, it becomes imperative for the dermatologists to be well versed with the cutaneous manifestations of these infections as they would give a quick clue to the underlying systemic, life-threatening infections for which treatment has to be started on an emergency note, so that the serious morbidity can be reduced and mortality prevented. Cutaneous lesions of systemic mycoses have a varied presentation; hence, a high degree of clinical suspicion is essential and a multidisciplinary approach is mandatory to treat patients with invasive fungal infections.

KEY POINTS

- Systemic fungal infections can commonly present as emergencies.
- They more commonly manifest in immunocompromised states.
- Systemic fungal infections can have early cutaneous features and they can be markers for early diagnosis and treatment.
- Candidiasis, Aspergillosis, Penicilliosis, Histoplasmosis, and Cryptococcosis are among the commonest systemic fungal infections.
- Amphotericin B, Voriconazole, Posaconazole, Itraconazole, and Echinocandins are the effective antifungals.

REFERENCES

1. Marcoux D, Jafarian F, Joncas V, Buteau C, Kokta V, Moghrabi A. Deep cutaneous fungal infections in immunocompromised children. *J Am Acad Dermatol* 2009;61:857–64.
2. Tessari G et al. Incidence and clinical predictors of primary opportunistic deep cutaneous mycoses in solid organ transplant recipients: A multicenter cohort study: Primary opportunistic deep cutaneous mycoses in solid organ transplant recipients. *Clin Transplant* 2009;24:328–33.
3. Tsai W-C et al. Cutaneous manifestations of subcutaneous and systemic fungal infections in tropical regions: A retrospective study from a referral center in southern Taiwan. *Int J Dermatol* 2017;56:623–9.
4. Shoham S, Marwaha S. Invasive fungal infections in the ICU. *J Intensive Care Med* 2010;25:78–92.
5. Tortorano AM et al. Invasive fungal infections in the intensive care unit: A multicentre, prospective, observational study in Italy (2006–2008): Fungal infections in intensive care unit. *Mycoses* 2012;55:73–9.
6. Denning DW, Stevens DA. Antifungal and surgical treatment of invasive aspergillosis: Review of 2,121 published cases. *Rev Infect Dis* 1990;12:1147–201.
7. Ostrosky-Zeichner L, Al-Obaidi M. Invasive fungal infections in the intensive care unit. *Infect Dis Clin North Am* 2017;31:475–87.
8. Reiss E, Shadomy JH, Lyon GM (Eds). Mucormycosis. In: *Fundamentals of Medical Mycology*. New York: Wiley-Blackwell; 2012:431–55.
9. Petrikkos G, Skiada A, Lortholary O, Roilides E, Walsh TJ, Kontoyiannis DP. Epidemiology and clinical manifestations of mucormycosis. *Clin Infect Dis* 2012;54(S1):S23–34.
10. Koh AY, Köhler JR, Coggshall KT, Van Rooijen N, Pier GB. Mucosal damage and neutropenia are required for *Candida albicans* dissemination. *PLOS Pathog [Internet]*. 2008 [cited 2018 August 27];4(2). Available from: https://www.ncbi.nlm.nih.gov/pmc/articles/PMC2242836
11. Pappo I, Polacheck I, Zmora O, Feigin E, Freund HR. Altered gut barrier function to *Candida* during parenteral nutrition. *Nutr Burbank Los Angel Cty Calif* 1994;10:151–4.
12. Shoham S, Levitz SM. The immune response to fungal infections. *Br J Haematol* 2005;129:569–82.
13. Shoham S, Han G, Granek T, Walsh T, Magee MF. Association between blood glucose levels and development of candidemia in hospitalized patients. *Endocr Pract* 2009;15:111–5.
14. Gibbons RA, Martinez OM, Garovoy MR. Altered monocyte function in uremia. *Clin Immunol Immunopathol* 1990;56:66–80.
15. Ibrahim AS, Edwards Jr JE, Filler SG. Zygomycoses. In: Dismukes WE, Pappas PG, Sobel JD (Eds), *Clinical*

Mycology. New York: Oxford University Press; 2003:241–51.

16. Kim MS et al. Clinical analysis of deep cutaneous mycoses: A 12-year experience at a single institution: Deep cutaneous mycoses in Korea. *Mycoses* 2012;55:501–6.

17. Bae GY et al. Clinicopathologic review of 19 patients with systemic candidiasis with skin lesions. *Int J Dermatol* 2005;44:550–5.

18. Taccone F et al. Epidemiology of invasive aspergillosis in critically ill patients: Clinical presentation, underlying conditions, and outcomes. *Crit Care* 2015;19:7.

19. van Burik J-AH, Colven R, Spach DH. Cutaneous aspergillosis. *J Clin Microbiol* 1998;36:3115–21.

20. Wald A, Leisenring W, van Burik JA, Bowden RA. Epidemiology of *Aspergillus* infections in a large cohort of patients undergoing bone marrow transplantation. *J Infect Dis* 1997;175:1459–66.

21. Martino R et al. Invasive fungal infections after allogeneic peripheral blood stem cell transplantation: Incidence and risk factors in 395 patients. *Br J Haematol* 2002;116:475–82.

22. Grow W et al. Late onset of invasive *Aspergillus* infection in bone marrow transplant patients at a university hospital. *Bone Marrow Transplant* 2002;29:15–9.

23. Roden MM et al. Epidemiology and outcome of Zygomycosis: A review of 929 reported cases. *Clin Infect Dis* 2005;41:634–53.

24. Nucci M, Anaissie E. Cutaneous infection by *Fusarium* species in healthy and immunocompromised hosts: Implications for diagnosis and management. *Clin Infect Dis* 2002;35:909–20.

25. Dignani MC, Anaissie E. Human fusariosis. *Clin Microbiol Infect* 2004;10:67–75.

26. Enoch DA. Invasive fungal infections: A review of epidemiology and management options. *J Med Microbiol* 2006;55:809–18.

27. Jaijakul S, Vazquez JA, Swanson RN, Ostrosky-Zeichner L. (1,3)-β-D-Glucan as a prognostic marker of treatment response in invasive candidiasis. *Clin Infect Dis* 2012;55:521–6.

28. Pickering JW, Sant HW, Bowles CAP, Roberts WL, Woods GL. Evaluation of a (1->3)-β-D-Glucan assay for diagnosis of invasive fungal infections. *J Clin Microbiol* 2005;43:5957–62.

29. Pappas PG et al. Clinical practice guideline for the management of candidiasis: 2016 update by the infectious diseases Society of America. *Clin Infect Dis Off Publ Infect Dis Soc Am* 2016;62:e1–50.

30. Donnelley MA, Zhu ES, Thompson GR3rd. Isavuconazole in the treatment of invasive aspergillosis and mucormycosis infections. *Infect Drug Resist* 2016;9:79–86.

31. Anaissie EJ. Pathogenic molds (including *Aspergillus* species) in hospital water distribution systems: A 3-year prospective study and clinical implications for patients with hematologic malignancies. *Blood* 2003;101:2542–6.

30

Dermatological emergencies in tropical infections and infestations

ANUP KUMAR TIWARY, NIHARIKA RANJAN LAL, AND PIYUSH KUMAR

INTRODUCTION

Tropical diseases are not limited to tropical regions alone in the present world due to increased travel opportunities and also due to environmental changes. Of note, some of these are life threatening and/or chronically debilitating and deserve prompt diagnosis and treatment to minimize the morbidity and mortality associated with such diseases. In this chapter, we discuss briefly the epidemiological and clinical aspects of tropical infections and infestations along with their appropriate management to guide physicians around the world.

BACTERIAL INFECTIONS

Chromobacterium violaceum

Chromobacterium violaceum is a gram-negative bacillus present in tropical and subtropical soil and stagnant water [1]. The infection mostly occurs in the summer months and can be rapidly fatal [2]. In most of the cases, the predominant portal of entry appears to be broken skin exposed to the organism through contaminated soil and water [3]. The infection begins with localized cellulitis at the site of trauma [4]. The clinical spectrum of *C. violaceum* infection is protean, including urinary tract infection, pneumonia, gastrointestinal infection, localized or metastatic abscesses, osteomyelitis, meningitis, peritonitis, brain abscess, endocarditis, hemophagocytic syndrome, respiratory distress syndrome, and fulminant sepsis [5].

Skin lesions may consist of diffuse pustular dermatitis [3], multiple nodules, hemorrhagic and pustular blebs with surrounding erythema, abscesses, cellulitis, and purpura scattered over the face, body, and extremities. Ecthyma gangrenosum also has been reported [2]. Metastatic abscesses could be the early clinical presentation of *C. violaceum* infection [1]. Rapid progression to life-threatening sepsis associated with metastatic abscess in *C. violaceum* infection is the most striking feature [5]. The infection has been reported to have a case fatality rate exceeding 50% and is typically observed in infants and children, sometimes with underlying conditions such as chronic granulomatous disease or glucose-6-phosphate dehydrogenase deficiency [1].

Diagnosis requires a high index of suspicion and is made on the basis of isolation of the organism from wounds and blood cultures [4]. Leukocytosis with left shift may be the only laboratory abnormality. Liver enzymes, platelet counts, and sedimentation rates may or may not be abnormal early in the course of infection [2].

Ciprofloxacin is the most effective antimicrobial *in vitro*, although other fluoroquinolones such as norfloxacin and pefloxacin are also very effective. The organism is also susceptible to imipenem, piperacillin, and mezlocillin [4]. In the absence of treatment, the prognosis is grave.

Vibrio vulnificus and parahaemolyticus

Vibrio vulnificus is a naturally occurring, gram-negative, halophilic bacterium of the noncholera group and free-living inhabitant of estuaries and marine environments throughout the world [6].

Hemorrhagic bullae at the site of inoculation comprise the most common feature of *V. vulnificus* wound infection. Metastatic spread of bacteria may occur and involve other parts of the skin [7]. Thirty-five percent of patients with wounds may become bacteremic, and 25% of cases with secondary bacteremia may be fatal [8]. Fatality is usually due to multiple-organ failure, acute respiratory distress syndrome (ARDS), or overwhelming sepsis [6].

Wound infections due to *V. parahaemolyticus* are usually minor infections. Though necrotizing soft-tissue infections are unusual, they can be life threatening, with rapid invasion and destruction of fascial planes and release of several cytotoxins [8,9].

Soft tissue infection by *V. vulnificus* represents a true surgical emergency. Early recognition and prompt aggressive débridement of all necrotic tissue are critical for survival. The combination of cefotaxime and minocycline is effective. More recently, fluoroquinolones have been demonstrated to be equally effective. The combination of quinolone plus cefotaxime has shown superior *in vitro* efficacy than either drug alone or the combination of minocycline plus cefotaxime [6].

Anthrax

Anthrax is a life-threatening zoonotic disease caused by the spore-forming bacterium *Bacillus anthracis* [10]. Infection occurs after cutaneous inoculation or inhalation of spores or after ingestion of infected material [11]. The most common type of human anthrax infection is cutaneous anthrax, which accounts for nearly 95% of all anthrax cases worldwide. Cutaneous anthrax occurs when either the spores or the bacteria itself enter the body through a cut or abrasion [11].

The primary lesion of cutaneous anthrax is a painless papule that usually develops approximately 7 days after inoculation of infected material. It most commonly occurs on the head, neck, or arms and develops central vesicle or bulla that becomes hemorrhagic as the lesion enlarges. The classic black central eschar is often surrounded by erythema and sometimes extreme edema. Localized lymphangitis and painful lymphadenopathy may occur [12].

Cutaneous anthrax can be self-limiting, and lesions resolve without complications or scarring in 80%–90% of cases with treatment. Extensive edema and toxemic shock due to massive edema, sepsis, meningitis, temporal artery inflammation, deep tissue necrosis, and secondary infection can be seen as rare and potentially life-threatening complications of cutaneous anthrax [13]. Cutaneous anthrax developing into renal failure requiring hemodialysis has also been reported [12].

Diagnosis is achieved by good history taking (occupation, exposure to animal), detecting the agent in Gram staining of the vesicle fluid, and/or detecting the growth of the microorganism in the culture. Penicillin G has been the drug of choice, while ciprofloxacin and doxycycline can be used as alternative treatments [10].

The prognosis of anthrax depends on the type of exposure. Many sources quote a mortality rate of up to 20% in untreated cutaneous anthrax usually due to septicemia and shock [11].

Plague

Plague, also known as Black Death, is caused by a bacterium named *Yersinia pestis* (*Pasteurella pestis*) [14]. These bacteria live in the bodies of rats and other rodents, causing among them highly lethal epidemics. When the infected *Xenopsylla cheopi* (rat flea) leaves the dead body of its rodent host, it goes on to bite any other suitable host, including humans.

The principal forms of plague are bubonic, septicemic, and pneumonic [15]. Bubonic plague occurs after inoculation of bacteria into skin or subcutaneous tissue of the host via the bite of a flea, usually after 2–8 days following inoculation [16]. Lymph nodes become inflamed and enlarged, and infection spreads via lymphatic channels, thoracic duct, and bloodstream, resulting in septicemia. Septicemia is almost always a lethal complication [16]. Other cutaneous features reported are purpuric lesions, erythema multiforme, petechiae, and diffuse erythematous pruritic papules [16].

Pneumonic plague is transmitted via aerosols. This is usually fatal without prompt treatment; bubonic plague has a mortality rate of 50%–60% if left untreated [15].

Drugs effective against plague include streptomycin and the tetracyclines [15]. Supportive therapy consists of volume resuscitation and management of sepsis syndrome [16].

Meningococcemia

Meningococcal disease is caused by a gram-negative diplococcus bacteria, *Neisseria meningitidis*, which is transmitted via droplets from patients or healthy carriers [17]. It may present with flu-like symptoms, purpuric rashes, septic fulminant meningitis, and multiorgan failure. The mortality rate is up to 90% if left untreated. Seasonal attacks in endemic areas are common in winter, mainly in children younger than 10 years [18]. Epidemic outbreaks depend on overcrowding, chronic nasopharyngeal carriage, smoking, preceding respiratory tract infection, virulent strains, and certain host factors (C_{5-9} complement deficiency, asplenia, immunosuppression) [19]. In the prodromal stage, the patient presents with self-limiting flu-like symptoms. With increasing bacterial load, endotoxemia ensues leading to hypotension and life-threatening acute adrenal hemorrhage (Waterhouse-Friderichsen syndrome) [20]. Maculopapular rashes and petechiae are the most common cutaneous lesions. Vesicles, purpura, ecchymosis, or gangrenous areas may also develop, known as purpura fulminans. After meningeal invasion, the patient presents with headache, projectile vomiting, photophobia, and mental obtundation along with meningeal signs. Seizures, cranial nerve palsies, and coma are other serious consequences [21]. Chronic meningococcemia may evolve into serious complications such as pneumonia, endocarditis, pericarditis, and cardiac tamponade.

Gram staining and culture for detection and isolation of organisms from blood, cerebrospinal fluid (CSF), skin, and synovial fluids should be done to confirm the diagnosis. Blood and CSF culture are highly sensitive in patients with meningococcemia, with or without meningitis. Latex agglutination, enzyme-linked immunosorbent assay (ELISA), and polymerase chain reaction (PCR) are alternative diagnostic methods for rapid identification [21].

Early institution of treatment is warranted to prevent complications. The drug of choice is penicillin G (4 million units IV/IM 4 hourly for 5–15 days). In case of resistance or allergy to penicillin, chloramphenicol or third-generation cephalosporins can also be given parenterally. Of note, rifampicin, azithromycin, and fluoroquinolones are tried to eradicate the nasal carriage in patients and healthy carriers [22].

Rhinoscleroma

Rhinoscleroma is a chronic granulomatous, slowly progressive but fatal disease caused by a gram-negative coccobacillus, Klebsiella rhinoscleromatis (Frisch bacillus). It is endemic in Central Europe, Africa, and Central and South America, but sporadic cases are seen all over the world [23]. Transmission is facilitated by direct or indirect contact with nasal exudates of an infected person [24]. It primarily affects the nose with a marked tendency to infiltrate the palate, pharynx, paranasal sinuses, orbit, larynx, and trachea, which may eventually result in their cicatricial obstruction and deformities [25].

In rhinoscleroma, granulomatous lesions start healing with dense fibrosis leading to stenosis and/or deformity of the involved structures such as Hebra nose (due to nasal cartilage destruction). Laryngotracheal stenosis may be life threatening, necessitating emergency tracheostomy.

Diagnosis is usually made by the clinical features and characteristic histopathological findings (on Giemsa or Warthin-Starry stain) of granulomatous infiltrate chiefly consisting of Mikulicz cells (large vacuolated foamy histiocyte) and plasma cells containing Russell bodies (eosinophilic aggregates of immunoglobulins within plasma cells) [26]. In doubtful cases, diagnosis can be confirmed by immunohistochemistry using a unique antigenic marker 02K3 [25].

The causative bacteria are usually sensitive to tetracycline, ciprofloxacin, co-trimoxazole, rifampicin, and aminoglycosides. Surgical, endoscopic, and laser treatments (carbon dioxide laser) can be done to correct the obstructive complications [25].

Nocardiosis

Nocardiosis is a suppurative infectious disease caused by aerobic, gram-positive, weakly acid-fast, branching, filamentous, opportunistic bacteria of genus Nocardia [27]. The lung is the most common primarily involved organ in immunocompromised patients usually presenting as pneumonia. Occasionally, it may disseminate hematogenously to other sites such as skin, eyes, and central nervous system (CNS), causing serious morbidity and mortality. Primary cutaneous involvement occurs rarely due to direct traumatic inoculation in immunocompetent individuals [28]. Pulmonary or disseminated forms, being more prevalent in developed countries, are commonly caused by Nocardia asteroides [29]. Primary cutaneous nocardiosis has three clinical forms: superficial infection such as cellulitis and abscess; lymphocutaneous or sporotrichoid spread of ulcerated papulonodular lesions on extremities with regional lymphadenopathy; and actinomycetoma with subcutaneous and deeper involvement. Pulmonary nocardiosis manifests as acute or chronic pneumonitis, abscess, pleural effusion, cavitation, or empyema [30]. The clinical presentation of disseminated cases depends on the organ involved such as meningitis, keratitis, endophthalmitis, and multiple noduloulcerative lesions [31].

Diagnosis can be made by seeing the characteristic morphology of nocardia and sulfur granules on direct microscopic examination of Gram, Grocott-silver, or acid-fast stained pus or sputum smears, but histopathological examination and culture are definitive [32]. Western blot assay, ELISA, and PCR are rapid diagnostic techniques. Plain chest radiography, computed tomography (CT) scanning, and magnetic resonance imaging (MRI) can also be done to look for pulmonary and brain involvement.

Cotrimoxazole is the most commonly employed drug in nocardiosis. Alternative drugs include potassium iodide (for lymphocutaneous form), dapsone, minocycline, amoxicillin clavulanate, ceftriaxone, erythromycin, linezolid, and amikacin. Surgical drainage and débridement are required for abscesses and necrotic areas.

Noma neonatorum

Noma neonatorum is a gangrenous and lethal infectious disease of neonates, caused by Pseudomonas aeruginosa [33]. The most commonly involved sites are mucocutaneous junctions of oral cavity, lips, nose, and perianal area, but scrotum and eyelids may also get affected. Without early diagnosis and proper treatment, it frequently leads to severe mutilating deformities and septicemia followed by death [34]. Onset of the disease has been reported up to 120 days of life, but most of the cases occur in the first 2 weeks of life starting after the third postnatal day [35]. It usually presents with erythematous induration of the oral cavity, lips, and nose [36]. In the presence of prematurity and very poor general health condition of the baby, it can be more fatal involving other distant sites, too. Of note, in the very short period of 2–3 days, mucocutaneous lesions turn into a gangrenous ulcer with blackish necrotic slough [37]. Systemic findings indicating septicemia are also associated, such as fever, hypotension, tachypnea, sclerema, hepatosplenomegaly, and respiratory insufficiency. Unfortunately, lack of early management of such cases ultimately results in severe tissue and bone loss with functional deformities leading to death.

Diagnosis should be confirmed in all of the clinically suspected cases by culture of blood, ulcerated tissues, CSF, or rectal swab along with antibiotic sensitivity so as to start the suitable drugs as early as possible.

Noma neonatorum should be treated aggressively with antipseudomonal antibiotics such as ceftazidime, ceftriaxone, piperacillin-tazobactam, gentamycin, and amikacin. Nutritional support, local wound care, and regular débridement (not too much) of devitalized tissue are equally important. Reconstructive surgery can be done 1 year after complete healing of the lesions [38].

Mycobacterium marinum

Mycobacterium marinum is a nontubercular photochromogenic mycobacterium and causes disease in many fish species and in humans handling fish or contaminated water. The infections in humans are usually limited to skin and soft tissues of a limb but may become invasive [39]. Disseminated infections involving internal organs are known to occur in immunocompromised persons and may be fatal, if untreated [40].

Exposure to virtually any type of aquatic environment, including fresh, salt, and brackish water, can lead to infection. The skin disease presents as ulcers, papules, pustules, nodules, warty lesions, abscesses, and cellulitis. Skin infection may spread via lymphatics, and nodular or ulcerating lesions may develop along the lymphatics, resulting in sporotrichoid forms.

Skin disease is usually limited to trauma-prone sites of one extremity, the upper extremity being affected more frequently than the lower. Dissemination may occur via blood, and patients develop nodules anywhere on body and manifestations secondary to bone and joints (tenosynovitis, septic arthritis, and osteomyelitis), bone marrow, and lung (and other visceral) involvement [41].

The optimal therapy for *M. marinum* infection has not yet been established. Localized disease may be treated with one antibiotic regimen, using minocycline or clarithromycin. Invasive and disseminated disease requires treatment with two antibiotic combinations. The most frequently used regimens are rifampicin and clarithromycin, rifampicin and ethambutol, doxycycline/minocycline and clarithromycin, and doxycycline/minocycline and rifampicin. Excision or surgical débridement is occasionally needed [42].

Bacillary angiomatosis

Bacillary angiomatosis is characterized by proliferative vascular lesions, is caused by *Bartonella henselae* and *B. quintana*, and is common in immunocompromised individuals. Domestic cat (*Felis domesticus*) and human body louse (*Pediculus humanus*) are the transmission vectors for *B. henselae* and *B. quintana*, respectively. Internal organ involvement may result in biliary obstruction and jaundice, gastrointestinal bleeding, encephalopathy, laryngeal obstruction, and asphyxiation. The illness responds well to antibiotic therapy but runs a chronic progressive course in untreated patients and may be fatal [43].

Flesh-colored papules, nodules, pedunculated lesions, and hyperkeratotic, indurated plaques are the usual cutaneous presentations and are usually multiple in number. The lesions may develop ulceration, discharge, crusting, and secondary infection.

Biopsy specimens of skin or mucosal lesions are diagnostic. Warthin-Starry silver or Grocott-silver methenamine stain is used to highlight bacteria. Blood culture, indirect immunofluorescent antibody studies, enzyme immunoassays, and PCR are other diagnostic methods. CT scan and MRI are done to identify internal organ involvement [44,45].

Erythromycin and tetracycline are the preferred antibiotics for treatment of bacillary angiomatosis. Usually, skin lesions are treated for a duration of 8–12 weeks. Osseous and liver lesions require at least 3 months of treatment. Recurrences are common in patients with HIV infection, and such patients may require lifelong therapy [46–48].

PARASITIC AND PROTOZOAL INFESTATIONS

Acanthamoeba

Several species cause severe human disease and include *Acanthamoeba* species, *Naegleria fowleri*, and *Balamuthia mandrillaris* [49]. Individuals prone to infection with *Acanthamoeba* are usually chronically ill, debilitated, diabetic, alcoholic, or immunosuppressed in some other way [50]. Cutaneous involvement can occur as primary cutaneous acanthamoebiasis and cutaneous involvement after dissemination [51].

The primary cutaneous lesions in patients with acanthamebiasis are polymorphic and are commonly described as intradermal or subcutaneous nodules that are erythematous or violaceous. Lesions can be pruritic, tender, or nontender, and they typically evolve through a course of enlargement, suppuration, and ulceration. A necrotic eschar may develop and then slough, thereby deepening the ulcer.

The diagnosis of *Acanthamoeba* infection requires visualization of amebic trophozoites and/or cysts, which may be found perivascularly [51]. Definitive identification to genus and species level can be obtained by immunofluorescence, culture method, or both. The prognosis of cutaneous acanthamebiasis is dismal, with a mortality rate of at least 74% in patients without CNS involvement and 100% in patients with CNS involvement. Patients with presumed or confirmed CNS involvement developed headaches, fever, altered mental status, hemiparesis, lethargy, spasticity, and seizures. Treatment for acanthamebiasis *in vivo* has not been available, although ketoconazole, flucytosine, pentamidine, sulfadiazine, and polymyxin B were known to be effective *in vitro* [50].

Schistosomiasis

Schistosomiasis (bilharziasis) is a serious systemic parasitic infestation by trematodes of the genus *Schistosoma* (blood flukes) [52]. The three species responsible are *Schistosoma mansoni*, *S. haematobium*, and *S. japonicum* [53]. During exposure to contaminated lakes/rivers in an endemic area, free-swimming cercariae penetrate the human skin and reach the venous circulation within 24 hours and via the portal system are carried to the veins around the rectum, colon (*S. mansoni* and *S. japonicum*), and pelvic and vesical veins (*S. haematobium*) where they lay eggs [54].

Cutaneous manifestations are common in schistosomiasis. Initially, it occurs during the penetration phase presenting as pruritic erythematous maculopapular eruptions (acute cercarial dermatitis) which last for hours to 1 week. After 4–8 weeks, ova-induced immune-complex-mediated urticarial eruptions associated with fever and gastrointestinal upset are seen, known as Katayama fever. Sometimes, ova embolize via the paravertebral venous plexus and get deposited in ectopic sites such as dermis, known as bilharziasis cutanea tarda [54]. Systemic complications arise once the ova initiate granulomatous inflammation in the tissues around veins. *S. mansoni* and *S. japonicum* form granuloma in the liver and large intestine causing hepatosplenomegaly, portal hypertension, esophageal varices, portal fibrosis (Symmers pipe stem fibrosis), hepatic failure, appendicitis, colitis, colonic polyps, and rectal prolapse. *S haematobium* affects the bladder leading to hematuria, hydronephrosis, and even carcinoma of bladder.

Eosinophilia supports the clinically suspected cases, but definitive diagnosis depends on the identification of eggs in stool or urine, biopsy (skin, rectal, or bladder), and serology. Abdominal ultrasonography, endoscopy, and barium enema play an integral role in hepatic and intestinal schistosomiasis [54]. The drug of choice is praziquantel (single dose of 40–60 mg/kg). Other available drugs are metrifonate for *S. haematobium* and oxamniquine for *S. mansoni* [55].

SPIROCHETES

Leptospirosis

Leptospirosis is a potentially fatal, waterborne zooanthroponosis caused by spirochete, *Leptospira interrogans*, acquired by direct or indirect contact with the urine of infected rodents (usually rats and pigs) [56]. It has a diverse array of cutaneous and life-threatening systemic manifestations such as ARDS, acute renal failure (ARF), and cardiogenic shock leading to death. It is more common in developing tropical countries with high rainfall and poor socioeconomic and sanitary conditions. Adult men engaged in recreational water activities or working in sewers, farms, and mines are more affected [57].

It enters into the blood circulation through abraded skin, mucous membranes, or the gastrointestinal tract [58]. Most of the leptospirotic infections are subclinical. In symptomatic cases, after an incubation period of 4–21 days, an acute nonspecific leptospiremic phase develops presenting with fever, myalgia, headache, flu-like symptoms, and conjunctival hyperemia that lasts for approximately 1 week [59]. Depending on the host immunity and serovars, the disease may progress further into one of two recognized

clinical forms: anicteric form and Weil disease. Weil disease is the severe form that has profound systemic manifestations such as hemorrhagic diathesis, uveitis, meningitis, cardiac arrhythmia, ARDS, severe hemolytic and cholestatic jaundice, and oligoanuric ARF [60]. Cutaneous lesions are morbilliform, scarlatiniform, or hemorrhagic, concentrated over the trunk. Desquamation, erythema nodosum, and infarcts may be seen on distal extremities in children. Characteristically, *L. interrogans autumnalis* may cause tender, erythematous papules on the shins on the fourth or fifth day of illness, called as pretibial fever or Fort Bragg fever.

Diagnosis requires a high index of suspicion based on history and physical examination. Diagnosis can be confirmed by culture on Ellinghausen-McCullough-Johnson-Harris medium, dark-field microscopy, immunostaining, ELISA, or PCR.

Early administration of suitable antibiotics, restoration of fluid, and correction of electrolytes, especially hypokalemia, are necessary to reduce mortality. Penicillin G is the drug of choice, and ampicillin, amoxicillin, and doxycycline are other alternatives. The prognosis is good if antibiotics are started within 4 days of onset of symptoms [58].

RICKETTSIAL INFECTIONS

Rocky Mountain spotted fever (RMSF)

This is a serious, life-threatening, but curable infectious disease caused by the bacteria *Rickettsia rickettsii* and is acquired by the bite of a tick harboring bacteria. The organism is endemic in parts of North, Central, and South America [61] and is prevalent in various parts of India [62]. It can present with wide variations in severity of clinical manifestations, and the mortality rate observed in untreated cases is around 20%–25%. The mean incubation period is 7 days (range 2–14 days), and initial features are nonspecific and include sudden onset of fever (usually greater than 38°C–39°C), and severe headache, usually accompanied by myalgia, anorexia, nausea, vomiting, abdominal pain, and photophobia. Rash appears 2–5 days after onset of fever, and then clinical triad as previously described may be seen in 60%–70% of cases during the second week of illness. Rash first appears on hands and feet as small, blanchable erythematous macules and spreads centripetally to involve extremities and trunk. Soon, macules develop central petechiae and may progress to skin necrosis and gangrene, requiring amputation [63]. Patients with RMSF develop various systemic features including cardiac (myocarditis, congestive heart failure, arrhythmias), pulmonary (pulmonary edema, pneumonitis), gastrointestinal (anorexia, diarrhea, abdominal pain and tenderness), renal (acute renal failure), neurological (altered mental status, photophobia, meningoencephalitis, cranial neuropathies, ataxia, hearing loss, hemiplegia, paraplegia, or complete paralysis, vertigo), ocular (petechial conjunctivitis, retinal hemorrhages, retinal ischemia), and musculoskeletal (myalgia and arthralgia) manifestations.

The diagnosis of RMSF requires a high index of suspicion and should be considered in patients presenting with febrile illness and history of possible tick exposure. Laboratory diagnosis is usually made by documenting a positive serological test for antirickettsial antibodies by indirect immunofluorescent antibody test, latex agglutination, or enzyme immunoassay. Seroconversion usually occurs by the second week of illness, and hence, serology has a limited role in initial treatment. Weil-Felix test is neither sensitive nor specific and is no longer recommended. PCR-based diagnosis is a useful technique but is not widely available. Immunohistochemical staining of a skin biopsy sample is another useful means of diagnosis and offers quick results [64].

The drug of choice for treatment is doxycycline at a dose of 100 mg twice daily for adults and 2.2 mg/kg twice daily for children. The treatment should be continued for 3 days after resolution of fever. Chloramphenicol is an alternative drug, but is less effective. Supportive management of systemic involvement is often required.

Epidemic typhus

Epidemic typhus is a potentially lethal, louse-borne, exanthematous disease caused by *Rickettsia prowazekii*. The infection is transmitted to human beings by the body louse *Pediculus humanus corporis*. The organisms cause damage to endothelial cells, resulting in multiorgan vasculitis. Involvement of end arteries may result in gangrene of the distal extremities, nose, earlobes, and genitalia. In severe cases, vasculitis may result in coma, multiorgan system failure, and death. The mortality rate in untreated, otherwise healthy patients may reach 20%, but may reach as high as 60% in elderly debilitated patients [65].

The patient develops abrupt onset of fever, headache, and skin rash. Other common associated findings include severe myalgias, arthralgias, and nonspecific constitutional symptoms (malaise, anorexia, chills). Central nervous system involvement is very common, and delirium, coma, and seizures may develop. A maculopapular and/or petechial rash is noted on days 4–7 and may begin on the axilla and trunk and spread centrifugally to involve extremities. Face, palms, and soles are typically spared, and eschars are absent [66].

The diagnosis of epidemic typhus rests on serology. Indirect immunofluorescence (IIF) assay or enzyme immunoassay (EIA) testing are used to detect rise in the specific immunoglobulin M (IgM) antibody titer, indicating an acute disease. Molecular studies like real-time PCR duplex are fast and can differentiate *R. prowazekii* from other rickettsiae. Early administration of doxycycline is recommended in patients with suspected epidemic typhus, even before confirming the diagnosis. The therapy should be continued for 2–4 days after defervescence. The patient should be investigated to assess severity of internal organs involvement and appropriate supportive therapy should be initiated. Prevention and treatment of louse infestations are the most important preventive measures [67].

CONCLUSION

Tropical infections and infestations include a wide range of conditions, and they are found in specific regions as suggested by the nomenclature. Suspicion of diagnosis is important when patients present with characteristic features in endemic regions.

KEY POINTS

- Tropical infections and infestations are varied in manifestations and include a variety of conditions occurring in tropical regions.
- Characteristic cutaneous features help in early diagnosis.
- Increasing global travel makes these diseases a must know for all concerned.

REFERENCES

1. Bottieau E et al. Fatal *Chromobacterium violaceum* bacteraemia in rural Bandundu, Democratic Republic of the Congo. *New Microbes New Infect* 2015;5:21–3.
2. Cindrich RB, Rudikoff D. Life-threatening bacterial skin infections. In: Wolf R, Parish LC, Parish JL (Eds), *Emergency Dermatology*. 2nd ed. New York: CRC Press; 2017:94.
3. Ray P et al. *Chromobacterium violaceum* septicaemia from north India. *Indian J Med Res* 2004;120:523–6.
4. Teoh AYB, Hui M, Ngo KY, Wong J, Lee KF, Lai PBS. Fatal septicaemia from *Chromobacterium violaceum*: Case reports and review of the literature. *Hong Kong Med J* 2006;12:228–31.
5. Yang CH, Li YH. *Chromobacterium violaceum* infection: A clinical review of an important but neglected infection. *J Chin Med Assoc* 2011;74:435–41.
6. Wolf R, Tüzün Y, Davidovici BB. Necrotizing soft tissue infections. In: Wolf R, Parish LC, Parish JL (Eds), *Emergency Dermatology*. 2nd ed. New York: CRC Press, Taylor and Francis Group; 2017:80–1.
7. Ruppert J et al. Two cases of severe sepsis due to *Vibrio vulnificus* wound infection acquired in the Baltic Sea. *Eur J Clin Microbiol Infect Dis* 2004;23:912–5.
8. Daniels NA, Shafaie A. A review of pathogenic *Vibrio* infections for clinicians. *Infect Med* 2000;17:665–85.
9. Tena D, Arias M, Álvarez BT, Mauleón C, Jiménez MP, Bisquert J. Fulminant necrotizing fasciitis due to *Vibrio parahaemolyticus*. *J Med Microbiol* 2010;59:235–8.
10. Chakraborty PP et al. Outbreak of cutaneous anthrax in a tribal village: A clinico-epidemiological study. *JAPI* 2012;60:11–4.

11. Cindrich RB, Rudikoff D. Life-threatening bacterial skin infections. In: Wolf R, Parish LC, Parish JL (Eds), *Emergency Dermatology*. 2nd ed. New York: CRC Press; 2017:89–90.

12. Akdeniz N, Calka O, Ozkol HU, Akdeniz H. Cutaneous anthrax resulting in renal failure with generalized tissue damage. *Cutan Ocul Toxicol* 2013;32:327–29.

13. Doganay M, Metan G, Alp E. A review of cutaneous anthrax and its outcome. *J Infect Public Health* 2010;3:98–101.

14. dos Santos Grácio J, Grácio MAA. Plague: A millenary infectious disease reemerging in the XXI century. *Bio Med Res Int* 2017, Article ID 5696542, 8 pages, 2017. doi: 10.1155/2017/5696542.

15. Human Plague—Four states, 2006. https://www.cdc.gov/mmwr/preview/mmwrhtml/mm5534a4.htm (accessed on 15 October 2017).

16. Cobbs CG, Chansolme DH. Plague. *Dermatol Clin* 2004;22:303–12.

17. Van Deuren M, Brandtzaeg P, van der Meer JWM. Update on meningococcal disease with emphasis on pathogenesis and clinical management. *Clin Microbiol Rev* 2000;13:144–66.

18. Stephens DS, Greenwood B, Brandtzaeg P. Epidemic meningitis, meningococcaemia, and *Neisseria* meningitis. *Lancet* 2007;369:2196.

19. Stephens DS. Unlocking the meningococcus: Dynamics of carriage and disease. *Lancet* 1999;353:941–2.

20. Betrosian AP, Berlet T, Agarwal B. Purpura fulminans in sepsis. *Am J Med Sci* 2006;332:339.

21. Johri S, Gorthi S, Anand A. Meningococcal meningitis. *Med J Armed Forces India* 2005;61:369–74.

22. Apicella MA. *Neisseria* meningitides. In: Mandell ML, Bennett JE, Dolin R (Eds), *Principles and Practices of Infectious Diseases*. 5th ed. Philadelphia: Churchill Livingstone; 2000:2228–42.

23. Okoth-Olende CA, Bjerregaard B. Scleroma in Africa: A review of cases from Kenya. *East Afr Med J* 1990;67:231.

24. Inamadar AC, Palit A, Kulkarni NH, Guggarigoudar SP, Yelikar BR. Nodulo-ulcerative lesions over the nose. *Indian J Dermatol Venereol Leprol* 2004;70:197–8.

25. Hay RJ, Adrians BM. Bacterial infections. In: Burns T, Breathnach S, Cox N, Griffiths C (Eds), *Rook's Textbook of Dermatology*. 8th ed. Edinburgh: Wiley-Blackwell; 2010:30.1–82.

26. Hoffman E, Loose LD, Harkin JC. The Mikulicz cell in rhinoscleroma. *Am J Pathol* 1973;73:47.

27. Li S et al. Clinical analysis of pulmonary nocardiosis in patients with autoimmune disease. *Medicine (Baltim)* 2015;94:e1561.

28. Soma S, Saha P, SenGupta M. Cutaneous *Nocardia brasiliensis* infection in an immunocompetent host after ovarian cystectomy: A case study. *Australas Med J* 2011;4:603–5.

29. Yang M et al. Clinical findings of 40 patients with nocardiosis: A retrospective analysis in a tertiary hospital. *Exp Ther Med* 2014;8:25–30.

30. Lai KW, Brodell LA, Lambert E, Menegus M, Scott GA, Tu JH. Primary cutaneous *Nocardia brasiliensis* infection isolated in an immunosuppressed patient: A case report. *Cutis* 2012;89:75–7.

31. Pradhan ZS, Jacob P, Korah S. Management of postoperative *Nocardia endophthalmitis*. *Indian J Med Microbiol* 2012;30:359–61.

32. Sharma NL, Mahajan VK, Agarwal S, Katoch VM, Das R, Kashyap M, Gupta P, Verma GK. Nocardial mycetoma: Diverse clinical presentations. *Indian J Dermatol Venereol Leprol* 2008;74:635–40.

33. Raimondi F et al. Noma neonatorum from multidrug-resistant *Pseudomonas aeruginosa*: An underestimated threat? *J Pediatr Infect Dis Soc* 2015;4:e25–7.

34. Lin JY, Wang DW, Peng CT, Tsai FJ, Chiou YM, Tsai CH. Noma neonatorum: An unusual case of noma involving a full term neonate. *Acta Pediatr* 1992;81:720–2.

35. Prajapati NC, Chaturvedi P, Bhowate RR, Mishra S. Noma neonatorum. *Indian Pediatr* 1995;32:1019–21.

36. Nayak PA, Nayak UA, Khandelwal V, Gupta A. Noma neonatorum. *BMJ Case Rep* 2013. doi: 10.1136/bcr-2013-009912.

37. Parikh TB, Nanavati RN, Udani RH. Noma neonatorum. *Indian J Pediatr* 2006;73:439–40.

38. Ghosal SP, Sen Gupta PC, Mukherjee AK, Choudhury M, Datta N, Sarkar AK. Noma neonatorum: Its etiopathogenesis. *Lancet* 1978;2:289–90.

39. Aubry A, Chosidow O, Caumes E, Robert J, Cambau E. Sixty-three cases of *Mycobacterium marinum* infection: Clinical features, treatment, and antibiotic susceptibility of causative isolates. *Arch Intern Med* 2002;162:1746–52.

40. Gould CV, Werth VP, Gluckman SJ. Fatal disseminated *Mycobacterium marinum* infection with bacteremia in a patient misdiagnosed as pyoderma gangrenosum. *Infect Dis Clin Pract* 2004;12:26–9.

41. Tchornobay AM, Claudy AL, Perrot JL, Levigne V, Denis M. Fatal disseminated *Mycobacterium marinum* infection. *Int J Dermatol* 1992;31(4):286–7.

42. Asakura T et al. Disseminated *Mycobacterium marinum* infection with a destructive nasal lesion mimicking extranodal NK/T cell lymphoma a case report. *Medicine* 95(11):e3131.

43. Sanchez Clemente N, Ugarte-Gil CA, Solórzano N, Maguiña C, Pachas P, Blazes D, Bailey R, Mabey D, Moore D. Bartonella bacilliformis: A systematic review of the literature to guide the research agenda for elimination. *PLOS Negl Trop Dis* 2012;6:e1819.

44. Minnick MF, Anderson BE, Lima A, Battisti JM, Lawyer PG, Birtles RJ. Oroya fever and verruga peruana: Bartonelloses unique to South America. *PLOS Negl Trop Dis* 2014;8:e2919.

45. Tarazona A, Maguiña C, de Guimaraes D-L, Montoya M, Pachas P. Terapia antibiótica para el manejo de la Bartonelosis o Enfermedad de Carrión en el Perú. *Rev Peru Med Exp Salud Publ* 2006;23:188–200.

46. Kaiser PO, Riess T, O'Rourke F, Linke D, Kempf VA. *Bartonella* spp.: Throwing light on uncommon human infections. *Int J Med Microbiol* 2011;301:7–15.

47. Maguiña C, Guerra H, Ventosilla P. Bartonellosis. *Clin Dermatol* 2009;27:271–80.

48. Mateen FJ, Newstead JC, McClean KL. Bacillary angiomatosis in an HIV-positive man with multiple risk factors: A clinical and epidemiological puzzle. *Can J Infect Dis Med Microbiol* 2005;16:249–52.

49. Morrison AO, Morris R, Shannon A, Lauer SR, Guarner J, Kraft CS. Disseminated *Acanthamoeba* infection presenting with cutaneous lesions in an immunocompromised patient: A case report, review of histomorphologic findings, and potential diagnostic pitfalls. *Am J Clin Pathol* 2016;145:266–70.

50. Park CH, Iyengar V, Hefter L, Pestaner JP, Vandel NM. Cutaneous acanthamoeba infection associated with acquired immunodeficiency syndrome. *Lab Med* 1994;25:386–8.

51. Paltiel M, Powell E, Lynch J, Baranowski B, Martins C. Disseminated cutaneous acanthamebiasis: A case report and review of the literature. *Cutis* 2004;73:241–5.

52. Vega-Lopez F, Hay RJ. Parasitic worms and protozoa. In: Breathnach S, Cox N, Griffiths C, Burns T (Eds), *Rook's Textbook of Dermatology*. 8th ed. Edinburgh: Wiley-Blackwell; 2010:37.1–26.

53. Elbaz T, Esmat T. Hepatic and intestinal schistosomiasis: Review. *J Adv Res* 2013;4:445–52.

54. Farrell AM et al. Ectopic cutaneous schistosomiasis: Extragenital involvement with progressive upward spread. *Br J Dermatol* 1996;135:110.

55. Davis-Reed L, Theis JH. Cutaneous schistosomiasis: Report of a case and review of the literature. *J Am Acad Dermatol* 2000;42:678–80.

56. Evangelista KV, Coburn J. Leptospira as an emerging pathogen: A review of its biology, pathogenesis and host immune responses. *Future Microbiol* 2010;5:1413–25.

57. Daher EF et al. Clinical presentation of leptospirosis: A retrospective study of 201 patients in a metropolitan city of Brazil. *Braz J Infect Dis* 2010;14:3–10.

58. Younes-Ibrahim M et al. Na,K-ATPase: A molecular target for *Leptospira interrogans* endotoxin. *Braz J Med Biol Res* 1997;30:213–23.

59. Mansour-Ghanaei F, Sarshad AII, Fallah MS, Pourhabibi A, Pourhabibi K, Yousefi-Mashhoor M. Leptospirosis in Guilan, a northern province of Iran: Assessment of the clinical presentation of 74 cases. *Med Sci Monit* 2005;11:219–23.

60. Izurieta R, Galwankar S, Clem A. Leptospirosis: The "mysterious" mimic. *J Emerg Trauma Shock* 2008;1:21–33.

61. Minniear TD, Buckingham SC. Managing Rocky Mountain spotted fever. *Expert Rev Anti Infect Ther* 2009;7:1131–7.

62. Rathi N, Rathi A. Rickettsial infections: Indian perspective. *Indian Pediatr* 2010;47:157–64.

63. Openshaw JJ, Swerdlow DL, Krebs JW, Holman RC, Mandel E, Harvey A, Haberling D, Massung RF, McQuiston JH. Rocky Mountain spotted fever in the United States, 2000–2007: Interpreting contemporary increases in incidence. *Am J Trop Med Hyg* 2010;83:174–82.

64. Dantas-Torres F. Rocky Mountain spotted fever. *Lancet Infect Dis* 2007;7:724–32.

65. Bechah Y, Capo C, Mege JL, Raoult D. Epidemic typhus. *Lancet Infect Dis* 2008;8:417–26.

66. Badiaga S, Brouqui P. Human louse-transmitted infectious diseases. *Clin Microbiol Infect* 2012;18:332–7.

67. Botelho-Nevers E, Socolovschi C, Raoult D, Parola P. Treatment of *Rickettsia* spp. infections: A review. *Expert Rev Anti Infect Ther* 2012;10:1425–37.

PART 8

Vasculitis

BIJU VASUDEVAN

31

Small vessel vasculitis

RENU GEORGE, ANKAN GUPTA, AND ASWIN M. NAIR

INTRODUCTION

Vasculitides are a heterogeneous group of disorders characterized by inflammation of blood vessels of varying sizes which leads to obstruction of the vascular lumen, thereby causing ischemia and infarction of the tissue supplied by them, which can result in manifestations ranging from benign cutaneous vasculitis to life-threatening multisystem involvement [1]. Skin manifestations often herald the onset of systemic involvement and can provide vital clues for an accurate diagnosis. Failure to diagnose it early can result in fatal consequences. This chapter focuses on the clinical features of vasculitis with emphasis on emergencies that are associated with primary small vessel vasculitides.

CLASSIFICATION

Classification of vasculitides has been revised over the years. Broadly, vasculitis can be divided into primary vasculitis and vasculitis secondary to systemic autoimmune disorders, infections, drugs, or malignancies. The gold standard previously was the classification advocated by the American College of Rheumatology (ACR) in 1990, but the present one is the nomenclature for vasculitides adopted at the International Chapel Hill Consensus Conference (CHCC) 2012 and is accepted worldwide [2,3]. It classifies vasculitis based on the size of the vessel involved as large, medium, and small vessel vasculitis as shown in Table 31.1. The aorta and its main branches at origin are called large vessels; vessels beyond the origin from aorta until they lose their muscle coat on their walls are called medium vessels; and further distally, the branches devoid of any muscle coat are called small vessels, which include small intraparenchymal arteries (except the initial penetrating branches), nonmuscular arterioles, capillaries, and postcapillary venules. Small vessel vasculitis contributes to most of the accounts of vasculitis documented historically [4].

Although most vasculitides affect children and adults, the clinical, epidemiological, etiological, and prognostic characteristics of pediatric vasculitides differ from adults and are discussed later [5].

ETIOPATHOGENESIS

The pathogenesis for vasculitis differs among the various types [1]. Several factors have been identified including drugs, infections, systemic diseases, malignancy, and rarely dietary factors [6]. The drugs most commonly implicated are ß-lactams, loop and thiazide-type diuretics, phenytoin, and allopurinol. Drugs such as minocycline, hydralazine, propylthiouracil, and montelukast have been implicated in the pathogenesis of antineutrophil cytoplasmic antibody (ANCA)–associated vasculitis (AAV). However, every new drug taken 7–10 days prior to the initiation of the appearance of symptoms should be deemed suspicious [6]. Certain infections, such as hepatitis B or C virus, human immunodeficiency virus (HIV), Epstein-Barr virus (EBV), and chronic bacteremias (e.g., infective endocarditis) may also be associated with vasculitis [7]. It is estimated that infections, medications, connective tissue diseases, and malignancy account for 23%, 20%, 12%, and 4% of cases of cutaneous vasculitis, respectively [8]. Small vessel cutaneous vasculitis may also occur following the use of cocaine adulterated with levamisole [6]. A search for malignancy is not warranted in all cases of vasculitis unless there is a high degree of suspicion [9]. Broadly, various triggers lead to breach of immune tolerance resulting in activation of humoral immunity predominantly in certain

Table 31.1 International Chapel Hill Consensus Conference 2012 classification

Large vessel vasculitis (LVV)	Takayasu arteritis
	Giant cell arteritis
Medium vessel vasculitis (MVV)	Classic polyarteritis nodosa
	Kawasaki disease
Small vessel vasculitis (SVV)	Antineutrophil cytoplasmic antibody (ANCA)–associated vasculitis (AAV)
	• Microscopic polyangiitis
	• Granulomatosis with polyangiitis (earlier known as Wegener granulomatosis)
	• Eosinophilic granulomatosis with polyangiitis (earlier known as Churg-Strauss syndrome)
	Immune complex SVV
	• Antiglomerular basement membrane disease
	• Cryoglobulinemic vasculitis
	• IgA vasculitis (earlier known as Henoch–Schönlein purpura)
	• Hypocomplementemic urticarial vasculitis (anti-C1q vasculitis)
Variable vessel vasculitis (VVV)	Behçet disease
	Cogan syndrome
Single-organ vasculitis	Cutaneous leukocytoclastic angiitis
	Cutaneous arteritis
	Primary central nervous system vasculitis
	Isolated aortitis
	Others
Vasculitis associated with systemic disease	Lupus vasculitis
	Rheumatoid vasculitis
	Sarcoid vasculitis
	Others
Vasculitis associated with probable etiology	Hepatitis C virus–associated cryoglobulinemic vasculitis
	Hepatitis B virus–associated vasculitis
	Syphilis-associated aortitis
	Drug-associated immune complex vasculitis
	Drug-associated AAV
	Cancer-associated vasculitis
	Others

Source: Jennette JC et al. Arthritis Rheum 2013;65:1–11.

vasculitis, such as ANCA-associated vasculitis, IgA vasculitis, and cryoglobulinemic vasculitis, and cell-mediated immunity in others. In addition, complement pathways are also activated as in the case of hypocomplementemic urticarial as well as secondary vasculitis. Innate immune cells, i.e., neutrophils, eosinophils, macrophages, and natural killer cells also play a role. These pathways ultimately lead to activation of pro-inflammatory cytokines, chemokines, and angiogenic factors and result in final transmural inflammation of small sized blood vessels in various organs with other features like granuloma in certain conditions (mainly AAV).

CLINICAL FEATURES

Cutaneous small vessel vasculitis

Cutaneous small vessel vasculitis (CSVV), by definition, has no visceral organ involvement [3]; however, patients with CSVV may develop systemic vasculitis over the course of their illness (Table 31.2).

CUTANEOUS MANIFESTATIONS

Palpable purpura (Figure 31.1) and/or petechiae (Figure 31.2) are the hallmarks of small vessel vasculitis. The lesions can, however, range from erythematous macules, papules, and nodules to necrotic ulcers (Figure 31.3). Severe inflammation may lead to hemorrhagic bullae (Figure 31.4), and vascular occlusion secondary to vasculitis may cause digital gangrene (Figure 31.5). The skin lesions usually occur symmetrically over the legs (Figure 31.6) and on areas of constrictive clothing and may be associated with pruritus, burning sensation, or pain. Systemic small vessel vasculitides such as AAV, CV, IgAV, and infective endocarditis, and medium vessel vasculitis such as polyarteritis nodosa may also present in a similar manner. Organs that merit attention in small vessel vasculitis include lungs, kidneys, gastrointestinal tract, peripheral and central nervous systems (PNS and CNS), and musculoskeletal system.

SYSTEMIC MANIFESTATIONS

Systemic manifestations and emergencies seen in association with SSV are listed in Table 31.2.

Table 31.2 Systemic manifestations and emergencies in small vessel vasculitis

System	Manifestations	Emergencies
Skin	Palpable purpura Subcutaneous nodules Livedo reticularis Wheals and angioedema	Hemorrhagic bullae Cutaneous necrosis Necrotic ulcers Acral gangrene
Lungs [10]	Cough Dyspnea Hemoptysis Pleural effusion Pulmonary edema Asthma Chronic obstructive pulmonary disease	Diffuse alveolar hemorrhage Pulmonary-renal syndrome
Kidneys [11]	Proteinuria Hematuria Secondary hypertension Chronic kidney disease	Rapidly progressing glomerulonephritis resulting in renal failure
Gastrointestinal tract	Colicky abdominal pain Melena Vomiting	Intussusception Gangrene of the gut Bowel perforation Gastrointestinal hemorrhage Acute pancreatitis
Peripheral nervous system, central nervous system	Mononeuritis multiplex Headache Cerebral vasculitis Seizures	Cerebrovascular accident
Musculoskeletal	Arthritis Arthralgia Jaccoud arthropathy Erosive deforming arthritis	
Cardiac	Myocarditis Pericarditis Pancarditis	Cardiac dysfunction and pulmonary edema
Eye	Conjunctivitis Uveitis Episcleritis Optic atrophy	Necrotizing scleritis
Ear, nose, throat	Nasal crusting Sinusitis Oral ulcers Otitis media Sensorineural deafness	Epistaxis Stridor, glottic, subglottic stenosis Septal perforation
Miscellaneous	Raynaud phenomenon Myalgia Unexplained weight loss	Painful scrotal edema Testicular hemorrhage Arterial and venous thrombosis

INVESTIGATIONS

Histopathology

It is best to biopsy a purpuric lesion of less than 48 hours duration (choose a bright red lesion) for routine histopathology and direct immunofluorescence (DIF). At least *two of three* of the following need to be present in the histopathology for a definite diagnosis of small vessel vasculitis [8,12]:

- Perivascular/angiocentric inflammatory infiltrates
- Disruption of vessel walls by the inflammatory infiltrate
- Fibrinoid necrosis

Other histopathologic features that suggest vasculitis (but are not diagnostic) include the presence of extravasated

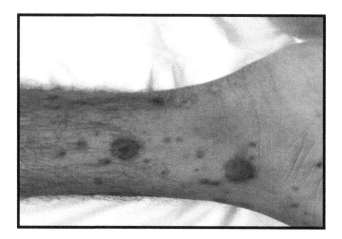

Figure 31.1 Palpable purpura over leg in a patient with cutaneous small vessel vasculitis.

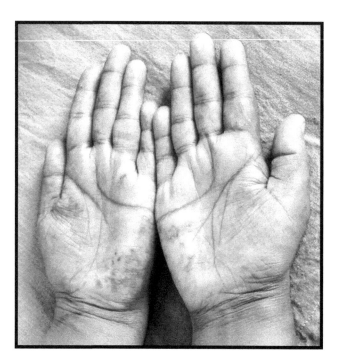

Figure 31.2 Palpable petechiae over the hypothenar eminence in a patient with small vessel vasculitis.

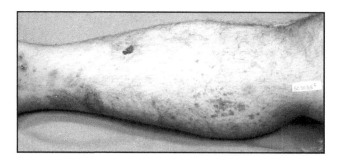

Figure 31.3 Necrotic ulcer with petechiae.

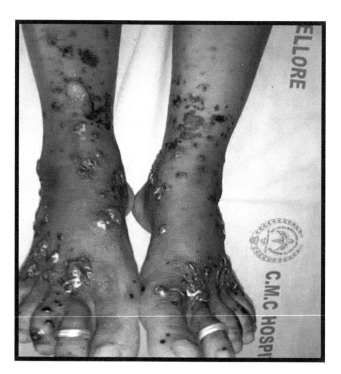

Figure 31.4 Hemorrhagic bullae bilaterally symmetrical over legs.

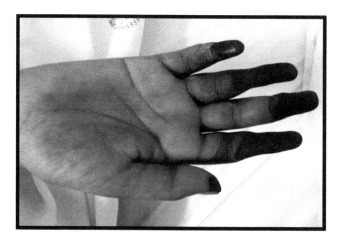

Figure 31.5 Digital gangrene.

erythrocytes, nuclear debris, endothelial cell swelling or necrosis, cutaneous ulceration, or necrosis. Granulomatous inflammation suggests granulomatosis with polyangiitis (GPA) or eosinophilic granulomatosis with polyangiitis (EGPA).

DIF assists in the diagnosis of conditions like Henoch-Schönlein purpura (IgAV). Deposits of immunoglobulin G (IgG), IgM, and/or complement are also seen with other immune complex SVV, whereas a negative immunofluorescence indicates a pauci-immune vasculitis (ANCA-associated vasculitis).

Laboratory tests

Laboratory tests are listed in Table 31.3. They help to determine systemic organ involvement as a result of vasculitis and may give a clue to the underlying etiology.

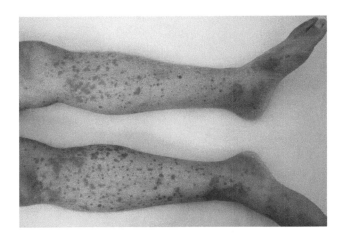

Figure 31.6 Symmetrical purpuric lesions on legs.

TREATMENT

Once systemic involvement has been excluded and the diagnosis of single-organ CSVV has been made, treatment is largely symptomatic. In those patients in whom drugs are considered to be the cause, discontinuation of the inciting drug leads to resolution in a few days. Systemic immunosuppressive therapy to arrest the disease process is usually reserved for the subset of patients who develop complications such as hemorrhagic bullae, ulceration, or chronic (duration of more than 4 weeks) or recurrent disease.

Treatment of acute uncomplicated cutaneous small vessel vasculitis

Rest, leg elevation, and use of compression stockings help in decreasing dependency and may decrease immune complex deposition, thereby decreasing the progression of vasculitis. Nonsteroidal anti-inflammatory drugs and antihistamines may be given for symptomatic relief.

Treatment of complicated or chronic cutaneous small vessel vasculitis

In complicated, chronic, or recurrent cases, initial management is usually with a short course of systemic steroids [16]. Second-line drugs like colchicine or dapsone may be added if

Table 31.3 Laboratory tests

Test	Remarks
Complete blood count with peripheral smear	• Normochromic normocytic anemia, leukocytosis, thrombocytosis may be seen with vasculitis • Thrombocytopenia may occur in sepsis; thrombocytopenic purpura is nonpalpable • Cytopenia suggests an underlying lupus, malignancy, or drug-induced etiology • Leukocytosis may be suggestive of an infection or hematologic malignancy • Peripheral eosinophilia is a criterion for eosinophilic granulomatosis with polyangiitis
Biochemistry panel including renal and hepatic function tests	• Organ involvement • To plan therapy
Bloodborne virus screening	A screening test for secondary vasculitides
Anti-streptolysin O titer	A positive test suggests antecedent upper respiratory tract streptococcal infection
Antinuclear antibody (ANA), serum complements, rheumatoid factor, serum cryoglobulins	• A positive ANA or rheumatoid factor, and low complements suggest evaluation for an underlying systemic connective tissue disease • Low complement levels may be a surrogate marker for cryoglobulinemic vasculitis; low complements are a requisite for diagnosing hypocomplementemic urticarial vasculitis syndrome
Antineutrophil cytoplasmic antibodies (ANCA) [15]	C-ANCA and P-ANCA are associated with ANCA-associated vasculitis
Urine microscopy and urine protein	The presence of proteinuria and hematuria with sediments suggests glomerulonephritis
Stool for presence of occult blood	A positive test may indicate upper or lower gastrointestinal bleed secondary to vasculitis
Chest x-ray	Predominantly perihilar region having fluffy opacities is suggestive of diffuse alveolar hemorrhage
Erythrocyte sedimentation rate and C-reactive protein	Inflammatory markers to guide the physician about the activity of the disease
Nerve conduction studies	Impaired in the presence of peripheral neuropathy
Malignancy screening (not always required)	Palpable purpura may be the presentation of a paraneoplastic process, e.g., hairy cell leukemia
Imaging studies as appropriate	

Table 31.4 Paediatric Rheumatology European Society/European League Against Rheumatism/Paediatric Rheumatology International Trials Organization classification

I. Predominantly large vessel vasculitis
  a. Takayasu arteritis
II. Predominantly medium-sized vessel vasculitis
  a. Childhood polyarteritis nodosa
  b. Cutaneous polyarteritis
  c. Kawasaki disease
III. Predominantly small vessels vasculitis
  a. Granulomatous
    i. Wegener granulomatosis
    ii. Churg-Strauss syndrome
  b. Nongranulomatous
    i. Microscopic polyangiitis
    ii. Henoch-Schönlein purpura
    iii. Isolated cutaneous leukocytoclastic vasculitis
    iv. Hypocomplementemic urticarial vasculitis
IV. Other vasculitides
  a. Behçet disease
  b. Vasculitis secondary to infection (including hepatitis B associated polyarteritis nodosa, malignancies, and drugs, including hypersensitivity vasculitis)
  c. Vasculitis associated with connective tissue diseases
  d. Isolated vasculitis of the central nervous system
  e. Cogan syndrome
V. Unclassified

lesions persist beyond 6 weeks and relapse on tapering steroids [17,18]. If the disease is refractory to steroids, then immunosuppressive therapy in the form of methotrexate, azathioprine, or mycophenolate mofetil may be tried. Other drugs used in recalcitrant cases include cyclosporine [19], rituximab [20], and IV immunoglobulin [21]. Drug therapy may be continued until no new lesions have developed for 2–3 months.

A treatment algorithm for chronic or complicated CSVV is presented in Table 31.4.

IMMUNE COMPLEX SMALL VESSEL VASCULITIS

Vasculitis associated with immune complex and/or complement deposition includes anti-GBM disease, cryoglobulinemic vasculitis, IgA vasculitis, and urticarial vasculitis. As compared to AAV, immune complex SVVs are associated with lesser arterial involvement [3].

Cryoglobulinemic vasculitis

Cryoglobulins (Cg) are immunoglobulins or a mixture of immunoglobulins and complement proteins that precipitate at a temperature less than 37°C [22]. Small or medium vessel

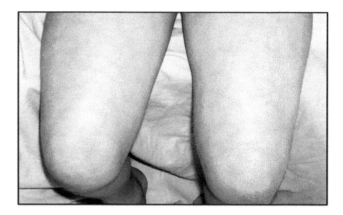

Figure 31.7 Livedo reticularis.

vasculitis occurring secondary to Cg containing immune complexes is labeled as cryoglobulinemic vasculitis [23].

CLINICAL FEATURES

Skin lesions in mixed cryoglobulinemia are indistinguishable from SVV [24]. Type I cryoglobulinemic vasculitis (CV) is related to an underlying B-cell lymphoproliferative disorder (typically Waldenström macroglobulinemia or multiple myeloma) and demonstrates monoclonal immunoglobulins (typically IgG or IgM, less commonly IgA). It may be associated with symptoms of hypercoagulability like Raynaud phenomenon and livedo reticularis (Figure 31.7). Some cases may have severe skin involvement with large necrotic ulceration (Figure 31.8) and digital gangrene [25]. Systemically, it mainly involves the kidneys [26], musculoskeletal system [27], and peripheral nervous system [28]. Types II and III, collectively called mixed cryoglobulinemia, are associated with viral infections, particularly hepatitis C virus and HIV and connective tissue disorders. Concurrent HCV infection is a poor prognostic indicator with associated severe liver fibrosis, CNS, and heart involvement [29]. CV has been classified on the basis of the clonality of Cg to rheumatoid factor binding activity [30,31].

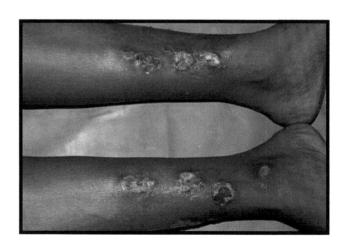

Figure 31.8 Large necrotic ulcers in cryoglobulinemic vasculitis

TREATMENT

Management consists of treating the underlying condition and specific treatment of vasculitis. Priority among these depends on the severity of vasculitis.

IgA vasculitis

IgA vasculitis is commonly seen in children and is discussed in detail in the section on "Small vessel vasculitis in the pediatric age group."

Urticarial vasculitis

Urticarial vasculitis (UV) is an immune complex mediated SVV that presents as persistent urticarial wheals. Based on complement levels and the presence and/or absence of specific systemic findings, UV has been classified into normocomplementemic urticarial vasculitis (NUV), hypocomplementemic urticarial vasculitis (HUV), and hypocomplementemic urticarial vasculitis syndrome (HUVS). Systemic involvement may be present in hypocomplementemic UV [32]. The hypocomplementemic form is also seen in association with connective tissue diseases like systemic lupus erythematosus.

CLINICAL FEATURES

The predominant cutaneous symptom is a long-lasting wheal associated with a burning sensation or tenderness that resolves with pigmentation. Other lesions seen include angioedema, purpura, erythema multiforme–like eruptions, bullous eruptions, Raynaud phenomenon, and/or livedo reticularis [33]. The systemic associations include musculoskeletal system, eye, lungs, and kidneys. Migratory, transient arthralgias and arthritis are the most common systemic manifestations. Jaccoud arthropathy is rarely seen and may be associated with aortic and mitral valvulopathy, requiring echocardiographic evaluation [34,35]. The renal involvement of UV tends to be more severe in children [36]. Rare complications include aseptic meningitis and cranial nerve palsies.

INVESTIGATIONS AND TREATMENT

The diagnosis can be confirmed by routine histopathology. Anti-C1q antibodies are associated with HUVS. DIF shows predominant IgG deposition along with complements and fibrin in the vessel walls and at the dermoepidermal junction [37]. There is no standard treatment algorithm for management, and symptomatology guides the therapy. Antihistamines mostly form the first line of therapy, especially if the predominant symptom is urticaria, and NSAIDs help for arthralgia but they do not modify the disease progress. With systemic involvement, systemic steroids with or without colchicine, dapsone, and hydroxychloroquine are the treatment options.

ANTINEUTROPHIL CYTOPLASMIC ANTIBODY-ASSOCIATED VASCULITIS

AAV includes a group of primary predominantly small vessel necrotizing vasculitis conditions that share common clinical features and organ involvement. They are associated with ANCAs specific for myeloperoxidase (P-ANCA) or proteinase 3 (C-ANCA) [38]. ANCA may be negative in some cases. C-ANCA is reasonably specific for GPA (75%–80%). This is seen in 25%–30% of microscopic polyangiitis (MPA) and 10%–15% patients of EGPA. P-ANCA is less specific, detected in MPA (50%–60%), EGPA (55%–60%), and GPA (10%–15%). If C-ANCA and P-ANCA coexist in a patient, drug-induced vasculitis should be suspected [39].

Clinical features

Skin lesions occur in 60% of patients with EGPA [40], 40% of patients with MPA [41], and 20% of patients with GPA [42]. Apart from the cutaneous vasculitic lesions like palpable purpura, livedo, and subcutaneous nodules, AAV may also present with nonvasculitic features such as pyoderma gangrenosum, erythema nodosum, or Sweet syndrome [43]. Urticaria and angioedema may be seen in EGPA.

Extracutaneous features

GRANULOMATOSIS WITH POLYANGIITIS

This entity tends to predominantly involve the upper and lower respiratory tract with variable renal involvement. Nearly 90% present with features of bloody rhinorrhea, sinusitis, nasal crusting, and recurrent otitis media leading to hearing loss and nasal septal perforation as well as collapse. Subglottic and tracheal stenosis, occurring as a sequel to the tracheal inflammation, can lead to airway narrowing requiring surgical dilations as well as intralesional glucocorticoid injection [44]. Patients can also present with rapidly rising creatinine, which is characterized histologically as pauci-immune crescentic glomerulonephritis. Other organ-threatening and life-threatening complications include necrotizing scleritis and diffuse alveolar hemorrhage (DAH).

MICROSCOPIC POLYANGIITIS

MPA is a pauci-immune necrotizing vasculitis affecting mostly the small vessels and occasionally the medium vessels [3]. Systemic involvement is mostly limited to kidneys with necrotizing glomerulonephritis being the most common presentation along with pulmonary capillaritis usually manifesting as cough, dyspnea, and hemoptysis [45]. Pulmonary hemorrhage has high mortality and may be associated with rapidly progressing glomerulonephritis (RPGN); the condition is then known as pulmonary-renal syndrome [46].

EOSINOPHILIC GRANULOMATOSIS WITH POLYANGIITIS

Like the other SVV subtypes, no confirmatory test exists for EGPA, and the diagnosis remains predominantly on clinical grounds. P-ANCA positivity is associated with higher incidence of life-threatening complications. Manifestations necessitating immediate intervention include mononeuritis (wrist/foot drop), alveolar hemorrhage (0%–4%), and rapidly progressive renal failure. Features associated with less favorable prognosis (original Five Factor Score) include elevated creatinine (>1.58 mg/dL), proteinuria >1 g/day, CNS, gastrointestinal, or myocardial involvement [47].

Investigations

Biopsy from a recent onset lesion demonstrates leukocytoclastic vasculitis in AAV. In GPA, a nonspecific perifollicular inflammation may be seen along with fibrinoid degeneration and foci of necrosis. A classical necrotizing vasculitis with granulomatous inflammation is seen in less than 20%, and occasionally it may mimic a neutrophilic dermatosis or show palisading granulomas [48]. In EGPA, we see either neutrophilic vasculitis or eosinophilic vasculitis, depending on the predominant inflammatory cells [49], which may later progress to a granulomatous stage wherein there are one or more extravascular palisading granulomas with central necrobiosis of collagen, neutrophil infiltration, and leukocytoclastic debris (known as Churg-Strauss granulomas) [50]. The absence of granulomatous inflammation on histopathology differentiates MPA from other AAV.

Treatment

Immediate treatment in life-threatening situations includes pulse steroids followed by high-dose prednisolone along with cyclophosphamide (CYC) as the preferred immunosuppressant. Rituximab is an option when CYC is contraindicated [51]. Azathioprine, mycophenolate mofetil, and methotrexate are long-term maintenance drugs [14,52]. Plasmapheresis and IVIg are used as an adjunct in life-threatening situations.

SMALL VESSEL VASCULITIS IN THE PEDIATRIC AGE GROUP

The most common vasculitis seen in the pediatric age group that present to dermatologists is Henoch-Schönlein purpura (HSP) and Kawaski disease (KD). Rarely, children may present with PAN or one of the AAV. The skin manifestations of vasculitis (with the exception of KD) in children are similar to adults and include symptomatic palpable purpuric lesions, hemorrhagic vesicles or bullae, nodules, ulcers associated with livedo reticularis, and rarely gangrene affecting predominantly the lower limbs. Purpuric lesions have to be differentiated from viral and rickettsial infections and meningococcemia. KD and polyarteritis nodosa (both medium vessel vasculitis) are not discussed in this chapter. The Paediatric Rheumatology European Society (PRES) in collaboration with the European League Against Rheumatism (EULAR) and the Paediatric Rheumatology International Trials Organization (PRINTO) have put forward a classification for childhood vasculitis as shown in Table 31.4 [54].

Henoch-Schönlein purpura (IgAV)

HSP is the most common systemic vasculitis in the pediatric age group occurring between 3 and 15 years of age. It has also been reported in infants [55]. The incidence is almost equal between the two genders [56].

ETIOPATHOGENESIS

Although HSP can follow any infection, the common triggers include streptococcal, staphylococcal, and parainfluenza infections [57]. Other triggers include vaccinations and medications. It has been found that in patients with HSP and IgA nephropathy, there is abnormal glycosylation of IgA1 molecules which results in the formation of large immune complexes, the clearance of which is impaired. They get deposited in small vessels of the affected organs activating the alternate complement pathway and an inflammatory response [57]. The 1990 ACR criteria continue to be widely used in adults (sensitivity: 87.1%; specificity: 87.7%). The EULAR/PRINTO/ PRES criteria (2010) proposed for HSP (sensitivity: 100%; specificity: 87%) include the presence of purpura or petechiae with lower limb predominance along with one or more of the following criteria: diffuse abdominal pain, arthritis or arthralgia, and histopathology showing leukocytoclastic vasculitis with IgA deposits or renal involvement [58].

CLINICAL FEATURES

HSP should be suspected in children presenting with symptomatic palpable purpura and petechiae on the lower limbs, gluteal region, and forearms. These lesions appear in crops often associated with pruritus, burning, and pain. Hemorrhagic vesicles, bullae, urticaria, targetoid lesions, and necrotic ulcers may also be present resulting in a polymorphous appearance. Edema of the hands, feet, periorbital area, and scrotum may also accompany the vasculitic lesions, especially in younger children [57].

The arthritis is usually oligoarticular and affects the large joints of the lower limbs. The periarticular skin is usually tender and erythematous. There is usually complete recovery with no residual deformity [57].

Abdominal pain is a result of edema and hemorrhage of the proximal small bowel wall secondary to the vasculitis and often results in colicky abdominal pain associated with vomiting. Intussusception occurs in 3%–4% of children and is one of the most severe of the gastrointestinal manifestations [58]. The other severe but rare manifestations include gangrene, bowel perforation, and massive hemorrhage. In one study, 17.6% of patients had overt gastrointestinal bleeding or had a positive test for the presence of stool occult blood [59]. They also found that the incidence of positive findings in imaging studies was higher when the stool occult blood was 3+ or 4+.

Pancreatitis has been reported to be a rare association of HSP in children. In one case it was the presenting feature, manifesting before development of palpable purpura [60]. The other intra-abdominal manifestations include hydrops of the gall bladder and pseudomembranous enterocolitis [61].

Renal manifestations vary from isolated hematuria with or without proteinuria to hypertension. The more severe cases may manifest as nephrotic syndrome with significant proteinuria or as acute glomerulonephritis. Nephritis occurs within a mean period of 2 weeks after the diagnosis of HSP is made and usually within a month in the majority of cases. The risk factors for developing nephritis are age older than 8 years, abdominal pain, and recurrence of HSP disease. It is recommended that weekly urine analysis be done for the first 2 months [62]. The prognosis of HSP is dependent on the severity of renal involvement. This can lead to chronic kidney disease in a small proportion of patients, even as late as 20 years after diagnosis [63]. Renal disease can mimic poststreptococcal glomerulonephritis or SLE nephritis. The C3 levels are normal in HSP nephritis as opposed to those of SLE with nephritis. The rare complications of HSP include cerebral vasculitis [64], scrotal or testicular hemorrhage [65], and interstitial pulmonary hemorrhage [66]. HSP nephritis with pulmonary findings may mimic AAV.

INVESTIGATIONS

The diagnosis can be established by the EULAR/PRINTO/PRES criteria [58]. The problem arises when the patient presents with systemic manifestations in the absence of skin lesions. The differential diagnosis of purpuric rash in children includes the ANCA-associated vasculitis, thrombocytopenia, septicemia, meningococcemia, CTD like SLE, infective endocarditis, and coagulopathies. However, the distinguishing features of the rash of HSP are that it is usually symptomatic, palpable, and present mainly on the lower limbs with normal bleeding parameters. Skin biopsy will show the presence of a small vessel leukocytoclastic vasculitis with deposits of IgA in the blood vessel wall. ANA and ANCA results will help to rule out CTD and AAV. Abdominal ultrasonography helps to diagnose most of the acute gastrointestinal emergencies.

TREATMENT

Management is largely supportive as most patients recover spontaneously [57]. Patients with painful hemorrhagic bullae, severe arthritis, abdominal symptoms, severe renal involvement, and/or testicular pain require hospitalization. Moderate pain resulting from arthritis or abdominal involvement can be managed by paracetamol or other NSAIDs provided there is no gastrointestinal bleed.

Blood transfusion is indicated if there is significant loss of blood, usually secondary to gastrointestinal bleeding. Hypertension, electrolyte imbalance, elevated creatinine, or massive proteinuria require close monitoring and prompt referral to the pediatric team. Patients with abdominal symptoms suggestive of intussusception, bowel infarction or perforation, and peritonitis should be referred to the surgeon for treatment.

The role of corticosteroids in the management of HSP remains controversial. However, a meta-analysis has shown that corticosteroid administration early in the course of disease may prove beneficial in the management of abdominal complications, prevent chronic renal disease, and reduce the duration of hospitalization [67]. The recommended dose of prednisolone varies from 1 to 2 mg/kg. Short-course steroids are indicated for severe skin involvement like hemorrhagic bullae, scrotal or testicular involvement, or abdominal pain and vomiting.

Granulomatosis with polyangiitis

The diagnosis in children is based on the EULAR/PRINTO/PRES GPA/WG classification criteria [58]. In one study involving 56 children, the organ systems involved were the ear/nose/throat (91%), constitutional (89%), respiratory (79%), mucosa and skin (64%), musculoskeletal (59%), and eye (35%). Hematuria/proteinuria were present in 50% of patients. Affected patients were predominantly female with a median age of onset being 7 years [68]. GPA should also be suspected in children presenting with a pulmonary-renal syndrome. Subglottic stenosis, tracheal and endobronchial stenosis, and thrombotic events have also been reported in GPA in children [69].

A comparative study of GPA versus MPA showed that patients with MPA were younger with more frequent gastrointestinal manifestations and more severe kidney disease and pulmonary manifestations were less frequent and severe [70]. Eye involvement is absent in MPA. The treatment options for these conditions include a combination of corticosteroids with cyclophosphamide (usually first line) with or without plasmapheresis, rituximab, methotrexate, azathioprine, and mycophenolate mofetil [70].

Eosinophilic granulomatosis with polyangiitis

This usually affects individuals with severe asthma or allergies. There are no specific criteria for the diagnosis in children. The common manifestations in children are asthma, eosinophilia, pulmonary infiltrates, sinusitis, and vasculitic skin rash. The other manifestations include cardiac disease, gastrointestinal involvement, peripheral neuropathy, and renal disease. Compared to adults with EGPA, children have a predominance of cardiopulmonary disease, lower rate of peripheral nerve involvement, and higher mortality [53].

Urticarial vasculitis

UV is extremely rare in children [13]. The entity in adults is described in detail in the section "Immune complex small vessel vasculitis," subsection "Urticarial vasculitis."

Acute hemorrhagic edema of infancy

It is a distinctive form of vasculitis occurring in infants and young children. The lesions are described as having a "cockade" (medallion) pattern, wherein the lesions appear as purpuric edematous annular or targetoid plaques with scalloped margins with a tendency to clear at the center. They may be

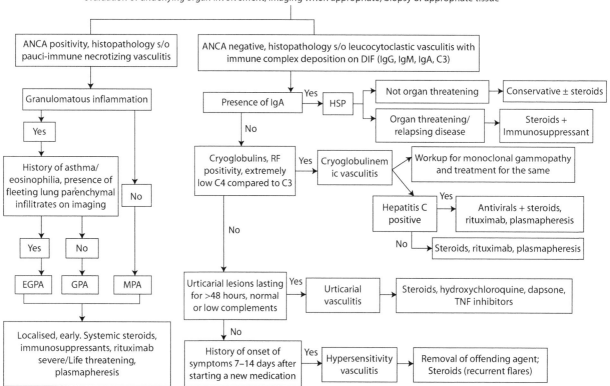

Algorithm for the management of suspected SVV (palpable purpura, scleritis, pulmonary-renal syndrome, neuropathy)

seen on the face, ears, or extremities. Facial edema may be present. The children are otherwise well. There may be a history of preceding upper respiratory or gastrointestinal infection [55]. Prognosis is good and children recover in 1–2 weeks. Symptomatic treatment with antihistamines and topical steroids helps to reduce the discomfort and hasten recovery.

CONCLUSION

Emergencies in small vessel vasculitis may be secondary to involvement of the gut, kidney, lung, respiratory system, musculoskeletal system, central and peripheral nervous systems, and sometimes the skin. Involvement of the skin with the classical lesions of palpable purpura facilitates rapid diagnosis, but in its absence, a high level of suspicion is required to arrive at a rapid diagnosis of SSV.

Following is an algorithm for the management of SSV.

KEY POINTS

- Small vessel vasculitis mainly involves the skin. However it too can have a variety of systemic manifestations as in medium vessel vasculitides.
- Palpable purpura symmetrically on the lower limbs is the hallmark.
- Urticaria, livedo, nodules and ulcers may also be resent.
- Lungs, kidneys, GI tract, heart, eye may also be variably involved.
- ANCA vasculitides have systemic involvement more predominantly.
- Oral corticosteroids, Pulse IV steroids and cyclophosphamide are the drugs of choice.
- Dapsone and colchicine are important second line dugs in CSSV.
- Prognosis depends on systemic involvement.

REFERENCES

1. Jennette JC, Falk RJ. Small-vessel vasculitis. *N Engl J Med* 1997;337:1512–23.
2. Hunder GG et al. The American College of Rheumatology 1990 criteria for the classification of vasculitis. Introduction. *Arthritis Rheum* 1990;33:1065–7.

3. Jennette JC et al. 2012 Revised International Chapel Hill Consensus Conference Nomenclature of Vasculitides. *Arthritis Rheum* 2013;65:1–11.

4. Iglesias Gamarra A, Matteson EL, Restrepo JF. Small vessel vasculitis. History, classification, etiology, histopathology, clinic, diagnosis and treatment. *Rev Colomb Reumatol* 2007;14:187–205.

5. Carlson JA, Cavaliere LF, Grant-Kels JM. Cutaneous vasculitis: Diagnosis and management. *Clin Dermatol* 2006;24:414–29.

6. Mullick FG, McAllister HA Jr, Wagner BM, Fenoglio JJ Jr. Drug related vasculitis. Clinicopathologic correlations in 30 patients. *Hum Pathol* 1979;10:313–25.

7. Blanco R, Martinez-Taboada VM, Rodriguez-Valverde V, Garcia-Fuentes M. Cutaneous vasculitis in children and adults. Associated diseases and etiologic factors in 303 patients. *Medicine (Baltim)* 1998;77:403–18.

8. Carlson JA, Ng BT, Chen KR. Cutaneous vasculitis update: Diagnostic criteria, classification, epidemiology, etiology, pathogenesis, evaluation and prognosis. *Am J Dermatopathol* 2005;27:504–28.

9. Bachmeyer C, Wetterwald E, Aractingi S. Cutaneous vasculitis in the course of hematologic malignancies. *Dermatology* 2005;210:8–14.

10. Krause ML, Cartin-Ceba R, Specks U, Peikert T. Update on diffuse alveolar hemorrhage and pulmonary vasculitis. *Immunol Allergy Clin North Am* 2012;32:587–600.

11. Greenhall GHB, Salama AD. What is new in the management of rapidly progressive glomerulonephritis? *Clin Kidney J* 2015;8:143–50.

12. Carlson JA. The histological assessment of cutaneous vasculitis. *Histopathology* 2010;56:3–23.

13. Alangari AA. Normocomplementemic urticarial vasculitis in a boy and his response to treatment. *Curr Pediatr Res* 2014;18:8–10.

14. Miller A, Chan M, Wiik A, Misbah SA, Luqmani RA. An approach to the diagnosis and management of systemic vasculitis revised version with tracked changes removed. *Clin Exp Immunol* 2010;160:143–60.

15. Savige J, Pollock W, Trevisin M. What do antineutrophil cytoplasmic antibodies (ANCA) tell us? *Best Pract Res Clin Rheumatol* 2005;19:263–76.

16. Management of adults with idiopathic cutaneous small vessel vasculitis. UpToDate. Available at: https://www.uptodate.com/contents/management-of-adults-with-idiopathic-cutaneous-small-vessel-vasculitis.

17. Sais G, Vidaller A, Jucgla A, Gallardo F, Peyri J. Colchicine in the treatment of cutaneous leukocytoclastic vasculitis. Results of a prospective, randomized controlled trial. *Arch Dermatol* 1995;131:1399–402.

18. Fredenberg MF, Malkinson FD. Sulfone therapy in the treatment of leukocytoclastic vasculitis. Report of three cases. *J Am Acad Dermatol* 1987;16:772–8.

19. Tosca AD, Ioannidou DJ, Katsantonis JC, Kyriakis KP. Cyclosporin A in the treatment of cutaneous vasculitis. Clinical and cellular effects. *J Eur Acad Dermatol Venereol* 1996;6:135–41.

20. El-Reshaid K, Madda JP. Rituximab therapy for severe cutaneous leukocytoclastic angiitis refractory to corticosteroids, cellcept and cyclophosphamide. *Case Rep Dermatol* 2013;5:115–9.

21. Ong CS, Benson EM. Successful treatment of chronic leucocytoclastic vasculitis and persistent ulceration with intravenous immunoglobulin. *Br J Dermatol* 2000;143:447–9.

22. Ramos-Casals M, Stone JH, Cid MC, Bosch X. The cryoglobulinaemias. *Lancet* 2012;379:348–60.

23. Lamprecht P, Gause A, Gross WL. Cryoglobulinemic vasculitis. *Arthritis Rheum* 1999;42:2507.

24. Giuggioli D, Manfredi A, Lumetti F, Sebastiani M, Ferri C. Cryoglobulinemic vasculitis and skin ulcers. Our therapeutic strategy and review of the literature. *Semin Arthritis Rheum* 2015;44:518.

25. Cohen SJ, Pittelkow MR, Su WP. Cutaneous manifestations of cryoglobulinemia: Clinical and histopathologic study of seventy-two patients. *J Am Acad Dermatol* 1991;25(1 Pt 1):21–7.

26. Tarantino A et al. Renal disease in essential mixed cryoglobulinaemia. Long-term follow-up of 44 patients. *Q J Med* 1981;50:1.

27. Weinberger A, Berliner S, Pinkhas J. Articular manifestations of essential cryoglobulinemia. *Semin Arthritis Rheum* 1981;10:224.

28. Ferri C, La Civita L, Cirafisi C, Siciliano G, Longombardo G, Bombardieri S, Rossi B. Peripheral neuropathy in mixed cryoglobulinemia: Clinical and electrophysiologic investigations. *J Rheumatol* 1992;19:889.

29. Pascual M, Perrin L, Giostra E, Schifferli JA. Hepatitis C virus in patients with cryoglobulinemia type II. *J Infect Dis* 1990;162:569.

30. Quartuccio L, Isola M, Corazza L, Ramos-Casals M, Retamozo S, Ragab GM et al. Validation of the classification criteria for cryoglobulinaemic vasculitis. *Rheumatology (Oxf)* 2014;53:2209.

31. Brouet JC, Clauvel JP, Danon F, Klein M, Seligmann M. Biologic and clinical significance of cryoglobulins. A report of 86 cases. *Am J Med* 1974;57:775–88.

32. McDuffie FC, Jr SW, Maldonado JE, Andreini PH, Conn DL, Samayoa EA. Hypocomplementemia with cutaneous vasculitis and arthritis. Possible immune complex syndrome. *Mayo Clin Proc* 1973;48:340.

33. Jachiet M et al. French Vasculitis Study Group. The clinical spectrum and therapeutic management of hypocomplementemic urticarial vasculitis: Data from a French nationwide study of fifty-seven patients. *Arthritis Rheumatol* 2015;67:527–34.

34. Houser SL, Askenase PW, Palazzo E, Bloch KJ. Valvular heart disease in patients with hypocomplementemic urticarial vasculitis syndrome associated

with Jaccoud's arthropathy. *Cardiovasc Pathol* 2002;11:210–6.

35. Ishikawa O, Miyachi Y, Watanabe H. Hypocomplementaemic urticarial vasculitis associated with Jaccoud's syndrome. *Br J Dermatol* 1997;137:804–7.

36. Cadnapaphornchai MA, Saulsbury FT, Norwood VF. Hypocomplementemic urticarial vasculitis: Report of a pediatric case. *Pediatr Nephrol* 2000;14:328–31.

37. Black AK. Urticarial vasculitis. *Clin Dermatol* 1999;17:565–9.

38. Falk RJ, Jennette JC. ANCA disease: Where is this field heading? *J Am Soc Nephrol* 2010;21:745–52.

39. Kallenberg CGM. Usefulness of antineutrophil cytoplasmic autoantibodies in diagnosing and managing systemic vasculitis. *Curr Opin Rheumatol* 2016;28:8–14.

40. Chen K-R, Carlson JA. Clinical approach to cutaneous vasculitis. *Am J Clin Dermatol* 2008;9:71–92.

41. Guillevin L et al. Microscopic polyangiitis: Clinical and laboratory findings in eighty-five patients. *Arthritis Rheum* 1999;42:421–30.

42. Duna GF, Galperin C, Hoffman GS. Wegener's granulomatosis. *Rheum Dis Clin North Am* 1995;21:949–86.

43. Chen K-R. Skin involvement in ANCA-associated vasculitis. *Clin Exp Nephrol* 2013;17:676–82.

44. Comarmond C, Cacoub P. Granulomatosis with polyangiitis (Wegener): Clinical aspects and treatment. *Autoimmun Rev* 2014;13:1121–5.

45. Kallenberg CGM. The diagnosis and classification of microscopic polyangiitis. *J Autoimmun* 2014;48,49:90–93.

46. Niles JL et al. The syndrome of lung hemorrhage and nephritis is usually an ANCA-associated condition. *Arch Intern Med* 1996;156:440e5.

47. Guillevin L et al. Prognostic factors in polyarteritis nodosa and Churg-Strauss syndrome. A prospective study in 342 patients. *Medicine (Baltimore)* 1996;75:17–28.

48. Patterson JW. *Weedon's Skin Pathology.* 4th ed. New York: Elsevier; 2015, Chapter 8, The vasculopathic reaction pattern: 195.

49. Ishibashi M, Kawahara Y, Chen KR. Spectrum of cutaneous vasculitis in eosinophilic granulomatosis with polyangiitis (Churg-Strauss): A case series. *Am J Dermatopathol* 2015;37:214–21.

50. Chu P, Connolly MK, LeBoit PE. The histopathologic spectrum of palisaded neutrophilic and granulomatous dermatitis in patients with collagen vascular disease. *Arch Dermatol* 1994;130:1278–83.

51. Yates M et al. EULAR/ERA-EDTA recommendations for the management of ANCA-associated vasculitis. *Ann Rheum Dis* 2016;75:1583–94.

52. Specks U et al. Efficacy of remission-induction regimens for ANCA-associated vasculitis. *N Engl J Med* 2013;369:414e27.

53. Zwerina J, Eger G, Englbrecht M, Manger B, Schett G. Churg-Strauss syndrome in childhood: A systematic literature review and clinical comparison with adult patients. *Semin Arthritis Rheum* 2009;39:108–15.

54. Ozen S et al. EULAR/PRES endorsed consensus criteria for the classification of childhood vasculitides. *Ann Rheum Dis* 2006;65:936–41.

55. Al-Sheyyab M, El-Shanti H, Ajlouni S, Sawalha D, Daoud A. The clinical spectrum of Henoch-Schönlein purpura in infants and children. *Eur J Pediatr* 1995;154:969–72.

56. Dolezalova P, Telekesova P, Nemcova D, Hoza J. Incidence of vasculitis in children in the Czech Republic: 2-year prospective epidemiology survey. *J Rheumatol* 2004;31:2295–9.

57. Trnka P. Henoch-Schönlein purpura in children. *J Pediatr Child Health* 2013;49:995–1003.

58. Ozen S, Pistorio A, Iusan SM, Bakkaloglu A, Herlin T, Brik R, Buoncompagni A; Paediatric Rheumatology International Trials Organisation (PRINTO). EULAR/PRINTO/PRES criteria for Henoch-Schönlein purpura, childhood polyarteritis nodosa, childhood Wegener granulomatosis and childhood Takayasu arteritis: Ankara 2008. Part II: Final classification criteria. *Ann Rheum Dis* 2010;69:798–806.

59. Chang WL, Yang YH, Lin YT, Chiang BL. Gastrointestinal manifestations of Henoch-Schönlein purpura. *Acta Paediatr* 2004;93:1427.

60. Soyer T, Egritas O, Atmaca E, Akman H, Ozturk H, Tezic T. Acute pancreatitis: A rare presenting feature of Henoch-Schönlein purpura. *J Paediatric Child Health* 2008;44:152–3.

61. Choong CK, Beasley SW. Intra-abdominal complications of Henoch-Schönlein purpura. *J Pediatr Child Health* 1998;34:405–9.

62. Jauhola O et al. Renal manifestations of Henoch-Schönlein purpura in a 6-month prospective study of 223 patients. *Arch Dis Child* 2010;95:877.

63. Davin JC, Coppo R. Henoch-Schönlein purpura nephritis in children. *Nat Rev Nephrol* 2014;10:563–73.

64. Belman AL, Leicher CR, Moshe SL, Mazey AP. Neurologic manifestations of Schönlein-Henoch purpura: Report of 3 cases and review of literature. *Pediatrics* 1985;75:687–92.

65. Ha TS, Lee JS. Scrotal involvement in childhood in Henoch-Schönlien purpura. *Acta Pediatr* 2007;96:552–5.

66. Vats KR, Vats A, Kim Y, Dassenko D, Sinaiko AR. Henoch-Schönlein purpura and pulmonary haemorrhage: A report and literature review. *Pediatr Nephrol* 1999;13:530–4.

67. Weiss PF, Feinstein JA, Feudtner C. Effects of corticosteroid on Henoch-Schönlein purpura: A systematic review. *Pediatrics* 2007;120:1079–87.

68. Bohm M et al. Clinical features of childhood granulomatosis with polyangiitis. *Pediatr Rheumatol* 2014;12:18.

69. Akikusa JD, Schneider R, Harvey EA, Hebert D, Thorner PS, Laxer RM, Silverman ED. Clinical features and outcome of pediatric Wegener's granulomatosis. *Arthrtis Rheum* 2007;57:837–44.

70. Cabral DA et al. Comparing presenting clinical features in 48 children with microscopic polyangiitis to 183 children who have granulomatosis with polyangiitis (Wegener's): An archive cohort study. *Arthritis Rheumatol* 2016;68:2514–26.

32

Medium vessel vasculitis

SUJAY KHANDPUR AND SUBUHI KAUL

INTRODUCTION

The Chapel Hill Consensus Conference 2012 (CHCC2012) defines medium vessels as main visceral arteries (and veins) and their initial branches and cutaneous vessels that contain a tunica media made of concentric layers of smooth muscles. These vessels in the skin are present either in deep reticular dermis of the septa or subcutaneous fat. The medium vessel vasculitides include polyarteritis nodosa (PAN) and Kawasaki disease (KD) [1,2]. However, it is important to note that two or more calibers of vessels may be affected in the same condition, i.e., combined small and medium vessel vasculitis, and it is the predominant type of vessel affected that forms the basis of this categorization [2].

Medium vessel vasculitis may only involve skin vasculature or manifest as a systemic vasculitis, and it is usually the latter that requires emergency management in an intensive care setting due to the occurrence of acute pulmonary insufficiency, renal or cardiac failure, or neurological and gastrointestinal (GI) complications [3].

POLYARTERITIS NODOSA

It may be a systemic necrotizing vasculitis (classic PAN) or a skin-limited disease (cutaneous PAN). Classic PAN is a multisystem necrotizing vasculitis, first described in 1866 by Kussmaul and Maier [4–6]. In 1903, the transmural nature of the inflammation was discovered by Ferrari, and he proposed the term *polyarteritis nodosa* [6]. It preferentially affects medium arteries of the kidneys, skin, GI tract, and nerves. Pulmonary capillaritis and glomerulonephritis are not features of PAN [3].

Epidemiology

The incidence of "classic" multisystem PAN ranges from 4–16 per million, and in approximately 10% of patients, the vasculitis is limited to the skin and referred to as *cutaneous PAN* (CPAN). PAN affects men four times more frequently than women. The most common population affected is middle-aged adults (40–60 years), although it can occur at any age [5].

Etiopathogenesis

The pathogenesis of PAN is heterogeneous and involves an interplay of antibodies against the endothelium, immune complex formation, cytokines, and adhesion molecules [3]. Classic findings of immune complex diseases, such as glomerulonephritis, and consumption of complement components are missing. Rather, renal involvement manifests as infarction or hemorrhage [7]. A recent study demonstrated the presence of antiphosphatidylserine–prothrombin complex IgM antibodies in 77.8% CPAN patients. This supports the hypothesis that an autoimmune response is elicited by prothrombin binding to apoptotic endothelial cells [6]. These antibodies can then activate the classical complement cascade giving rise to CPAN.

CPAN is associated with streptococcal infection, inflammatory bowel disease, minocycline therapy, and less commonly, hepatitis B virus (HBV), mycobacterial, and *Parvoviris B19* infections [6–8]. Classic PAN is associated with HBV infection in 7%–10% of patients [3,5]. Other infectious triggers of classic PAN are hepatitis C virus (HCV), human immunodeficiency virus (HIV), cytomegalovirus (CMV), and *Parvovirus B19* [9–12]. PAN is also associated with inflammatory diseases, drugs, and malignancies (e.g., hairy cell leukemia) [5].

Cutaneous polyarteritis nodosa

CLINICAL FEATURES

CPAN represents a skin-limited disease and accounts for 10% of cases [5]. The most frequent features are tender subcutaneous nodules, livedo reticularis, and ulcers. The nodules are often the first manifestation and are multiple, reddish-purple, and tender, ranging in size from 0.5 to 3 cm and with or without superimposed ulceration (Figure 32.1). Petechiae, palpable purpura, gangrene, and autoamputations may rarely be seen. An area of livedo reticularis surrounding an ulcer is characteristic of CPAN but may not be seen in every case (Figure 32.2). The most common site affected is the legs and less commonly the arms, forearms,

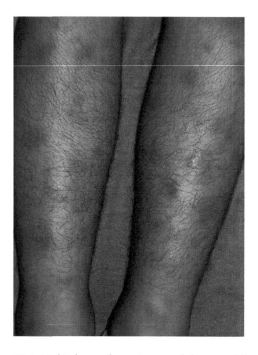

Figure 32.1 Multiple erythematous nodules over bilateral legs and feet suggestive of medium vessel vasculitis.

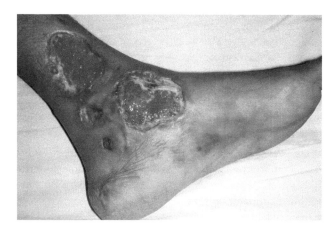

Figure 32.2 Multiple small and large punched-out ulcers with background livedo reticularis suggestive of medium vessel vasculitis.

trunk, head, and neck [6]. It may be accompanied by fever and constitutional symptoms and even neuropathy. A recent study found the prevalence of mononeuritis multiplex to be 22%, diagnosed by electromyoneurography in those complaining of paresthesia [8]. CPAN comprises a larger proportion of polyarteritis cases in children, approximately 30%, and is often preceded by streptococcal infections. It has a chronic relapsing course and rarely progresses to systemic PAN [5,6,13].

INVESTIGATIONS

A diagnosis of CPAN can be made based on clinical and histopathological features after ruling out systemic involvement. Since most cases of CPAN do not progress to classic PAN, it is imperative that a correct diagnosis is made, since treatment, disease course, and prognosis vary significantly [6].

A complete blood count; renal and liver function tests; urine analysis including urine routine and microscopy to look for dysmorphic red blood cells, proteinuria, and casts; a 24-hour urine protein analysis; and stool examination for occult blood should be done at baseline. The erythrocyte sedimentation rate (ESR) is raised in approximately 60% of patients. Hepatitis B surface antigen, anti-HCV antibody, HIV serology, and antistreptolysin-O titers are undertaken to evaluate any underlying etiological trigger [6].

Immunological workup includes tests for antineutrophil cytoplasmic antibodies (ANCAs), antinuclear antibodies (ANAs), rheumatoid factor, cryoglobulins, and complement levels. A negative immunological workup rules out other vasculitides, including systemic vasculitis and connective tissue diseases.

A negative test for ANCA and serological or microbiological evidence of streptococcal infection were added by European League Against Rheumatism (EULAR)/Paediatric Rheumatology European Society (PReS) in 2005 as criteria to diagnose CPAN [14,15].

Skin biopsies should be deep to include the subcutaneous tissue. Histopathological examination reveals necrotizing nongranulomatous vasculitis with fibrinoid necrosis of the arteriolar wall, fibrin thrombi in the lumen and predominantly neutrophilic infiltrate, karyorrhexis, and red blood cell extravasation involving the lower dermis and subcutaneous fat [6,15]. A Verhoeff-Van Gieson stain highlights the internal elastic lamina suggesting a medium vessel arteriolitis, but sometimes it may be partially destroyed or completely absent. CPAN must be differentiated from superficial thrombophlebitis (involvement of medium-caliber vein), since management profiles of the two entities differ.

TREATMENT

The course of CPAN varies from months to several years with several episodes of relapses and remissions. Mild cases respond well to nonsteroidal anti-inflammatory drugs (NSAIDs), colchicines, or dapsone [7]. Severe cases with cutaneous ulceration, associated nerve involvement and constitutional features warrant a course of oral corticosteroids: Prednisolone at a dose of 30 mg/day is usually effective; however, up to 1 mg/kg/day may be required to achieve remission. In those cases showing frequent relapses and requiring long-term systemic corticosteroids, an adjuvant may be added to prevent relapse after tapering steroids and to offset the adverse effects of high-dose/long-term steroids. Several steroid-sparing agents have been used: colchicine, hydroxychloroquine, NSAIDs, dapsone, azathioprine, methotrexate, cyclophosphamide, mycophenolate mofetil, and IV immunoglobulin [6,16]. Etanercept was recently reported to be effective in a case of refractory CPAN, but further studies are required [17].

Classic polyarteritis nodosa

CLINICAL FEATURES

PAN usually presents with constitutional symptoms of fever, malaise, myalgia, and weight loss along with features of multisystem involvement. The presentation varies widely: it may run an indolent course or lead to abrupt onset of life-threatening complications [18].

The peripheral nervous system and skin are most commonly affected [19,20]. Common cutaneous features include painful nodules located chiefly on the lower limbs, palpable purpura, retiform purpura, livedo racemosa, necrotic punched-out ulcers, and gangrene [3,5,18–21]. Neurological involvement frequently manifests as mononeuritis multiplex, which may present as paresthesias, wrist or foot drop, and uncommonly as symmetrical polyneuropathy [3]. Renal involvement typically manifests as hypertension and/or renal failure [5]. Less commonly, acute renal hemorrhage can occur, presenting with flank mass, acute flank pain, and hypovolemic shock (Lenk triad—a representation of Wünderlich syndrome) [21–24]. Several cases have been reported where spontaneous aneurysmal rupture with renal/perirenal hemorrhage and life-threatening shock were the presenting features in cases of undiagnosed PAN [23,25–27]. In fact, a meta-analysis found that the most common vascular cause of spontaneous perirenal hemorrhage was PAN [28]. These cases require immediate medical and surgical intervention, as untreated cases have significant mortality. GI involvement manifests as mesenteric ischemia or infarction, bowel perforation or hemorrhage, cholecystitis, pancreatitis, and appendicitis and is found in 14%–65% cases. The most common GI symptom encountered is postprandial abdominal pain due to mesenteric ischemia [21,29–31]. An acute surgical abdomen presentation requiring emergency intervention, in up to one-third of cases, may occur in patients who develop small intestine hemorrhage or perforation [7]. Hepatitis manifests as an elevation in transaminases and is usually clinically silent [29]. Cerebral infarcts due to vasculitic occlusion or thrombotic microangiopathy are a rare complication [5]. Orchitis manifesting as testicular pain and cardiomyopathy causing dyspnea are seen more commonly in those with HBV-associated disease [9]. Cardiac involvement is due to myocardial damage secondary to coronary artery vasculitis

or secondary uncontrolled hypertension. Cardiac failure is the most common manifestation, whereas myocardial infarction is rare [32]. Less commonly, involvement of the lower limbs in the form of myositis or acute compartment syndrome due to ruptured aneurysms has been reported [33–37]. These patients present with abrupt-onset leg pain with an inability to walk. Other organs are rarely involved, and the lungs are usually spared [5,21]. The clinical features of PAN are summarized in Table 32.1.

Table 32.1 Clinical manifestations in polyarteritis nodosa

Clinical feature	Frequency (%)
Constitutional symptoms	93.1
• Fever	
• Weight loss	
• Myalgia	
• Arthralgia	
Neurologic	40–88.9
• Mononeuritis	
• Polyneuropathy	
Cutaneous	28–58
• Nodules	
• Livedo	
• Purpura	
• Ulcers	
Gastrointestinal	14–44
• Ischemia	
• Perforation	
Renal	8–66
• Hypertension	
• Infarction	
• Hemorrhage	
Testes	2–18
• Orchitis	
Ophthalmologic	3–44
• Retinal exudates	
• Keratitis	
• Uveitis	
Vascular malformation	6
• Ischemia	
• Necrosis	
• Claudication	
Cardiac	4–30
• Cardiomyopathy	
• Pericarditis	
Central nervous system	2–28
• Cerebral infarcts	
• Confusion	
Respiratory	3–5
• Pleurisy	
• Pleural effusion	

Source: Pagnoux C et al. *Arthritis Rheum* 2010;62(2):616–26; Hernández-Rodríguez J et al. *J Autoimmun* 2014;48-49:84–9; Sharma A et al. *Int J Rheum Dis* 2017;20(3):390–7; Matsuo S et al. *Intern Med* 2017;56(11):1435–8.

DIFFERENTIAL DIAGNOSIS

The clinical differentials of PAN include ANCA-associated vasculitis, erythema nodosum (EN), erythema induratum, autoimmune connective tissue disease, and cryoglobulinemic vasculitis. Thromboembolic conditions such as antiphospholipid syndrome, cholesterol emboli, and infective endocarditis should be excluded [5].

A diagnosis based on clinical findings alone is challenging, and ANCA serology, laboratory tests for renal involvement, and chest imaging are required to rule out ANCA-associated vasculitides [38].

Erythema nodosum is not associated with livedo, retiform purpura, or ulceration, and the presence of such lesions should raise suspicion of a vasculitic process. Histopathology helps rule out this condition, as septal panniculitis without vasculitis is observed in EN [6]. Erythema induratum (nodular vasculitis) may or may not ulcerate and can mimic PAN. Histopathology shows evidence of granulomatous lobular panniculitis with vasculitis [39].

In hypercoagulable states a complete coagulation profile including prothrombin time, aPTT, proteins C and S activity, homocysteine level, lupus anticoagulant, anticardiolipin, β-2-glycoprotein-1, factor V Leiden, and anti-thrombin III genetic test are required to differentiate them [40].

PROGNOSIS

The prognosis of PAN in patients on treatment has improved, with the 5-year survival being 80%. The 5-year survival for untreated cases is 13% [41,42].

The prognosis for those with HBV-associated disease is lower. With fulminant or multiorgan disease, 5-year survival is lower than 15% [21]. GI involvement in the form of mesenteric ischemia has a poor prognosis with a 50% 1-year survival rate [5].

The French Vasculitis Study Group (FVSG) developed a "Five Factor Score" (FFS) as a prognostic tool for the evaluation of patients with various types of vasculitis, including PAN [7]. A revised FFS based on additional data was proposed in 2011, and for PAN comprises only four factors that are associated with greater mortality [43]:

1. Age more than 65 years
2. Cardiac symptoms
3. GI involvement
4. Renal dysfunction (plasma creatinine >1.7 mg/dL)

INVESTIGATIONS AND DIAGNOSIS

There are no diagnostic laboratory tests for PAN. These laboratory tests can aid in determining the degree of organ involvement and excluding the differential diagnoses.

Laboratory tests that should be done are as follows:

1. Serum creatinine and blood urea nitrogen (BUN)
2. Muscle enzyme concentrations
3. Liver function studies
4. Viral markers—HIV, HBV, and HCV serologies
5. Urine analysis
6. Acute-phase proteins—ESR and CRP
7. Blood culture—to exclude infective endocarditis
8. ANCA
9. Antinuclear antibody, Anti-Sm
10. Complement level—C3, C4
11. Cryoglobulins
12. Serum electrophoresis—Rule out monoclonal gammopathy

Characteristic changes on angiography aid in the diagnosis of PAN. Cross-sectional imaging and arteriography may be used in place of histopathology for diagnosis of classic PAN and are usually performed on the renal or mesenteric circulation [33]. Angiographic findings, namely, aneurysms, ectasias, and occlusive arterial disease, are found in 40%–90% of patients, coincident with the onset of clinical symptoms [45].

A rapid diagnosis is necessary in cases with life-threatening complications, i.e., renal/perirenal hemorrhage, acute renal failure, hepatic infarct, cardiac failure, and GI hemorrhage or perforation [21].

Noninvasive modalities such as computed tomography (CT) and magnetic resonance imaging (MRI) can identify infarcts and delineate hemorrhages. These may be preferred in patients with decreased glomerular filtration rate, in whom use of contrast for angiography is contraindicated [21,45].

In 1990, the American College of Rheumatology established 10 criteria for classifying PAN based on the clinical and laboratory features. These are tabulated in Table 32.2. They found that the presence of 3 out of 10 features had a sensitivity of 82.2% and specificity of 86.6% [21,44].

TREATMENT

The severity of disease with regard to organs involved and associated dysfunction guides the management. Glucocorticoids are the mainstay of treatment with remission rates of 50%. Mild forms of classic PAN are often treated

Table 32.2 The American College of Rheumatology classification criteria for polyarteritis nodosa

Clinical features	Laboratory-based findings
• Livedo reticularis	• Diastolic blood pressure >90 mm Hg
• Myalgias	• Blood urea nitrogen >40 mg/dL or serum creatinine >1.5 mg/dL
• Testicular pain/tenderness	• Positive hepatitis B virus serology
• Mononeuropathy or polyneuropathy	• Histopathology showing presence of neutrophilic or mixed leukocytic infiltration of arterial walls
• Involuntary weight loss of 4 kg or more	• Abnormalities on arteriography

Source: Howard T et al. Tech Vasc Interv Radiol 2014;17(4):247–51.

with 1 mg/kg/day followed by tapering, with a minimal dose being continued for 9–12 months [3,7]. Other adjuvants used are azathioprine (2 mg/kg/day), mycophenolate mofetil (2–3 g/day), or methotrexate (20–25 mg/week) [3,47].

The use of cyclophosphamide in addition has increased the remission rate to nearly 90% [21]. It must be considered in all cases with critical organ involvement or severe disease [3,7]. According to the EULAR recommendations, for primary medium vessel vasculitis, combined use of cyclophosphamide and glucocorticoid achieves better disease control and longer remission as compared to glucocorticoid alone. However, there is no appreciable effect on long-term survival [46]. Cyclophosphamide can be administered either intravenously or orally. IV pulse cyclophosphamide is commonly used at a dose of 600 mg/m^2 (up to 1.2 g) at intervals of 2–4 weeks, while oral cyclophosphamide is administered at 2 mg/kg/day (up to 200 mg/day) with dose adjustments made for age [7]. Reduction of cyclophosphamide dose by 25% for those above 60 years and by 50% for patients above 75 years of age is recommended [46].

Refractory disease has been successfully treated with several biological agents, including infliximab, etanercept, tocilizumab, and rituximab [17,48,50–53].

The treatment of HBV-associated PAN requires the addition of lamivudine and a short duration of corticosteroids. Plasmapheresis aids in the control of more severe cases [7]. PAN associated with HCV has been managed with ribavirin, pegylated interferon-α, along with immunosuppressive agents including corticosteroids, cyclophosphamide, and rituximab [47].

KAWASAKI DISEASE

Introduction

Kawasaki disease (KD), also known as mucocutaneous lymph node syndrome, is a medium vessel vasculitis with an uncertain etiology. In 1967, Tomisaku Kawasaki first described this vasculitic syndrome in Japanese children [54]. The main complication of KD is coronary artery aneurysms, and it is the most common acquired cause of pediatric cardiac disease in the developed world [5,55]. A recent Japanese study found acute cardiac events, i.e., myocardial infarction and coronary artery revascularization or death, in 21% of KD patients [56]. However, with prompt treatment, the risk of coronary artery aneurysms is reduced to approximately 5% [57]. This highlights the need for a correct and rapid diagnosis to decrease cardiovascular complications.

Epidemiology

KD is a disease of childhood; nearly 75%–88% of affected cases are less than 5 years of age [55]. Cases that have been reported in adolescents and adults are associated with higher morbidity and mortality [58]. It is slightly more common in males, with a male-to-female ratio of 1.5:1 [54].

The incidence varies widely with ethnicities and geographical location. Currently, the incidence of KD reported from North America, Europe, and Australia is 4–25 per 100,000 children below 5 years, whereas a much higher incidence was found in Japan at 265/100,000 [54,57]. Its incidence in the United States was found to be the highest among Asians and Pacific Islanders, followed by African Americans and Hispanics, and was the lowest in Caucasians [55,58].

Etiopathogenesis

Although the exact etiology of KD is unknown, several factors suggest an infectious agent, with a resultant cascade of immune responses leading to the disease. Seasonal variation and clustering of KD cases have been extensively studied over a 14-year period in Japan. There is marked increase in incidence during the winter and spring months [59]. The typical clinical presentation of fever with rash resembling other infectious childhood illnesses, its low recurrence rate, and the tendency to affect infants older than 6 months point toward an environmental trigger [54,59].

Both viral and bacterial agents have been implicated as triggers. Multiple viruses are suggested pathogens: Ebstein-Barr, varicella zoster, parainfluenza, CMV, chikungunya, human metapneumonia, and coxsackie [60].

Bacterial superantigens have also been thought to act as triggers, due to the presence of genes encoding superantigens in the stool of 70% patients versus 26% in healthy controls [5,61].

KD patients have a genetic predisposition to the development of the disease and its complications [54]. Multiple studies have identified single nucleotide polymorphisms that have an immunoregulatory function and are associated with susceptibility to KD, coronary artery aneurysms, and resistance to IV immunoglobulin [54]. Genome-wide association studies found an activating IgG receptor, FcgRIIa or CD32a, a protein on an antigen-presenting cell surface, CD40, and a tyrosine kinase encoding gene, BLK, to have a significant association with KD. Another recent and significant polymorphism found to be associated with predisposition to KD is inositol 1,4,5-triphosphate 3-kinase C gene (ITPKC) [5,54].

Clinical features

KD should be suspected in any child presenting with unexplained and prolonged fever associated with cutaneous changes. The pyrexia is usually high grade and spiking (>39°C/102°F) and may be resistant to antipyretics that lasts from 1 to 3 weeks if untreated [62].

The cutaneous exanthem, often manifesting as a diffusely maculopapular (morbilliform) rash (Figures 32.3 and 32.4) occurs in greater than 80% of patients. Uncommonly, scarlatiniform erythroderma, erythema multiforme–like, urticarial or pustular lesions may also be present [5]. The rash usually begins within 5 days of the onset of fever. Involvement of the trunk and extremities with desquamation in the groin area is an early and characteristic finding [5,62].

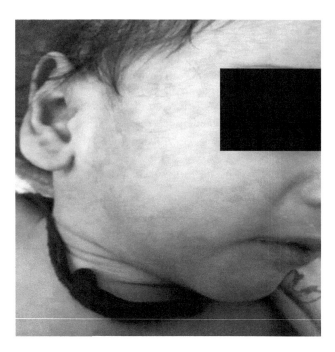

Figure 32.3 Maculopapular eruption on face of a child with Kawasaki disease.

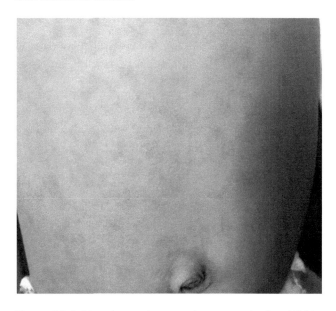

Figure 32.4 Maculopapular eruption on trunk of a child in a case of Kawasaki disease.

The bulbar conjunctiva is diffusely congested with sparing of the perilimbal area, and anterior uveitis may be evident on slit-lamp examination, usually in the first week of fever. Erythema, dryness, fissuring of the lips, and an erythematous tongue with prominence of fungiform papillae (strawberry tongue) are characteristic oral changes. There may also be diffuse erythema of the oropharyngeal mucosa.

The most infrequent but important clinical feature is cervical lymphadenopathy. Usually there is nonsuppurative, unilateral lymphadenopathy with multiple lymph node enlargement, present in the anterior cervical triangle with size more than 1.5 cm in diameter.

Table 32.3 Criteria for diagnosis of Kawasaki disease

Required criterion	At least four of five principal features

Fever lasting 5 or more days	1. Polymorphous exanthem
	2. Acral changes
	    Early: Erythema/edema of hands and feet
	    Late: Desquamation of hands and feet
	3. Cervical lymphadenopathy (commonly unilateral)
	4. Bilateral nonexudative conjunctival congestion
	5. Oropharyngeal changes
	    Strawberry tongue
	    Lip dryness, cracking, fissures, and bleeding
	    Diffuse mucosal erythema

Source: Wei YJ et al. Echocardiography 2016;33(5):764–70.

The diagnosis of "classic" KD is made clinically and is based on the presence of fever and principal features (Table 32.3).

In those with fever of less than 5 days (3–4 days), a diagnosis of classic KD may still be made when ≥4 principal clinical features, especially acral changes, are present. A diagnosis of incomplete KD may be made even if a few or none of the principal features are present. Prolonged fever of ≥5 days with coronary artery abnormalities are considered confirmatory [62].

Cardiovascular manifestations during the acute/subacute phase or after convalescence are the main contributors to morbidity and mortality and make prompt diagnosis and treatment essential. During the acute episode, all three layers of the heart, i.e., the pericardium, myocardium, and endocardium, may be inflamed. A hyperdynamic precordium with tachycardia, systolic flow murmurs, and a gallop rhythm due to decreased ventricular compliance as a result of myocardial inflammation may be present in the acute phase. Myocarditis has been demonstrated in 50%–70% of KD patients [62].

Coronary artery abnormalities in the acute phase of KD are aneurysmal dilations that are usually evident on echocardiography by the 10th day of fever. The incidence of coronary artery abnormalities ranges from 2.9% to 13% [63]. Even with extensive or large aneurysms, patients become symptomatic only if myocardial ischemia develops due to luminal obstruction/thrombosis [62]. Giant coronary aneurysms, which are the most severe cardiac manifestation of KD, occur in 0.2% cases. They are associated with coronary stenosis, a higher incidence of myocardial infarction, and sudden death [64]. Rarely, during the acute illness, coronary artery rupture resulting in myocardial ischemia, fatal arrythmias, and cardiac tamponade have been reported [63]. Symptoms/signs of myocardial ischemia and infarction in infants may go unrecognized; thus, urgent echocardiography in all suspected cases of KD is mandatory.

Aneurysms of other medium-sized arteries, e.g., axillary, brachial, femoral, and mesenteric arteries, may occur in those with severe coronary artery abnormalities. Rarely, involvement of extremity arteries can result in peripheral gangrene and, consequently, loss of digits [62].

Valve dysfunction, especially mitral valve involvement, occurs in 23%–27% of patients leading to regurgitant murmurs. These however are transient, mild, to moderate in severity and resolve as the acute episode abates [62].

Kawasaki disease shock syndrome (KDSS) is a potentially fatal manifestation of myocarditis and must be managed urgently. In KDSS, hypotensive shock occurs, necessitating administration of volume expanders, vasoactive agents, and intensive care [65–67].

Central nervous system involvement manifests as irritability, hearing loss, facial nerve palsy, or aseptic meningitis. Diarrhea, abdominal pain, vomiting, jaundice, and pancreatitis are signs and symptoms of GI involvement. Pulmonary nodules or infiltrates may be found on chest x-ray. Arthralgias or arthritis and urethritis or hydrocele are other relatively uncommon associated features [62].

The term *atypical KD* has often been used interchangeably with *incomplete KD*, but this should be reserved for cases that present with uncommon or rare findings, such as transient sensorineural hearing loss, transient lower motor neuron facial nerve palsy, hepatomegaly with jaundice, and acalculous gallbladder enlargement [68].

Differential diagnoses

There are several febrile childhood illnesses that may present a diagnostic challenge, especially early in the course of KD or in the absence of the complete clinical picture. The following conditions may resemble KD and need to be ruled out:

- *Viral infections*: Measles, adenoviral and enteroviral infections
- *Bacterial toxin-mediated disease*: Scarlet fever, staphylococcal or streptococcal toxic shock syndrome
- *Stevens-Johnson syndrome and other drug hypersensitivity exanthems*
- *Systemic-onset juvenile idiopathic arthritis*
- *Rickettsial fever*, e.g., Rocky Mountain spotted fever
- *Leptospirosis*

Investigations

Diagnosis is based on fulfillment of the KD criteria. Laboratory data may act as supportive evidence in case of incomplete or atypical KD. Erythrocyte sedimentation rate and C-reactive protein are almost always raised, and normal levels are unlikely in true KD. Similarly, thrombocytosis after 1 week of fever and leukocytosis supports a diagnosis of KD [62,68].

SUPPLEMENTAL LABORATORY TESTS

- Hemoglobin < reference range for age [68]
- Raised leukocyte count (>15,000/mm^3 with granulocyte predominance)
- Thrombocytosis after 1 week of fever (>4,50,000 cells/mm^3)
- Raised alanine transaminase (greater than the reference range)
- Hypoalbuminemia (<3 mg/dL)
- Sterile pyuria (>10 WBC/high-power field)

Thrombocytosis is a late feature and can be seen in the second week of illness; it usually resolves in 1–2 months. Anemia is frequently present and is normocytic normochromic. Of the markers of inflammation, ESR increases with IV immunoglobulin (IVIg); therefore, CRP is considered a better marker of treatment response.

ECHOCARDIOGRAPHY

Echocardiography is the primary noninvasive tool for cardiac assessment in KD, during both the acute phase and long-term follow-up [49,54]. A baseline echocardiogram establishes a baseline to enable long-term follow-up of coronary artery morphology, valvular abnormalities, left ventricular wall motion, and pericardial effusion [54]. In uncomplicated cases, the echocardiogram should be repeated after 1–2 weeks of treatment and after 4–6 weeks after treatment. More frequent, twice weekly, monitoring is recommended for those with severe involvement and should be continued until there is arrest of progression [62].

OTHER IMAGING TECHNIQUES

Conventional angiography is the gold standard for visualization of the coronary vasculature; however, it is invasive and causes children to be exposed to radiation. CT angiography and cardiac MRI are alternatives [54]. These imaging techniques are not routinely used in the diagnosis and management of KD [62].

Treatment

Early diagnosis and treatment with a single, high dose of IVIg (2 g/kg) reduces the occurrence of coronary artery disease in KD, which has been corroborated by meta-analyses [69]. IVIg should be administered as soon as the diagnosis is made or within 10 days of onset [62]. Beyond the 10th day, IVIg should be administered only if there is evidence of ongoing inflammation—persistent fever, coronary artery abnormalities, and raised inflammatory markers (ESR and CRP). Posttreatment elevations in ESR alone should not be considered to indicate IVIg resistance [62].

Aspirin, administered for its antiplatelet and anti-inflammatory action, is used at doses varying from 30 mg/kg/day to 100 mg/kg/day during the acute phase of KD. Usually, this high dose is continued until 48–72 hours after fever subsides, following which a low dose of 3–5 mg/kg/day is maintained up to 2 months of fever onset. In cases with persistent coronary artery abnormalities, aspirin is continued indefinitely [62].

A recent meta-analysis on the use of corticosteroids (IV prednisolone 2 mg/kg/day for 5 days followed by tapering oral doses for a few weeks) in KD found that, if administered as an adjuvant along with IVIg, corticosteroids decreased the risk of development of coronary artery abnormalities [49].

In cases with IVIg resistance, characterized by persistence or recurrence of fever after 36 hours of IVIg, a second dose of IVIg can be administered. Other options are adjuvant corticosteroids, infliximab, etanercept, anakinra, cyclosporine, cyclophosphamide, or plasma exchange [62].

CONCLUSION

Medium vessel vasculitis (PAN) may be skin limited or be associated with systemic involvement. A complete workup of each patient based on clinical signs and symptoms is mandatory. Patients must be followed closely as this entity may evolve and progress over a period of time. Sometimes the first skin biopsy may not be helpful, and subsequent biopsies from well-established lesions may clinch the diagnosis. Treatment and prognosis differ significantly in skin-limited versus classic PAN.

Prolonged high-grade pyrexia associated with exanthemata and acral/mucosal changes, in children less than 5 years, should arouse suspicion of Kawasaki disease, which requires urgent echocardiography and prompt treatment.

KEY POINTS

- Characteristic cutaneous features of PAN are tender nodules, livedo reticularis, and punched-out ulcers. Consider systemic involvement in any case with unexplained abdominal pain, uncontrolled hypertension, renal dysfunction, focal neurologic deficits, or shortness of breath.
- Rule out systemic involvement at baseline.
- Rule out possible underlying conditions, e.g., connective tissue disorder and infections.
- Treatment is determined by the extent of involvement, severity of cutaneous disease, and presence of underlying conditions.
- Suspect Kawasaki disease in children with prolonged high-grade fever with characteristic mucocutaneous changes.
- Baseline and follow-up echocardiography is a must in all cases of Kawasaki disease.
- Prompt initiation of IV immunoglobin and aspirin reduces morbidity and mortality.
- Corticosteroids may be used as an adjuvant to reduce the risk of coronary artery abnormalities.

REFERENCES

1. Goldsmith LA, Katz S, Gilchrest BA, Paller AS, Leffell DJ WK. *Fitzpatrick's Dermatology in General Medicine*. 8th ed. Singapore: McGraw-Hill; 2012:2013–29.

2. Jennette JC et al. 2012 Revised International Chapel Hill Consensus Conference Nomenclature of Vasculitides. *Arthritis Rheum* 2013;65(1):1–11.
3. Wolff R, Parish LC. *Dermatology, Emergency*. 2nd ed. Boca Raton, FL: CRC Press, Taylor and Francis Group; 2017:226–35.
4. Erden A et al. Comparing polyarteritis nodosa in children and adults: A single center study. *Int J Rheum Dis* 2017;20(8):1016–22.
5. Bolognia JL, Jorizzo JL, Schaffer J V. *Dermatology*. 3rd ed. China: Elsevier Health Sciences; 2012:385–409.
6. Morgan AJ, Schwartz RA. Cutaneous polyarteritis nodosa: A comprehensive review. *Int J Dermatol* 2010;49(7):750–6.
7. De Virgilio A et al. Polyarteritis nodosa: A contemporary overview. *Autoimmun Rev* 2016;15(6):564–70.
8. Criado PR, Marques GF, Morita TC, de Carvalho JF. Epidemiological, clinical and laboratory profiles of cutaneous polyarteritis nodosa patients: Report of 22 cases and literature review. *Autoimmun Rev* 2016;15(6):558–63.
9. Pagnoux C et al. Clinical features and outcomes in 348 patients with polyarteritis nodosa: A systematic retrospective study of patients diagnosed between 1963 and 2005 and entered into the French Vasculitis Study Group Database. *Arthritis Rheum* 2010;62(2):616–26.
10. Calabrese LH. Vasculitis and infection with the human immunodeficiency virus. *Rheum Dis Clin North Am* 1991;17(1):131–47.
11. Corman LC, Dolson DJ. Polyarteritis nodosa and *Parvovirus B19* infection. *Lancet* 1992;339(8791):491.
12. Pagnoux C, Cohen P, Guillevin L. Vasculitides secondary to infections. *Clin Exp Rheumatol* 2006;24(2 Suppl. 41):71–81.
13. Ozen S. The changing face of polyarteritis nodosa and necrotizing vasculitis. *Nat Rev Rheumatol* 2017 11;13(6):381–6.
14. Ozen S et al. EULAR/PReS endorsed consensus criteria for the classification of childhood vasculitides. *Ann Rheum Dis* 2006;65:936–41.
15. Matteoda MA, Stefano PC, Bocián M, Katsicas MM, Sala J, Cervini AB. Cutaneous polyarteritis nodosa. *An Bras Dermatol* 2015;90:S188–90.
16. Parperis K, Rast F. Inner peace: Cutaneous polyarteritis nodosa. *Am J Med* 2017;130(7):796–8.
17. Inoue N, Shimizu M, Mizuta M, Ikawa Y, Yachie A. Refractory cutaneous polyarteritis nodosa: Successful treatment with etanercept. *Pediatr Int* 2017;59(6):751–2.
18. Hernández-Rodríguez J, Alba MA, Prieto-González S, Cid MC. Diagnosis and classification of polyarteritis nodosa. *J Autoimmun* 2014;48-49:84–9.
19. Shimojima Y, Ishii W, Kishida D, Fukushima K, Ikeda S-I. Imbalanced expression of dysfunctional regulatory T cells and T-helper cells relates

to immunopathogenesis in polyarteritis nodosa. *Mod Rheumatol* 2017;27(1):102–9.

20. Sharma A et al. Polyarteritis nodosa in north India: Clinical manifestations and outcomes. *Int J Rheum Dis* 2017;20(3):390–7.

21. Howard T, Ahmad K, Swanson JA, Misra S. Polyarteritis nodosa. *Tech Vasc Interv Radiol* 2014;17(4):247–51.

22. Katabathina VS, Katre R, Prasad SR, Surabhi VR, Shanbhogue AKP, Sunnapwar A. Wunderlich syndrome: Cross-sectional imaging review. *J Comput Assist Tomogr* 2011;35(4):425–33.23.

23. Beirão P, Teixeira L, Pereira P, Coelho ML. Wunderlich's syndrome as a manifestation of polyarteritis nodosa. *BMJ Case Rep* 2017;2017:bcr2016218478.

24. Chandrakantan A, Kaufman J. Renal hemorrhage in polyarteritis nodosa: Diagnosis and management. *Am J Kidney Dis* 1999;33(6):e8.

25. Sautter T, Trinkler FB, Sulser T, Schöpke W, Hauri D. Spontaneous perirenal hemorrhage after rupture of an aneurysm in case of polyarteritis nodosa along with anuric renal failure. Case report and review of the literature. *Urol Int* 1997;59(3):188–90.

26. Smith DL, Wernick R. Spontaneous rupture of a renal artery aneurysm in polyarteritis nodosa: Critical review of the literature and report of a case. *Am J Med* 1989;87(4):464–7.

27. Choi H-I et al. Bilateral spontaneous perirenal hemorrhage due to initial presentation of polyarteritis nodosa. *Case Rep Med* 2015;1–4.

28. Zhang JQ, Fielding JR, Zou KH. Etiology of spontaneous perirenal hemorrhage: A meta-analysis. *J Urol* 2002;167(4):1593–6.

29. Ebert EC, Hagspiel KD, Nagar M, Schlesinger N. Gastrointestinal involvement in polyarteritis nodosa. *Clin Gastroenterol Hepatol* 2008;6(9):960–6.

30. Fernandes SRM, Samara AM, Magalhães EP, Sachetto Z, Metze K. Acute cholecystitis at initial presentation of polyarteritis nodosa. *Clin Rheumatol* 2005;24(6):625–7.

31. Suresh E, Beadles W, Welsby P, Luqmani R. Acute pancreatitis with pseudocyst formation in a patient with polyarteritis nodosa. *J Rheumatol* 2005;32(2):386–8.

32. Chasset F, Francès C. Cutaneous manifestations of medium- and large-vessel vasculitis. *Clin Rev Allergy Immunol* 2017;53(3):452–68.

33. Gago R, Shum LM, Vilá LM. Right upper quadrant abdominal pain as the initial presentation of polyarteritis nodosa. *BMJ Case Rep* 2017 22;2017:bcr2016218019.

34. Calvo R, Negri M, Ortiz A, Roverano S, Paira S. Myositis as the initial presentation of panarteritis nodosa. *Rheumatol Clin* 2017. pii: S1699-258X(17)30169-9. doi: 10.1016/j.reuma.2017.06.010. [Epub ahead of print].

35. Hasaniya N, Katzen JT. Acute compartment syndrome of both lower legs caused by ruptured tibial

artery aneurysm in a patient with polyarteritis nodosa: A case report and review of literature. *J Vasc Surg* 1993;18(2):295–8.

36. Yang SN, Cho NS, Choi HS, Choi SJ, Yoon E-S, Kim DH. Muscular polyarteritis nodosa. *J Clin Rheumatol* 2012;18(5):249–52.

37. Balbir-Gurman A, Nahir AM, Braun-Moscovici Y. Intravenous immunoglobulins in polyarteritis nodosa restricted to the limbs: Case reports and review of the literature. *Clin Exp Rheumatol* 2007;25(1 Suppl. 44):S28–30.

38. Marzano AV, Raimondo MG, Berti E, Meroni PL, Ingegnoli F. Cutaneous manifestations of ANCA associated small vessels vasculitis. *Clin Rev Allergy Immunol* 2017;53(3):428–38.

39. Kazandjieva J, Antonov D, Kamarashev J, Tsankov N. Acrally distributed dermatoses: Vascular dermatoses (purpura and vasculitis). *Clin Dermatol* 2017;35(1):68–80.

40. Dabiri G, Damstetter E, Chang Y, Baiyee Ebot E, Powers JG, Phillips T. Coagulation disorders and their cutaneous presentations: Diagnostic work-up and treatment. *J Am Acad Dermatol* 2016;74(5):795–804.

41. Frohnert PP, Sheps SG. Long-term follow-up study of periarteritis nodosa. *Am J Med* 1967;43(1):8–14.

42. Balow JE. Renal vasculitis. *Kidney Int* 1985;27(6):954–64.

43. Guillevin L et al. The five-factor score revisited: Assessment of prognoses of systemic necrotizing vasculitides based on the French Vasculitis Study Group (FVSG) cohort. *Medicine (Baltim)* 2011;90(1):19–27.

44. Lightfoot RW et al. The American College of Rheumatology 1990 criteria for the classification of polyarteritis nodosa. *Arthritis Rheum* 1990;33(8):1088–93.

45. Stanson AW et al. Polyarteritis nodosa: Spectrum of angiographic findings. *Radiographics* 2001;21(1): 151–9.

46. Mukhtyar C et al. EULAR recommendations for the management of primary small and medium vessel vasculitis. *Ann Rheum Dis* 2009;68(3):310–7.

47. Forbess L, Bannykh S. Polyarteritis nodosa. *Rheum Dis Clin North Am* 2015;41(1):33–46.

48. Matsuo S et al. The successful treatment of refractory polyarteritis nodosa using infliximab. *Intern Med* 2017;56(11):1435–8.

49. Campanilho-Marques R, Ramos F, Canhão H, Fonseca JE. Remission induced by infliximab in childhood polyarteritis nodosa refractory to conventional immunosuppression and rituximab. *Jt Bone Spine* 2014;81(3):277–8.

50. Mori M, Miyamae T, Imagawa T, Katakura S, Kimura K, Yokota S. Meta-analysis of the results of intravenous gamma globulin treatment of coronary artery lesions in Kawasaki disease. *Mod Rheumatol* 2004;14(5):361–6.

51. Saunier A, Issa N, Vandenhende M-A, Morlat P, Doutre M-S, Bonnet F. Treatment of polyarteritis nodosa with tocilizumab: A new therapeutic approach? *RMD Open* 2017;3(1):e000446.

52. Seri Y et al. A case of refractory polyarteritis nodosa successfully treated with rituximab. *Mod Rheumatol* 2017;27(4):696–8.

53. Ribeiro E et al. Rituximab efficacy during a refractory polyarteritis nodosa flare. *Case Rep Med* 2009; 2009:738293. Published online 2010.

54. Dietz SM et al. Dissecting Kawasaki disease: A state-of-the-art review. *Eur J Pediatr* 2017;176(8):995–1009.

55. Uehara R, Belay ED. Epidemiology of Kawasaki disease in Asia, Europe, and the United States. *J Epidemiol* 2012;22(2):79–85.

56. Tsuda E, Tsujii N, Hayama Y. Cardiac events and the maximum diameter of coronary artery aneurysms in Kawasaki disease. *J Pediatr* 2017;188:70–4.

57. Singh S, Vignesh P, Burgner D. The epidemiology of Kawasaki disease: A global update. *Arch Dis Child* 2015;100(11):1084–8.

58. Newburger JW et al. Diagnosis, treatment, and long-term management of Kawasaki disease: A statement for health professionals from the Committee on Rheumatic Fever, Endocarditis and Kawasaki Disease, Council on Cardiovascular Disease in the Young, American Heart Association. *Circulation* [Internet] 2004;110(17):2747–71.

59. Burns JC et al. Seasonality and temporal clustering of Kawasaki syndrome. *Epidemiology* 2005;16(2):220–5.

60. Rowley AH et al. Ultrastructural, immunofluorescence, and RNA evidence support the hypothesis of a "New" virus associated with Kawasaki disease. *J Infect Dis* 2011;203(7):1021–30.

61. Suenaga T, Suzuki H, Shibuta S, Takeuchi T, Yoshikawa N. Detection of multiple superantigen genes in stools of patients with Kawasaki disease. *J Pediatr* 2009;155(2):266–70.

62. McCrindle BW et al. Diagnosis, treatment, and long-term management of Kawasaki disease: A scientific statement for health professionals from the American Heart Association. *Circulation* 2017;135(17):927–99.

63. Wei YJ, Zhao XL, Liu BM, Niu H, Li Q. Cardiac complications in 38 cases of Kawasaki disease with coronary artery aneurysm diagnosed by echocardiography. *Echocardiography* 2016;33(5):764–70.

64. Fukazawa R et al. Nationwide survey of patients with giant coronary aneurysm secondary to Kawasaki disease 1999–2010 in Japan. *Circ J* 2017;82(1): 239–46.

65. Lin M-T, Fu C-M, Huang S-K, Huang S-C, Wu M-H. Population-based study of Kawasaki disease shock syndrome in Taiwan. *Pediatr Infect Dis J* 2013;32(12):1384–6.

66. Yang H-F, Chen W-L, Chang C-N, Chen S-J, Fan H-C. Kawasaki disease shock syndrome: Case report. *Paediatr Int Child Health* 2016 2;36(1):76–8.

67. Sinhabahu VP, Suntharesan J, Wijesekara DS. Kawasaki shock syndrome in a 12-year-old girl mimicking septic shock. *Case Rep Infect Dis* 2016;2016:4949036.

68. Zhu FH, Ang JY. The clinical diagnosis and management of Kawasaki disease: A review and update. *Curr Infect Dis Rep* 2016;18(10):32.

69. Altman CA. Clinical assessment of coronary arteries in Kawasaki disease: Focus on echocardiographic assessment. *Congenit Heart Dis* 2017;12(5):636–40.

70. Freeman AF, Shulman ST. Kawasaki Disease: Summary of the American Heart Association Guidelines. *Am Fam Physician* 2006;74: 1141–8.

33

Vasculitis mimics

DEBDEEP MITRA, AJAY CHOPRA, AND NEERJA SARASWAT

INTRODUCTION

The vasculitides are defined by histological inflammation of blood vessels seen in various tissues. Multiorgan involvement is a unique feature of this group of disorders.

Cutaneous involvement in cases of vasculitis is very common due to its rich vasculature. It may be a primary event, reflector of a fatal systemic disease, or evidence of association with some other systemic disorder. Skin involvement may vary from subtle cutaneous lesions and predominant systemic involvement to widespread cutaneous necrosis and ulceration. Cases with predominant systemic involvement may present initially to other specialties, depending on the major organ of manifestation. In such cases misdiagnosis is frequent; cases of acute abdomen, undergoing emergency exploratory laparotomy, later diagnosed as cutaneous small vessel vasculitis (CSVV), is not uncommon.

There are a wide variety of conditions that can mimic true vasculitis clinically, based on laboratory investigations, radiographically and histopathologically. It is extremely important to distinguish vascular inflammation from non-vasculitic disorders as it has significant therapeutic implications, since immunosuppressive therapy that is directed at the primary systemic vasculitides may be associated with significant toxicities, and a failure to recognize a vasculitis mimic may delay the initiation of effective therapy for the disorder in question.

For understanding purposes, the term *mimic* in this chapter includes conditions that may or may not result in true vascular inflammation (*vasculitis*) but present similarly to the defined primary systemic vasculitides. The chapter also attempts to make note of key categories of disease that may mimic the primary vasculitides, focusing on a few important entities in each category.

CONDITIONS MIMICKING CUTANEOUS AND SYSTEMIC VASCULITIS

There are a wide variety of conditions that can mimic vasculitis clinically, radiologically, and on histopathology. Table 33.1 tabulates a few of these conditions mimicking vasculitis [1]. Important causes of vasculitis can be remembered with the help of the pneumonic: *MEDICAL* which refers to *m*alignancies, *e*ndocarditis, *d*rugs, *i*nfections, *c*ollagen disorders, and *a*ntiphospholipid antibody syndrome.

WHEN TO SUSPECT VASCULITIS MIMICS

It is very important to take a proper history and to carefully examine the patient of suspected vasculitis. In general, there are two important case scenarios to be kept in mind while dealing with a case of suspected vasculitis: (1) unexplained ischemia such as claudication, angina, limb ischemia, stroke, transient ischemic attack, angina, and cutaneous ischemia and (2) multiple organ involvement in a systemically ill patient, especially in the presence of other suggestive clinical features with constitutional symptoms.

Once vasculitis is suspected based on these factors, it is important to keep in mind the following factors that raise the suspicion of the presence of a vasculitis mimic:

- Extremes of age
- Immunocompromised patients
- Acute onset of symptoms with rapid deterioration of symptoms

- Patients on drugs known to cause vasculitis, i.e., hydralazine, propylthiouracil, carbimazole, etc.
- Underlying established malignancies
- Comorbidities like hepatic or renal disorders

INFECTIONS

A wide variety of infections caused by bacteria, viruses, and fungi may have vasculitis as an initial clinical presentation. The insult to the vasculature can either be by direct invasion of the endothelium by the organism or because of immune-mediated hypersensitivity response, mainly type III.

Direct injury to the endothelium of the blood vessel can be seen in case of cytomegalovirus, herpes simplex, Rickettsiae, some fungi, and bacteria. *Candida* polysaccharides and fragments of gram-positive and gram-negative organisms can also activate the alternate pathway and result in an inflammatory reaction that is characteristic of vasculitis [2]. Staphylococcus and streptococcus can lead to vascular injury because of release of factors such as tumor necrosis factor and inflammatory cytokines.

Bacterial infections

Important bacterial species causing vasculitis mimics and their mechanisms include the following:

- Direct invasion by the bacteria leading to the formation of mycotic aneurysms are seen in staphylococcus, streptococcus, and salmonella infections.
- Tropism for vascular endothelium is a feature of rickettsial species (Figure 33.1). This results in widespread leak from the microvasculature, formation of thrombi in the region, eventually leading to widespread organ involvement.
- *Neisseria* species is associated with small vessel vasculitis. This is the reason for pustule formation seen in *Neisseria gonorrhea* infection. *Neisseria meningitidis* can also result in skin and gastrointestinal tract endothelium damage showing necrosis and thrombosis.

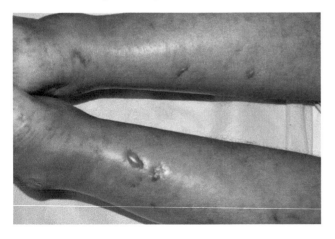

Figure 33.1 Bullous lesions as part of rickettsial infection.

Viral infection

a. *Hepatitis C virus*: The patient presents with a triad of arthritis, palpable purpura, and type II cryoglobulinemia. It leads to small vessel leukocytoclastic vasculitis of the skin. Lower extremities are predominantly affected and are cold on examination. However, medium and small vessels may also be involved.

b. *Hepatitis B virus*: It leads to immune complex mediated disease. Vasculitis of small vessels may lead to "urticaria-arthritis syndrome."

c. *Human T-lymphotrophic virus*: This can result in cutaneous, retinal, and central nervous system (CNS) vasculitis involvement.

d. *Varicella zoster virus and cytomegalovirus*: These infections act in several ways to result in vasculitis.

e. *Parvovirus B19*: This virus has been reported to cause polyarteritis nodosa in some case reports.

f. *Others*: Rubella virus, adenovirus, echovirus, coxsackie virus, parainfluenza virus, herpes simplex, and hepatitis A virus infection.

Infective endocarditis

Infective endocarditis (IE) can mimic the entire spectrum of vasculitides clinically, radiologically, and at histopathology. IE can result in mycotic (infected) aneurysms affecting the aorta and its branches and pulmonary arteries, as well as small vessel inflammation in various organs because of direct infection (septic vasculitis), through immune complex mediated (purpura, glomerulonephritis [GN]) or embolic phenomenon.

Splinter hemorrhages may also be seen in both IE and small vessel vasculitis. The prevalence of mycotic aneurysms in one series of patients was 2.3% [2]. Mycotic aneurysms can occur in any arterial location, resulting in symptoms related to organ-specific or multiorgan ischemia and inflammation. Aneurysms can occur at major branches of the aorta, most frequently the femoral artery and abdominal aorta, followed by the thoracoabdominal and thoracic aorta. Blood cultures are useful in identifying the responsible organism.

VASCULAR DISORDERS

Pityriasis lichenoides

Pityriasis lichenoides (PL) is thought to be an overlap of vasculitis and an immune complex mediated pathomechanism. There is evidence to suggest that the entities that make up pityriasis lichenoides represent cytotoxic CD8 T-cell proliferation that can occur in different settings. Infective triggers have also been implicated in many cases. Clinically the milder variant of PLC is unlikely to be confused with vasculitis, but severe and necrotic lesions of pityriasis lichenoides et varioliformis acuta (PLEVA) may clinically resemble vasculitis.

Clinically the lesions of PLEVA are edematous papules and nodules that have central vesiculation and hemorrhagic necrosis (Figure 33.2). In addition to the cutaneous lesions

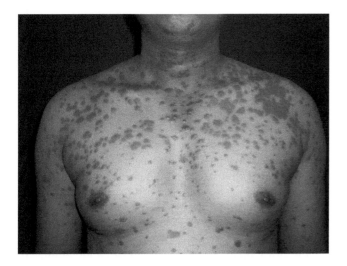

Figure 33.2 Pityriasis lichenoides et varioliformis acuta manifesting as papules with vesiculation on trunk.

that simulate vasculitis, the presence of constitutional symptoms also gives a confusing picture.

Histologically there are features of vasculitis in inflammatory or necrotic lesions. There is extravasation of erythrocytes with features of endothelial proliferation.

Treatment of pityriasis chronica includes systemic corticosteroids, dapsone, cyclosporine, and IV immunoglobulin.

VASCULAR OCCLUSIVE DISORDERS

Antiphospholipid syndrome

This is an autoimmune hypercoagulable disorder, characterized by recurrent arterial and venous thrombosis, loss of pregnancy, thrombocytopenia, and persistently positive anticardiolipin or lupus anticoagulant antibodies.

Pathogenetic mechanisms leading to thrombosis include activation of endothelial cells, monocytes or platelets, complement activation, and inhibition of protein C. Multifocal thrombotic events with angiographic appearances of arterial narrowing secondary to luminal thrombi can mimic the clinical and angiographic appearance of vasculitis.

Antiphospholipid syndrome can occur as a primary disorder or in association with diseases such as systemic lupus erythematosus. Diagnosis of antiphospholipid antibody syndrome can be confirmed by serial testing for antiphospholipid antibodies in the right clinical context.

Behçet disease

Presently, Behçet disease is classified as a vasculitis, though it formed a major vasculitic mimic until recently (Figures 33.3 through 33.5).

EMBOLIC CONDITIONS

Embolic conditions like Sneddon syndrome and cholesterol embolism can result in conditions mimicking vasculitis.

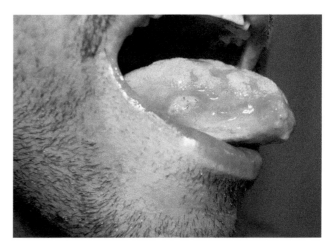

Figure 33.3 Oral ulcer of Behçet disease.

Sneddon syndrome is a rare, arterio-occlusive disorder associated with generalized livedo racemosa and cerebrovascular ischemic attack. The condition involves small and medium-sized arteries.

Clinically there is associated livedo racemosa mainly seen on the upper and lower extremities. However, other areas like the trunk and face may also be involved. This syndrome is usually seen in women of childbearing age.

Livedo racemosa involves persistent irreversible skin lesions that are red or bluish in color with irregular margins. It is worsened by cold exposure and pregnancy.

There is no effective therapy available for the management of this disorder; however, anticoagulants and agents inhibiting platelet aggregation are the most widely accepted modalities. Avoiding smoking, obesity, and oral contraceptive pills including estrogen is recommended.

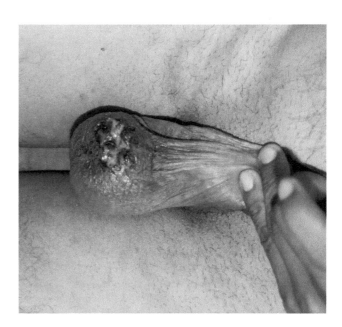

Figure 33.4 Scrotal ulcer in Behçet disease.

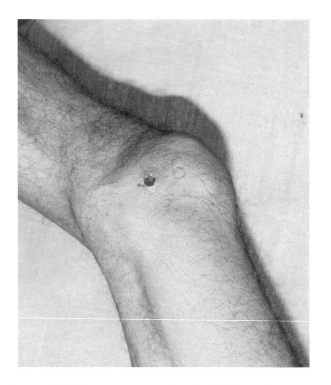

Figure 33.5 Cutaneous vasculopathy in Behçet disease.

Cholesterol emboli

Cholesterol embolization (atheroembolism) can occur from the arterial wall because of trauma from catheter manipulation, direct trauma, surgery, anticoagulation, or thrombolysis. Extremities are more commonly affected. The patient presents with limb ischemia with a livedo reticularis-like rash and normal pulses. Other cutaneous presentations include purpura, ulcers, nodules, cyanosis, and frank gangrene [3]. Other sites of embolization include the gastrointestinal tract and CNS. Bedsides, ophthalmoscopy may reveal retinal cholesterol emboli.

A deep skin biopsy would show cholesterol crystals (identified by "cholesterol clefts") in the cutaneous microvessels.

Left atrial myxomas

Cardiac myxomas are the most common primary cardiac tumors that are benign, occur mostly in the left atrium, and can produce symptoms due to valvular obstruction, embolization, or paraneoplastic effects.

This condition is most commonly observed in middle-aged females. Paraneoplastic manifestations of myxomas include fever, arthralgias, and weight loss that can mimic the constitutional symptoms seen with systemic vasculitis. Recurrent embolic phenomena can lead to tissue infarction with digital ischemia, cutaneous infarcts, limb claudication, hemoptysis (pulmonary infarction), hematuria (renal infarction), and stroke (cerebral infarction) [4].

DRUGS

A wide variety of drugs may result in mimics of vasculitis or can cause a true vasculitis. Common drugs implicated are minocycline and hydralazine and carbamazepine. These drugs may be associated with positive antineutrophil cytoplasmic antibody (ANCA) testing and, in some cases, may be associated with a vasculitic syndrome [5]. Use of cocaine results in nasal mucosal irritation and necrosis, intense vasoconstriction which leads to nasal septal perforation, and collapse with a saddle-nose deformity. This can result in a particularly elusive mimic of Wegener granulomatosis (WG). The patient presents with facial pain, epistaxis, and constitutional symptoms. In addition, the patient may have a classical ANCA pattern on immunofluorescence and positive antiproteinase 3 (PR3) testing by immunoassay, compounding the diagnostic confusion with WG [6]. Multisystem involvement goes in favor of WG.

DERMATOSES

Schamberg disease

Schamberg purpura (SP), also known as progressive pigmentary dermatoses of Schamberg, purpura pigmentosa progressive is the most common variety of pigmented purpuric dermatoses. This entity was first reported by a dermatologist from Philadelphia, Jay Frank Schamberg, in 1901.

Schamberg purpura is prevalent across all age groups and affects males more commonly than females. Various pathogenetic mechanisms reported in the literature include genetic, medications, venous hypertension, gravitational dependency, capillary fragility, contact allergy to wool or clothing dye, exercise, and trauma.

It most commonly affects the legs. However, it can involve other areas of the body, distributed irregularly on both sides. Clinically it presents as multiple polysized irregular plaques and patches with a peculiar orange-brown color. Over the period, some of the lesions can darken while a few of the lesions disappear. There is a characteristic "cayenne pepper" appearance within the edges of old macules.

MALIGNANCIES

A large variety of malignancies are associated with vasculitis. These are mostly hematological malignancies rather than solid tumors. A close association in the temporal profile between carcinoma and vasculitis suggests that vasculitis may be a paraneoplastic syndrome. The etiopathogenesis of vasculitis in malignancy patients is not known. The evidence of autoantibodies, immune complex, and complement consumption is absent on investigation, and histopathology reveals leukocytoclastic vasculitis. Malignancy-associated vasculitis typically does not respond to conventional therapy.

Table 33.1 Conditions mimicking vasculitis

- Infections:
  - Bacterial, fungal, and viral
- Vascular disorders:
  - Pityriasis lichenoides chronica
  - Perniosis
- Vascular occlusive disease:
  - Disseminated intravascular coagulation
  - Thrombocythemia
  - Thrombotic thrombocytopenic purpura
  - Homocystinuria
  - Antiphospholipid antibody syndrome
- Embolic states:
  - Sneddon syndrome
  - Cholesterol embolism
  - Left atrial myxoma
- Purpura:
  - Platelet deficiency
  - Drug induced
- Dermatoses:
  - Schamberg disease
- Malignancies:
  - Lymphomas
  - Leukemias
- Miscellaneous:
  - Insect bite reaction

MANAGEMENT

As discussed earlier in the chapter, there are several conditions that mimic vasculitis, and they need to be considered in the differential diagnosis depending on clinical presentation. It is important to differentiate vasculitis from vasculitis mimics (Table 33.1; Figure 33.6) [2]. Prompt evaluation is necessary, as delay in the diagnosis and treatment of many of these etiologies can lead to significant mortality or morbidity. A complete history and physical examination are essential to observe patterns to help discern causative agents or disease characteristics. Careful attention to drug ingestion, inclusive of "homeopathic" medications, is important. A review of possible exposures (i.e., contact, infectious, chemical) and travel history may also elucidate an occult cause.

First, infection is a great mimic of vasculitis. There are several clinical and laboratory features common to both vasculitis and infection. Constitutional symptoms like fever, malaise, arthralgia, myalgia, and weight loss, and laboratory features such as normocytic normochromic anemia, peripheral blood leucocytosis, thrombocytosis, raised erythrocyte sedimentation rate, and C-reactive protein are encountered in both. Because treatment of vasculitis entails the use of immunosuppressive drugs, the consequences of not recognizing infection would be disastrous. Thus, it is prudent to carry out a full and appropriate infection screen in all patients with suspected vasculitis, especially those presenting with systemic inflammatory features. Procalcitonin levels are raised in patients with infection but not in noninfective inflammatory conditions, but this test is not widely available.

Treatment depends on the underlying condition that mimics vasculitis. The infectious causes, if suspected, need to be treated promptly with appropriate antibiotics or antivirals along with supportive therapy. The offending drug should be stopped if a drug is likely to be the cause of vasculitis. Likewise, the treatment of underlying malignancy, inflammation, and thrombotic condition is required if it is associated with vasculitis.

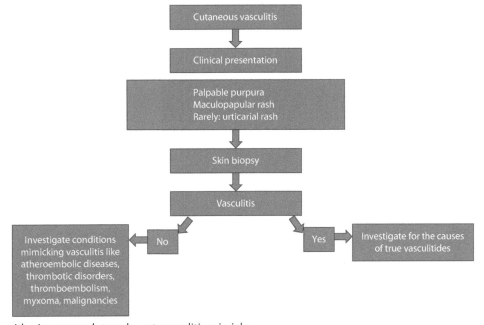

Figure 33.6 Algorithmic approach to rule out vasculitis mimicks.

KEY POINTS

- Infections, malignancies, drugs, few vascular disorders and certain occlusion disorders form the main causes of vasculitis mimics
- Rickettsial infections, cholesterol emboli, pigmented purpuric dermatoses and pityriasis lichenoides are common mimics.
- Minocycline, carbamazepine and hydrlazine are the causative drugs for vasculitis mimicks.
- It is important to rule out theses causes before labeling a case as actual vasculitis.

REFERENCES

1. Witort-Serraglini E et al. Endothelial injury in vasculitides. *Clin Dermatol* 1999;17:587.

2. Chen IM, Chang HH, Hsu CP, Lai ST, Shih CC. Ten-year experience with surgical repair of mycotic aortic aneurysms. *J Chin Med Assoc* 2005;68(6):265–71.

3. Carlson JA, Chen KR. Cutaneous pseudovasculitis. *Am J Dermatopathol* 2007;29(1):44–55.

4. Nishio Y, Ito Y, Iguchi Y, Sato H. MPO-ANCA-associated pseudovasculitis in cardiac myxoma. *Eur J Neurol* 2005;12(8):619–20.

5. Wiik A. Drug-induced vasculitis. *Curr Opin Rheumatol* 2008;20(1):35–9.

6. Wiesner O et al. Antineutrophil cytoplasmic antibodies reacting with human neutrophil elastase as a diagnostic marker for cocaine-induced midline destructive lesions but not autoimmune vasculitis. *Arthritis Rheum* 2004;50(9):2954–65.

34

Purpura fulminans

RAJAN KAPOOR, A. P. DUBEY, AND ANURADHA MONGA

INTRODUCTION

Purpura fulminans (PF), described first by Guelliot in 1884, is a rare, potentially disabling and life-threatening emergency, characterized pathologically by progressive hemorrhagic infarction, tissue necrosis, and intravascular thrombosis typically involving small dermal vessels [1]. Clinically it is usually accompanied by features of sepsis, such as hypotension and disseminated intravascular coagulation (DIC). Most of the cases are seen in the pediatric age group [2]. It can progress to multiorgan failure and severe large vessel thrombosis, thereby causing high mortality up to 42% in the setting of sepsis during the initial stages, and it results in long-term morbidity in survivors. Therefore, early recognition, diagnosis, and management of the initiating cause of PF can help avert these very adverse outcomes.

PF predominantly occurs in three clinical settings:

- Neonatal purpura fulminans
- Postinfectious
- Idiopathic

Each of these clinical settings is associated with different etiology (Table 34.1), pathophysiology, clinical presentation, and management strategy. All of them, however, have a rapidly progressive clinical course associated with hemodynamic collapse and DIC [3].

NEONATAL PURPURA FULMINANS

Etiopathogenesis

It can be inherited or acquired. Neonatal PF is associated with inherited deficiency of naturally occurring anticoagulants such as protein C, protein S, as well as antithrombin III. Protein C and S exert its anticoagulant activity primarily through inactivation of coagulation factors Va and VIIIa, which are required for factor X activation and thrombin

Table 34.1 Etiology of purpura fulminans

Inherited	Acquired
Neonatal PF	
i) Protein C deficiency	i) Increased consumption
	a) Infection
	b) DIC
	c) Acute Venous Thrombosis
ii) Protein S deficiency	ii) Decreased Synthesis
	a) Hepatic Failure
	b) Vit K Deficiency
	c) Warfarin Therapy
Acute Infectious PF	
i) Neissera Meningitidis	
ii) Streptococcus Pneumoniae	
iii) Group B Stretococcus	
iv) Haemophilus Influenza Type b	
v) Staphylococcus Aureus	
Idiopathic PF	
i) Varicella	
ii) Scarlet Fever	
iii) Viral Exanthem	
iv) Non-infectious causes	

generation, whereas antithrombin III directly inhibits thrombin. Antithrombin III and protein C are exclusively synthesized by the liver, whereas protein S is synthesized by hepatocytes as well as kidneys, megakaryocytes, and endothelial cells. Inherited deficiencies of protein C or protein S resulting either from homozygous or heterozygous mutations or coinheritance with other inherited forms of thrombophilia can result in PF and severe coagulopathies [4]. Pathological mutations in *PROC* and *PROS1* genes, respectively, are found to cause inherited protein C and protein S deficiencies.

Antithrombin III deficiency occurs in three distinct forms; type I antithrombin III (AT III) deficient patients have both the reduced levels as well as the function, whereas type II and type III patients have normal levels with functional defects. Patients with AT III deficiency present with both arterial and venous thromboembolic episodes manifesting since adulthood, and neonates with homozygous deficiency present with PF with embolic lesions in skin.

Acquired cases are more common and result from consumptive coagulopathy caused by severe infections (especially streptococcus), DIC, hepatic dysfunction or failure, and coexisting relative deficiency of protein C or protein S [5,6].

Pathophysiology and coagulation cascade are depicted as a flowchart in Figures 34.1 and 34.2, respectively.

Clinical features

Neonatal PF usually presents 2–12 hours after birth, and most of the cases occur within 72 hours after birth, with rapidly progressive purpuric skin lesions and DIC [7]. However, infants with delayed onset of presentation up to 6–12 months have also been reported [8]. Typically, lesions are seen over the perineal region, flexor aspect of the thigh, skin over the anterior abdominal wall, male genitalia, previous sites of trauma such as cannulation sites, and also sites of friction including heels and buttocks (Figure 34.3).

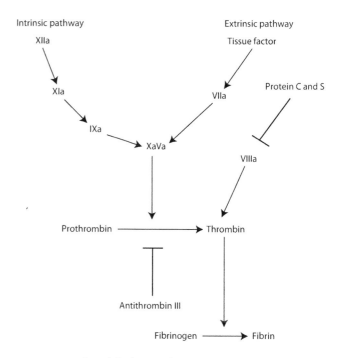

Figure 34.2 Simplified coagulation cascade.

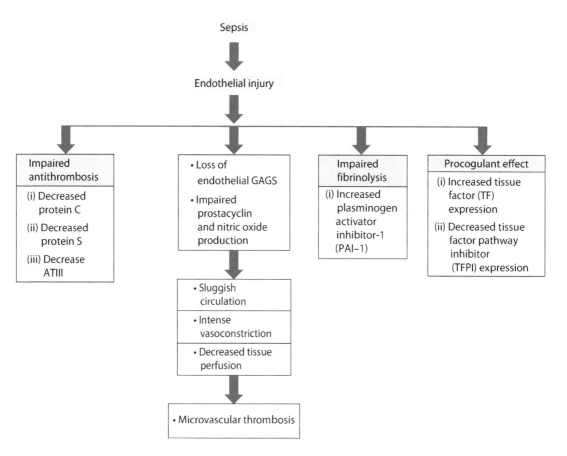

Figure 34.1 Pathophysiology of infectious purpura fulminans.

Clinical severity depends on the underlying etiology. The skin lesions appear first as erythematous well-demarcated large macules that then rapidly enlarge to become dark red or bluish areas and may become vesiculated forming hemorrhagic bullae. They later develop black hemorrhagic crusting with subsequent necrosis and gangrene leading to loss of extremities and sepsis (Figure 34.4 through 34.6) [9]. A margin of erythema may be present around the areas of necrosis, and bleeding into the necrotic area can lead to severe pain. Severe protein C deficiency is also associated with cerebral venous thrombosis (CVT), and antenatal events such as vitreous hemorrhage and retinal detachment have been reported [10]. The affected neonates may also show significant neurological involvement due to antenatal/postnatal CVT with periventricular hemorrhagic infarction and also hydrocephalus. Vitreal bleeding, thrombosis of the retinal vein or artery or vitreal vein thrombosis is also associated with retinal detachment.

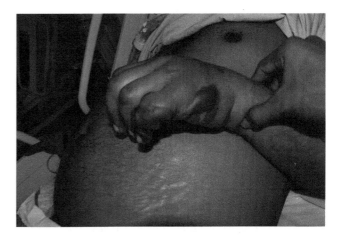

Figure 34.5 Hemorrhagic blisters with necrosis on dorsum hands.

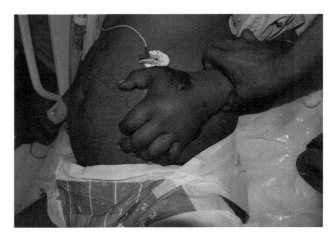

Figure 34.6 Large hemorrhagic blister on dorsum of hands.

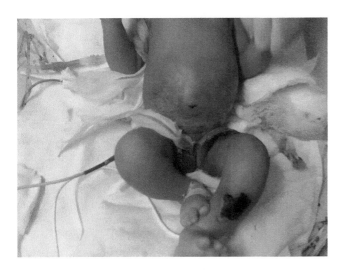

Figure 34.3 Neonatal purpura fulminans in a neonate with severe protein C deficiency. (Photo courtesy of Col Karthik Rammohan, Neonatologist Command Hospital Kolkata.)

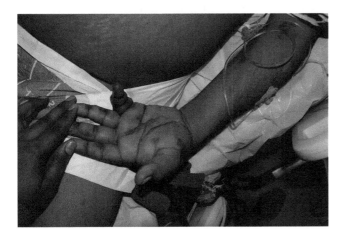

Figure 34.4 Hemorrhagic blisters with necrosis on palms of hands in an infant.

Diagnosis

The diagnosis of neonatal PF is based on the clinical picture, strong family history of thrombotic events which may be present, demonstration of undetectable levels of protein C or protein S, and a lower level of these natural anticoagulants in parents [11]. During the acute phase of the illness, findings of DIC predominate, such as low platelet count, increased prothrombin time, and activated partial thromboplastin time.

Genetic testing of the child and the parents is useful to distinguish between congenital and acquired deficiency of proteins C and S, but it is carried out in research laboratories and not available for clinical use. Functional assays are present for initial screening. It is important to understand that levels of protein C and S will be reduced during acute thrombosis and inflammation, thereby reducing the utility of these tests in the acute setting. If the test has been done in an acute setting, it should be repeated after complete recovery from the acute event [12].

Thus, in the setting of acute thrombosis, it is difficult to differentiate whether neonatal PF is inherited or acquired. In the absence of signs and symptoms of generalized septicemia, inherited deficiency of protein C or S is to be considered. Blood samples from the infant and parents should be drawn for assessing antigen and activity levels of proteins C and S.

Treatment

Based on provisional diagnosis, treatment of PF should be started without any delay. Fresh frozen plasma (FFP) or cryoprecipitate should be used as initial replacement therapy until protein C concentrate is available [5]. FFP should be started at the rate of 10–20 mg/kg every 6–12 hours along with injectable enoxaparin (2 mg/kg) [13]. One mL/kg of FFP will increase the plasma protein C concentration by 1 IU/dL, and the aim is to maintain a rough protein C activity of >10 IU/dL [14]. FFP administration at this dosing can lead to hyperproteinemia, hypertension, loss of venous access, and potential for exposure to infectious viral agents. Protein C concentrates have limited availability worldwide and are presently not available for use in India. Protein C concentrates should be started at doses of 100 IU/kg followed by 50 IU/kg every 6 hours. Both human plasma derived and viral inactivated protein C concentrates are recommended for treatment, whereas recombinant activated protein C is not indicated due to reports of increased risk of bleeding in such patients [15,16]. The treatment should continue until all the lesions in the skin, CNS, and eyes resolve. Apart from treatment of PF, sepsis and DIC are to be managed based on clinical and laboratory parameters with component support and broad-spectrum antibiotics.

Anticoagulation therapy, initially with unfractionated heparin (UFH) or low molecular weight heparin (LMWH), is to be started concurrently with administration of protein C. Initiation of warfarin should commence after a few days of anticoagulation with UFH or LMWH and to be overlapped initially to prevent warfarin-induced skin necrosis and other thrombotic complications. As protein C synthesis is vitamin K dependent, levels may reduce if warfarin is initiated alone and may trigger paradoxical thrombosis.

Warfarin either alone or concurrently with protein C concentrates if available should be given as maintenance therapy to maintain a target international normalized ratio (INR). If used as single-agent maintenance therapy, a target INR between 2.5 and 3.5 is to be aimed at, whereas if protein C concentrates are used as prophylaxis along with warfarin, a target INR of 1.5–2.5 is recommended [14]. Rarely liver transplantation has been carried out in severe homozygous protein C deficiency.

Early PF lesions are reversible with treatment, but once lesions get established, they progress rapidly within 24–48 hours to cause full-thickness skin necrosis and also extensive soft tissue necrosis. This may require surgical débridement and even fasciotomies or amputation. This also correlates with histological appearance initially of occlusion of the small dermal vessels with microthrombi leading to capillary dilation and also red cell congestion in early stages of PF. Later stages are characterized by irreversible ischemic injury to the endothelium along with extravasation of red blood cells into the dermis and leading to gangrenous necrosis.

ACUTE INFECTIOUS PURPURA FULMINANS

Introduction

Acute infectious PF can occur in conjunction with acute illness or through endotoxin-mediated sepsis. This critical setting results in disturbance of normal hemostasis, shifting a quiescent state favoring anticoagulation to a procoagulant disease state resulting in overwhelming coagulopathy.

Etiopathogenesis

Acute infectious PF occurs in around 15%–25% of those with meningococcemia, and the majority of cases occur in the pediatric age group. Though it can occur with infection with any meningococcal serogroup, it appears to be associated in high frequency with serogroup C isolates [17–19].

Pathogenesis of acute infectious PF can be well explained on the basis of Schwartzman reaction, which is a hemorrhagic and necrotizing response produced by injection of the endotoxin of gram-negative organisms. Endotoxin from *Neisseria meningitidis* is more potent in eliciting such a response than endotoxin from other gram-negative organisms [20,21].

The coagulation and complement pathways are systemically activated leading to endothelial dysfunction and DIC. Widespread activation of coagulation can lead to consumption of platelets and the circulating coagulation factors leading to bleeding. The sudden loss of various anti-inflammatory and anticoagulant proteins (such as protein C) can lead to extensive thrombus formation, inhibition of fibrinolysis, and further activation of the inflammatory pathways. In DIC complicating sepsis caused by some organisms such as meningococcus, there is also a local defect in protein C activation on the endothelium of the small vessels causing loss of anticoagulant and anti-inflammatory protein C activity, locally leading to microvascular thrombosis in the dermal vessels leading to PF [22–24].

Also in patients with acute infectious PF, there is endotoxin-mediated acquired deficiency of proteins C and S, and increased consumption of antithrombin III [25–27].

Few reports have recently reported association with *Staphylococcus* [28]. Common infectious agents leading to PF are listed in Table 34.1.

Clinical presentation

The four primary characteristic features of this syndrome are as follows:

- Large, purpuric skin lesions
- Fever
- Hemodynamic instability
- DIC

Lesions of PF are similar irrespective of the etiology, which initially starts with a burning sensation, followed by development of erythematous and petechial lesions with or without edema and rapid progression to painful, well-defined purpuric lesions. Later these lesions evolve into vesicles or bullae, followed by development of hemorrhagic crusts, necrosis, and gangrene. The pathology often extends into subcutaneous tissues, muscles, and/or bones. In contrast to neonatal or idiopathic PF, where the lesions typically involve the skin of the thighs, buttocks, and lower trunk, lesions in acute infectious PF involve distal extremities in symmetrical fashion and progressively involve proximal parts over the course of the illness, especially in severe sepsis. This is probably due to the greater impact of circulatory collapse on distal extremities due to paucity of collaterals for tissue perfusion. This may also be due to site-specific variation in the release of cytokines, heterogeneity in endothelial cell expression of the procoagulant and anticoagulant factors, cytokine receptors, physical properties of the skin such as variation of temperature, and tissue perfusion [29].

PF due to severe sepsis is usually accompanied by microvascular thrombosis and hemorrhagic infarction in the lungs, kidneys, CNS, and adrenal glands. This can cause rapidly progressive multiorgan failure and a high mortality rate.

Treatment

Initial treatment of acute infectious PF consists of prompt restoration of circulation and respiratory support as impaired tissue perfusion will result in further ischemic damage of endothelial cells and favor thrombosis resulting in a vicious cycle of hypoperfusion. Furthermore, hypoperfusion due to shock results in increased levels of catecholamines, thereby shunting blood away from the liver, resulting in decreased synthesis of proteins required for normal hemostatic balance and reduced clearance of activated clotting factors. Apart from maintaining hemodynamics, patients should be started on broad-spectrum parenteral antibiotics not only against N. meningitidis but also against streptococci and staphylococci.

Other therapeutic interventions include vitamin K and FFP to correct existing deficiencies of vitamin K dependent clotting factors, such as protein C, S, and AT III. Continued use of FFP should be guided by regular measurements of protein C, protein S, and antithrombin III levels. Though it is not known what the precise effective factor levels are, recommendations are to maintain antithrombin III above 50% of normal and protein C and S at least 25% of normal values [27]. Heparin is useful in patients of PF who develop skin necrosis during the course of illness, particularly those with thrombophilic states. Heparin acts through inhibition of clotting, as well as maintains hemostasis by interrupting the consumption of anticoagulant factors, and/or inhibiting the procoagulant and antifibrinolytic effects of thrombin [31].

Other experimental modalities of treatment being attempted in the treatment of acute infectious PF include protein C and AT III concentrate, prostacyclin, tissue plasminogen activator, and vasodilation. The role of plasmapheresis and double volume exchange transfusion is controversial, and they have been used in rare instances to remove circulating cytokines, autoantibodies, and endotoxins [32–34].

IDIOPATHIC PURPURA FULMINANS

Idiopathic PF is a rare entity occurring during the postinfectious convalescent phase of acute illness [30,35]. Most of the cases are preceded by infections such as varicella, group A streptococcus, or a nonspecific viral exanthematous illness, though cases following noninfectious illness have also been reported. The disorder follows a biphasic course, i.e., after recovering from an otherwise uncomplicated childhood illness, the patient develops purpuric skin lesions over proximal regions like the thigh and buttocks, which may rapidly evolve into extensive areas of necrosis and gangrene. The scrotum and penis may also be involved in males. The condition typically spares the distal extremities. Acquired deficiency of protein C or S, which may be autoantibody mediated, is the postulated pathogenesis of this disorder. It differs from acute infectious PF in the manner that extracutaneous manifestations involving other organs are rare, distal extremities are generally spared, and hemodynamic collapse, multiorgan failure, and large vessel thrombosis are uncommon (Table 34.2). These differences account for lower mortality rates in idiopathic PF as compared to acute infectious PF. Management is similar to that of infectious PF. Supportive treatment and replacement of deficient blood components, FFP, and clotting factors is the mainstay of therapy along with early recognition and treatment of secondary infection.

Differential diagnosis

Differential diagnoses include traumatic bleeding, immune thrombocytopenic purpura, thrombotic thrombocytopenic purpura, and Henoch–Schönlein purpura.

KEY POINTS

- Purpura fulminans is a rare, life-threatening dermatological emergency characterized by progressive hemorrhagic infarction, tissue necrosis, and intravascular thrombosis typically involving small dermal vessels, secondary to deficiency of natural anticoagulants like proteins C, S, and antithrombin.
- Acquired forms secondary to fulminant bacterial infections are much more common than inherited deficiencies of natural anticoagulants.
- Key to successful management is early clinical suspicion, early institution of replacement of deficient proteins by fresh frozen plasma, and management of associated sepsis and disseminated intravascular coagulation.
- Inherited forms may require lifelong anticoagulation and replacement therapy for the deficient protein.

Table 34.2 Differentiating features between acute infectious PF and idiopathic PF

Etiology	• N. Menigitidis • S. Pneumonia • H. Influenza	• Varicella • Viral exanthem • Non-infectious causes
Age	Any age	Children and Adolescents
Site of lesion	• Distal Extremeties • Symmetric Involvement	• Proximal Extremities • Asymmetric Involvement
Clinical Presentation	• Acute Febrile illness • Haemodynamic Instability • Multiorgan Failure	• Preceded by Febrile illness • Hypotension rare • Other organ rare involved
Pathogenesis	• Endothelial Dysfunction • Anticoagulants Dysfunction • Coagulation activation	• Acquired protein C and S deficiency • Autoantibody mediated • Other mechanism
Prognosis	Mortality > 40%	Mortality <15%

REFERENCES

1. Nolan J, Sinclair R. Review of management of purpura fulminans and two case reports. *Br J Anaesth* 2001;86:581–6.
2. Andreasen TJ, Green SD, Childers BJ. Massive infectious soft tissue injury: Diagnosis and management of necrotizing fascitis and purpura fulminans. *Plast Reconstr Surg* 2001;107:1025–34.
3. D'Cruz D, Cervera R, Olcay Aydintug A, Ahmed T, Font J, Hughes GR. Systemic lupus erythematosus evolving into systemic vasculitis: A report of five cases. *Br J Rheumatol* 1993;32:154–7.
4. Rietsma PH et al. Protein C deficiency: A database of mutations, 1995 update. On behalf of Subcommittee on Plasma Coagulation Inhibitors of the Scientific and Standardization Committee of ISTH. *Thromb Haemost* 1995;73:876–9.
5. Zenciroglu A, Karagol BS, Ipek MS, Okumus N, Yarali N, Aydin M. Neonatal purpura fulminans secondary to group B streptococcal infection. *Pediatr Hematol Oncol* 2010;27:620–5.
6. Issacman SH, Heroman WM, Lightsey AL. Purpura fulminans following late-onset group B beta-hemolytic streptococcal sepsis. *Am J Dis Child* 1984;138:915–6.
7. Mahasandana C et al. Homozygous protein C deficiency in an infant with purpura fulminans. *J Paediatr* 1990;117:750–3.
8. Tuddenham EG et al. Homozygous protein C deficiency with delayed onset of symptoms at 7 to 10 months. *Thromb Res J* 1989;89:475–84.
9. Manco-Johnson MJ, Abshire TC, Jacobson LJ, Marlar RA. Severe neonatal protein C deficiency: Prevalence and thrombotic risk. *J Paediatr* 1991;119:793–8.
10. Hattenbach LO, Beeg T, Kreuz W, Zubcov A. Ophthalmic manifestations of congenital protein C deficiency. *J AAPOS* 1993;3:188–90.
11. Estelles A et al. Severe inherited "homozygous" protein C deficiency in a newborn infant. *Thromb Haemost* 1984;52:53–6.
12. Goodwin AJ, Rosendaal FR, Kottke-Marchant K, Bovill EG. A review of the technical, diagnostic, and epidemiologic considerations for protein S assays. *Arch Pathol Lab Med* 2002;126:1349–66.
13. Cardo PR, Bernardelli IM, Rivitti EA, Sotto MN, Vilella MA, Valente NY, Martins JE. Childhood onset skin necrosis resulting protein C deficiency. *J Eur Acad Dermatol Venerol* 2007;24:537–9.
14. Goldenberg NA, Manco-Johnson MJ. Protein C deficiency. *Haemophilia* 2008;14:1214–21.
15. Veldman A et al. Human protein C concentrate in the treatment of purpura fulminans: A retrospective analysis of safety and outcome in 94 pediatric patients. *Crit Care* 2010;14:R156.
16. Nadel S et al. Drotrecogin alfa (activated) in children with severe sepsis: A multicentre phase III randomised controlled trial. *Lancet* 2007;369:836–43.
17. Wong VK, Hitchcock W, Mason WH. Meningococcal infections in children: A review of 100 cases. *Pediatr Infect Dis J* 1989;8:224–7.
18. Andersen BM. Endotoxin release from *Neisseria meningitidis*. Relationship between key bacterial characteristics and meningococcal disease. *Scand J Infect Dis Suppl* 1989;64:143.
19. Powars D et al. Epidemic meningococcemia and purpura fulminans with induced protein C deficiency. *Clin Infect Dis* 1993;17:254–61.
20. Periappuram M, Taylor MRH, Keane CT. Rapid detection of meningococci from petechiae in acute meningococcal infection. *J Infect* 1995;31:201–3.
21. Bronza JP. Shwartzman reaction. *Semin Thromb Hemost* 1990;16:326–33.
22. Esmon CT. Blood coagulation. In: Nathan DG, Orkin SH (Eds), *Nathan and Oski's Hematology of Infancy and Childhood*. 5th ed. Philadelphia: WB Saunders; 1998:1531–56.
23. Brox JH, Osterud B, Bjorklid E, Fenton JW. Production and availability of thromboplastin in endothelial cells: The effect of thrombin, endotoxin and platelets. *Br J Haematol* 1984;57:239–46.

24. Conkling PR, Greenberg CS, Weinberg JB. Tumor necrosis factor induces tissue factor-like activity in human leukemia cell line U937 and peripheral blood monocytes. *Blood* 1988;72:128–33.

25. Cobcroft R, Henderson A. Meningococcal purpura fulminans treated with antithrombin III concentrate: What is the optimal replacement therapy? *Aust NZ J Med* 1994;24.

26. Fijnvandraat K et al. Coagulation activation and tissue necrosis in meningococcal septic shock: Severely reduced protein C levels predict a high mortality. *Thromb Haemost* 1995;73:15–20.

27. Rivard GE, David M, Farrell C, Schwarz HP. Treatment of purpura fulminans in meningococcemia with protein C concentrate. *J Pediatr* 1995;126:646–52.

28. Kravitz GR, Dries DJ, Peterson ML, Schlievert PM. Purpura fulminans due to *Staphylococcus aureus*. *CID* 2005;40:948–50.

29. Adcock DM, Bronza J, Marlar RA. Proposed classification and pathologic mechanism of purpura fulminans and skin necrosis. *Semin Thromb Hemost* 1990;16:333–40.

30. Hjort PF, Rapaport SI, Jorgensen L. Purpura fulminans. Report of a case successfully treated with heparin and hydrocortisone. Review of 50 cases from the literature. *Scand J Haematol* 1964;1:169–92.

31. Manco-Johnson MJ et al. Lupus anticoagulant and protein S deficiency in children with post-varicella purpura fulminans or thrombosis. *J Pediatr* 1996;128:319–23.

32. Brandtzaeg P et al. Plasmapheresis in the treatment of severe meningococcal or pneumococcal septicaemia with DIC and fibrinolysis. Preliminary data on eight patients. *Scand J Clin Lab Invest* 1985;45:53–5.

33. Bjorvatn B et al. Meningococcal septicaemia treated with combined plasmapheresis and leucapheresis or with blood exchange. *Br Med J (Clin Res Ed)* 1984;288:439–41.

34. Togari H et al. Endotoxin clearance by exchange blood transfusion in septic shock neonates. *Acta Paediatr Scand* 1983;72:87–91.

35. Francis RB. Acquired purpura fulminans. *Semin Thromb Hemost* 1990;16:310–25.

Approach to purpura

MANAS CHATTERJEE AND RUCHI HEMDANI

INTRODUCTION

Purpura is defined as extravasation of red blood cells resulting in discoloration of the skin or mucous membranes secondary to any disturbance of the normal physiological mechanisms that normally prevent blood from escaping from the vessels, or from damage or lack of support to the vasculature. It is an important and easily recognizable sign and can occur isolated or as part of a systemic disorder. The causes of purpura range from trivial (actinic/senile purpura) to extremely alarming and life-threatening conditions (vasculitis) that need to be diagnosed and treated early. The most common causes of purpura are due to platelet and coagulation disorders, which are generally dealt with by hematologists. For dermatologists, two major disease groups presenting with purpura are vasculitis affecting small and medium-sized cutaneous vessels and cutaneous vascular occlusion syndromes. Microvascular occlusion syndromes are important to recognize because they may mimic vasculitis but require a different approach to diagnosis and therapy [1].

An easy clinical differentiation from intravascular causes of erythema can be made by diascopy where purpura do not show any blanching on being pressed by a slide, which is present in cases of erythema. Management of purpura is generally multidisciplinary involving the dermatologist, hematologist, rheumatologist, nephrologist, and other relevant specialists for life-threatening causes.

CLASSIFICATION

Classifying purpura is difficult as there is overlap among the various causes for different clinical patterns. A broad classification exists that divides purpura into primary purpura,

where the hemorrhage is an integral part of lesion formation, and secondary purpura in which hemorrhage occurs into established lesions of nonpurpuric dermatoses (e.g., stasis dermatitis or dependent cellulitis) [2]. Another classification is a morphological classification based on the morphology of purpuric lesions, which has its own limitations (Table 35.1). An etiological classification based on intravascular, vascular, and extravascular causes is also present (Table 35.2). However, etiology in most cases of purpura is difficult to determine.

A separate classification for vasculitis called the 2012 International Chapel Hill Consensus Conference classification is described in Chapter 31, where primary vasculitis is discussed [3]. The causes of secondary vasculitis are as follows:

1. Vasculitis associated with systemic disease
   a. Lupus vasculitis
   b. Rheumatoid vasculitis
   c. Others
2. Vasculitis associated with probable etiology
   a. Cancer-associated vasculitis
   b. Infections associated (e.g., hepatitis C, hepatitis B, and syphilis)
   c. Drug-associated vasculitis
   d. Others

Other dermatologically relevant causes of purpura

- Inherited defects affecting structural components of dermis/vessel wall (Ehlers–Danlos syndrome, Marfan syndrome, osteogenesis imperfecta, pseudoxanthoma elasticum)

- Hemangiomatous disorders (cavernous hemangioma, hereditary hemorrhagic telangiectasia)
- Biochemical (homocystinuria, hyperhomocystinemia, diabetes, Cushing syndrome)
- Physical (trauma, venous rupture, chemical and mechanical contact irritants)
- Others (malignant hypertension)

PATHOGENESIS

A number of complex and interdependent mechanisms exist for the normal physiological function of preventing escape of blood from vessels. These include an intact vascular bed with adequate connective tissue support, formation of platelet plugs, and an intact coagulation pathway [4]. Abnormalities in any of these mechanisms can lead to purpura formation.

Pathogenic mechanisms of purpura include simple hemorrhage, inflammatory hemorrhage (vessel directed inflammation), and occlusive hemorrhage (minimal inflammation).

Table 35.1 Morphological classification of purpura

Petechiae	Pinhead-sized (<4 mm) bright red round hemorrhagic macules that eventually become rust colored; generally seen in disorders of platelets
Macular purpura	Reddish-blue hemorrhagic macule varying in size from 4 mm to 1 cm
Ecchymoses	Reddish blue or purplish or bluish-black macule measuring >1 cm, deep extravasations seen commonly in coagulation disorders
Palpable Purpura	Raised, partially blanchable lesions that can range in size from a few millimeters to several centimeters in diameter, characteristically seen in leukocytoclastic vasculitis (LCV)
Noninflammatory retiform purpura	Reticulate pattern of whole lesion or its edges and vary in size;[a] most typical presentation of microvascular occlusion syndromes
Inflammatory retiform purpura	Reticulate pattern of whole lesion or its edges and vary in size;[a] early lesions typically exhibit prominent erythema

Source: Warren P. Dermatology. 2nd ed. Spain: Elsevier; 2008: 321–30.

[a] Morphology of retiform purpura is composed of "puzzle pieces" of the livedo reticularis pattern. Some lesions are riverine or serpentine purpura, and some are branching purpura. Very few of these lesions are stellate, i.e., characterized by a central area of necrosis or hemorrhage with radiating extensions.

Purpura generally have a very simple evolution, from initial hemorrhage to steady clearing of red blood cells and hemoglobin clinically seen as fading of lesions and transition of color from red to blue or purple to green, yellow, or brown before complete fading, which is easily appreciated in larger lesions.

Immune complex–mediated vasculitis has a different pathogenetic mechanism of purpura formation as follows [5]:

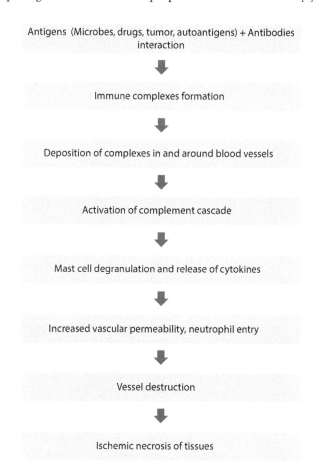

Antigens (Microbes, drugs, tumor, autoantigens) + Antibodies interaction

⬇

Immune complexes formation

⬇

Deposition of complexes in and around blood vessels

⬇

Activation of complement cascade

⬇

Mast cell degranulation and release of cytokines

⬇

Increased vascular permeability, neutrophil entry

⬇

Vessel destruction

⬇

Ischemic necrosis of tissues

EVALUATION OF PATIENTS WITH PURPURA

Our aim is to evaluate and classify patients presenting with this important dermatologic sign in order to recognize patients whose purpura is a sign of a life-threatening disease, and would therefore require detailed laboratory investigations and prompt management.

History

Detailed history is of paramount importance and includes details regarding the onset of purpura (sudden/insidious), duration, progress, preceding history of infection, drug intake, trauma, stress, associated mucocutaneous symptoms, constitutional and systemic symptoms, bleeding from

Table 35.2 Etiological classification of purpura

A. Intravascular causes
1. Platelet disorders
   a. Thrombocytopenia
   b. Platelet function disorders
   c. Thrombocytosis
2. Coagulation disorders
   a. Inherited disorders (e.g., hemophilia, Von Willebrand disease)
   b. Acquired disorders
      i. Drugs (e.g., anticoagulants)
      ii. Metabolic (vitamin K deficiency, liver disease)
      iii. Disseminated intravascular coagulation and purpura fulminans
      iv. Thrombophilias (protein C, protein S deficiency)
      v. Localized (heparin injection sites, some insect bites)
      vi. Secondary to systemic disease (often multifactorial, e.g., macrophage activation syndrome)
3. Intravascular pressure spikes
   a. Straining during childbirth
   b. Valsalva maneuver
   c. Vigorous repetitive coughing or retching or crying in children
   d. Tourniquet stasis
4. Purpura with microvasculature occlusion
   a. Embolic (e.g., septic, fat, cholesterol, crystal, myxoma)
   b. Cryoproteins (e.g., cryoglobulinemia, cryofibrinogenemia)
   c. Infective (e.g., ecthyma gangrenosum, disseminated strongyloidiasis)
   d. Platelet plugs (e.g., thrombotic thrombocytopenic purpura, myeloproliferative disorders)
   e. Dysproteinemias (Waldenstrom macroglobulinemia)

B. Vessel wall causes
1. Associated with inflammation
   a. Toxin and drug induced
   b. Capillaritis (pigmented purpuric dermatoses) [14–20]
   c. Vasculitis
   d. Infections
2. Non inflammatory/Direct vascular damage:
   a. Toxin and drug mediated (e.g., aspirin, barbiturates, carbromal)
   b. Systemic amyloidosis
   c. Fibrin clot occlusion
   d. Cryoglobulin gel occlusion

C. Extravascular causes
1. Decreased vascular support (e.g., actinic purpura, steroid purpura, scurvy, Ehlers–Danlos syndrome, amyloidosis)
2. Abnormal vessels (e.g., acroangiodermatitis)
3. Purpura around vascular lesions (targetoid hemosiderotic hemangioma, aneurysmal fibrous histiocytoma, tufted hemangioma)

D. Miscellaneous
1. Purpura in otherwise nonpurpuric dermatoses (e.g., lichen sclerosus, pityriasis rosea, lichen nitidus, erythema multiforme, pityriasis lichenoides group) [28–35]
2. Painful bruising syndrome (Gardner-Diamond syndrome)
3. Physical and artifactual purpura
4. Contact purpura
5. Stigmata
6. Paroxysmal finger hematoma
7. Easy bruising syndrome and purpura simplex

other sites, and family and past history of bleeding tendencies. Drug history is particularly important if a new drug has been started. Also, history of a recent blood transfusion may be relevant as posttransfusion purpura is a rare but serious complication, characterized by severe thrombocytopenia 5–10 days after transfusion [6]. In case of women of reproductive age, the obstetric history becomes important with regard to pregnancy loss.

Examination

Thorough clinical examination of the lesions has to be done to identify purpura based on morphological traits, number, size, distribution, site (Table 35.3) [2], palpability, and associated features like pustules, nodules, necrosis, and ulceration. Particular attention has to be paid to determine systemic associations (associated constitutional symptoms: fever, arthralgia, malaise). There are certain warning signs (Box 35.1) [2] that indicate that thorough investigation in the patient is required. At times there is an overlap of clinical presentations. A detailed and careful examination of early lesions in such cases can determine whether there is a substantial inflammatory component and thus greatly aid in focusing on the differential diagnosis, thereby directing appropriate evaluation. Also, evaluation can be greatly facilitated on the basis of morphologic subsets as the differential diagnoses of purpura are extensive (Table 5.4) [1,7].

Table 35.3 Sites of purpura that can aid diagnosis

Site	Cause of purpura
Eyelids	Increased venous pressure classically during Valsalva, severe coughing/vomiting after endoscopy [22], Panda sign in amyloidosis, ecchymosis related to neuroblastoma
Ears	Cryoglobulinemia, other hyperviscosity disorders, antineutrophil cytoplasmic antibody positive vasculitis, drugs such as propylthiouracil, levamisole
Face, ears, acral areas	Acute hemorrhagic edema of infancy, cryoglobulinemia, other hyperviscosity disorders, embolic causes, rickettsial infection
Friction sites	Clothing contact purpura, some cases of capillaritis, Henoch–Schönlein purpura, Ehlers–Danlos syndrome
Intraoral	Thrombocytopenia, amyloidosis, myelomonocytic leukemia, angina bullosa hemorrhagica

Source: Mittal A, Gupta LK. In: Sacchidanand S, Oberai C, Inamadar AC (Eds), *IADVL Textbook of Dermatology*. 4th ed. Mumbai: Bhalani; 2015:1187–203.

Based on history and clinical examination, a general approach to purpura is as follows [7]:

Identify the primary morphology

Determine the likely pathophysiology

Consider possible differentials

Appropriate workup accordingly

LABORATORY TESTS

Investigations for purpura depend on clinical differentials as revealed by history and clinical examination. These include the following:

1. Complete blood count, with differential count.
2. Routine hemogram may provide clues to hematologic abnormalities leading to purpura.
3. Peripheral blood smear to assess the morphology and number of platelets. It also screens for schistocytes (seen in DIC) to rule out myeloproliferative disease.
4. Platelet count is the most important test in the evaluation of nonpalpable purpura. Purpura due to thrombocytopenia usually occurs below a count of 50,000/mm^3.
5. Platelet function abnormalities can be assessed by *in vitro* tests. Bleeding time is a useful screening tool for it. The normal bleeding time is 3–6 minutes, which may be prolonged in thrombocytopenia and platelet function disorders but is normal in coagulation disorders. Bleeding time nowadays is less commonly preferred to platelet function analysis (PFA-100), which has greater

Table 35.4 Differential diagnosis based on morphologic subsets

A. Petechiae (<4 mm)

1. Hemostatically relevant thrombocytopenia (<20,000/mm^3)
   a. Thrombocytopenia
      i. Immune thrombocytopenic purpura
      ii. Thrombotic thrombocytopenic purpura [12]
      iii. Disseminated intravascular coagulation
      iv. Heparin-induced thrombocytopenia
   b. Drugs (causing peripheral destruction, e.g., quinine, quinidine; causing decreased production and causing bone marrow fibrosis, e.g., chemotherapy)
   c. Leukemia/bone marrow failure
   d. Hemolytic uremic syndrome
   e. Liver cirrhosis

2. Abnormal platelet function
   a. Congenital/hereditary
      i. Von Willebrand disease
      ii. Glanzmann thromboaesthenia
      iii. Storage pool disease
   b. Acquired (aspirin, NSAIDs, renal insufficiency, monoclonal gammopathy)
   c. Thrombocytosis
   d. Myeloproliferative diseases
   e. Renal insufficiency

3. Nonplatelet etiologies
   a. Raised intravascular pressure (Valsalva, seizure)
   b. Mild inflammatory conditions
      i. Pigmented purpuric dermatosis
      ii. Hypergammaglobulinemic purpura, Waldenstrom)
   c. Amyloidosis
   d. Steroid (topical/systemic) induced atrophy
   e. Fragility syndromes (Ehlers–Danlos syndrome)
   f. Scurvy (perifollicular)
   g. Graft versus host disease
   h. Infection
      i. Early Rocky Mountain spotted fever
      ii. Parvovirus
      iii. Epstein-Barr virus
   i. Trauma (linear mostly)
   j. Fixed increased pressure (stasis, ligatures)
   k. Early leukocytoclastic vasculitis
   l. Actinic damage

B. Nonpalpable purpura/macular purpura (4–10 mm)

1. Hypergammaglobulinemic purpura (Waldenstrom)
2. Infections/inflammation/trauma in patients with abnormal platelet function
3. Infections/inflammation/trauma in patients with thrombocytopenia or immune compromise
4. Abnormal coagulation + Trauma
   a. Disseminated intravascular coagulation
   b. Renal or hepatic dysfunction
   c. Anticoagulant medications
   d. Vitamin K deficiency
5. Early lesions of vasculitis (leukocytoclastic vasculitis), pauci-immune complex vasculitis (usually in dependent distribution)
6. Poor dermal support + Trauma
   a. Actinic damage
   b. Amyloid
   c. Steroid atrophy
   d. Fragility syndromes
   e. Trauma
   f. Scurvy
7. Others
   a. Contact dermatitis
   b. Emboli

C. Macular ecchymoses (≥1 cm)

1. Procoagulant defect plus minor trauma
   a. Anticoagulant use
   b. Hepatic insufficiency with poor procoagulant synthesis
   c. Vitamin K deficiency
   d. Disseminated intravascular coagulation (some)

(Continued)

Table 35.4 *(Continued)* Differential diagnosis based on morphologic subsets

2. Poor dermal support of vessels plus minor trauma	a. Actinic (solar, senile) purpura b. Corticosteroid therapy, topical or systemic c. Vitamin C deficiency (scurvy) d. Systemic amyloidosis (light chain related, some familial types) e. Hereditary: Ehlers–Danlos syndrome
3. Platelet problems plus minor trauma	a. Platelet function defects, including von Willebrand disease and those induced by medications and metabolic diseases b. Acquired or congenital thrombocytopenia
4. Other causes	a. Hypergammaglobulinemic purpura (Waldenstrom) b. Capillaritis c. Easy bruising syndrome, purpura simplex d. Physical and artifactual causes e. Stigmata f. Painful bruising syndrome

D. Inflammatory palpable purpura with prominent early erythema

1. Leukocytoclastic vasculitis due to immune complex disease
   a. Small vessels only
      i. Idiopathic (45%–55%), infection (15%–20%), inflammatory diseases (15%–20%), drug (10%–15%), malignancy (5%) associated IgG or IgM complexes
      ii. Idiopathic IgA complexes (HSP), or IgA complexes associated with drugs or infection
      iii. Hypergammaglobulinemic purpura of Waldenström
      iv. Urticarial vasculitis: often minimally purpuric
      v. Pustular vasculitis (e.g., bowel bypass syndrome)
   b. Small and medium-sized (macroscopic) vessels involved
      i. Mixed cryoglobulinemia
      ii. Rheumatic vasculitides (lupus erythematosus, rheumatoid arthritis)
      iii. Behçet disease

2. Pauci-immune leukocytoclastic vasculitis
   a. Antineutrophil cytoplasmic antibody associated
      i. Granulomatosis with polyangiitis (Wegener granulomatosis)
      ii. Microscopic polyangiitis
      iii. Eosinophilic granulomatosis with polyangiitis (Churg-Strauss syndrome)
   b. Other
      i. Erythema elevatum diutinum
      ii. Sweet syndrome (vasculitis unusual)
      iii. Levamisole vasculitis
      iv. Leukemic vasculitis

3. Not leukocytoclastic vasculitis
   a. Small vessels only
      i. Erythema multiforme (classic target lesion, can also be seen in small vessel vasculitis especially IgA associated)
      ii. Pityriasis lichenoides et varioliformis acuta
      iii. Pigmented purpuric eruptions
      iv. Hypergammaglobulinemic purpura of Waldenstrom (some lesions may have histologic evidence of leukocytoclastic vasculitis)
   b. Other
      i. Papular and purpuric eruption due to cytarabine
      ii. Parvovirus B-19 infection (follicular and purpuric papules, popular and purpuric gloves and socks)

E. Noninflammatory retiform purpura

1. Occlusion primarily due to microvascular platelet plugs	a. Heparin necrosis b. Thrombocytosis secondary to myeloproliferative disorders c. Paroxysmal nocturnal hemoglobinuria d. Thrombotic thrombocytopenic purpura (though platelet plugs form primarily in visceral vessels, and skin hemorrhage is due more often to thrombocytopenia)
2. Cold-related gelling or agglutination	a. Cryoglobulinemia, monoclonal (early lesions of mixed cryoglobulinemia are often inflammatory and leukocytoclastic due to immune complex deposition)

(Continued)

Table 35.4 (*Continued*) Differential diagnosis based on morphologic subsets

	b. Cryofibrinogenemia (though most cryofibrinogens are incidental findings in hospitalized patients)
	c. Cold agglutinins (rarely cause occlusion; usually cause hemolysis or are asymptomatic)
3. Occlusion due to organisms growing in vessels	a. Vessel-invasive fungi (mucormycosis, Aspergillus usually in immunocompromised patients)
	b. Ecthyma gangrenosum (often Pseudomonas or other gram-negative bacilli proliferating in adventitia of subcutaneous arterioles)
	c. Disseminated strongyloidiasis
	d. Lucio phenomenon in leprosy
4. Systemic alteration in control of coagulation	a. Proteins C and S related
	i. Homozygous protein C or protein S deficiency
	ii. Acquired protein C deficiency (some patients with sepsis-associated DIC)
	iii. Coumadin necrosis (protein C dysfunction)
	iv. Postinfectious purpura fulminans (protein S dysfunction)
	b. Antiphospholipid antibody, lupus anticoagulant
5. Vascular coagulopathy	a. Livedoid vasculopathy/atrophie blanche (may also have a systemic prothrombotic component)
	b. Malignant atrophic papulosis/Degos disease (antiphospholipid antibody syndrome can mimic this disease)
	c. Sneddon syndrome (in some patients, related to antiphospholipid antibody syndrome)
6. Embolization or crystal deposition	a. Cholesterol emboli
	b. Oxalate crystal deposition (rare)
	c. Marantic endocarditis, atrial myxoma, crystal globulins hypereosinophilic syndrome (all rare)
7. Reticulocyte, red blood cell occlusion	a. High reticulocyte states:
	i. Sickle cell disease; occlusion worsened by red cell sickling
	ii. Other severe hemolytic anemias
8. Miscellaneous	a. Calciphylaxis

F. Inflammatory retiform purpura

Vasculitis	a. Primarily dermal vessels
	i. IgA vasculitis
	b. Dermal and subcutaneous vessels usually involved
	i. Mixed cryoglobulinemia
	ii. Rheumatic vasculitides (lupus erythematosus, rheumatoid arthritis)
	iii. Polyarteritis nodosa
	iv. Microscopic polyangiitis
	v. Wegener granulomatosis
	vi. Churg-Strauss syndrome
Dermal vessel inflammation/occlusion/constriction	a. Livedoid vasculopathy
	b. Septic vasculitis
	c. Chilblains (pernio)
	d. Pyoderma gangrenosum

Source: Warren P. *Dermatology.* 2nd ed. Spain: Elsevier; 2008:321–30; Arakaki R, Fox L. *Curr Derm Rep* 2017;6:55–62.

Table 35.5 Investigations depending on morphology of purpura

Petechiae	Macular purpura	Palpable purpura	Retiform purpura
Complete blood count with differential	Complete blood count with differential	Complete blood count with differential	Complete blood count with differential
Liver function test	Liver function test	Liver function test	Peripheral blood smear and blood culture
Renal function test	Renal function test	Renal function test	Complement
Coagulation studies	Coagulation studies	Urinalysis	Echocardiogram
Rule out drug as etiology		ASO titer	Urine toxicology screen
Platelet function study	Rule out drug as etiology	Complement	Biopsy for hematoxylin and eosin (H&E), culture, and direct immunofluorescence (DIF)
Evaluate for fragility syndromes	Evaluate for fragility syndromes	Echocardiogram	Antineutrophil cytoplasmic antibody, rheumatoid factor, cryoglobulins
Other tests as required	Other tests as required	Hepatitis serologies	Hypercoagulability workup
		Biopsy for H&E, culture and DIF	Serum calcium, phosphate
		Other tests as required	Serum immunoelectrophoresis

Source: Arakaki R, Fox L. Curr Derm Rep 2017;6:55–62.

sensitivity and reproducibility than the bleeding time test [8].

6. Coagulation profile, which includes clotting time, prothrombin time, and fibrinogen level, may detect coagulation factor abnormalities. Protein C and protein S levels are special tests done if occlusion syndromes are suspected.

7. Capillary resistance test (Hess test) depends on the principle that if capillary pressure is made to sufficiently exceed tissue pressure, leakage of blood may occur, producing petechiae. In the Hess test, the sphygmomanometer cuff is inflated around the upper arm and kept at 80 mm Hg for 5 minutes. The appearance of more than five petechiae over an area of 5 cm diameter just below the antecubital fossa is considered a positive test. This test can be positive in purpura due to thrombocytopenia or vascular defects.

8. Occult blood tests of urine and stool are employed to detect hemorrhage from body sites other than the skin.

9. Histopathology of biopsy specimens of early lesions is required especially if vasculitis is thought of as a cause. The evolution and clearing of lesions are complicated in vasculitis and in microvascular occlusion and with later lesions having overlapping histopathology. Histopathology must be interpreted with respect to the lesion's age and clinical setting. Histopathology of cutaneous lesions in purpura fulminans shows cutaneous necrosis without evidence of inflammation and occlusion of blood vessels with platelet-fibrin thrombi [9].

10. Other serological tests like antiphospholipid antibody syndrome panel, antinuclear antibody, serum protein electrophoresis, immunoelectrophoresis, SS-A and SS-B levels, and rheumatoid factor, should be undertaken when indicated and should focus on finding the nature and extent of the underlying cause.

11. Immunofluorescence studies for immune complexes if vasculitis is suspected (Table 35.5).

MANAGEMENT

Management primarily deals with identifying the correct etiology and treating it along with simultaneous initiation of nonspecific treatment in the form of rest to limb, compression hosiery, pain relief, and ulcer care wherever applicable. Oral immunosuppressives are required in most cases of vasculitis. Specific treatment is further detailed in Table 35.6.

CONCLUSION

Purpura is an important cutaneous clinical sign with myriad of causes ranging from trivial to life-threatening disorders. Prompt identification of this sign and approaching the patient based on thorough history and clinical examination can be significant as early diagnosis and treatment initiation can save the life of a patient in cases with purpura secondary to causes with significant mortality.

Table 35.6 Treatment of important conditions manifesting as purpura

Condition	Specific treatment
Purpura due to platelet disorders	
Immune thrombocytopenic purpura [10,11]	Systemic steroids: Prednisolone (1–1.5 mg/kg body weight per day) in severe cases followed by IV immunoglobulins (IVIg) if platelet counts remain below 5000 per cm^3; ongoing bleed requires platelet infusion, splenectomy; avoid activities that predispose to trauma and medications that impair platelet function; chronic refractory cases: immunosuppressives (azathioprine, cyclophosphamide, or cyclosporine in addition to steroids), anti-D IgG; rituximab can be utilized
Thrombotic thrombocytopenic purpura (TTP)	Acquired acute TTP: Daily plasma exchange followed by glucocorticoids or splenectomy; familial TTP: Infusion of platelet-poor fresh frozen plasma, cryoprecipitate-poor plasma (cryosupernatant)
Disseminated intravascular coagulation	Management of the precipitating cause along with supportive measures: Replacement of blood products and anticoagulants
Purpura fulminans	Treatment is supportive, with treatment of the underlying disease with antibiotics and anticoagulation with replacement of fresh frozen plasma [13]; protein C and antithrombin therapy may be instituted; plasma exchange in sepsis with multiple organ dysfunction (if facilities are available); for severe necrotic lesions of the extremities, amputation may be needed
Pigmented purpuric dermatoses	Persistent lesions do not respond well to therapy; reassurance and supportive hosiery; topical steroids may reduce symptoms of pruritus and lighten the pigment; some beneficial therapeutics include pentoxifylline, psoralen plus ultraviolet A therapy, ascorbic acid, griseofulvin, and cyclosporine; methotrexate has been used in case of Majocchi disease
Purpura mediated by drugs and toxins	Withdrawal of implicated agent
Purpura associated with infections	Treat the underlying infection
Purpura from raised intravascular pressure [21]	Measures to reduce intravascular pressure
Purpura from decreased vascular support	
a. Actinic/senile purpura	No treatment is required; reassure the patient; topical therapy with retinol, alpha hydroxy acids, ceramides, arnica oil, niacinamide, and phytonadione have also been tried individually or in combination with benefits in only a few patients [23]
b. Steroid purpura [24]	Stop usage of steroids; topical retinoids have been used with little benefit
c. Scurvy [25,26]	Vitamin C replenishment
Disorders of connective tissue	
Acroangiodermatitis of Mali [27]	Correction of the underlying vascular pathology; compression stockings for venous stasis and local wound care for ulcers; various medical modalities of therapy include oral erythromycin 500 mg four times a day or dapsone 50 mg twice a day for 3 months along with topical corticosteroid preparations; surgical treatment for underlying arteriovenous malformations; laser: pulsed-dye laser has been used with some success for clearing few lesions
Dermatoses associated with purpura	Treatment as per the underlying dermatoses
Painful bruising syndrome (synonyms: psychogenic purpura, Gardner-Diamond syndrome, autoerythrocyte sensitization syndrome)	There is no definitive treatment; symptomatic therapy is initiated for severe general symptoms; several approaches including antihistamines, corticosteroids, antidepressants, hormones, and vitamins have met with variable success [36]; psychotherapy, which is most effective when initiated early in the disease, is recommended [37].

(Continued)

Table 35.6 (*Continued*) Treatment of important conditions manifesting as purpura

Condition	Specific treatment
Physical and artifactual purpura	Counsel the patient; avoid trauma
Contact purpura [38]	Avoid contact with offending agent
Paroxysmal finger hematoma (synonyms: Achenbach syndrome) [39]	Avoid trauma to extremities
Stigmata [40]	Psychotherapy with particular attention to the sociocultural background of patient and patient's family
Vasculitis	Discussed in Chapter 31

REFERENCES

1. Warren P. Purpura: Mechanisms and differential diagnosis. In: Bolognia JL, Jorizzo JL, Rapini RP (Eds), *Dermatology*. 2nd ed. Spain: Elsevier; 2008:321–30.
2. Mittal A, Gupta LK. Purpura. In: Sacchidanand S, Oberai C, Inamdar AC (Eds), *IADVL Textbook of Dermatology*. 4th ed. Mumbai: Bhalani Publishing; 2015:1187–203.
3. Jennette JC et al. 2012 Revised International Chapel Hill Consensus Conference Nomenclature of Vasculitides. *Arthritis Rheum* 2013;65(1):1–11.
4. Bandyopadhyay D. Pupura, vasculitis, and neutrophilic dermatoses. In: Valia RG, Valia AR (Eds), *IADVL Textbook of Dermatology*. 3rd ed. Mumbai: Bhalani Publishing; 2010:681–715.
5. Sneller MC, Langford CA, Fauci AS. The vasculitis syndromes. In: Kasper DL et al. (Eds), *Harrison's Principles of Internal Medicine*. 16th ed. New York: McGraw-Hill; 2005:2002–17.
6. Thomas AE, Baird SF, Anderson J. Purpuric and petechial rashes in adults and children: Initial assessment. *BMJ* 2016;352:1285.
7. Arakaki R, Fox L. Updates in the approach to the patient with purpura. *Curr Derm Rep* 2017;6:55–62.
8. Posan E, McBane RD, Grill DE, Motsko CL, Nichols WL. Comparison of PFA-100 testing and bleeding time for detecting platelet hypofunction and von Willebrand disease in clinical practice. *Thromb Haemost* 2003;90(3):483–90.
9. Adcock DM, Hicks MJ. Dermatopathology of skin necrosis associated with purpura fulminans. *Semin Thromb Hemost* 1990;16(4):283–92.
10. Carcao MD et al. Short course oral prednisone therapy in children presenting with acute immune thrombocytopenic purpura (immune thrombocytopenic purpura). *Acta Paediatr Suppl* 1998;424:71–4.
11. Dickerhoff R, von Ruecker A. The clinical course of immune thrombocytopenic purpura in children who did not receive intravenous immunoglobulins or sustained prednisone treatment. *J Pediatr* 2000;137(5):629–32.
12. Galbusera M, Noris M, Remuzzi G. Thrombotic thrombocytopenic purpura—Then and now. *Semin Thromb Hemost* 2006;32(2):81–9.
13. Chalmers E et al. Purpura fulminans: Recognition, diagnosis and management. *Arch Dis Child* 2011;96(11):1066–71.
14. Kanwar AJ, Thami GP. Familial Schamberg's disease. *Dermatology* 1999;198:175–6.
15. Hoesley FJ, Huerter CJ, Shehan JM. Purpura annularis telangiectodes of Majocchi: Case report and review of the literature. *Int J Dermatol* 2009;48:1129–33.
16. Babilas P, Roesch A, Szeimies RM, Landthaler M, Vogt T. Zosteriform pigmented purpura of Schamberg: Case report and differential diagnosis of zosteriform skin lesions. *J Dtsch Dermatol Ges.* 2004;2(11):931–4.
17. Mishra D, Maheshwari V. Segmental lichen aureus in a child. *Int J Dermatol.* 1991;30:654–55.
18. Robert I, Rudolph MD. Lichen aureus. *J Am Acad Dermatol* 1983;8:722–4.
19. Kems MJ, Mallatt BD, Shamma HN. Granulomatous pigmented purpura: Unusual histological variant. *Am J Dermatopathol* 2009;31(1):77–80.
20. Sathiasekar AC, Deepti DA Sekar GSS. Drug-induced thrombocytopenic purpura. *J Pharm Bioallied Sci* 2015;7(2):S827–9.
21. Kravitz P. The clinical picture of "cough purpura," benign and non-thrombocytopenic eruption. *Va Med* 1979;106(5):373–4.
22. Kaliyadan F, Kuruvilla JP. Post vomiting purpura. *Indian Dermatol Online J* 2016;7(5):456–7.
23. Ceilley RI. Treatment of actinic purpura. *J Clin Aesthet Dermatol* 2017;10(6):44–50.
24. Abraham A, Roga G. Topical steroid-damaged skin. *Indian J Dermatol* 2014;59(5):456–9.
25. Mintsoulis D, Milman N, Fahim S. A case of scurvy-uncommon disease—Presenting as panniculitis, purpura, and oligoarthritis. *J Cutan Med Surg* 2016;20(6):592–5.
26. Christensen AF, Clemmensen O, Junker P. Case report—Palpable purpura with an unexpected outcome. *Case Rep Rheumatol* 2013;15:1–3.
27. Mehta AA, Pereira RR, Nayak CS. Dhurat. Acroangiodermatitis of Mali: A rare vascular phenomenon. *IJDVL* 2010;76(5):553–6.
28. Pierson JC, Dijkstra JW, Elston DM. Purpuric pityriasis rosea. *J Am Acad Dermatol* 1993;28:1021.

29. Yanez S, Val-Bernal JF. Purpuric generalized lichen nitidus: An unusual eruption simulating pigmented purpuric dermatosis. *Dermatology* 2004;208:167–70.

30. Lewis M, Mercurio MG. Genital purpura as the presenting sign of lichen sclerosus. *JAAD* 2016;75(5):e97–8.

31. Limb J, Binning A. Thrombosis associated with varicella zoster in an adult. *Int J Infect Dis* 2009;13:e498–500.

32. Nikkels AF et al. Simultaneous reactivation of herpes simplex virus and varicella zoster virus in a patient with idiopathic thrombocytopenic purpura. *Dermatology* 1999;199(4):361–4.

33. Karatsun V et al. Autoerythrocyte sensitization (Gardner-Diamond) syndrome mimicking compartment syndrome. *Arch Orthop Trauma Surg* 2003;123:370–1.

34. Ingen–Housz–Oro S et al. Painful bruising syndrome mimicking cellulitis of the leg. *Ann Dermatol Venereol* 2002;129:1029–32.

35. Vivekanandh K, Dash G, Mohanty P. Gardner-Diamond syndrome: A psychogenic purpura. *Indian Dermatol Online J* 2017;8(6):521–2.

36. Jafferany M, Bhattacharya G. Psychogenic purpura (Gardner-Diamond syndrome). *Prim Care Companion CNS Disord* 2015;17(1):1–49.

37. Ring HC, Miller IM, Benfeldt E, Jemec GB. Artefactual skin lesions in children and adolescents: Review of the literature and two cases of factitious purpura. *Int J Dermatol* 2015;54(1):e27–32.

38. Bonamonte D, Foti C, Vestita M, Angelini G. Noneczematous contact dermatitis. *ISRN Allergy* 2013;2013Article ID 361746, 10 . https://doi.org/10.1155/2013/361746.

39. Layton AM, Cotterill JA. A case of Achenbach's syndrome. *Clin Exp Dermatol* 1993;18:60–1.

40. Verstraete M. Psychogenic haemorrhage. *Verh K acadgeneeskdbelg* 1991;53(1):5–28.

PART 9

Skin Malignancies Presenting as Emergencies

VINAY GERA

36

Dermatological manifestations of malignancies and dermatological emergencies due to malignancy

TANUMAY ROYCHOWDHURY

INTRODUCTION

Patients with malignant hemopathies such as leukemias and lymphomas often present to a dermatologist with emergencies that require immediate attention. These referrals could range from severe pruritus or rash to localized cutaneous lesions to systemic emergencies, and it is a difficult task for the clinician to distinguish common causes versus those caused by the primary disease or features resulting from ongoing drugs or procedures such as bone marrow transplantation that might have been performed.

This review aims at helping the reader understand some common causes for emergencies in this subset of patients with leukemias and lymphomas and also creating an algorithmic approach to rash/pruritus in such patients.

The etiologies for urgent presentation to a dermatology outpatient department or referral for an inpatient in case of malignancies could be broadly classified as follows:

1. Extramedullary cutaneous localizations of primary disease
   a. Leukemia cutis
   b. Secondary cutaneous lymphomas
2. Primary cutaneous lymphomas
3. Cutaneous infections of affected skin
4. Adverse cutaneous reactions to anticancer drugs
5. Paraneoplastic manifestations

EXTRAMEDULLARY CUTANEOUS LOCALIZATIONS OF PRIMARY DISEASE: LEUKEMIA CUTIS/GRANULOCYTIC SARCOMA

Extramedullary (EM) involvement of leukemias can occur in the presence or absence of bone marrow involvement. The spectrum of EM leukemia ranges from leukemia cutis (LC) to granulocytic sarcoma (GS), also known as chloroma, myeloid sarcoma, or myeloblastoma, which may overlap. LC can infiltrate the epidermis, dermis, and subcutis and present accordingly. LC is now used as an umbrella term for any cutaneous infiltration of leukemia. Further classification of lymphoid LC or myeloid LC is sometimes done depending on the cell type.

A dermatologist has an important role in the diagnosis of leukemia cutis since it has immense prognostic significance. Leukemia cutis could occur prior to systemic involvement, signify relapse, signify blast transformation, or correlate with other extramedullary sites of involvement.

Epidemiology

Since LC is a rare diagnosis, the true incidence is not known. Its incidence is higher in places endemic for HTLV-1 infection such as Japan and the Caribbean; hence, chances of cutaneous manifestations of HTLV-1 associated adult T-cell leukemia/lymphoma (ATLL) are higher in these areas. LC is higher among children, and up to 25% of cases of congenital leukemias can present with LC, without any prognostic significance. In up to 7% of LC, skin involvement precedes bone marrow disease or systemic symptoms.

Extramedullary involvement is most common in acute myeloid leukemia (AML), especially AML type 4 and monoblastic AML type 5, but it is also seen in myelodysplastic syndrome (MDS), chronic myeloid leukemia (CML), chronic lymphocytic leukemia (CLL), chronic myelomonocytic leukemia (CMML), and acute lymphocytic leukemia (ALL). In AML, <10% of GS and <5% of LC have been observed.

MDS represents a heterogenous group of clonal hematopoietic disorders characterized by ineffective hemopoiesis and cytopenias. The median age is 60–75 years and can be primary (*de novo*) or secondary (postcytotoxic therapy or radiotherapy). It carries a 30%–40% risk of transformation to AML.

Etiopathogenesis

Leukemic cells, usually myeloblasts, can invade through the bloodstream into nonhematopoeitic tissue such as skin. EM involvement usually occurs concurrently with bone marrow involvement, although before and after presentations are also reported. EM can sometimes be the only initial presenting feature and hence poses an emergency if recognized early by the dermatologist. GC almost always progresses to systemic disease, though aleukemic LC is known to occur. Aleukemic LC (LC without systemic involvement) is managed like systemic disease. LC and GS can also be presenting features of relapse in those without extramedullary involvement at primary diagnosis.

Clinical features

LC typically presents as erythematous to brown or violaceous infiltrated subcutaneous papules or nodules (Figure 36.1). Irrespective of the type of primary leukemia, they have similar papulonodular morphology and have a tendency to arise at sites of prior or current inflammation, notably on the back, trunk, face, and extremities.

Usually secondary epidermal changes of scaling, vesicles, or erosions are not seen. Grouped lesions with polymorphous manifestations including purpuric macules, papules, nodules, and plaques with necrosis or crusting with a hemorrhagic red or bluish halo can be found. Numbers can range from solitary to multiple lesions, and firm hemorrhagic infiltrative papulonodular eruption developing over a short duration of days to weeks leads the clinician suspect metastatic infiltration.

Investigations

The first step is to do a complete blood count and a peripheral blood picture if a hemogenic malignancy is suspected. Skin biopsy is the only conclusive way to diagnose LC. Histologically a Grenz zone spares the papillary dermis.

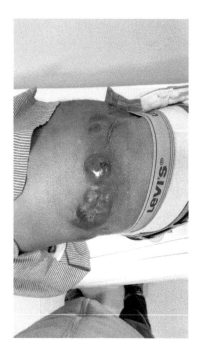

Figure 36.1 Leukemia cutis.

When atypical infiltrates are observed, phenotyping is done by immunohistochemistry/flow cytometry.

Prognosis and treatment

Prognosis is poor as with other extramedullary involvement in leukemias, whether AML or CML. In CLL, the prognosis is dependent on large cell transformation or systemic involvement rather than cutaneous infiltration.

Treatment of leukemia cutis is aggressive systemic chemotherapy or bone marrow transplant in first remission since it often indicates poor prognosis. The role of a dermatologist is in the suspicion of this condition and performance of a biopsy to make an early diagnosis.

EXTRAMEDULLARY CUTANEOUS LOCALIZATIONS OF PRIMARY DISEASE: SECONDARY CUTANEOUS LYMPHOMAS

Secondary cutaneous lymphomas, depending on the cell type, localization, and subtype, have various clinical morphologies. The more common subtypes include peripheral T-cell lymphoma, NK/T-cell lymphoma, anaplastic large cell lymphoma, angioimmunoblastic lymphoma, and ATLL under the T-cell lineage. B-cell lineage lymphomas include diffuse large B-cell lymphoma (most common), Burkitt lymphoma, and others.

Epidemiology

Secondary cutaneous lymphomas, although not uncommon in practice, have been reported in very few studies as compared to primary cutaneous lymphomas. In three comparative studies from Korea and Japan, 20%–50% of

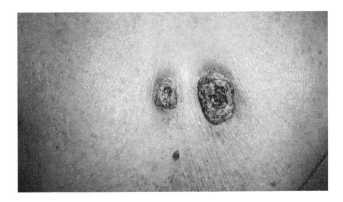

Figure 36.2 NK/T-cell lymphoma.

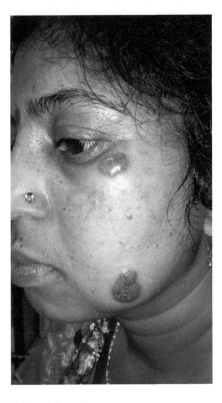

Figure 36.3 B-cell lymphoma.

all cutaneous lymphomas can be secondary. Secondary B-cell lymphomas are more common than primary B-cell lymphomas.

Clinical features

NK/T-cell secondary lymphomas commonly present as inflamed cellulitic/indurated plaques that ulcerate (Figure 36.2). Other T-cell lineage lesions can present as patches, plaques, or nodules and are often multiple and disseminated. Angioimmunoblastic lymphomas can present as disseminated macules or patches. Lesions are usually seen on extremities in the T-cell lineage.

B-cell lesions present as solitary or a few plaques or tumescent nodules, and are often located over the head, neck, trunk, or less frequently on the extremities (Figure 36.3).

Investigations

A skin biopsy with immunohistochemistry and T-cell receptor rearrangement for clonality helps to confirm diagnosis. Lactate dehdrogenase (LDH) levels, systemic examination, imaging including positron emission tomography–computed tomography (PET-CT) scan, blood/bone marrow examination, and lymph node biopsies/splenic biopsies/suspected primary site biopsies help in making an appropriate diagnosis.

Treatment and prognosis

Evidence of skin lesions within 6 months of diagnosis of the primary lymphoma is associated with a poor prognosis. Usually a secondary cutaneous lymphoma portends a poorer prognosis with an estimated 5-year survival rate around 30%. Early diagnosis is therefore of paramount importance. The treatment is mostly with single-agent to multiagent chemotherapy depending on the cell type and staging of the primary disease. The dermatologist's role is mainly to identify a cutaneous lymphoma and look for primaries elsewhere and help determine whether this is a primary or secondary skin manifestation.

PRIMARY CUTANEOUS LYMPHOMAS

The most common primary cutaneous lymphomas are mycosis fungoides (MF) and lymphomatoid papulosis that have an indolent course and do not present as emergencies. However, certain T-cell subtypes such as Sézary syndrome that presents with erythroderma or advanced-stage mycosis fungoides, extranodal NK/T-cell lymphoma, nasal type (ENKTCLNT) and other Epstein-Barr virus (EBV)–associated neoplasms, ATLL, primary cutaneous aggressive epidermotropic CD8+ cytotoxic T-cell lymphoma (AECTCL), and primary cutaneous γδ T-cell lymphoma (PCGDTCL) can have a fatal course.

MF that has undergone large cell transformation or folliculotropic MF can be aggressive with ulceration. Subcutaneous panniculitis such as T-cell lymphoma with hemophagocytosis is potentially aggressive as well and presents as an emergency. It is important to recognize these particular subtypes when tailoring therapy, which is broadly guided by the stage of the disease.

Sézary syndrome

Sézary syndrome is a leukemic variant of CTCL, with significant blood involvement (B2) under evaluation of the skin (T), lymph nodes (N), visceral involvement (M), and blood (B) (TNMB) classification, and has a very aggressive course, similar to visceral involvement with a poor prognosis (Figure 36.4). Assessment of peripheral blood for tumor burden by clonality and evaluation of the peripheral blood for Sézary cells in erythroderma is important in addition to noting age, male gender, and LDH levels.

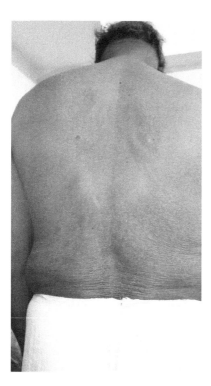

Figure 36.4 Sézary syndrome.

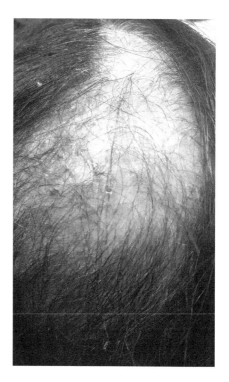

Figure 36.6 Folliculotropic mycosis fungoides.

Large cell transformation

Large cell transformation (LCT) is defined histologically by the presence of lymphocytes four times the size of a normal lymphocyte, present as micronodules or representing 25% of the infiltrate. LCT usually indicates a switch from the typically prolonged indolent course of patch/plaque disease to an accelerated and more aggressive clinical course with decreased survival. Transformation usually is observed in the skin but may occur in lymph nodes, visceral organs, the oronasal mucosal region, including maxillary sinus, and the central nervous system. Clinically there will be a sudden change in a plaque to a tumoral lesion or spontaneous ulceration which suggests an urgent biopsy to look for LCT (Figure 36.5). CD30 can be expressed in usually less than 75% of T cells, but if it exceeds this, it is important to differentiate it from a CD30+ Anaplastic large cell lymphoma (ALCL) arising in MF.

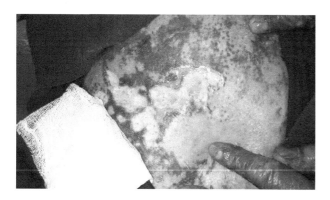

Figure 36.5 Large cell transformation.

Folliculotropic mycosis fungoides

Folliculotropic MF (FMF) is a distinct clinicopathologic subtype with extracutaneous spread to peripheral blood, marrow, and viscera, such as the central nervous system, lungs, and oronasal mucosa, and has a 10-year survival of patients with advanced stage skin-limited disease as low as 28%. FMF distribution is concentrated on the head and neck and hair-bearing regions, associated with alopecia (especially the eyebrows), follicular papules, and acneiform or cystic lesions, in addition to patches, plaques, tumors, and/or erythroderma (Figure 36.6). The atypical lymphocytes are folliculocentric and folliculotropic, in contrast to the epidermotropism of classic MF. Age older than 60 years, extensive secondary bacterial infection at the time of diagnosis, and large cell transformation were found to be independent risk factors. Those with indurated/infiltrated plaques and tumors, typically on the head and neck and pruritic, and histologically presenting with a greater perifollicular lymphocytic density, frequently with eosinophils, extending deeper into the reticular dermis, have a poorer outcome and hence need to be managed aggressively.

Adult T-cell leukemia/lymphoma

ATLL is a rare but aggressive peripheral T-cell lymphoma that is associated with the retrovirus human T-cell lymphotropic virus type-1 (HTLV-1). It is included in the World Health Organization-European Organisation for Research and Treatment of Cancer (WHO-EORTC) classification of cutaneous lymphomas, yet cutaneous disease is often a manifestation of disseminated disease. ATLL may mimic

MF and Sézary syndrome, warranting a brief discussion of this subtype. HTLV-1 infection is endemic in southwestern Japan, the Caribbean, Central and South America, and Africa, but is also becoming more prominent in other nonendemic countries, such as India and Bangladesh.

ATLL is usually seen in adults (mean age mid-40s to mid-60s) depending on demographic populations. ATLL is clinically heterogeneous, with acute, lymphomatous, chronic, and smoldering forms, and we discuss the acute and lymphomatous states under emergencies. The acute form includes patients with the classical features of leukemia, hypercalcemia, and systemic disease, with multiple organ involvement. Acute ATLL is the most common subtype seen in Japan, whereas lymphomatous presentations are more common in the Western hemisphere. ATLL skin lesions may mimic a variety of inflammatory dermatoses including psoriasis, drug eruptions, viral eruptions, and MF/Sézary syndrome (Figure 36.7).

Diagnosis of cutaneous ATLL is made by documenting the T-cell lymphoma or by documenting 5% or more atypical multilobated atypical cells in peripheral blood, and a positive HTLV-1 serology. Histologically, biopsies of ATLL may show varying degrees of epidermal, dermal, and subcutaneous infiltration, including cases of massive panniculitic infiltrates. ATLL typically shows an immunophenotype that is CD3+/CD5+/CD4+/CD25+. Erythrodermic and purpuric variants have a mean survival of 3–4.4 months, so it is an emergency once diagnosed. An unusual rapid progress should prompt HTLV-1 serology and a high index of suspicion in patients from endemic and emerging status countries and planned for stem cell transplant when not responding to chemotherapy.

Extranodal NK/T-cell lymphoma, nasal type (Figure 36.8), primary cutaneous aggressive epidermotropic CD8+ cytotoxic T-cell lymphoma (Figure 36.9), primary cutaneous γδ T-cell lymphoma (Figure 36.10) panniculitic tumor may be seen. Immunohistochemistry (IHC) stains

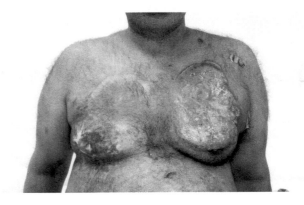

Figure 36.8 Extranodal NK/T-cell lymphoma, nasal type.

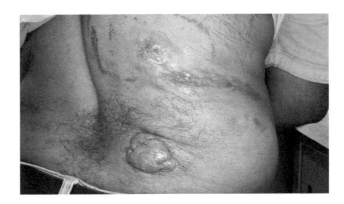

Figure 36.9 Primary cutaneous aggressive epidermotropic CD8+ cytotoxic T-cell lymphoma.

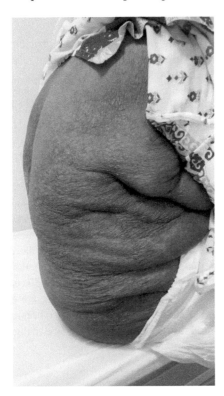

Figure 36.7 Adult T-cell leukemia.

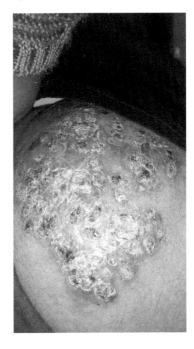

Figure 36.10 Primary cutaneous γ/δ T-cell lymphoma.

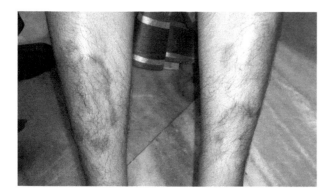

Figure 36.11 Subcutaneous panniculitis like T-cell lymphoma.

negatively for ß-F1 and positive for γδ, subcutaneous panniculitis like T-cell lymphoma (Figure 36.11) and primary cutaneous diffuse large B-cell lymphoma, leg type are the other important primary cutaneous lymphomas that can manifest as emergencies.

CUTANEOUS INFECTIONS IN INFILTRATED SKIN

In infiltrated skin, the skin barrier function is compromised and patients are at an increased risk of developing cutaneous infections with which they get referred to a dermatologist. Disseminated herpes simplex infections and staphylococcal infections presenting with oozy, crusted, and inflamed skin are the two common problems faced by a dermatologist dealing with patients with malignant hemopathies/lymphoproliferative disorders; delay in recognition and treatment can have fatal outcomes. Primary pyodermas, cellulitis to staphylococcal sepsis have also been reported.

Swabs for culture and sensitivity should be done on oozing skin, and even though it might be difficult to differentiate between colonization and infection, they need to be started on empirical antibiotics and antivirals under appropriate clinical suspicion. Patients also benefit from chlorhexidine baths, dilute potassium permanganate, or sodium hypochlorite (bleach) baths to prevent secondary infection in altered barrier status such as erythrodermic CTCL.

Other common infections and infestations include scabies and dermatophytosis in countries endemic for such infections, and these should be suspected in those with severe pruritus and confirmed with appropriate examination and investigations.

Fusarium, aspergillosis, candidiasis, *Macrophomina*, and such other rare opportunistic infections can occur in the setting of immunocompromised status because of bone marrow hypoplasia or chemotherapy-induced neutropenia/lymphopenia.

Uncommon viral reactivation such as cytomegalovirus (CMV) or EBV can also present with maculopapular rashes and needs to be suspected. Clinicians should consider possible septicemia when facing a patient with monomorphic disseminated lesions, especially on the hands or feet.

Faint erythematous macules and papules in a sick patient could even be candidal septicemia, and a biopsy is more likely to help diagnose rather than aerobic blood cultures.

Persistent indurated plaques could be manifestation of underlying necrotizing cellulitis or early ecthyma gangrenosum. Repeated biopsies and blood and tissue cultures are important when the diagnosis is uncertain.

ADVERSE CUTANEOUS REACTIONS TO ANTICANCER DRUGS

Drug reactions are among the most common reasons for which the dermatologist's opinion is sought by a treating hemato-oncologist, and the drugs range from trial drugs to older drugs like imatinib. The severe cutaneous adverse reaction (SCAR) pattern, drug list, and concomitant differential count in peripheral blood help narrow the causes. The Naranjo score and algorithm of drug causality in epidermal necrolysis are considered the standard assessment tools to evaluate the causality of adverse drug reactions and Stevens-Johnson syndrome/toxic epidermal necrolysis (SJS/TEN), respectively.

Imatinib in CML, rituximab for B-cell leukemia/lymphomas and denileukin and brentuximab vedotin for lymphomas are standard licensed drugs and all are reported to be associated with SJS/TEN. Imatinib has been majorly associated with drug reaction with eosinophilia and systemic symptoms and acute generalized exanthematous pustulosis.

Severe mucositis or oral ulceration from cyclical neutropenia or drug-induced mucositis can be a cause for emergency and requires multispecialty involvement for pain relief and management.

The other drug-related emergency is anaphylactoid or severe urticarial reactions, and they can occur with L-asparginase or cisplatin/carboplatin. Rechallenge is best avoided.

Digital necrosis has been reported with bleomycin and interferon therapy and requires urgent withdrawal. Last, an iatrogenic cause of extravasation reactions from inlying catheters can cause severe cutaneous necrosis and need to be kept in mind for localized reactions and managed actively.

PARANEOPLASTIC MANIFESTATIONS

Mucocutaneous paraneoplastic manifestations are classified as per predominant pathological change and include the following categories: dermal depositions, neutrophilic dermatoses, papulosquamous disorders, proliferative reactions, reactive erythemas, vacuolar degeneration of the basal layer, vasculitis, and vesiculobullous disorders. Most of these are emergencies because of the rapidity and severity and also because they may occur prior to knowledge of the hematologic malignancy.

Dermal deposits

They usually refer to systemic amyloidosis in the setting of multiple myeloma. Amyloidosis is characterized by purpura, papules, hyperpigmentation, macroglossia, tongue papules, periocular purpura, and alopecia. A biopsy of clinically involved skin with special staining will yield a diagnosis in almost 100% of patients. Paraneoplastic amyloidosis carries a poor prognosis, with a mean survival of less than 1 year.

Neutrophilic dermatosis

This includes pyoderma gangrenosum (PG), Sweet syndrome, and neutrophilic eccrine hidradenitis. Bullous or atypical PG is associated with an underlying hematological malignancy (acute myelogenous leukemia, myelodysplasia, myeloproliferative disorders, and multiple myeloma) in 7% of cases; hence, workup for PG includes ruling out for these malignancies. Paraneoplastic Sweet syndrome is most commonly associated with acute myelogenous leukemia. Both can respond to systemic steroids and management of the underlying malignancy.

Pruritus of unknown origin

This is a persistent severe itching that can lead to excoriations, prurigo nodularis, and lichen simplex chronicus. An underlying malignancy is the etiology in 11% of pruritus patients. Polycythemia vera is the malignancy most commonly associated with paraneoplastic pruritus, followed by Hodgkin lymphoma, multiple myeloma, cutaneous T-cell lymphoma, Sézary syndrome, and other leukemias. Aprepitant, thalidomide, gabapentin/pregabalin, and phototherapy are drugs that are useful in severe intractable pruritus besides liberal moisturizing and sometimes, potent topical steroids and topical anesthetic agents like pramoxine. It is important to rule out drug-related events here as well besides senile pruritus and common infestations like scabies.

Reactive erythemas

They present as emergencies including erythroderma and exfoliative dermatitis and are associated with malignancy in 8%–23% of cases. Reactive erythemas are most often linked to lymphoma (cutaneous T-cell and Hodgkin) or leukemia but have also been seen in cases of solid organ cancers. The manifestations can include generalized erythema with or without scaling, alopecia, nail dystrophy, lymphadenopathy, pruritus, and fever. Skin biopsies are frequently nonspecific. Treatment is targeted at the underlying malignancy with supportive skin care with wet, wrap therapy, narrow-band ultraviolet B (UVB) phototherapy, topical emollients and corticosteroids, as well as antihistamines, as indicated. It is important to maintain fluid and electrolytes, prevent secondary infections, and control body temperature to reduce morbidity and mortality.

Adult-onset erythromelalgia

This is related to a myeloproliferative disorder with thrombocytosis in 20% of cases preceding malignancy. Erythromelalgia is defined by severe attacks of burning pain, erythema, and warmth of the distal extremities that can be relieved by cold exposure and/or elevation of the extremities. Since intravascular platelet activation and aggregation cause the distal arterioles to become occluded, antiplatelet agents like high-dose aspirin are useful.

Paraneoplastic vasculitis

This most commonly presents as leukocytoclastic vasculitis. Associated cutaneous lesions are polymorphous and include nonblanchable purpura, erythematous papules and nodules, ulcers, and pruritic plaques with 18% of patients having an underlying malignancy. Cutaneous small vessel vasculitis is associated with hairy cell leukemia, chronic myelogenous leukemia, myeloma, lymphoma, and myelodysplastic syndrome among hematologic malignancies. Dermatologist interventions range from topical steroids and antihistamines to methylprednisolone, prednisone, dapsone, colchicine, methotrexate, and azathioprine depending on the severity, duration, and systemic involvement of vasculitis.

Autoimmune vesiculobullous reaction

This pattern includes paraneoplastic pemphigus (PNP), epidermolysis bullosa acquisita, and linear IgA dermatoses. PNP is diagnosed with Anhalt criteria and is proposed to be named as paraneoplastic autoimmune multiorgan syndrome because the condition affects multiple organ systems such as gastrointestinal tract involvement or bronchiolitis obliterans in the lung. A wide variety of lesions (florid oral mucosal lesions, a generalized polymorphous cutaneous eruption, and pulmonary involvement) may occur with severe stomatitis often being the presenting feature. Investigations to diagnose PNP should include checking for systemic complications (to identify tumor), skin biopsies (for histopathological and immunofluorescence studies), and serum immunological studies. Investigations to diagnose PNP should include checking for systemic complications (to identify tumor), skin biopsies (for histopathological and immunofluorescence studies), and serum immunological studies. High-dose steroids, steroid-sparing agents, rituximab, and IVIg have been used in management but the key lies in managing the primary underlying disease. Often the prognosis is poor because of eventual progression of malignancy and aggressive immunosuppression therapy resulting in infectious complications.

MISCELLANEOUS MANIFESTATIONS

Secondary hemophagocytic lymphohistiocytosis (HLH)

This has been reported with NK/T-cell lymphomas, SPTCL, ALCL, ALL, Hodgkin lymphoma, multiple myeloma, etc. The pathomechanism in malignancy-associated HLH may be the impairment of the cytotoxic pathway by the neoplasm through neoplastic changes in the cytotoxic cell itself or through malignancy-associated immune dysregulation. The strong association with NK/T-cell lymphomas and other EBV-related malignant neoplasms points to a possible common mechanism shared by cases of nonmalignant EBV-associated HLH. HLH is a medical emergency, whether in children or adults, and presents as a purpuric morbilliform rash or erythroderma and unexplained sudden onset of a systemic inflammatory response syndrome (SIRS), including fever, malaise, hepatosplenomegaly, jaundice, generalized lymphadenopathy, and cytopenias. The diagnostic criteria include fever; splenomegaly; cytopenias affecting at least two of three lineages in the peripheral blood; hyperferritinemia greater than 10,000 μg/L; hypertriglyceridemia and/or hypofibrinogenemia; hemophagocytosis in the bone marrow, spleen, or lymph nodes; low or absent NK-cell activity determined by the 51-Cr release assay; and high levels of soluble CD25. The therapy of HLH aims to suppress the exaggerated immune response through the use of immunosuppressive agents. The 2004 treatment protocol formulated at the second international meeting of the Histiocyte Society recommends an 8-week induction therapy with corticosteroids, etoposide, and cyclosporine A as the backbone of HLH treatment plus urgent treatment of the underlying malignancy.

Graft versus host disease

Graft versus host disease occurs in posttransplant patients and is classified as acute and chronic depending on the arbitrary 100-day cut-off posttransplant and has been discussed in Chapter 53.

CONCLUSION

A dermatologist needs to have a high index of suspicion for any patient with an underlying malignant hemopathy or lymphoproliferative disorder and needs to be willing to biopsy and investigate the patient presenting with cutaneous conditions.

KEY POINTS

- Cutaneous manifestations could be the earliest manifestation of malignancies which can present as emergencies, e.g., Leukemia cutis.
- Secondary cutaneous lymphomas which can present as emergencies include AK/T-cell lymphoma, peripheral T-cell lymphoma, anaplastic large cell lymphoma and angioimmunoblastic lymphoma.
- Sezary syndrome and Mycosis fungoides can present as emergencies among primary cutaneous lymphomas.
- Drug reactions to anticancer drugs can present as emergencies.

37

Melanoma-associated emergencies

VIDYA KHARKAR AND M. R. L. SUJATA

INTRODUCTION

Melanoma, also known as malignant melanoma, is a type of cancer that develops from the pigment-containing cells known as melanocytes [1]. Its incidence and overall mortality rates have been rising in recent decades [2]. Melanoma is the most serious form of skin cancer. Melanoma represents 4% of skin cancers but accounts for 80% of skin cancer deaths. Up to one-fifth of patients develop metastatic disease, which usually is associated with death. Early detection combined with improved diagnostic tools and new immunologic and molecularly targeted treatments for advanced stages of the disease influence the disease outcome.

EPIDEMIOLOGY

Global incidence of invasive melanoma is about 160,000 new cases per year with 48,000 deaths [3]. The higher incidence rates are recorded in Australia and New Zealand with up to 60 cases per 100,000 inhabitants per year, whereas the lowest rates are found in Asia and Africa [4,5].

Annual incidence rates have increased among all populations, ranging from 3% to 7%, which results in a doubling every 10–20 years [6]. Recent data from the United States have shown an increase of melanoma in young females (with the peak difference in the 20–24-year-old age group) [7]. Increasing rates of melanoma are also observed in the age group older than 60 years, particularly in males [8].

ETIOPATHOGENESIS

This includes risk factors, environmental factors, and genetic factors.

Risk factors

MELANOMA PRECURSORS

About 75%–80% of cutaneous melanomas (CMs) originate from normal skin. Only 20%–25% of melanomas develop in a cutaneous melanocytic nevus [9].

Congenital nevi

The risk of malignant transformation in congenital melanocytic nevi (CMN) depends on the size of the lesion. For large CMN (largest diameter >20 cm), lifetime risk of melanoma transformation is between 5% and 15% [10,11]. Malignant transformation most often occurs during childhood [10,12,13]. The risk of transformation of small CMN is between 2.6% and 4.9% in CMN <4.5 cm in diameter [14].

Common nevi

The annual risk of transformation of a nevus into a melanoma is very low. It is about 1/200,000 before the age of 40 in both sexes and 1/30,000 for men older than 60 [15]. For a 20-year-old individual, the lifetime risk of transformation of a mole is 1/3,000 for males and 1/10,000 for females.

Atypical/dysplastic nevi

Atypical/dysplastic nevus (AN/DN) are acquired pigmented lesions. These are differentiated from common acquired nevi by either pathological ("dysplastic nevi") or clinical features ("atypical nevi"). AN are characterized by a large size (>5 mm) with irregularly distributed colors and a tendency to emerge after a young age. These features are clinically suspicious of melanoma and often require excision. The risk of melanoma increases with the number of DN in the same patient [16–19]. However, the risk of melanoma transformation of an AN/DN is very low and varies with the grade of atypia [20]. The annual rate of transformation of AN/DN is approximately 1 in 30,000 moles and 1 in 40,000 moles for males and females, respectively [15].

Environmental factors

ULTRAVIOLET RADIATION

Studies have shown that a major risk factor for melanoma development is exposure to ultraviolet (UV) radiation. One or more blistering sunburns during childhood or adolescence doubles the risk for melanoma in later life [21]. UV radiation frequently leads to DNA mutations such as the formation of pyrimidine dimers or deamination of cytosine into thymidine. Individuals who have a history of familial melanoma, which contributes to 8%–12% of melanoma cases, demonstrate a high sensitivity to UV [22]. These individuals are likely to develop melanoma earlier in age and to develop multiple melanoma lesions. Patients with fair complexions (light skin types) are at a greater risk of developing a melanoma [23]. Melanoma risk is mainly related to intermittent sun exposure and sunburn history [24,25].

ARTIFICIAL SOURCES OF ULTRAVIOLET: SUNBEDS AND THERAPEUTIC ULTRAVIOLET USE

A meta-analysis extended to studies published up to May 2012 shows a relative risk of melanoma around 1.2 for the use of artificial UV sources [26]. The risk increases by 1.8% for each additional session of sunbed use per year and is 42% in cases of intensive use. The first use of sunbeds before the age of 35 years is associated with a higher risk. Therapeutic UV can be involved in melanoma risk. An increased risk for melanoma was first reported in a 16-center prospective study of 1,380 patients treated with high cumulative dosages of psoralen plus ultraviolet A (PUVA) [27].

Genetic factors

A large number of genes are being investigated for their role in melanoma, including inherited genes and genetic defects that are acquired due to environment factors, such as excessive sun exposure. A number of rare mutations, often running in families, greatly increase melanoma susceptibility. The best understood melanoma susceptibility gene is *CDKN2A* on chromosome 9. Hereditary mutations in this gene underlie susceptibility to melanoma in 40% of families with three or more cases of melanoma [28]. Studies have shown that around 40%–60% of all melanoma cases exhibit an activated *BRAF* mutation [29]. The V600E missense mutation that changes valine into glutamic acid is the most common *BRAF* alteration and constitutes about 90% of *BRAF* activating mutations or about 50% of all metastatic melanomas [29–31]. Another source of molecular changes that may allow for melanoma initiation or propagation is found in the NRAS GTPase or neuroblastoma RAS oncogene. NRAS GTPase mutations are found in 15%–20% of melanoma patients [32]. Mutations or chromosomal duplication in the *c-KIT* gene have been detected in about 23% of

acral melanomas and in less than 2% of cutaneous melanomas [33]. Melanocortin 1 receptor (MC1R) polymorphisms may also be involved in a few cases [34]. When melanoma is transitioning from a primary tumor into a metastatic variant, it appears to undergo epithelial to mesenchymal transition (EMT) [35]. One of the changes in the EMT is the switch in the expression of E-cadherin to N-cadherin by the melanoma cells. The newly increased N-cadherin expression facilitates melanoma migration into the dermis and interactions with dermal fibroblasts and vascular endothelial cells. This sequence of events allows the melanoma to spread out of its epidermal origin [36]. The N-cadherin-containing melanoma cells also adhere to vascular endothelial cells, which may provide the melanoma access to enter the blood vessel and metastasize throughout the body [36].

CLINICAL FEATURES

Melanoma can be classified into four different clinical subtypes: superficial spreading malignant melanoma (SSMM), lentigo maligna melanoma, nodular melanoma, and acral lentiginous melanoma (characterized by the site of origin; palm, sole, or subungual). Malignant melanoma *in situ* and lentigo maligna are considered premalignant lesions.

Superficial spreading melanoma

This commonly displays the ABCDE warning signs [37]. It tends to present as a flat or slightly elevated brown lesion with variegated pigmentation (i.e., black, blue, pink, or white discoloration) with an irregular shape often >6 mm.

ABCDEs OF MELANOMA

A	Asymmetry
B	Border irregularity
C	Color variation
D	Diameter >6 mm
E	Evolving (changing)

Lentigo maligna (lentigo maligna melanoma)

Lentigo maligna melanoma presents as a slowing growing or changing patch of discolored skin with variegated shape and color. They often show slow progressive changes from *in situ* lentigo maligna (LM) to invasive LMM and may be detected using the ABCDE rule.

Nodular melanoma

A nodular melanoma may arise on any site but is most common on exposed areas of the head and neck and usually presents as a rapidly enlarging lump (weeks to months)

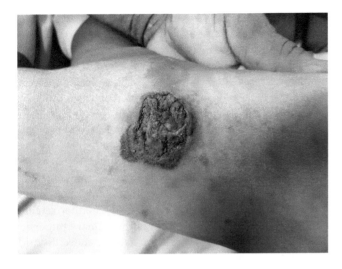

Figure 37.1 Nodular melanoma on forearm.

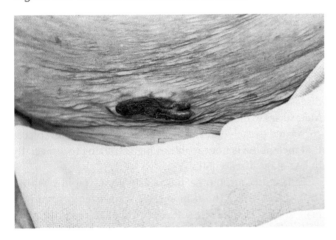

Figure 37.2 Nodular melanoma on abdomen.

(Figures 37.1 and 37.2). One-third of nodular melanomas are amelanotic, i.e., nonpigmented and may be ulcerated. This can often lead to diagnostic difficulty. However, any new ulcerated nodular skin lesion should alert the clinician to the high possibility of skin cancer.

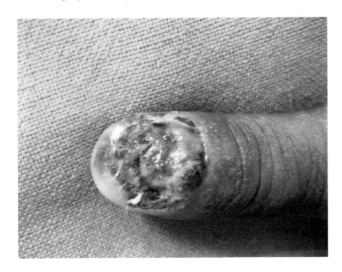

Figure 37.3 Subungual melanoma.

Acral lentiginous melanoma

This type of melanoma starts as a slowly enlarging flat patch of discolored skin and tends to follow the ABCDE rule. Although initially smooth at first, it later becomes thicker with an irregular surface. Subungual melanoma is a part of acral lentiginous melanoma (Figure 37.3).

SSMM is by far the most common clinical subtype of melanoma in white skin and accounts for approximately 70% of cases diagnosed. In contrast, acral lentiginous melanoma is the least common subtype in white patients, more often seen in patients with African American skin types.

Other variants

AMELANOTIC MELANOMA

All melanoma subtypes may present as amelanotic or hypomelanotic lesions clinically, commonly observed with nodular and desmoplastic subtypes. It is less common than clinically pigmented melanoma, approximately 2%–8% of cases; it poses serious diagnostic challenges for patients and clinicians alike. Lesions may present as pink or red macules, plaques, or nodules, often with well-defined borders [38]. Some tumors may present a subtle light-brown pigmentation. Amelanotic melanomas are often clinically confused with benign lesions (e.g., melanocytic nevus, inflamed seborrheic keratosis, hemangioma, pyogenic granuloma), often leading to considerable delay in the diagnosis and potential worse prognosis.

SPITZOID MELANOMA

The term *spitzoid melanoma* has been used to indicate a subset of melanomas that have a morphologic resemblance to Spitz tumors, both clinically and histologically. These lesions usually present as faintly erythematous growing papules or nodules. They can be amelanotic or have a brown, black, or blue color. Spitzoid melanomas generally have more severe histologic atypia than atypical Spitz tumors.

DESMOPLASTIC MELANOMA

Desmoplastic melanoma is a rare but histologically and clinically distinct variant of melanoma [39]. It presents as a slowly growing plaque, nodule, or scar-like growth, and it is usually amelanotic and located in chronically sun-exposed areas of older patients. It may clinically simulate a scar, or nonmelanoma skin cancer (e.g., basal cell or squamous cell carcinoma).

PIGMENT SYNTHESIZING (ANIMAL-TYPE) MELANOMA

Pigment synthesizing (animal-type) melanoma (also termed *melanocytoma*) is a rare subtype of melanoma composed of heavily pigmented dermal epithelioid and spindled melanocytes [40]. It presents as a blue-black or blue, slow-growing nodule most frequently located on the extremities and, less commonly, on the head/neck and trunk. It is an indolent type of melanoma, with low

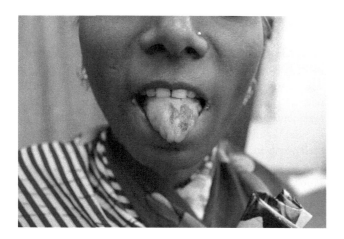

Figure 37.4 Mucosal melanoma.

incidence of metastasis and low mortality rate, but it has a high frequency of positive sentinel lymph nodes. The histopathologic diagnosis may be difficult due to overlapping features with other dermal melanocytic proliferations, such as common blue nevus, cellular blue nevus, malignant blue nevus, and Spitz nevus.

MUCOSA

Rarely, mucosal melanomas can occur (Figure 37.4).

Metastatic melanomas

After formation of a primary tumor, melanoma cells enter the lymphatic vessels, traverse to the lymph node, and subsequently enter into the systemic circulation via the thoracic duct. After reaching systemic circulation, cells adhere to the microvasculature of a target organ, extravasate, and subsequently proliferate in order to form a clinically relevant metastasis.

While melanomas rarely recur locally at the site of excision, they often recur as metastases at distant sites [41]. Even in stage IA melanoma patients, who have a 20-year survival rate of at least 90%, recurrences of disease still occur, often a decade or more after removal of the primary tumor [42].

Melanoma metastases cause the vast majority of morbidity and mortality associated with this disease.

The presence of metastasis to visceral sites predicts poor outcome in melanoma [43]. The 1-year survival rates in melanoma patients with clinically apparent metastasis to one, two, or three different visceral sites is 36%, 13%, and 1%, respectively. The most important tumor intrinsic variable that can predict metastatic recurrence in early melanomas is the thickness of the tumor [44]. Prognosis is inversely proportional to tumor thickness. Strikingly, differences of only 1–2 mm in the thickness can alter prognosis substantially.

Sentinel lymph node dissection is generally offered to patients with melanomas exceeding 1 mm in depth. The sentinel node is the first lymph node encountered by fluid draining from the cutaneous site of the primary tumor and is thought to represent the first noncontiguous site tumor

cells will spread to [45–47]. The presence or absence of tumor cells in the sentinel node has very important prognostic implications. In fact, histological evidence of tumor cells in the lymph node is probably the best indication that subclinical spread of melanoma cells has already occurred.

Male sex, age, and anatomic location can also influence recurrence rates. Factors such as the presence of ulceration, microscopic satellite lesions, and increased mitoses per high-power field all predict poor outcome.

Melanomas are capable of metastasizing to both regional and distant sites. The most common sites of regional metastasis are nearby skin, subcutaneous tissue, and lymph nodes [48]. Metastases to skin are referred to as either satellite lesions (if they are relatively close to the primary tumor) or in-transit metastases (if they are relatively more distant), though they do not differentially influence melanoma staging. Metastasis to the skin may be the first external clue that lymphatic or hematogenous spread has occurred [49].

The most common clinically apparent sites of distant metastases in melanoma patients are skin, lung, brain, liver, bone, and intestine. Metastasis to lung is common and often the first clinically apparent site of visceral metastasis. Other sites of metastasis such as bone and intestines occur later in disease progression and are rarely the first site of detection. Metastases to other sites such as liver and brain are inversely correlated to each other. In fact, it seems there are few places that melanoma is not capable of metastasizing to, especially in late-stage disease [50].

Cutaneous melanoma metastasis grows rapidly within the skin or under the skin surface. Consistency usually is firm to hard but may be soft. They are often red or black in color. They may ulcerate or bleed.

Epidermotropic metastatic melanoma is rare. It is often misdiagnosed as primary melanoma. Epidermotropic metastatic melanoma should be considered if multiple lesions arise with similar pathology. Subcutaneous metastatic melanoma presents as skin-colored or bluish swellings that are usually painless.

Tumor in lymph nodes may cause swelling of the extremities and enlarged glands. Lymphedema can result from obstruction of lymphatic vessels due to melanoma in lymph node or surgical removal of lymph glands. Tumor in the lungs may cause shortness of breath, cough, and bloody sputum. Tumor in the brain may cause headaches, dizziness, and seizures. Tumor metastasis into the liver may cause weight loss, nausea, a swollen liver, and abnormal blood tests. Tumor in bone may cause bone pain or unusual fractures. Intra-abdominal dissemination of melanoma can manifest with weight loss, vague abdominal pain, and/or anemia. Patients can also present in the emergency setting with bowel intussusception, obstruction, bleeding, or perforation.

Melanoma of the uveal tract is a cancer that arises from neuroectodermal melanocytes of the iris, ciliary body, or choroid. It is the most common intraocular malignant tumor in Caucasians, with a high potential for hematogenous dissemination. Clinical features of melanoma-associated retinopathy (MAR) include shimmering, flickering, or pulsating photopsias, night blindness, and loss of peripheral vision [51–54]. Patients with any form of melanoma (cutaneous, choroidal, ciliary body, or choroidal nevi) may have eye involvement, usually in the context of metastatic disease [51,52]. Vision loss typically stabilizes or progresses slowly.

INVESTIGATIONS

Suspicious skin and subcutaneous lesions should be biopsied. A sentinel node biopsy is sometimes performed after a primary melanoma is diagnosed. Fine needle aspiration or core biopsy of the lymph node lesion usually is adequate for tissue diagnosis. Immunohistochemical studies include immunoreactivity for S-100, vimentin, and HMB-45. Electron microscopy studies are recommended to look for melanosomes or premelanosomes, if the findings are equivocal.

Blood tests include the serum LDH that is a marker for progressive metastatic disease at distant sites. When it is elevated it confers a worse prognosis.

Chest x-ray may detect lung metastases. Plain x-ray of the abdomen can show multiple dilated loops of small bowel.

Ultrasound scanning can reveal liver and lymph node metastases. Computed tomography and magnetic resonance imaging can show metastatic deposits in most body sites. Positron emission tomography scanning has good diagnostic accuracy for metastatic melanoma. "Hot spots" of tissue are seen.

Other investigations

Ophthalmologic examinations should be reserved for patients who have Melanoma with unknown primary (MUP) with visceral metastases, primarily of the liver. Funduscopic examination of MAR is usually normal at onset, with retinal arterial attenuation seen later. Cerebrospinal fluid analysis is generally normal. Otorhinolaryngologic examination is done to look for metastases to the head and neck region. Proctoscopy and gynecologic examinations are done if inguinal lymph node metastases are present.

STAGING AND GRADING

Microstaging

Breslow tumor thickness (depth of invasion) is the strongest predictor of survival in a primary melanoma. Melanoma thickness is measured in millimeters from the top of the granular cell layer of the epidermis (or base of an ulcer) to the deepest point of tumor penetration. The other features to be noted are ulceration, Clark level of invasion, presence of tumor infiltrating lymphocytes, mitoses/mm^2, regression, vascular invasion, and microscopic satellites.

Tumor thickness and ulceration are major determinants of T stage in the current staging system.

Clark levels relate the depth of invasion of melanoma cells to the different anatomic layers of the skin: level I is confined to the epidermis (*in situ*), level II invades the papillary dermis, level III fills the papillary dermis to the junction with the superficial reticular dermis, level IV invades the reticular dermis, and level V invades the fat. In the current staging system, the Clark level is used to distinguish between stage Ia and Ib lesions.

Melanoma stages are 5-year survival rates [55] based on the classification of the American Joint Committee on Cancer (AJCC). The stages classify 5-year survival from initial melanoma diagnosis with proper treatment.

- *Stage 0*: Melanoma *in situ* (Clark Level I), 99.9% survival
- *Stage I/II*: Invasive melanoma, 89%–95% survival
  - T1a: Less than 1.0 mm primary tumor thickness, without ulceration, and mitosis $<1/mm^2$
  - T1b: Less than 1.0 mm primary tumor thickness, with ulceration or mitoses $\geq 1/mm^2$
  - T2a: 1.01–2.0 mm primary tumor thickness, without ulceration
- *Stage II*: High-risk melanoma, 45%–79% survival
  - T2b: 1.01–2.0 mm primary tumor thickness, with ulceration
  - T3a: 2.01–4.0 mm primary tumor thickness, without ulceration
  - T3b: 2.01–4.0 mm primary tumor thickness, with ulceration
  - T4a: Greater than 4.0 mm primary tumor thickness, without ulceration
  - T4b: Greater than 4.0 mm primary tumor thickness, with ulceration
- *Stage III*: Regional metastasis, 24%–70% survival
  - N1: Single positive lymph node
  - N2: Two to three positive lymph nodes *or* regional skin/in-transit metastasis
  - N3: Four positive lymph nodes *or* one lymph node and regional skin/in-transit metastases
- *Stage IV*: Distant metastasis, 7%–19% survival
  - M1a: Distant skin metastasis, normal lactate dehydrogenase (LDH)
  - M1b: Lung metastasis, normal LDH
  - M1c: Other distant metastasis *or* any distant metastasis with elevated LDH

TREATMENT

Primary melanomas are typically treated with surgical excision, which yields a high survival rate. However, following metastasis, surgical excision of the tumor yields only about a 10% 5-year survival rate [56].

Excisional biopsies remove the tumor. Further surgery is often necessary to reduce the risk of recurrence. The standard treatment is complete surgical excision with adequate surgical margins. Assessment is done for the presence of detectable metastatic disease. This is done by a wide local excision (WLE) with 1–2 cm margins. Melanoma *in situ* and lentigo malignas are treated with narrower surgical margins, usually 0.2–0.5 cm.

Only 5% of patients with lentigo maligna progress to lentigo maligna melanoma after several years. Various therapeutic methods are used to treat lentigo maligna. These include cryotherapy, superficial radiation, and surgical excision with mapping and modified Mohs surgery.

Approaches to metastatic melanoma include surgical metastasectomy, immunotherapy, targeted inhibition of the mitogen activated protein kinase (MAPK) pathway, and radiation therapy to symptomatic sites of metastases. Radiation therapy has also proven to be ineffective for treating metastatic melanoma [56]. Thus, metastatic melanomas are medically managed by chemotherapeutics, and dacarbazine has been used for this purpose. Dacarbazine, dimethyltriazeno-imidazolcarboxamide (DTIC), is an alkylating agent. This is the monochemotherapy approved by the U.S. Food and Drug Administration (FDA) for treating melanomas and is the best option for treating metastatic melanoma [56,57].

Interleukin-2 (IL-2) and interferon-alpha (IFN-α) are two immunotherapies used to alter a patient's own immune activity to target melanoma cells [58]. IL-2 therapy gives a response rate of 16%–17% but is associated with increased morbidity and toxicities. IFN-α is an FDA-approved adjuvant therapy. It is given after surgery to help prevent any remaining melanoma cells from proliferating. IFN-α treatment leads to a long-lasting immune response, and the combination of immunotherapeutic agents, such as IL-2 and IFN-α, has a response rate of 31% [59,60].

Newer therapeutic approaches

VEMURAFENIB

Vemurafenib (PLX4032) is a BRAF kinase inhibitor. Vemurafenib inhibits the mutant BRAF and thus confers a degree of specificity toward melanoma harboring mutant form BRAF. Vemurafenib was approved by the FDA in August 2011 for unresectable stages III and IV or metastatic melanomas that harbor BRAFV600 mutations. It is prescribed at a dose of 960 mg twice a day orally. Treatment is continued until disease progresses or unacceptable side effects develop. Vemurafenib is contraindicated for melanomas that harbor wild-type BRAF. It is also contraindicated in electrolyte abnormalities, long QT syndrome with drugs that cause prolongation of QT interval.

DABRAFENIB

Dabrafenib is the next-generation agent similar to vemurafenib. The FDA approved dabrafenib in 2013 for BRAFV600-positive unresectable or metastatic melanomas. The dose is 150 mg twice a day orally. Dabrafenib is contraindicated in melanoma harboring wild-type BRAF.

TRAMETINIB

Trametinib was approved by the FDA in May 2013 for BRAFV600E or BRAFV600 K positive unresectable or metastatic melanomas. Its mechanism of action is different from that of vemurafenib or dabrafenib. Trametinib inhibits MEK, i.e., the extracellular signal-regulated kinase that is downstream of BRAF. Its dose is 2 mg orally once daily. The contraindications include melanoma harboring wild-type BRAF and patients previously treated with BRAF inhibitors. In January 2014, the FDA granted approval to a combination of dabrafenib and trametinib for unresectable or metastatic melanoma with BRAFV600 mutations. Dabrafenib and trametinib in combination improve survival significantly compared to vemurafenib alone in BRAFV600 mutant metastatic melanomas [61]. A combination of BRAF and MEK inhibitors appears to be superior to monotherapy.

IPILIMUMAB

Ipilimumab is a humanized monoclonal antibody that prevents T-cell activation via inhibition of cytotoxic T-lymphocyte antigen-4 (CTLA-4) [62]. It was approved by the FDA in March 2011 for late-stage metastatic melanoma. It boosts antitumor immunity [63,64].

PEMBROLIZUMAB

Pembrolizumab is a humanized monoclonal IgG4 antibody. It targets human cell surface receptor PD-1 (programmed cell death-1) and interferes with PD-1 ligand binding. This interference results in activation of T-cell-mediated response against tumors. The FDA approved pembrolizumab for the management of advanced or unresectable melanomas that are refractory to other therapeutics.

NIVOLUMAB

Nivolumab is a fully human monoclonal antibody that targets PD-1. It functions in a manner similar to pembrolizumab. The FDA granted approval in December 2014 for treatment of metastatic melanomas that do not respond to other forms of treatment.

Emergency surgery for metastatic melanoma

Melanoma of the gastrointestinal tract can cause acute abdominal pain rarely and may require emergency surgery on the small bowel, especially in cases of intestinal obstruction, perforation, intussusceptions, and intractable bleeding [65]. Generally, intestinal metastasis of melanoma is difficult to diagnose and when encountered it reflects advanced disease and dismal outcome [65–67].

Spontaneous splenic rupture is a rare cause of major nontraumatic hemorrhage. Splenectomy is to be done. The adrenal can be a site of solitary metastasis from melanoma [68]. Complete adrenal resection and adjuvant treatment are to be given. Rare reports of metastatic melanoma to the stomach, colon, and rectum/anal canal have also been reported [69–76]. Metastatic melanoma to the gastrointestinal tract or to another solid organ should be suspected in any patient with a history of cutaneous melanoma and a new onset of abdominal symptoms.

Treatment of metastases in organs

Patients with disease that has metastasized to the brain have poor prognosis and generally ineffective treatment options. Recently, ipilimumab and vemurafenib are promising treatment options for patients with melanoma and central nervous system involvement. Radical metastasectomy for pulmonary metastases should be performed early for patients who have solitary or a minimal number of pulmonary metastases without extrathoracic involvement. Inhalative IL-2 therapy in combination with DTIC is an effective and nontoxic treatment of lung metastasis of malignant melanoma. Hepatic resection for metastatic melanoma of liver significantly improves survival over medical treatment alone. The metastatic disease is stabilized with systemic therapy prior to surgery. Treatment of bone metastases of malignant melanoma can be curative or palliative. The options include surgery, chemotherapy, radiotherapy, biological therapy, and combination therapy (chemotherapy combined with biological agents). Combination therapy, as an initial treatment, gives a higher response rate and long-term remissions [77].

Tumor lysis syndrome (TLS)

Tumor lysis syndrome (TLS) is a well-known oncologic emergency that is characterized by severe metabolic derangements. As the consequence of tumor dissolution, TLS causes the massive release of intracellular components into the blood. The release of intracellular products (e.g., uric acid, phosphates, calcium, and potassium) overwhelms the body's homeostasis mechanisms. TLS occurs in patients with malignancies who are exposed to chemotherapy, radiation, or corticosteroids. It usually presents within 1–5 days of initiating treatment.

The syndrome is characterized by the rapid development of hyperuricemia, hyperkalemia, hyperphosphatemia, hypocalcemia, metabolic acidosis, and acute renal failure [78]. The electrolyte imbalances and severe metabolic acidosis can lead to serious and potentially fatal arrhythmias. Treatment of TLS includes inpatient monitoring, vigorous fluid resuscitation, allopurinol or urate oxidase therapy to lower uric acid levels, urinary alkalinization, and hemodialysis.

CONCLUSION: WHY IS MALIGNANT MELANOMA AN EMERGENCY?

Malignant melanoma causes 80% of skin cancer deaths. It is the most common type of cancers in developed countries. Up to one-fifth of patients develop metastatic disease which is usually associated with death. Early detection and appropriate excision result in a cure rate of more than 90% in low-risk (less than 1 mm Breslow depth) melanoma patients.

Metastatic melanoma may present with acute abdominal pain, sudden decrease in visual acuity, headache, dizziness, seizures, dyspnea, severe backache, bone pain, and fractures depending on the organ involved. These warrant prompt diagnosis and emergency management.

KEY POINTS

- Malignant melanoma, a malignancy arising from melanocytes, is showing an increasing incidence and mortality rates in recent decades.
- Early detection of the melanoma and prompt treatment with knowledge of the recent advances are essential for better prognosis.
- Awareness of the various symptoms of metastatic melanoma for accurate diagnosis and management is of paramount importance to deal with this dreaded disease.

REFERENCES

1. Melanoma Treatment—Health profession version (PDQ®). National Cancer Institute. http://www.cancer.gov/types/skin/hp/melanoma-treatment-pdq (accessed on June 26, 2015).
2. Lens MB, Dawes M. Global perspectives of contemporary epidemiological trends of cutaneous malignant melanoma. *Br J Dermatol* 2004;150(2):179–85.
3. Eggermont AM, Spatz A, Robert C. Cutaneous melanoma. *Lancet* 2014;383(9919):816–27.
4. de Vries E, Coebergh JW. Cutaneous malignant melanoma in Europe. *Eur J Cancer* 2004;40(16):2355–66.
5. MacLennan R, Green AC, McLeod GR, Martin NG. Increasing incidence of cutaneous melanoma in Queensland, Australia. *JNCI* 1992;84(18):1427–32.
6. Garbe C, Leiter U. Melanoma epidemiology and trends. *Clin Dermatol* 2009;27(1):3–9.
7. Purdue MP, Freeman LB, Anderson WF, Tucker MA. Recent trends in incidence of cutaneous melanoma among US Caucasian young adults. *J Invest Dermatol* 2008;128(12):2905.
8. Nikolaou V, Stratigos AJ. Emerging trends in the epidemiology of melanoma. *Br J Dermatol* 2014;170(1):11–9.
9. Noto G. On the clinical significance of cutaneous melanoma's precursors. *Indian Dermatol Online J* 2012;3(2):83.
10. Tannous ZS, Mihm MC, Sober AJ, Duncan LM. Congenital melanocytic nevi: Clinical and histopathologic features, risk of melanoma, and clinical management. *J Am Acad Dermatol* 2005;52(2):197–203.
11. Ruiz-Maldonado R, de la Luz Orozco-Covarrubias M. Malignant melanoma in children: A review. *Arch Dermatol* 1997;133(3):363–71.
12. Krengel S, Hauschild A, Schäfer T. Melanoma risk in congenital melanocytic naevi: A systematic review. *Br J Dermatol* 2006;155(1):1–8.
13. Vourc'h-Jourdain M, Martin L, Barbarot S. Large congenital melanocytic nevi: Therapeutic management and melanoma risk: A systematic review. *J Am Acad Dermatol* 2013;68(3):493–8.

14. Rhodes AR, Melski JW. Small congenital nevocellular nevi and the risk of cutaneous melanoma. *J Pediatr* 1982;100(2):219–24.

15. Tsao H, Bevona C, Goggins W, Quinn T. The transformation rate of moles (melanocytic nevi) into cutaneous melanoma: A population-based estimate. *Arch Dermatol* 2003;139(3):282–8.

16. Clark WH, Elder DE, Guerry D, Epstein MN, Greene MH, Van Horn M. A study of tumor progression: The precursor lesions of superficial spreading and nodular melanoma. *Hum Pathol* 1984;15(12):1147–65.

17. Kath R, Rodeck U, Menssen HD, Mancianti ML, Linnenbach AJ, Elder DE, Herlyn M. Tumor progression in the human melanocytic system. *Anticancer Res* 1989;9(4):865–72.

18. Bataille V, Bishop JA, Sasieni P, Swerdlow AJ, Pinney E, Griffiths K, Cuzick J. Risk of cutaneous melanoma in relation to the numbers, types and sites of naevi: A case-control study. *Br J Cancer* 1996;73(12):1605.

19. Tucker MA, Halpern A, Holly EA, Hartge P, Elder DE, Sagebiel RW, Guerry D, Clark WH. Clinically recognized dysplastic nevi: A central risk factor for cutaneous melanoma. *JAMA* 1997;277(18):1439–44.

20. Reddy KK, Farber MJ, Bhawan J, Geronemus RG, Rogers GS. Atypical (dysplastic) nevi: Outcomes of surgical excision and association with melanoma. *JAMA Dermatol* 2013;149(8):928–34.

21. Weinstock MA, Colditz GA, Willett WC, Stampfer MJ, Bronstein BA, Mihm MC, Speizer FE. Nonfamilial cutaneous melanoma incidence in women associated with sun exposure before 20 years of age. *Pediatrics* 1989;84(2):199–204.

22. Soufir N, Avril MF, Chompret A, Demenais F, Bombled J, Spatz A, Stoppa-Lyonnet D, French Familial Melanoma Study Group, Bénard J, Bressac-de Paillerets B. Prevalence of p16 and CDK4 germline mutations in 48 melanoma-prone families in France. *Hum Mol Genet* 1998;7(2):209–16.

23. Gandini S, Sera F, Cattaruzza MS, Pasquini P, Zanetti R, Masini C, Boyle P, Melchi CF. Meta-analysis of risk factors for cutaneous melanoma: III. Family history, actinic damage and phenotypic factors. *Eur J Cancer* 2005;41(14):2040–59.

24. Gandini S, Sera F, Cattaruzza MS, Pasquini P, Picconi O, Boyle P, Melchi CF. Meta-analysis of risk factors for cutaneous melanoma: II. Sun exposure. *Eur J Cancer* 2005;41(1):45–60.

25. Hodis E et al. A landscape of driver mutations in melanoma. *Cell* 2012;150(2):251–63.

26. Boniol M, Autier P, Boyle P, Gandini S. Cutaneous melanoma attributable to sunbed use: Systematic review and meta-analysis. *BMJ* 2012;345:e4757.

27. Stern RS, Nichols KT, Väkevä LH. Malignant melanoma in patients treated for psoriasis with methoxsalen (psoralen) and ultraviolet A radiation (PUVA). *N Engl J Med* 1997;336(15):1041–5.

28. Goldstein AM et al. Features associated with germline CDKN2A mutations: A GenoMEL study of melanoma-prone families from three continents. *J Med Genet* 2007;44(2):99–106.

29. Flaherty KT et al. Inhibition of mutated, activated BRAF in metastatic melanoma. *N Engl J Med* 2010;363(9):809–19.

30. Chapman PB et al. Improved survival with vemurafenib in melanoma with BRAF V600E mutation. *N Engl J Med* 2011;364(26):2507–16.

31. Dong J, Phelps RG, Qiao R, Yao S, Benard O, Ronai Z, Aaronson SA. BRAF oncogenic mutations correlate with progression rather than initiation of human melanoma. *Cancer Res* 2003;63(14):3883–5.

32. Kelleher FC, McArthur GA. Targeting NRAS in melanoma. *Cancer J* 2012;18(2):132–6.

33. Beadling C et al. KIT gene mutations and copy number in melanoma subtypes. *Clin Cancer Res* 2008;14(21):6821–8.

34. Palmer JS, Duffy DL, Box NF, Aitken JF, O'Gorman LE, Green AC, Hayward NK, Martin NG, Sturm RA. Melanocortin-1 receptor polymorphisms and risk of melanoma: Is the association explained solely by pigmentation phenotype? *Am J Hum Genet* 2000;66(1):176–86.

35. Hao L, Ha JR, Kuzel P, Garcia E, Persad S. Cadherin switch from E-to N-cadherin in melanoma progression is regulated by the PI3K/PTEN pathway through Twist and Snail. *Br J Dermatol* 2012;166(6):1184–97.

36. Li G, Satyamoorthy K, Herlyn M. N-cadherin-mediated intercellular interactions promote survival and migration of melanoma cells. *Cancer Res* 2001;61(9):3819–25.

37. Abbasi NR, Shaw HM, Rigel DS, Friedman RJ, McCarthy WH, Osman I, Kopf AW, Polsky D. Early diagnosis of cutaneous melanoma: Revisiting the ABCD criteria. *JAMA* 2004;292(22):2771–6.

38. Pizzichetta MA, Talamini R, Stanganelli I, Puddu P, Bono R, Argenziano G, Veronesi A, Trevisan G, Rabinovitz H, Soyer HP. Amelanotic/hypomelanotic melanoma: Clinical and dermoscopic features. *Br J Dermatol* 2004;150(6):1117–24.

39. Chen LL, Jaimes N, Barker CA, Busam KJ, Marghoob AA. Desmoplastic melanoma: A review. *J Am Acad Dermatol* 2013;68(5):825–33.

40. Bax MJ, Brown MD, Rothberg PG, Laughlin TS, Scott GA. Pigmented epithelioid melanocytoma (animal type melanoma): An institutional experience. *J Am Acad Dermatol* 2017;77(2):328–32.

41. Balch CM, Urist MM, Karakousis CP, Smith TJ, Temple WJ, Drzewiecki K, Jewell WR, Bartolucci AA, Mihm Jr MC, Barnhill R. Efficacy of 2-cm surgical margins for intermediate-thickness melanomas (1–4 mm). Results of a multi-institutional randomized surgical trial. *Ann Surg* 1993;218(3):262–9.

42. Balch CM et al. Final version of 2009 AJCC melanoma staging and classification. *J Clin Oncol* 2009;27(36):6199–206.

43. Balch CM et al. Prognostic factors analysis of 17,600 melanoma patients: Validation of the American Joint Committee on Cancer melanoma staging system. *J Clin Oncol* 2001;19(16):3622–34.

44. McCarthy WH, Shaw HM, Thompson JF, Milton GW. Time and frequency of recurrence of cutaneous stage I malignant melanoma with guidelines for follow-up study. *Am J Hum Genet* 1988;166(6):497–502.

45. Nathanson SD. Insights into the mechanisms of lymph node metastasis. *Cancer* 2003;98(2):413–23.

46. Wong SL et al. Melanoma patients with positive sentinel nodes who did not undergo completion lymphadenectomy: A multi-institutional study. *Ann Surg Oncol* 2006;13(6):809–16.

47. Kingham TP, Panageas KS, Ariyan CE, Busam KJ, Brady MS, Coit DG. Outcome of patients with a positive sentinel lymph node who do not undergo completion lymphadenectomy. *Ann Surg Oncol* 2010;17(2):514–20.

48. Gimotty PA, Guerry D, Ming ME, Elenitsas R, Xu X, Czerniecki B, Spitz F, Schuchter L, Elder D. Thin primary cutaneous malignant melanoma: A prognostic tree for 10-year metastasis is more accurate than American Joint Committee on Cancer staging. *J Clin Oncol* 2004;22(18):3668–76.

49. Wolf IH, Richtig E, Kopera D, Kerl H. Locoregional cutaneous metastases of malignant melanoma and their management. *Dermatol Surg* 2004;30(s2):244–7.

50. Patel JK, Didolkar MS, Pickren JW, Moore RH. Metastatic pattern of malignant melanoma: A study of 216 autopsy cases. *Am J Surg* 1978;135(6):807–10.

51. Boeck K, Hofmann S, Klopfer M, Ian U, Schmidt T, Engst R, Thirkill CE, Ring J. Melanoma-associated paraneoplastic retinopathy: Case report and review of the literature. *Br J Dermatol* 1997;137(3):457–60.

52. Lu Y, Jia L, He S, Hurley MC, Leys MJ, Jayasundera T, Heckenlively JR. Melanoma-associated retinopathy: A paraneoplastic autoimmune complication. *Arch Ophthalmol* 2009;127(12):1572–80.

53. Berson EL, Lessell S. Paraneoplastic night blindness with malignant melanoma. *Am J Ophthalmol* 1988;106(3):307–11.

54. Keltner JL, Thirkill CE, Yip PT. Clinical and immunologic characteristics of melanoma-associated retinopathy syndrome: Eleven new cases and a review of 51 previously published cases. *J Neuroophthalmol* 2001;21(3):173–87.

55. Balch CM et al. Final version of the American Joint Committee on Cancer staging system for cutaneous melanoma. *J Clin Oncol* 2001;19(16):3635–48.

56. Bhatia S, Tykodi SS, Thompson JA. Treatment of metastatic melanoma: An overview. *Oncology (Williston Park, NY)* 2009;23(6):488–96.

57. Gogas H, Bafaloukos D, Bedikian AY. The role of taxanes in the treatment of metastatic melanoma. *Melanoma Res* 2004;14(5):415–20.

58. Parmiani G, Castelli C, Rivoltini L, Casati C, Tully GA, Novellino L, Patuzzo A, Tosi D, Anichini A, Santinami M. Immunotherapy of melanoma. *Semin Cancer Biol* 2003;13(6):391–400.

59. Tompkins WA. Immunomodulation and therapeutic effects of the oral use of interferon-alpha: Mechanism of action. *J Interferon Cytokine Res* 1999;19(8):817–28.

60. Bajetta E et al. Multicenter phase III randomized trial of polychemotherapy (CVD regimen) versus the same chemotherapy (CT) plus subcutaneous interleukin-2 and interferon-α2b in metastatic melanoma. *Ann Oncol* 2006;17(4):571–7.

61. Robert C et al. Improved overall survival in melanoma with combined dabrafenib and trametinib. *N Engl J Med* 2015;372(1):30–9.

62. O'day SJ et al. Efficacy and safety of ipilimumab monotherapy in patients with pretreated advanced melanoma: A multicenter single-arm phase II study. *Ann Oncol* 2010;21(8):1712–7.

63. Hodi FS et al. Improved survival with ipilimumab in patients with metastatic melanoma. *N Engl J Med* 2010;2010(363):711–23.

64. Wolchok JD et al. Ipilimumab monotherapy in patients with pretreated advanced melanoma: A randomised, double-blind, multicentre, phase 2, dose-ranging study. *Lancet Oncol* 2010;11(2):155–64.

65. Shpitz B, Kaufman Z, Gildor A, Dinbar A. Metastatic malignant melanoma of the small bowel as a surgical emergency. *Harefuah* 1990;119(11):364–5.

66. Catena F, Ansaloni L, Gazzotti F, Gagliardi S, Di Saverio S, De Cataldis A, Taffurelli M. Small bowel tumours in emergency surgery: Specificity of clinical presentation. *ANZ J Surg* 2005;75(11):997–9.

67. Giacobbe A, Facciorusso D, Modola G, Andriulli A. Metastatic melanoma: Endoscopy as aid to earlier *in vivo* diagnosis of gastrointestinal involvement. A case report. *Minerva Gastroenterologica E Dietologica* 1996;42(3):169–71.

68. Wantz M, Antonicelli F, Derancourt C, Bernard P, Avril MF, Grange F. Survie prolongée et régression tumorale spontanée au cours d'un mélanome de stade IV: rôles possibles de la surrénalectomie et de la libération massive d'antigènes tumoraux. *InAnnales de Dermatologie et de Vénéréologie* 2010;137(6):464–7.

69. Shenoy S, Cassim R. Metastatic melanoma to the gastrointestinal tract: Role of surgery as palliative treatment. *WV Med J* 2013;109(1):30–4.

70. Namikawa T, Hanazaki K. Clinicopathological features and treatment outcomes of metastatic tumors in the stomach. *Surg Today* 2014;44(8):1392–9.

71. Mourra N, Jouret-Mourin A, Lazure T, Audard V, Albiges L, Malbois M, Bouzourene H, Duvillard P. Metastatic tumors to the colon and rectum: A multi-institutional study. *Arch Pathol Lab Med* 2012;136(11):1397–401.

72. Damato B, Eleuteri A, Taktak AF, Coupland SE. Estimating prognosis for survival after treatment of choroidal melanoma. *Prog Retin Eye Res* 2011;30(5):285–95.

73. Triozzi PL, Eng C, Singh AD. Targeted therapy for uveal melanoma. *Cancer Treat Rev* 2008;34(3):247–58.

74. An J et al. A comparative transcriptomic analysis of uveal melanoma and normal uveal melanocyte. *PLOS ONE* 2011;6(1):e16516.

75. Bishop KD, Olszewski AJ. Epidemiology and survival outcomes of ocular and mucosal melanomas: A population-based analysis. *Int J Cancer* 2014;134(12):2961–71.

76. Huang X, Wang L, Zhang H, Wang H, Zhao X, Qian G, Hu J, Ge S, Fan X. Therapeutic efficacy by targeting correction of Notch1-induced aberrants in uveal tumors. *PLOS ONE* 2012;7(8):e44301.

77. Rigel DS, Carucci JA. Malignant melanoma: Prevention, early detection, and treatment in the 21st century. *CA Cancer J Clin* 2000;50(4):215–36.

78. Cairo MS, Bishop M. Tumour lysis syndrome: New therapeutic strategies and classification. *Br J Haematol* 2004;127(1):3–11.

38

Hemophagocytic lymphohistiocytosis

ARADHANA SOOD, DEEP KUMAR RAMAN, AND PANKAJ DAS

INTRODUCTION

Hemophagocytic lymphohistiocytosis (HLH) is a rare, potentially life-threatening condition characterized by uncontrolled and ineffective immune activation. It was first described in 1939 [1] as histiocytic medullary reticulosis; subsequently, the familial form was described in 1952 [2]. Though more common in the pediatric age group, it can be seen in all ages. Both familial and sporadic forms of the disease can be triggered by infections; Epstein-Barr virus (EBV) is implicated in most. These patients may present to the dermatologist, as skin rash is seen in almost 65% of HLH cases. Early diagnosis and prompt treatment can be lifesaving; however, diagnosis can pose a challenge due to variable clinical presentations and a lack of specific markers.

EPIDEMIOLOGY

HLH is primarily a disease of the pediatric population but can be seen in any age group. Familial hemophagocytic lymphohistiocytosis (FLH) is usually seen from birth to 18 months. The estimated incidence of familial HLH is 1 in 50,000 live births. The male-to-female ratio is 1:1, though some studies have reported an increased incidence in males [3,4]. Ethnic preponderance is noted in some forms with familial HLH 2 (FLH2) being more common in the African American community and FLH3 in the Turkish/ Kurdish population.

CLASSIFICATION

HLH has been classified as primary and secondary [5,6], where *primary HLH* denotes the presence of an underlying genetic defect and *secondary HLH* is a HLH phenomenon occurring due to any other condition; however, a genetic predisposition in secondary HLH cannot be ruled out. Some authors prefer to classify HLH into inherited and acquired forms (Table 38.1).

PATHOPHYSIOLOGY

HLH is a syndrome of excessive inflammation and tissue destruction resulting from abnormal immune activation caused by a lack of normal downregulation of activated macrophages and lymphocytes.

Macrophage activation

The primary mediator for tissue damage in HLH is increased cytokine production by macrophages, natural killer (NK) cells, and cytotoxic cells (CTLs). In HLH the elimination of activated macrophages by NK cells and CTLs using the perforindependent cytotoxicity and granzyme B-dependent pathway is defective. Decreased NK cell activity leads to sustained T-cell activation and release of inflammatory cytokines. Levels of interferon gamma (IFNγ); tumor necrosis factor alpha (TNFα), interleukins (IL)6, IL10, and IL12; and the soluble IL2 receptor (CD25) are grossly elevated in patients of HLH [7–9]. Some studies have reported increased levels of IL18 in secondary HLH [10]. This cytokine storm is responsible for the multiorgan involvement and high mortality in these patients.

Hemophagocytosis

Hemophagocytosis is the presence of red blood cells, platelets, or white blood cells (or fragments of these cells) within

Table 38.1 Classification of hemophagocytic lymphohistiocytosis

1. **Primary/Inherited hemophagocytic lymphohistiocytosis (HLH)**
   a. Familial HLH
      i. Known genetic defects
         1. PRF1/Perforin (FHL2)
         2. UNC13D/Munc13-4 (FHL3)
         3. STX11/Syntaxin 11 (FHL4)
         4. STXBP2/Munc18-2 (FHL5)
      ii. Unknown genetic defects (FHL1)
   b. Immune deficiency syndromes
      i. Chediak-Higashi syndrome
      ii. Griscelli syndrome
      iii. X-linked lymphoproliferative syndrome

2. **Secondary/Acquired HLH**
   a. Exogenous triggers
      i. Infection-associated hemophagocytic syndrome (IAHS)
      ii. Toxin associated
   b. Endogenous triggers
      i. Macrophage activation syndrome
      ii. Malignancy associated

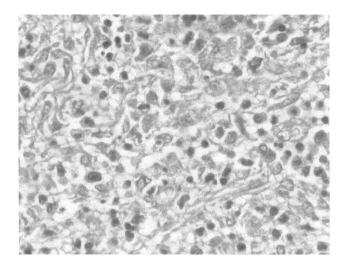

Figure 38.1 Hemophagocytosis in spleen.

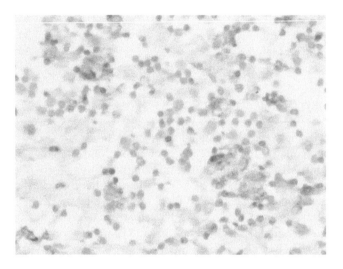

Figure 38.2 Immunohistochemistry for CD68 showing hemophagocytosis in spleen.

the cytoplasm of macrophages. It can be seen in HLH in bone marrow/liver/spleen (Figures 38.1 and 38.2) and lymph nodes; however, it is not pathognomic of HLH.

Role of toll-like receptors

Toll-like receptors (TLRs) are non-antigen-specific receptors on the surface of NK cells, which can be activated by various infective agents. Genes regulating TLRs are upregulated in patients with macrophage activation syndrome (MAS) and juvenile idiopathic arthritis.

Genotype/phenotype correlation

Patients with PRF1 mutation present much earlier in life than those with STX11 mutation. Adults with PRF1, MUNC134, and STXBP2 mutations tend to have more indolent disease [11].

Triggering factors

IMMUNE ACTIVATION TRIGGERS

The most common trigger that causes immune activation both in familial and sporadic cases is infection. Viral infections are the leading trigger among infections, with EBV being most commonly implicated [12]. Other viruses known to precipitate HLH are cytomegalovirus, parvovirus, herpes simplex virus, varicella zoster virus, measles virus, human herpes virus8, H1N1 influenza virus, and

HIV [4]. Other infectious agents such as bacteria (e.g., *Brucella*, gram-negative bacteria, tuberculosis), parasites (e.g., leishmaniasis, malaria), and fungi are less commonly implicated [13].

IMMUNODEFICIENCY TRIGGERS

Malignancy, rheumatologic disorders, inherited syndromes, and HIV infection are the common immunodeficiency triggers. Hematological malignancies such as T, NK, and anaplastic large cell lymphomas, and leukemias are commonly associated with HLH [14]. HLH in association with rheumatological diseases is known as MAS. The common association of MAS in the pediatric age group is sJIA, whereas in adults, autoimmune and rheumatologic associations such as rheumatoid arthritis, Still disease, lupus erythematosus, mixed connective tissue disease, systemic sclerosis, pulmonary sarcoidosis and polyarteritis nodosa, and Sjögren syndrome have been reported [15].

CLINICAL FEATURES

HLH presents clinically as a febrile illness with multiorgan involvement. The fever is high grade, seen in more than 90% of cases, and is associated with hepatosplenomegaly, lymphadenopathy, skin rash. and neurologic symptoms.

Frequency of clinical signs in hemophagocytic lymphohistiocytosis

The rash associated with HLH is usually diffuse and erythematous (Figure 38.3); however, petechial and purpuric rashes are not uncommon [4,7,15] (Table 38.2). Central nervous system (CNS) involvement may present as seizures, altered sensorium, ataxia, hemiplegia, and at times may precede other symptoms [16,17]. There may be features of fulminant hepatic failure and coagulopathy. Pulmonary involvement is seen in approximately 40% of cases and may be due to infection or acute respiratory distress syndrome requiring ventilatory support. Renal involvement is seen in about 16% and presents as hyponatremia or renal failure [4]. Severe hypotension requiring vasopressors may occur.

LABORATORY EVALUATION

Baseline investigations

A complete hemogram reveals cytopenias in over 80% of HLH cases. In MAS, the counts may be initially elevated followed by delayed-onset cytopenia [18]. Liver function tests show raised bilirubin and elevated levels of liver enzymes aspartate

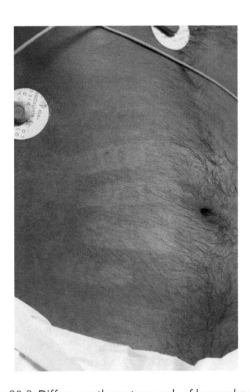

Figure 38.3 Diffuse erythematous rash of hemophagocytic lymphohistiocytosis.

Table 38.2 Frequency of main clinical features in hemophagocytic lymphohistiocytosis

Clinical sign	Frequency (%)
Fever	60–100
Hepatomegaly	39–97
Splenomegaly	35–100
Skin rash	3–65
Lymphadenopathy	17–52
Neurological signs	7–47

amino transferase (AST), alanine aminotransferase (ALT), gamma glutamyl transferase (GGT), lactate dehydrogenase (LDH), and hypoalbuminemia. Coagulation parameters such as prothrombin time, activated partial thromboplastin time (aPTT), fibrinogen, and D-dimer are deranged. Other important biochemical markers for HLH are ferritin and triglycerides, both of which are elevated. Decreased fibrinogen levels and raised serum neopterin are additional indicators of HLH [19]. Cultures from blood, marrow, urine, and cerebrospinal fluid (CSF) must be carried out, and if available, viral titers and polymerase chain reaction for EBV, cytomegalovirus, and other adenoviruses should be done if available.

Bone marrow studies

Bone marrow studies are mandatory in suspected HLH cases to detect hemophagocytosis and to rule out other causes of cytopenias and malignancies. The cellularity of the marrow is variable, and hemophagocytosis is seen in 25%–100% of HLH but may not be evident in the initial stage of the disease [20]. Macrophages can be highlighted by CD163 staining.

Cerebrospinal fluid studies

CSF studies show pleocytosis and raised proteins, but hemophagocytosis is rare. Cultures and viral studies should be carried out on the CSF too.

Imaging

Imaging studies like x-ray chest, ultrasound abdomen, echocardiography, and CT scan are carried out to rule out systemic involvement and malignancies.

Special investigations

IMMUNOLOGICAL TESTS

The following tests help in diagnosing HLH by establishing the hyperimmune state.

- Levels of soluble IL2 receptor alpha (sCD25)
- Soluble levels of the hemoglobinhaptoglobin scavenger receptor (sCD163)

- Immunoglobulin levels (IgM, IgG, IgA)
- Flowcytometric analysis for cell surface expression of
  - Lysosomalassociated membrane protein 1 (LAMP1, or CD107 alpha) for NK cell function
  - Perforin and granzyme B proteins
  - Sap and XIAP in males
  - Lymphocyte subset analysis

Elevated soluble IL2 receptor alpha, reduced cell surface expression of CD107-α, elevated sCD163; and reduced perforin, SAP, or XIAP are consistent with a diagnosis of HLH. Peripheral blood T-cell subsets normal helper/suppressor ratio of peripheral T cells, with low B cells and variable immunoglobulin levels are seen [21]. Elevated granzyme B has been found and is a marker of lymphocyte activation.

GENETIC STUDIES

Genetic testing should be carried out in children born to consanguineous parents or those with positive family history and relapsing or refractive disease.

DIAGNOSIS

Currently the diagnosis of HLH is based on the 2004 criteria [22]. Early cases of HLH may be missed by using this criteria, as all may not fulfill the five out of eight requisites for diagnosis; hence, a revised criteria for diagnosis was proposed by the HLH Society in 2009 [23]. Clinical judgment should be used in initiating the treatment in cases that do not meet the diagnostic criteria for HLH.

HLH 2004 diagnostic criteria

1. Molecular diagnosis consistent with HLH. Pathologic mutations of PRF1, MUNC13D, or STX11 are identified.

   or

2. Fulfillment of five of eight of the following criteria:
   a. Fever
   b. Splenomegaly
   c. Cytopenias (affecting at least two of three lineages in the peripheral blood): hemoglobin <9 g/100 mL (in infants <4 weeks: hemoglobin <10 g/100 mL); platelets <100 × 103/mL; neutrophils <1 × 103/mL
   d. Hypertriglyceridemia (fasting, ≥265 mg/100 mL) and/or hypofibrinogenemia (≤150 mg/100 mL)
   e. Hemophagocytosis in BM, spleen, or lymph nodes
   f. Low or absent NK cell activity
   g. Ferritin ≥500 ng/mL
   h. Soluble CD25 (soluble IL-2 receptor) >2400 U/mL (or per local reference laboratory)

Proposed HLH diagnostic criteria 2009

1. Molecular diagnosis consistent with HLH or X-linked lymphoproliferative syndrome.

   or

2. Fulfillment of at least three of four of the following criteria
   a. Fever
   b. Splenomegaly
   c. Cytopenias (minimum two cell lines reduced)
   d. Hepatitis

3. Fulfillment of at least one of four of the following criteria
   a. Hemophagocytosis
   b. ↑ Ferritin
   c. ↑ sIL2Rα (age based)
   d. Absent or very decreased NK function

4. Other supportive diagnostic features

   a. Hypertriglyceridemia
   b. Hypofibrinogenemia
   c. Hyponatremia

Though hemophagocytosis and elevated ferritin levels are helpful in the diagnosis of HLH, neither are pathognomic of the disease and diagnosis; hence, management should not be solely based on these.

DIFFERENTIAL DIAGNOSIS

The differential diagnosis of HLH includes all of those conditions that manifest with fever, cytopenias, liver involvement, and/or neurological findings. The common illnesses that may simulate HLH are sepsis and multiorgan dysfunction, MAS, drug reaction with eosinophilia and systemic symptoms, liver failure, autoimmune lymphoproliferative syndrome, encephalitis, and transfusion-associated graft versus host disease.

MANAGEMENT

The key to successful management of HLH lies in early diagnosis and prompt initiation of therapy. The aim of treatment is to control the precipitating infection and arrest proliferation and activation of T cells and the cytokine storm [24].

Specific management

Steroids are the mainstay of management of HLH. Dexamethasone in the dose of 10 mg/m²/day is the drug of choice in most secondary HLH, as it has better CNS penetration; however, severe forms of familial or secondary HLH require additional treatment with etoposide (150 mg/m²/twice a week) or cyclosporine (6 mg/kg/day).

Intrathecal methotrexate can be added in case of CNS involvement.

IVIg has been found useful only when given early in the disease. In familial HLH, stem cell transplant can replace the defective immune system. Monoclonal antibodies such as infliximab alemtuzumab and daclizumab have been tried with variable success [5,25]. Alemtuzumab targets the CD52 antigen, which is expressed on most lymphocytes, monocytes, macrophages, and dendritic cells. Infliximab and daclizumab target TNF and CD52, respectively. Rituximab has been used in EBV-triggered HLH. Splenectomy and liver transplant are reserved for refractory cases.

Supportive management

Supportive management is directed at controlling infection and providing cardiorespiratory support. Transfusion and dialysis may be required in severe cases.

CONCLUSION

HLH is a potentially fatal condition that is often misdiagnosed. It should be considered a differential in all cases presenting with fever with rash, which have hepatosplenomegaly, pancytopenia, and liver dysfunction. Though a diagnostic criterion exists, therapy should not be withheld for want of fulfillment of these criteria. Energetic and timely initiation of treatment is lifesaving. The outcome is favorable in secondary HLH cases in comparison to primary/familial HLH.

KEY POINTS

- HLH is a potentially fatal illness that presents with fever, cytopenias, organomegaly, and rash, with or without CNS involvement.
- These patients may have an underlying genetic or immunological defect.
- Hemophagocytosis, though present, is not pathognomic of the disease.
- The mainstay of treatment is control of triggering infection and containing the immune activation.

REFERENCES

1. Scott R, Robb-Smith A. Histiocytic medullary reticulosis. *Lancet* 1939;2:194–8.
2. Farquhar J, Claireaux A. Familial hemophagocytic reticulosis. *Arch Dis Child* 1952;27:519–25.
3. Henter JI, Elinder G, Söder O, Ost A. Incidence in Sweden and clinical features of familial hemophagocytic lymphohistiocytosis. *Acta Paediatr Scand* 1991;80:428.
4. RamosCasals M et al. Adult haemophagocytic syndrome. *Lancet* 2014;383:1503.
5. Siddaiahgari SR, Agarwal S, Madukuri P, Moodahadu LS. Hemophagocytic lymphohistiocytosis: A review. *J Blood Disord Transfus* 2016;7:363.
6. Bhattacharya M, Ghosh MK. Hemophagocytic lymphohistiocytosis—Recent concept. *JAPI* 2008;453–7.
7. Aricò M, Danesino C, Pende D, Moretta L. Pathogenesis of haemophagocytic lymphohistiocytosis. *Br J Haematol* 2001;114:761.
8. Komp DM, McNamara J, Buckley P. Elevated soluble interleukin2 receptor in childhood hemophagocytic histiocytic syndromes. *Blood* 1989;73:2128.
9. Tang Y et al. Early diagnostic and prognostic significance of a specific Th1/Th2 cytokine pattern in children with haemophagocytic syndrome. *Br J Haematol* 2008;143:84.
10. Mazodier K et al. Severe imbalance of IL18/IL18BP in patients with secondary hemophagocytic syndrome. *Blood* 2005;106:3483.
11. Horne A et al. Characterization of PRF1, STX11 and UNC13D genotypephenotype correlations in familial hemophagocytic lymphohistiocytosis. *Br J Haematol* 2008;143:75.
12. McClain K et al. Virusassociated histiocytic proliferations in children. Frequent association with EpsteinBarr virus and congenital or acquired immunodeficiencies. *Am J Pediatr Hematol Oncol* 1988;10:196.
13. Risdall RJ, Brunning RD, Hernandez JI, Gordon DH. Bacteriaassociated hemophagocytic syndrome. *Cancer* 1984;54:2968.
14. Miyahara M et al. B-cell lymphoma-associated hemophagocytic syndrome: Clinicopathological characteristics. *Ann Hematol* 2000;79:378.
15. Otrock ZK, Eby CS. Clinical characteristics, prognostic factors, and outcomes of adult patients with hemophagocytic lymphohistiocytosis. *Am J Hematol* 2015;90:220.
16. Jovanovic A et al. Central nervous system involvement in hemophagocytic lymphohistiocytosis: A singlecenter experience. *Pediatr Neurol* 2014;50:233.
17. Haddad E et al. Frequency and severity of central nervous system lesions in hemophagocytic lymphohistiocytosis. *Blood* 1997;89:794.
18. Rosado FG, Kim AS. Hemophagocytic lymphohistiocytosis: An update on diagnosis and pathogenesis. *Am J Clin Pathol* 2013;139:713–27.
19. Ibarra MF et al. Serum neopterin levels as a diagnostic marker of hemophagocytic lymphohistiocytosis syndrome. *Clin Vaccine Immunol* 2011;18:609–14.
20. Rivière S et al. Reactive hemophagocytic syndrome in adults: A retrospective analysis of 162 patients. *Am J Med* 2014;127:1118.
21. Egeler RM, Shapiro R, Loechelt B, Filipovich A. Characteristic immune abnormalities in hemophagocytic lymphohistiocytosis. *J Pediatr Hematol Oncol* 1996;18:340.

22. Henter JI et al. HLH-2004: Diagnostic and therapeutic guidelines for hemophagocytic lymphohistiocytosis. *Pediatr Blood Cancer* 2007;48:124–31.

23. Filipovich AH. Hemophagocytic lymphohistiocytosis (HLH) and related disorders. *Hematology Am Soc Hematol Educ Program* 2009:127–31.

24. Bode SF et al. Recent advances in the diagnosis and treatment of hemophagocytic lymphohistiocytosis. *Arthritis Res* 2012;14:213.

25. Marsh RA et al. Salvage therapy of refractory hemophagocytic lymphohistiocytosis with alemtuzumab. *Pediatr Blood Cancer* 2013;60:101–9.

39

Hypereosinophilic syndrome

PREEMA SINHA AND SUNMEET SANDHU

INTRODUCTION

The hypereosinophilic syndrome (HES) is a group of rare disorders occurring worldwide, spanning all age groups and characterized by elevated eosinophil counts greater than 1.5×10^9/L for greater than 6 months with eosinophil-mediated organ damage and/or dysfunction, provided other potential causes for the damage have been excluded. The disease can affect multiple organs with a multitude of clinical presentations. Skin lesions can be the presenting symptom affecting up to 50% of patients with HES [1].

DEFINITION

HES was defined by Chusid et al. [2], who proposed three diagnostic criteria (Table 39.1) [2,3]:

1. Persistent eosinophilia of 1.5×10^9 eosinophils/L of blood for longer than 6 months (or death before 6 months associated with signs and symptoms of hypereosinophilic disease).
2. Lack of evidence for parasitic, allergic, or other known causes of eosinophilia.
3. Presumptive signs and symptoms of organ involvement, including hepatosplenomegaly, organic heart murmur, congestive heart failure, diffuse or focal nervous system abnormalities, pulmonary fibrosis, fever, weight loss, and anemia.

Modification—Patients with marked eosinophilia and obvious marked tissue damage like cardiac involvement should not be observed for 6 months before diagnosis and vigorous therapy is initiated.

CLASSIFICATION

HESs are subclassified according to the pathogenic mechanisms resulting in eosinophil expansion: primary, secondary, and idiopathic [3,4].

- *Primary (or neoplastic) HES*: Eosinophilic expansion occurs in the setting of an underlying stem cell, myeloid, or eosinophilic neoplasm, and is considered (or proven) clonal.
- *Secondary (or reactive) HES*: Eosinophilic expansion occurs due to overproduction of eosinophilopoietic cytokines by other cell types and is polyclonal. Generally encountered in parasitic infections, certain solid tumors, and T-cell lymphoma.
  - Lymphocytic variant HES (L-HES) is a subvariant.
- *Idiopathic HES*: The underlying cause of hypereosinophilia (HE) remains unknown despite extensive etiologic workup.

HYPEREOSINOPHILIC SYNDROME VARIANTS

HES has also been subdivided into several clinically relevant variants [3,4]:

1. *Myeloid variants of HES (M-HES)*: More typical features of myeloproliferative disorders are present with raised serum vitamin B12 levels, anemia, thrombocytopenia, hepatosplenomegaly, and eosinophilic tissue damage and/or fibrosis [5,6].
   - This variant is resistant to treatment with glucocorticosteroids.

Table 39.1 Diagnostic criteria for hypereosinophilic syndrome

- Peripheral blood eosinophilia of at least 1500 eosinophils/µL
  - Longer than 6 months
  - Less than 6 months with evidence of organ damage
- Signs and symptoms of multiorgan involvement
- No evidence of parasitic or allergic disease or other known causes of peripheral blood eosinophilia

- Myeloproliferative features in the setting of marked eosinophilia and clinical manifestations of HES have been associated with the presence of the *FIP1L1/PDGFRA* fusion gene [7].
- These patients show marked clinical improvement with imatinib, a tyrosinase kinase inhibitor [7].
- Most of the clinical manifestations improve with imatinib treatment; however, structural damage, including cardiac valve abnormalities and ischemic injury, are permanent.
- Hence, imatinib treatment should be initiated as soon as possible after the diagnosis is made.

2. *T-lymphocytic variants of HES (L-HES)*: Lymphocytic variant HES (L-HES) is characterized predominantly by skin and soft tissue involvement [8,9].
   - Cardiovascular, pulmonary, and rheumatological involvement, are also seen frequently.
   - Although end-organ complications of hypereosinophilia are generally benign, with mainly cutaneous manifestations, long-term prognosis is overshadowed by an increased risk of developing T-cell lymphoma, as a result of malignant transformation of aberrant T cells years after HES diagnosis.
   - The frequently reported abnormal T-cell phenotype in L-HES is CD3−CD4+. The presence of large irregular cells allows these lymphocyte populations to be identified via T-cell receptor rearrangement studies and flow cytometric analysis [10].
   - The majority of patients have elevated serum immunoglobulin E (IgE), skin involvement, and lymphadenopathy.
   - High IL-5 levels are implicated in the generation of eosinophilia; however, increased IL-5 levels neither correlate with the presence of L-HES nor predict the response to treatment [10].

3. *Familial HES*: Autosomal dominant transmission of marked eosinophilia is reported in successive generations [11].
   - Eosinophilia begins at birth and most family members remain asymptomatic, although progression with fatal endomyocardial fibrosis and neurologic abnormalities are known to occur in a few.
   - The exact cause is unknown, but the responsible gene has been mapped onto 5q31-q33, in the region of the cytokine gene cluster. This area also contains genes encoding IL-3, IL-5, and GM-CSF, which are important for eosinophil development and function.

4. *Idiopathic HES (IHES)*: Despite careful evaluation of HE, the etiology in as many as 75% of cases of presumed HES remains undefined.

5. *Organ-restricted hypereosinophilic conditions*: This term is applied to disorders with blood eosinophilia ≥1500/mL in the setting of a single organ involvement.
   - Overlap disorders include a wide variety of single organ-restricted eosinophilic disorders, such as eosinophilic gastrointestinal disorders, chronic eosinophilic pneumonia, and Wells syndrome.

6. *Specific/defined syndromes associated with HE*: This term is applied to disorders with blood eosinophilia ≥1500/mL in association with a distinct diagnosis, wherein the role of eosinophils in disease complications and clinical manifestations remains inconclusive.
   - Examples include collagen vascular diseases, sarcoidosis, ulcerative colitis, autoimmune lymphoproliferative syndrome, human immunodeficiency virus (HIV) infection, hyperimmunoglobulin E syndromes (e.g., dedicator of cytokinesis 8 [DOCK8] deficiency), and caspase recruitment domain-containing protein 9 (CARD9) deficiency.
   - *Episodic angioedema with eosinophilia (Gleich syndrome)*: It is a rare disorder characterized by recurrent episodes of urticaria, fever, angioedema, weight gain, oliguria, elevated serum immunoglobulin M (IgM), and dramatic eosinophilia that occurs at 3–4-week intervals and resolves with spontaneous diuresis in the absence of therapy [12].
     - Cyclic elevations of serum interleukin (IL)-5 preceding the rise in eosinophilia, increased numbers of activated T cells, and eosinophilic degranulation in the dermis during symptomatic episodes are seen.
   - *Eosinophilic granulomatosis with polyangiitis*: Eosinophilic granulomatosis with polyangiitis (EGPA, formerly called Churg-Strauss) is difficult to categorize, particularly in the absence of documented eosinophilic vasculitis on tissue biopsy. Clinical manifestations can involve the sinuses, lungs, skin, heart, peripheral nerves, and other structures [13].

7. *Hypereosinophilia of undetermined significance or benign eosinophilia (HE_US)*: Describes patients with persistent unexplained HE, but without apparent complications related to tissue eosinophilia. The persistent hypereosinophilia that generally does not result in significant clinical manifestations cannot be explained, and there is difficulty in predicting whether the patient will eventually develop clinical manifestations related to eosinophilic organ infiltration, and thus progress to HES.

EPIDEMIOLOGY

HES is a very rare condition [2,3].

- Estimated prevalence is between 0.36 and 6.3 per 100,000.
- Patients are commonly diagnosed between the ages of 20 and 50 years.
- In a child with a suspected diagnosis of HES, a careful evaluation for clonal abnormalities should be performed.
- Ninety percent of patients with myeloproliferative HES are male, but lymphocytic variant has equal gender distribution.

PATHOPHYSIOLOGY

The basic pathology of HES is the sequestration of eosinophils in organ tissues or systems [1–3].

- Eosinophil-derived neurotoxin, eosinophil cationic protein, and major basic protein are enzymes released by eosinophils that cause endothelial damage and promote fibrosis, thrombosis, and infarction.
- Common target organs include the skin, lung, gastrointestinal tract, cardiovascular system, and brain.
- Clinical improvement parallels a decrease in eosinophil count.

CLINICAL PRESENTATIONS OF HYPEREOSINOPHILIC SYNDROME

HES generally presents with blood, heart, nervous system, lung, and especially, skin involvement (Table 39.2). Signs and symptoms relate to organ systems infiltrated by eosinophils.

Cutaneous features

HES conditions may present with varied cutaneous abnormalities [2,3,4].

Table 39.2 Common mucocutaneous findings in hypereosinophilic syndrome

- Angioedema
- Eczema
- Erythema annulare centrifugum
- Erythroderma
- Livedo reticularis
- Mucosal (oral and genital) ulcers
- Nail fold infarcts
- Necrotizing vasculitis
- Purpuric papules
- Splinter haemorrhages
- Urticaria
- Vasculitis
- Wells syndrome (eosinophilic cellulitis)

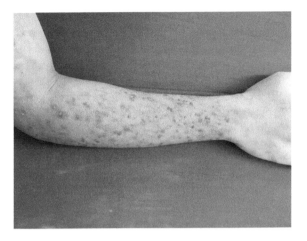

Figure 39.1 Extensive highly pruritic papulonodular lesions over upper extremity in a patient of lymphocytic variant of HES.

- Over 50% of HES patients have skin lesions of the trunk and/or extremities as the first manifestation of HES, including pruritic erythematous macules, papules, plaques, wheals, and nodules (Figures 39.1 and 39.2).
- Splinter hemorrhages and/or nail fold infarcts may herald the onset of thromboembolic disease [1].
- Eczematous lesions (involving hands, flexural areas, or dispersed plaques), erythroderma, and generalized thickening of the skin are also common.
- Urticaria and angioedema occur in all HES subtypes and are characteristic of certain variants, especially lymphocytic HES.

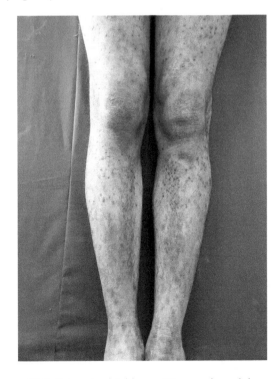

Figure 39.2 Extensive highly pruritic papulonodular lesions over lower extremity in a patient of lymphocytic variant of HES.

- Mucosal ulcers of the oropharynx and anogenital portend an aggressive clinical course, and death is likely within 2 years of presentation if the disorder is untreated. Mucosal ulcers may characterize myeloproliferative *FIP1L1-PDGFRA*-positive HES [14].
- Other various cutaneous disorders seen include erythema annulare centrifugum, necrotizing vasculitis, livedo reticularis, purpuric papules, and Wells syndrome (eosinophilic cellulitis). A diagnosis of HES may be delayed or missed because an association between skin findings and HES is not appreciated.
- Lymphocytic variant (L-HES) has predominant cutaneous features in the form of urticaria, erythroderma, and plaques. Patients with cutaneous symptoms should be investigated for the presence of abnormal T cells to exclude cutaneous T-cell lymphoma [15].
- The presence of lymphomatoid papulosis should prompt a search for *FIPILI-PDGFRA* mutation [16].

Pulmonary disease

Pulmonary involvement can be seen in 40%–60% of cases [17,18].

- Pulmonary involvement is common in HES and may result from eosinophilic infiltration of the lung with subsequent fibrosis, heart failure, or pulmonary emboli.
- The most common presenting symptoms are dyspnea, cough, and wheezing.
- Lung involvement results in nocturnal cough, productive sputum, wheezing, and dyspnea, which raises the suspicion of bronchial hyperreactivity. Patients may be misdiagnosed as having asthma. However, pulmonary function tests typically reveal no airflow limitation.
- Pulmonary involvement may also be secondary to congestive heart failure or emboli originating from right ventricular thrombi.

Gastrointestinal disorders

Eosinophilic gastritis, enteritis, and/or colitis may occur secondary to HES and cause weight loss, abdominal pain, vomiting, and/or severe diarrhea [19].

- Hepatic involvement may take the form of chronic active hepatitis, focal hepatic lesions, eosinophilic cholangitis, or the Budd-Chiari syndrome.

Cardiac involvement

Seen in nearly 60% of patients with HES, with endomyocardial fibrosis being most common [18,19].

- Endocardial clot formation often leads to valve dysfunction, reduced cardiac output, and embolization to brain, viscera, and limbs.
- Presence of splinter hemorrhages in the nail beds indicates ongoing embolization [1].

- Any patient with marked eosinophilia who satisfies the criteria for HES, and splinter nail bed hemorrhages should be considered a medical emergency and aggressively treated.
- Eosinophilic myocarditis is a major cause of morbidity and mortality among patients with HES.
- Platelet-derived growth factor receptor alpha (*PDGFRA*)–associated HES has an increased incidence of incapacitating and potentially lethal cardiac involvement in the absence of therapy.
- Although cardiac involvement is best diagnosed by means of endomyocardial biopsy, this technique can have a high morbidity and mortality and be difficult to perform. Instead, a noninvasive procedure such as transesophageal echocardiography is valuable for detecting thrombus formation.
- Significant arrhythmia with chronic heart failure is often found in the late stages of HES.
- The development of cardiac disease in HES is unpredictable.
- Cardiac involvement does, however, appear to be more common in patients with the Fip1-like1-platelet-derived growth factor receptor alpha (*FIP1L1-PDGFRA*) fusion.

Neuropsychiatric disease

Common in HES with patients often presenting with loss of intellect, depressed mood, and poor coordination [20,21].

- HES may be complicated by cerebral thromboemboli, encephalopathy, peripheral neuropathy, and sinus thrombosis.
- Neurologic complaints, particularly those associated with cerebral thromboemboli, are occasionally the presenting symptoms of HES.
- Cerebral thromboemboli can arise from intracardiac thrombi and manifest as embolic strokes or transient ischemic episodes.
- Encephalopathy can present with behavioral changes, confusion, ataxia, and memory loss.
- Affected patients may also have signs of upper motor neuron injury, such as increased muscle tone, heightened deep tendon reflexes, and a positive Babinski response.
- Peripheral neuropathy can also occur as mononeuritis multiplex or radiculopathy.

Thrombotic complications

Venous and arterial blood vessels may be damaged in HES, although the mechanisms remain largely unknown [22,23].

- Patients have been reported to develop femoral artery occlusion, intracranial sinus thrombosis, or digital gangrene in the setting of progressive Raynaud phenomenon.

Table 39.3 Indicators of medical emergency in hypereosinophilic syndrome (HES)

- Embolic events constitute a medical emergency.
- Any patient with marked eosinophilia who satisfies the criteria for HES, and with splinter nail bed hemorrhages should be considered a medical emergency and be treated aggressively.
- Mucosal ulcers of the oropharynx and anogenital region portend an aggressive clinical course; death is likely within 2 years of presentation if the disorder is untreated.
- Eosinophilic endomyocardial disease is common in patients with prolonged peripheral blood eosinophilia from any cause.

Ocular manifestations

Ocular symptoms, particularly blurred vision, may be related to microemboli or local thrombosis. Adie syndrome (pupillotonia), keratoconjunctivitis sicca, and scleritis are the other main forms of ocular involvement [24,25].

The indicators for various complications in HES are given in Table 39.3.

LABORATORY TESTS

Key criterion for diagnosis is peripheral blood eosinophilia.

- Other causes of eosinophilia to be ruled out such as allergic and parasitic diseases.
- Tests to detect target organ involvement, especially liver enzymes, serum troponin, and rarely, increased blood urea nitrogen and creatinine levels.
- As eosinophilic endomyocardial disease is an emergency and can develop in any patient with prolonged hypereosinophilia, periodic echocardiography is important.
- Pulmonary function test, chest radiograph, and computed tomography (CT) may be required to evaluate the pulmonary complications.
- Levels of immunoglobulin E (IgE) are high in L-HES.
- In myeloproliferative HES levels of vitamin B12 and tryptase are increased.
- Chic2 fluorescent *in situ* hybridization assay or polymerase chain reaction assay to detect the *FIP1L1PDGFRA* gene product.
- Testing for other clonal cytogenetic abnormalities or abnormal clonal T-cell populations.
- Cutaneous histopathologic features of HES varys with the type of lesion, e.g., biopsy from urticarial lesions resembles idiopathic urticaria. Features of vasculitis are generally associated with only Churg-Strauss syndrome.

DIFFERENTIAL DIAGNOSIS

A variety of conditions can be associated with secondary blood or tissue eosinophilia and clinical manifestations of HES, which include the following:

- Leukemias and lymphomas.
- Paraneoplastic syndromes.
- KIT mutation-associated systemic mastocytosis with eosinophilia.
- Drug hypersensitivity reactions.
- Parasitic infections and infestations.
- HES with episodic angioedema may resemble hereditary angioedema.
- Pruritic eczematoid lesions of lymphocytic HES may resemble those of atopic dermatitis, drug reaction, fungal reaction, and T-cell lymphoma.
- Patients with oro-genital lesions and those having thrombosis need to be differentiated from syndromes like Behçet syndrome, Crohn disease, Reiter syndrome, and ulcerative colitis.
- The relationships among HES, acute leukemias, chronic eosinophilic leukemias (CELs), and myelodysplastic syndromes continue to be refined. Patients with HES can develop T-cell lymphomas or acute lymphoblastic leukemia, and patients with acute lymphocytic leukemia (ALL), especially those with pre-B-cell ALL, can present clinically with HES.

TREATMENT

- The goal of the treatment is to relieve the signs and symptoms and to improve the organ function while keeping peripheral blood eosinophils at 1000–2000/μL and minimizing treatment side effects.
- In myeloproliferative-HES patients with the mutant gene *FIP1L1-PDGFRA*, imatinib mesylate is indicated, and it usually induces remission, but endomyocardial disease can worsen during the first few days of treatment. Hence, levels of troponin should be measured during the initial days of treatment. Systemic corticosteroids given before and with the treatment can improve overall cardiac function [26,27].
- Patients with no gene mutation respond to prednisolone as first-line therapy [28].
- Interferon-α (IFN-α) is also useful in treating myeloid and lymphocytic HES [29].
- Other treatments with reported benefits include hydroxyurea, dapsone, vincristine sulfate, cyclophosphamide, methotrexate, 6-thioguanine, 2-chlorodeoxyadenosine and cytarabine combination therapy, cyclosporine, IV immunoglobulin, etoposide, pulsed chlorambucil, and psoralen plus ultraviolet A phototherapy [30].
- Extracorporeal photophoresis alone or in combination with IFN-α has also been tried [30].
- Monoclonal antibodies (mepolizumab) against human IL-5 have been associated with clinical improvement and reductions in peripheral blood and dermal eosinophils. This has proven to be useful in lymphocytic HES [31].
- Alemtuzumab, a monoclonal antibody to CD52 approved for use in T- and B-cell leukemias, has been used in isolated cases.

Table 39.4 Salient features of hypereosinophilic syndrome (HES)

- HES is a heterogeneous group of rare disorders with different etiologies.
- The clinical manifestations of HES may be indistinguishable from those of secondary eosinophilia.
- Steroids remain the mainstay of treatment for most patients with HES.
- Treatment with tyrosine kinase inhibitors like imatinib is indicated for patients with proven myeloid variants of HES.
- Novel monoclonal antibody therapies like mepolizumab, especially those targeting eosinophils, show promise for the treatment of HES.

- Bone marrow transplantation (BMT), including non-myeloablative peripheral stem cell transplantation, has been used successfully in the treatment of HES. BMT, because of high morbidity and mortality, should be reserved for patients with M-HES resistant to tyrosine kinase inhibitor therapy and patients with other forms of HES in whom end-organ damage is severe and progressive despite aggressive therapy [32].

CONCLUSION

The salient features of HES are summarized in Table 39.4.

KEY POINTS

- Rare group of diseases associated with persistent eosinophilia and multiorgan involvement.
- Skin, heart, central nervous system and respiratory tract are most commonly affected.
- Primary, secondary and idiopathic variants exist.
- Corticosteroids and imatinib are the usual treatment modalities.

REFERENCES

1. Gleich GJ, Leiferman KM. The hypereosinophilic syndromes: Current concepts and treatments. Br J Haematol 2009;145:271–85.
2. Chusid MJ, Dale DC, West BC, Wolff SM. The hypereosinophilic syndrome: Analysis of fourteen cases with review of the literature. Medicine (Baltim) 1975;54:127.
3. Simon H-U et al. Refining the definition of hypereosinophilic syndrome. J Allergy Clin Immunol 2010;126:45–9.
4. Valent P et al. Contemporary consensus proposal on criteria and classification of eosinophilic disorders and related syndromes. J Allergy Clin Immunol 2012;130:607–12.
5. Pardanani A et al. FIP1L1-PDGFRA fusion: Prevalence and clinicopathologic correlates in 89 consecutive patients with moderate to severe eosinophilia. Blood 2004;104:3038–45.
6. Metzgeroth G et al. Recurrent finding of the FIP1L1PDGFRA fusion gene in eosinophilia-associated acute myeloid leukemia and lymphoblastic T-cell lymphoma. Leukemia 2007;21:1183–8.
7. Cools J et al. A tyrosine kinase created by fusion of the PDGFRA and FIP1L1 genes as a therapeutic target of imatinib in idiopathic hypereosinophilic syndrome. N Engl J Med 2003;348:1201–14.
8. Roufosse F, Cogan E, Goldman M. Lymphocytic variant hypereosinophilic syndromes. Immunol Allergy Clin North Am 2007;27:389–413.
9. Simon HU, Plotz SG, Dummer R, Blaser K. Abnormal clones of T cells producing interleukin-5 in idiopathic eosinophilia. N Engl J Med 1999;341:1112–20.
10. Ravoet M et al. Molecular profiling of CD3-CD4+ T cells from patients with the lymphocytic variant of hypereosinophilic syndrome reveals targeting of growth control pathways. Blood 2009;114:2969–83.
11. Rioux JD et al. Familial eosinophilia maps to the cytokine gene cluster on human chromosomal region 5q31-q33. Am. J. Hum. Genet 1998;63:1086–94.
12. Morgan SJ et al. Clonal T-helper lymphocytes and elevated IL-5 levels in episodic angioedema and eosinophilia (Gleich's syndrome). Leuk Lymph 2003;44:1623–25.
13. Manganelli P et al. Familial vasculitides: Churg-Strauss syndrome and Wegener's granulomatosis in 2 first-degree relatives. J Rheumatol 2003;30:618–21.
14. Ionescu MA, Murata H, Janin A. Oral mucosal lesions in hypereosinophilic syndrome—An update. 2008;14:115–22.
15. Kazmierowski JA, Chusid MJ, Parrillo JE, Fauci AS, Wolff SM. Dermatologic manifestations of the hypereosinophilic syndrome. Arch Dermatol 1978;114:531–5.
16. McPherson T, Cowen EW, McBurney E, Klion AD. Platelet-derived growth factor receptor-alpha-associated hypereosinophilic syndrome and lymphomatoid papulosis. Br J Dermatol 2006;155:824–6.
17. Nair P et al. The identification of eosinophilic gastroenteritis in prednisone-dependent eosinophilic bronchitis and asthma. Allergy Asthma Clin Immunol 2011;7:4.
18. Ogbogu P, Rosing DR, Horne MK. Cardiovascular manifestations of hypereosinophilic syndromes. Immunol Allergy Clin North Am 2007;27:457–75.
19. Zientek DM, King DL, Dewan SJ, Harford PH, Youman DJ, Hines TR. Hypereosinophilic syndrome with rapid progression of cardiac involvement and early echocardiographic abnormalities. Am Heart J 1995;130:1295–8.
20. Karnak D, Kayacan O, Beder S, Delibalta M. Hypereosinophilic syndrome with pulmonary and cardiac involvement in a patient with asthma. CMAJ 2003;168:172–5.

21. Spry CJ. The hypereosinophilic syndrome: Clinical features, laboratory findings and treatment. *Allergy* 1982;37:539–51.

22. Mukai HY, Ninomiya H, Mitsuhashi S, Hasegewa Y, Nagasawa T, Abe T. Thromboembolism in a patient with transient eosinophilia. *Ann Hematol* 1996;72:93–5.

23. Kojima K, Sasaki T. Veno-occlusive disease in hypereosinophilic syndrome. *Intern Med* 1995;34(12):1194–7.

24. Bozkir N, Stern GA. Ocular manifestations of the idiopathic hypereosinophilic syndrome. *Am J Opthalmol* 1992;113:456.

25. Catalano L, Scala A, Rotoli B. Adie's syndrome (benign pupillotonia) and hypereosinophilic syndrome. *Haematologica* 1988;73:549.

26. Gleich GJ, Leiferman KM, Pardanani A, Tefferi A, Butterfield JH. Treatment of hypereosinophilic syndrome with imatinib mesylate. *Lancet* 2002;359:1577–8.

27. Metzgeroth G et al. Safety and efficacy of imatinib in chronic eosinophilic leukaemia and hypereosinophilic syndrome: A phase-II study. *Br J Haematol* 2008;143:707–15.

28. Butterfield JH, Sharkey SW. Control of hypereosinophilic syndrome-associated recalcitrant coronary artery spasm by combined treatment prednisone, imatinib mesylate and hydroxyurea. *Exp Clin Cardiol* 2006;11:25–8.

29. Schandene L et al. Interferon alpha prevents spontaneous apoptosis of clonal Th2 cells associated with chronic hypereosinophilia. *Blood* 2000;96:4285–92.

30. Klion AD. How I treat hypereosinophilic syndromes. *Blood* 2015;126:1069–77.

31. Rothenberg ME et al. Treatment of patients with the hypereosinophilic syndrome with mepolizumab. *N Engl J Med* 2008;358:1215–28.

32. Bergua JM et al. Resolution of left and right ventricular thrombosis secondary to hypereosinophilic syndrome (lymphoproliferative variant) with reduced intensity conditioning allogenic stem cell transplantation. *Ann Hematol* 2008;87:937–8.

PART 10

Emergencies in Connective Tissue Disorders

BIJU VASUDEVAN

40

Emergencies in systemic lupus erythematosus

VISHALAKSHI VISWANATH AND RASHMI MODAK

INTRODUCTION

Systemic lupus erythematosus (SLE) is a systemic autoimmune disorder involving multiple organ systems and is characterized by excess production of various antibodies that form immune complexes and cause organ damage. A patient of SLE often presents in different phases during the disease process, and acute/severe phases of worsening symptoms often present in the emergency department (ED). A dermatologist is often the first point of contact during these phases or is often called up by the internist when the patient presents with a fever with cutaneous rash with or without multiorgan involvement. This chapter provides a brief overview of SLE with emphasis on the emergencies encountered in LE.

EPIDEMIOLOGY

SLE is an uncommon disease. The overall prevalence has ranged from 15 to 144 per 100,000, and the incidence has ranged from 1.8 to 23.2 cases per 100,000 per year [1,2]. The prevalence ratio of females to males is 9:1 and younger age of onset is seen in females compared to males [3].

Skin manifestations are seen in almost 80% cases of SLE. The cutaneous manifestations have been classified into chronic cutaneous LE (CCLE), discoid LE (DLE), subacute cutaneous LE (SCLE), and acute cutaneous LE (ACLE) [4]. Any of these forms can appear in patients with SLE. ACLE rash may be seen in 51%, SCLE lesions in 7%, and DLE in 25% of cases of SLE [5]. The risk of progression of a localized and generalized DLE to SLE is 5% and 20%, respectively. Lupus panniculitis may have a 35% chance of a preceding, concurrent, or subsequent progression to SLE, whereas 50% of SCLE patients can develop SLE, albeit with lower risk of organ involvement [6]. Among the systemic organs, renal disease is seen in up to 50% of cases of SLE and is the chief predictor of overall morbidity and mortality in LE patients [7].

ETIOPATHOGENESIS

The etiopathogenesis of SLE is complex, and a brief overview is provided [6,8,9]. Multifactorial interactions among genetic and environmental factors are responsible. Multiple genes contribute to disease susceptibility, and it is modified by the interaction of sex, hormonal milieu, and environmental factors that can initiate the disease process and influence the clinical expression. Environmental factors associated with onset of SLE include exposure to sunlight and ultraviolet radiation, smoking, infections, and medications such as hydralazine and tumor necrosis factor (TNF) inhibitors.

Multiorgan inflammation is the hallmark of SLE. Inflammation or tissue injury is triggered by the production of pathogenic autoantibodies that are directed against nucleic acids and their binding proteins, reflecting a global loss of self-tolerance. The loss of immune tolerance, increased antigenic load, defective B-cell suppression, and shift in Th1 to Th2 immune responses lead to B-cell hyperactivity and the production of pathogenic autoantibodies. Defective immune regulatory mechanisms, such as clearance of apoptotic cells and immune complexes, also contribute to development of SLE. The autoantibodies are not organ specific, and a wide range of autoantibodies are produced, some being disease specific (anti-dsDNA and anti-Sm), whereas some are more common (antinuclear antibody [ANA] and anti-Ro antibodies). The primary pathophysiologic findings in various organs include fibrinoid necrosis, collagen sclerosis, necrosis, basophilic body formation, and vascular endothelial thickening.

CLINICAL MANIFESTATIONS

The clinical manifestations in SLE are diverse and can affect most systems. Fever, joint involvement, and skin rash are the classical features. The cutaneous manifestations can be specific and nonspecific (Box 40.1) [6,10]. Table 40.1 summarizes the salient aspects of organ involvement in SLE [6,10]. Based on clinical manifestations (cutaneous/systemic) and immunologic criteria, the current diagnostic criteria followed for SLE are the Systemic Lupus International Collaborating Clinics (SLICC) criteria (Box 40.2) [11].

BOX 40.1: Cutaneous lupus erythematosus subtypes: Salient clinical features

SPECIFIC MANIFESTATIONS

Chronic cutaneous lupus erythematosus (CCLE)

- Clinical prototype—Discoid LE (DLE)
- Variants: Hypertrophic, mucosal, LE profundus/panniculitis, LE tumidus, chilblain LE, LE/lichen planus overlap

Subacute cutaneous lupus erythematosus (SCLE)

- Morphological types:
  - Papulosquamous or psoriasiform lesions
  - Annular lesions with polycyclic margins

Acute cutaneous lupus erythematosus (ACLE)

- Erythema in form of malar rash on face or diffuse morbilliform rash on trunk
- Facial edema
- Bullous lesions (resembling toxic epidermal necrolysis [TEN])

NONSPECIFIC MANIFESTATIONS

- Vascular changes
  - Vasculitis: Leukocytoclastic vasculitis, urticarial vasculitis, gangrene, periungual infarcts, splinter hemorrhages
  - Vasculopathy: Raynaud phenomenon, gangrene, purpura, infarcts, ulcers, livedo reticularis, atrophie blanche, erythromelalgia, thrombophlebitis
- Alopecia
  - Nonscarring alopecia: Lupus hair (coarse, dry, and fragile hair along the peripheral hairline), telogen effluvium (diffuse hair loss), alopecia aerate (patchy hair loss)
  - Scarring alopecia secondary to DLE
- Mucosal changes: Painless palatal ulcers is the hallmark, ulcers may develop on the buccal mucosa or nasopharynx.
- Pigmentary changes: Hypopigmentation due to DLE or SCLE, drug-induced bluish-black pigmentation
- Nail changes: Nail fold erythema, splinter hemorrhages, red lunulae, nail fold hyperkeratosis
- Urticaria: Urticarial wheals, chronic urticaria, or hypocomplementemic urticarial vasculitis
- Bullous lesions: Can occur in three clinical settings:
  - Bullous lesions in ACLE (resembling TEN) or SCLE (Rowell syndrome)
  - Bullous SLE seen as widespread blistering with subepidermal blisters and neutrophilic infiltrates
  - SLE in association with other autoimmune bullous disease including pemphigus erythematosus (Senear-Usher syndrome), pemphigus foliaceus, paraneoplastic pemphigus, bullous pemphigoid, pseudoporphyria, epidermolysis bullosa acquisita, dermatitis herpetiformis, and IgA disease
- Miscellaneous: Calcinosis cutis, papulonodular mucinosis, rheumatoid nodules, sclerodactyly, cutis laxa

---

Table 40.1 Salient features of organ involvement in systemic lupus erythematosus

System involved	Salient features
Neuropsychiatric	Seizures, psychosis, encephalopathy, peripheral neuropathy, Guillain-Barré syndrome, brain infarcts
Cardiovascular	Pericarditis, myocarditis, endocarditis, congestive cardiac failure
Pulmonary	Pneumonitis, acute respiratory distress syndrome, pleurisy, pleural effusion, pulmonary hypertension
Renal	Glomerulonephritis (World Health Organization class II–V), proteinuria, hypertension, nephrotic syndrome
Gastrointestinal	Acute pancreatitis, peritonitis, ascites, hepatitis, bowel infarcts secondary to mesenteric vasculitis
Hematologic	Anemia, leukopenia, thrombocytopenia
Musculoskeletal	Arthralgia, arthritis, myositis, myalgia, tendinitis, avascular bone necrosis
Ocular	Conjunctivitis, episcleritis, retinal artery occlusion, keratoconjunctivitis sicca
Others	Fever, malaise, weight loss, lymphadenopathy, infection/sepsis, hypertensive crisis

CLINICAL CRITERIA

Acute cutaneous lupus

Malar rash
Subacute cutaneous lupus (nonindurated psoriasiform and/or annular polycyclic lesions)

Chronic cutaneous lupus

Classical discoid rash-localized or generalized
Verrucous DLE, lupus panniculitis, mucosal DLE, lupus tumidus, chilblain lupus, discoid lupus-lichen planus overlap

Oral ulcers

Palate, buccal, tongue, or nasal ulcers (in the absence of other causes)

Nonscarring alopecia

Diffuse thinning or hair fragility with visible broken hairs (in the absence of other causes)

Synovitis involving >2 joints

Serositis

Pleurisy, pleural effusions, pleural rub
Typical pericardial pain, pericardial effusion, pericardial rub, pericarditis by electrocardiogram

Renal manifestations

Urine protein/creatinine (or 24-hour urine protein) representing 500 mg of protein in 24 hours or red blood cell casts

Neurological manifestations

Seizures, psychosis, mononeuritis multiplex, myelitis, peripheral or cranial neuropathy, acute confusional state

LABORATORY CRITERIA

Hemolytic anemia
Leukopenia/lymphopenia

Leukopenia <4000 mm³
Lymphopenia <1000 mm³
Thrombocytopenia

<100,000 mm³

IMMUNOLOGICAL CRITERIA

Antinuclear antibodies (ANAs)
Anti-dsDNA
Anti-Sm

Antiphospholipid antibody

Lupus anticoagulant, false-positive rapid plasma reagin, medium or high titer anticardiolipin, and ß-2-glycoprotein I

Low complement

Low C3, C4, or CH50

Direct Coombs test

In the absence of hemolytic anemia
Classify a patient as having SLE if
a. The patient satisfies four of the criteria, including at least one clinical criterion and one immunologic criterion or
b. The patient has biopsy-proven nephritis compatible with SLE and with ANA or anti-dsDNA antibodies

EMERGENCIES IN SYSTEMIC LUPUS ERYTHEMATOSUS

Recent-onset (duration of disease ≤3 months) SLE accounts for 32.1% of the patients in emergency, and this group showed a distinctive pattern of younger age with higher frequencies of neuropsychiatric and hematologic manifestations. Causes of mortality in LE emergencies are usually related to infections and antiphospholipid syndrome (APS). In addition, extent of organ damage rather than the disease activity determines the mortality in SLE emergencies [12]. Risk factors predicting poor outcome of emergencies in SLE patients include the following:

- Older age group (≥45 years)
- Longer duration of disease
- Presence of renal insufficiency
- Presence of pulmonary hypertension
- Invasive infections

The subset of LE patients presenting in the ED may present with cutaneous lesions and life-threatening organ involvement; this may pose difficulties in specific population groups or may be a consequence of the various medications used in LE. These are summarized in Box 40.3.

Dermatological emergencies in lupus erythematosus

Both LE-specific and nonspecific cutaneous manifestations can present in the ED. The clinical scenarios and cutaneous mimickers that can pose diagnostic difficulties are discussed.

BOX 40.3: Emergencies in lupus erythematosus (LE): Clinical scenarios

- Emergencies due to cutaneous manifestations
  - LE-specific skin lesions
  - ACLE (morbilliform rash, facial edema, toxic epidermal necrolysis–like lesions)
  - Subacute cutaneous LE (Rowells, erythema multiforme with annular lesions)
  - Discoid LE (chilblain, LE panniculitis)
  - Bullous eruptions
  - Vascular involvement (vasculitis, vasculopathy)
  - Urticaria/angioedema
  - Unusual manifestations (erythroderma, calciphylaxis, calcinosis cutis, pyoderma gangrenosum)
  - Drug-induced LE
- Emergencies due to systemic involvement
  - Antiphospholipid syndrome
  - Hematologic
  - Renal
  - Gastrointestinal
  - Cardiovascular
  - Pulmonary
  - Neuropsychiatric
  - Rheumatologic
- Emergencies in specific population group
  - Neonatal and childhood LE
  - Pregnancy
- Emergencies due to medications used in LE
  - Side effects due to prolonged or high-dose corticosteroids
  - Side effects due to disease-modifying anti-rheumatic drugs and immunosuppressives

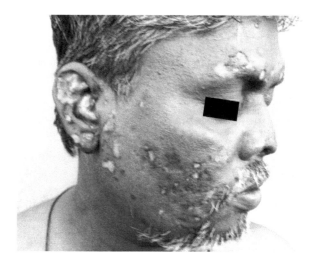

Figure 40.1 Classical discoid lupus erythematosus lesions localized on face and ears.

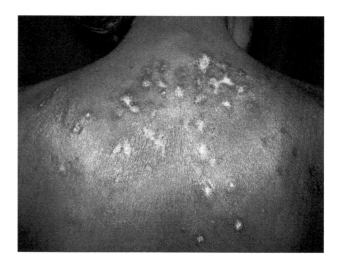

Figure 40.2 Disseminated discoid lupus erythematosus lesions on trunk.

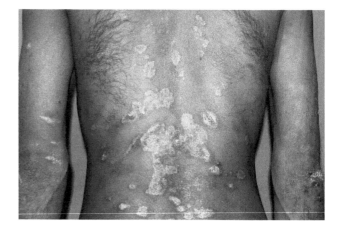

Figure 40.3 Psoriasiform lesions in subacute cutaneous lupus erythematosus.

LUPUS ERYTHEMATOSUS–SPECIFIC CUTANEOUS LESIONS

Fever, arthralgia, and skin rash is the classical manifestation of SLE in the ED. Although the ACLE type of skin rash is commonly seen in the ED, patients with organ involvement may have concomitant CCLE (Figures 40.1 and 40.2) or SCLE (Figure 40.3) type of skin rash. ACLE lesions may present as malar rash (Figure 40.4) or as facial edema over the butterfly area of the face, sparing the nasolabial folds. This may be confused with dermatomyositis, erysipelas, or contact dermatitis. Diffuse erythema may be seen over photoexposed areas and upper trunk and extremities, and morbilliform rash can mimic a viral exanthem or a drug reaction. Epidermal necrosis resembling toxic epidermal necrolysis (TEN) may be seen, and there is often a diagnostic dilemma to differentiate it from drug-induced TEN [13].

Widespread lesions resembling erythema multiforme (EM) may be seen in ACLE (Figure 40.5a and b). EM concomitant with annular lesions of SCLE is seen in Rowell

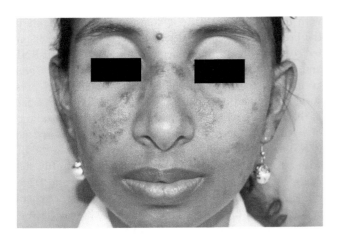

Figure 40.4 Localized malar rash in acute cutaneous lupus erythematosus.

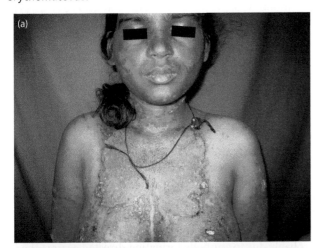

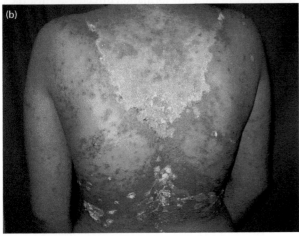

Figure 40.5 (a and b) Extensive rash in systemic lupus erythematosus.

syndrome. Erosions on the palate are characteristic in SLE (Figure 40.6). Perniotic lesions of chilblain or LE profundus may occasionally ulcerate and present in the ED. LE profundus needs to be differentiated from panniculitis due to other connective tissue diseases, such as dermatomyositis and scleroderma and from Weber-Christian disease and erythema nodosum [14].

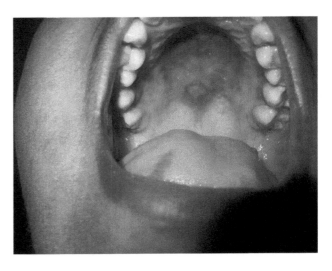

Figure 40.6 Palatal erosion.

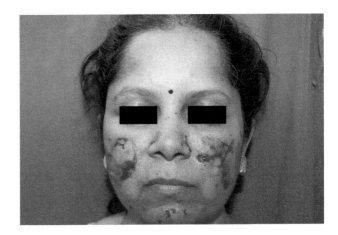

Figure 40.7 Bullous lupus erythematosus.

BULLOUS ERUPTIONS

Bullous lesions are not common; these may resemble TEN/EM, or may occur in association with other autoimmune bullous disorders or as bullous SLE (BSLE), a distinct entity. BSLE can be diagnosed in a patient of SLE with vesiculobullous eruptions all over the body, including the non-sun-exposed areas (Figure 40.7); histopathology findings of subepidermal blisters and neutrophilic dermal infiltrate; and direct immunofluorescence showing linear IgG deposits at the basement membrane zone [6]. The differential diagnosis includes epidermolysis bullosa acquisita (EBA), dermatitis herpetiformis (DH), bullous pemphigoid (BP), and linear IgA bullous dermatosis [15].

VASCULAR INVOLVEMENT

Vascular involvement in SLE can be due to vasculitis or vasculopathy. Vasculitis is caused by primary inflammation of vessel walls with secondary occlusion by fibrin, whereas in vasculopathy narrowing of the vessel walls is noninflammatory due to ischemic causes or thromboembolic phenomenon [6]. Cutaneous manifestations of vascular involvement in SLE can resemble vasculitis or vasculopathy due to varied causes such as infections, drugs, connective tissue diseases, and other systemic diseases.

Cutaneous lesions in vasculitis present as palpable purpura when small vessels are involved and as stellate purpura with or without necrosis and ulceration when medium and/or large vessels are involved. Gangrene of fingers and toes, periungual infarcts, and splinter hemorrhages are some of the other manifestations of vasculitis. Palpable purpura with ulceration and necrosis in severe cases may also be seen due to the presence of cryoglobulins.

Vasculopathy presenting as Raynaud phenomenon, livedo reticularis, livedoid vasculopathy (Figure 40.8), ulcerated purpuric plaques, ecchymosis, digital gangrene (Figure 40.9), and thrombophlebitis may be seen as the clinical presentation of SLE in the ED. Raynaud phenomenon

with impending gangrene is common in SLE patients in the presence of periungual telangiectasias, ice-pick or pitted scarring of pulps of fingers, and high ANA, anti-RNP, and nucleolar antibodies [6]. Livedo reticularis is seen as mottled bluish-red discoloration, blanching on pressure, distributed over buttocks, legs, and the outer aspect of the arms. In patients with SLE and APS, the appearance of livedo reticularis may herald central nervous system (CNS) involvement [6]. The patient may present to the ED with atrophie-blanche-like lesions, including painful, stellate white scars seen over the lower extremities and Degos disease-like lesions (white atrophic macules with peripheral erythema) [6]. Erythromelalgia, which is characterized by burning pain and erythema of hands and feet, increasing on dependence and exposure to heat, may be seen due to microvascular arteriovenous shunting in SLE patients with or without APS. Purpura fulminans may also be an atypical manifestation in SLE along with APS [16].

URTICARIA/ANGIOEDEMA

Urticaria and angioedema constitute one of the most common dermatology referrals in the ED. SLE patients may rarely present to the ED with urticaria, urticarial vasculitis, or angioedema. Chronic autoimmune urticaria may be a rare initial manifestation in LE patients [17]. Urticarial vasculitis presents as painful urticarial lesions lasting for greater than 24 hours, leaving a characteristic postinflammatory hyperpigmentation, characterized by leukocytoclastic vasculitis and hypocomplementemia (Figure 40.10). Few cases of angioedema are reported in SLE. It may be the result of an acquired type of C1 inhibitor deficiency, most probably due to antibody formation directed against the C1 inhibitor molecule [18].

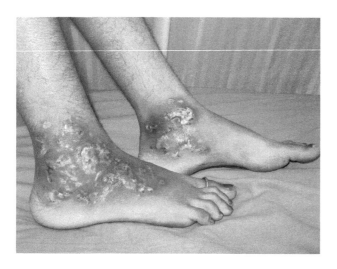

Figure 40.8 Livedoid vasculopathy.

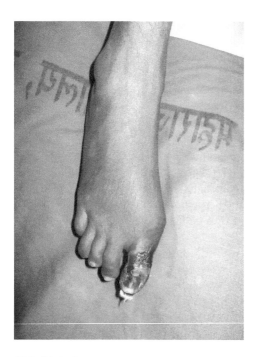

Figure 40.9 Digital gangrene.

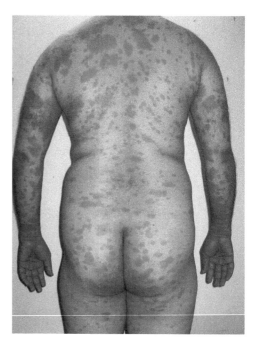

Figure 40.10 Urticarial vasculitis.

UNUSUAL MANIFESTATIONS

Erythroderma is an uncommon manifestation reported in SCLE patients, or exfoliative dermatitis may occur as an adverse effect of the medications used in SLE (Figure 40.11a and b) [19].

Calciphylaxis may be seen in SLE patients with end-stage renal disease or can occur in patients with normal renal function [20,21]. The disease manifests as violaceous lesions with cutaneous necrosis and ulcerations and can mimic APS and be associated with a high mortality. Calcinosis cutis in SLE may be localized or generalized or can occur in association with lupus panniculitis [22,23]. Lesions present as subcutaneous nodules over the buttocks and extremities which may ulcerate, leading to extrusion of a chalky-white material. Pyoderma gangrenosum may be an uncommon manifestation in LE and present in the ED [24]. Leg ulcers in SLE may occur due to vasculitis, vasculopathy, APS, pyoderma gangrenosum, or calcinosis cutis (Figure 40.12) [25].

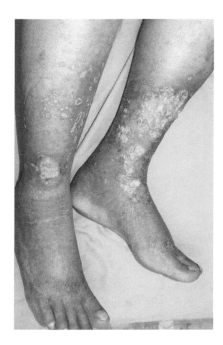

Figure 40.12 Leg ulcers in systemic lupus erythematosus.

DRUG-INDUCED LUPUS ERYTHEMATOSUS

Cutaneous involvement in drug-induced SLE may be vasculitic, bullous lesions, erythema multiforme-like lesions, or may resemble pyoderma gangrenosum [6]. Drug-induced SLE differs from SLE in that it occurs in an older age group, renal and central nervous system involvement are infrequent, antihistone antibodies are frequent, anti-DNA antibodies are absent, and the serum complement is normal. Procainamide, hydralazine, minocycline, isoniazid, and phenytoin are commonly used agents that can cause LE. TNF-α inhibitors produce ANAs, and in this subset of patients arthritis predominates over cutaneous symptoms.

Emergencies due to lupus erythematosus in various organ systems

ANTIPHOSPHOLIPID SYNDROME

APS is characterized by symptoms occurring due to the presence of antiphospholipid antibodies (APAs), namely, lupus anticoagulant, anticardiolipin antibodies, and anti-ß-2 glycoprotein antibodies. APS presents with clinical features of thrombosis (venous, arterial, and microvascular) and pregnancy-related complications. The signs and symptoms leading to life-threatening situations in APS are mainly due to vascular thrombi resulting in cerebrovascular events, pulmonary embolisms, arterial occlusions, and myocardial infarction or microangiopathic hemolysis. Pregnancy-related APS may present as stillbirths and spontaneous abortions due to fatal APS-related disorders including eclampsia, preeclampsia, and HELLP (hemolysis, elevated liver enzymes, low platelet count) syndrome [26]. Cutaneous lesions include thrombophlebitis, purpura (Figure 40.13a and b) and ecchymoses, livedo reticularis, leg

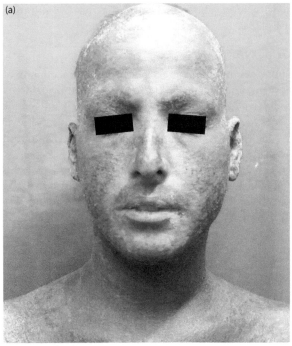

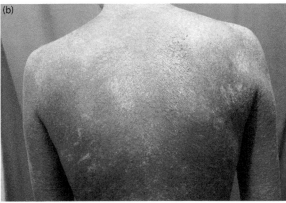

Figure 40.11 (a and b) Erythroderma in subacuteous lupus erythematosus.

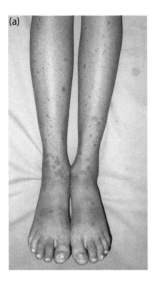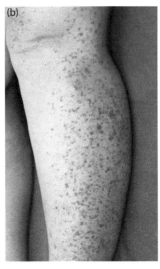

Figure 40.13 (a and b) Vasculitis manifesting as purpura on legs.

ulcers, cutaneous necrosis, gangrene, and subungual splinter hemorrhages. APS may be catastrophic in association with development of disseminated intravascular coagulation and purpura fulminans. Catastrophic APS (CAPS) is seen in less than 1% of patients but has a high mortality of almost 50% [27]. CAPS is a rare manifestation of APS. About 40% of CAPS patients have SLE, 10% another rheumatic disease, and 50% no history of autoimmune disease. Common precipitants include infection, surgery, trauma, pregnancy, oral contraceptives, and cessation of warfarin in an APS patient. The diagnosis of CAPS is made on the basis of

- Evidence of thrombosis in at least three organs
- Histological finding of small-vessel occlusion in at least one organ
- Laboratory confirmation of APA
- Rapid development of clinical features

Adrenal insufficiency in CAPS is due to adrenal venous infarction and presents acutely with flank pain, nausea, vomiting, hypotension, and electrolyte abnormalities.

HEMATOLOGIC

Manifestations in SLE include leukopenia, lymphopenia, thrombocytopenia, autoimmune hemolytic anemia (AIHA), thrombotic thrombocytopenic purpura (TTP), and myelofibrosis [28].

These can occur as a manifestation of SLE, a consequence of SLE treatment, or a part of another blood dyscrasia, and can often present in the ED.

RENAL

Almost 50% of SLE patients develop lupus nephritis, increasing the morbidity and mortality [29]. Lupus nephritis comprises a spectrum of vascular, glomerular, and tubulointerstitial lesions. Glomerulonephritis is the most fundamental factor causing renal impairment. SLE-associated tubulointerstitial injury may be primary or secondary depending on its association with glomerulonephritis. Primary tubulointerstitial nephritis is rare and may present as acute kidney injury with no or mild proteinuria [30]. It is usually associated with secondary Sjögren disease and anti-Ro/anti-La positivity [31]. Renal thrombotic microangiopathy is a major cause of acute renal failure in SLE, especially when associated with APS [32]. Focal proliferative and diffuse proliferative lupus nephritis present with severe systemic symptoms and as an acute complication in the ED. Patients present with hypertension, peripheral edema, and cardiac compromise, such as tamponade and heart failure.

GASTROINTESTINAL

Emergencies include intestinal pseudo-obstruction, spontaneous bacterial peritonitis, pancreatitis, liver dysfunction, and intestinal vasculitis. Mesenteric vasculitis and pancreatitis are life-threatening complications, and patients present with fever, abdominal pain, diarrhea, vomiting, and sepsis [28].

PULMONARY

Lupus pneumonitis is a rare but potential infection in SLE, and it manifests with fever, breathlessness, pleuritic pain, productive cough, central cyanosis, and basal crepitus. A chest x-ray may show bilateral patchy infiltrates [33]. Alveolar hemorrhage is another rare and fatal complication and manifests as dyspnea, fever, hemoptysis, and chest pain [34]. A patient presenting with tachypnea, hypoxemia, and a drop in hemoglobin with or without hemoptysis may evolve to acute respiratory distress syndrome [31]. Acute reversible hypoxemia (ARH), another entity presenting in the ED, is characterized by abnormal arterial blood gases (ABGs) and elevated plasma complement (C3a) without obvious parenchymal lung disease [35,36]. Pulmonary hypertension manifesting with severe dyspnea can occur due to thromboembolic disease or disease activity and has a poor prognosis.

CARDIOVASCULAR

SLE can involve all components of the heart, including the valves, pericardium, myocardium, and coronary arteries.

Valvular insufficiency (mitral more common than aortic) may occur due to valvular vegetations (Libman-Sacks endocarditis) [37]. Embolic stroke secondary to endocarditis has been reported [38]. Pericarditis along with other serositis has been reported in active SLE. It is usually asymptomatic [39] but may present with sharp stabbing pain behind the sternum [3]. Pericardial tamponade is rare and may present with ascites and edema. Myocardial dysfunction with cardiomegaly may present with tachycardia or arrhythmia. Acute myocarditis is usually seen with pericarditis [40].

Coronary artery disease is the most common cause of death in patients with long-standing SLE. Atherosclerotic diseases are more prevalent in SLE patients than in the general population. In young women with SLE, the risk of myocardial infarction is increased 50-fold [41]. Risk factors for atherosclerosis genesis in SLE include disease activity, APS, and drug-related adverse effects [42].

CENTRAL NERVOUS SYSTEM

The prevalence of CNS impairment/involvement ranges from 10% in early stages to 80% in later stages of SLE [43]. A strong association between cerebral infarction, presenting as classical stroke or as transient ischemic attack, and APAs has been noted [44]. These events can lead to a significant cognitive disorder and increase the chances of sudden death. A patient may present to the ED with generalized/partial seizures, with negative findings on computed tomography, magnetic resonance imaging, or angiogram, as a primary symptom of SLE. Seizures can occur due to inflammatory damage resulting from existing vasculopathy or due to APAs [31,45]. Longitudinal myelitis in SLE can occur in two forms, one affecting gray matter (acute catastrophic form) and one involving white matter (resembling neuromyelitis optica) [28]. Myelitis presents as pain, weakness, and sphincteric defects.

Neuropsychiatric manifestations seen in SLE patients are collectively termed as *neuropsychiatric systemic lupus erythematosus* (NPSLE). Mild to moderate cognitive dysfunction with a benign course is usually seen; however, 3%–5% of patients may have severe dysfunction. Chorea in SLE patients is associated with APS. Lupus psychosis with delusions, hallucinations, and acute confusional episodes may present in ED [46].

RHEUMATOLOGIC

Severe polyarthralgias and myalgias can be seen in SLE or in overlap cases with rheumatoid arthritis. Proximal interphalangeal and metacarpophalangeal joints involvement that is not erosive may be present. Due to chronic steroids and predisposition to weaker tendons, these patients may present with tenosynovitis and tendon rupture in the ED. SLE patients can have concomitant fibromyalgia [47]. Acute hip pain may be due to avascular necrosis of the femoral head, and the risk factors include corticosteroid use, presence of the Raynaud phenomenon, vasculitis, and APS [6].

Emergencies in special population subsets

NEONATAL AND CHILDHOOD LUPUS ERYTHEMATOSUS

Neonatal lupus occurs due to passive transfer of maternal anti-SSA antibodies. Ro/SSA antibodies are present in 82%–100% of infants and 92%–100% of mothers [6]. Ultraviolet exposure and phototherapy may precipitate the cutaneous rash. About 15%–20% SLE patients may have the onset of SLE in childhood [6].

Neonatal LE may present with cardiac and noncardiac manifestation. The major cardiac finding is heart block with or without cardiomyopathy. Cardiac neonatal lupus is a life-threatening condition with a 20% mortality rate, and 70% require pacemaker implantation. Noncardiac

manifestations include rash, cytopenia, and hepatic abnormalities that usually resolve within 6–12 months [48]. Cutaneous manifestations simulate SCLE rash and may present as annular or scaly erythematous rash on the face and periorbital area (raccoon sign) [49]. A recent systematic review has reported that maternal SLE is associated with learning disabilities, autism spectrum disorders, attention deficit disorders, and speech problems in the offspring [50].

The average age of onset of childhood SLE is between 12 and 14 years and rarely before 5 years. They tend to have a severe clinical course compared to adults and may present in the ED. Higher percentages of renal involvement, hematological manifestations, seizures, ocular manifestations, and vasculitis are seen as compared to adults [51,52]. SLE may also present to the ED with unusual manifestations such as the inability to walk or talk, intermittent pain and swelling of joints, generalized edema, and dyspnea [53].

LUPUS ERYTHEMATOSUS IN PREGNANCY

A flare-up of lupus is common in pregnancy and the postpartum period [54]. Reported rates of disease flares range from 13.5% to 65% of pregnancies [55]. Approximately 15%–30% of patients with lupus flare have severe

Table 40.2 Adverse effects of systemic lupus erythematosus (SLE) medications and emergency presentation

SLE medications	Adverse effects— Presentation in emergency department
Corticosteroids	Immunosuppression
	Infections
	Avascular necrosis of femur
	Osteopenia
	Diabetes
	Adrenal insufficiency
Hydroxychloroquine	Ophthalmological adverse events—loss of vision
	Anemia in G6PD deficient
Nonsteroidal anti-inflammatory drugs	Gastritis
	Renal compromise
Azathioprine	Immunosuppression
	Liver toxicity
	Pancreatitis
Methotrexate	Immunosuppression
	Liver toxicity
	Mucocutaneous toxicity
Cyclophosphamide	Immunosuppression
	Bladder toxicity
Dapsone	In G6 PD deficient patients, hemolysis, methemoglobinemia
	Dapsone syndrome
Thalidomide	Peripheral neuropathy
Biologicals	Infections

Table 40.3 Investigations and clinical relevance in emergencies

Investigation	Clinical relevance in emergency department
A. Laboratory tests	
Complete blood count	Cell count abnormalities—hematologic emergencies, disease activity, drug toxicities
Liver function tests	Liver dysfunction, preeclampsia, drug toxicities
Renal function tests	Nephritis
Urine analysis	Nephritis, preeclampsia
24-hour urine analysis—protein/creatinine	
Cardiac enzymes	Myocarditis, pulmonary embolism, myocardial infarction
Lipase levels	Pancreatitis
Lactate	Vasculitis and for severity of disease
Blood culture/pus swabs	Infections (due to immunosuppression)
Paracentesis	Spontaneous bacterial peritonitis
B. Imaging studies	
X-rays	
Chest	Pleural effusion, pneumonitis, enlarged cardiac silhouette
Pelvis/hips	Avascular necrosis of femur head
Long bones	Pathologic fractures due to steroids
Dual-energy x-ray absorptiometry scan	Osteoporosis, osteopenia
Computed tomography	
Chest	Pulmonary fibrosis, empyema
Head	Stroke, intracranial hemorrhage
Abdomen	Perforation, pancreatitis, mesenteric vasculitis
Long bones	Pathologic/occult fractures due to steroids
Magnetic resonance imaging	
Brain	Stroke, vasculitis
Hips	Avascular necrosis of femur head grading
Echocardiogram	Pericardial effusion, cardiac tamponade, cardiac failure, endocarditis, pulmonary hypertension
C. Immunological tests	
Antinuclear antibody, ds DNA, Sm, Ro/La	Disease confirmation
Complement C3, C4, CH50	Disease activity
Antiphospholipid antibodies Coomb test	Suspected antiphospholipid syndrome, pregnancy Autoimmune hemolytic anemia
D. Tissue biopsies	
Skin biopsy, lupus band test	Disease confirmation
Kidney biopsy	Disease activity and grading

Table 40.4 Systemic agents in systemic lupus erythematosus

Drug	Dosage
Antimalarials	Hydroxychloroquine 200–400 mg Chloroquine 200–400 mg
Corticosteroids	Low-dose oral prednisolone (0.1–0.2 mg/kg)—mild disease and musculoskeletal manifestations High doses of oral prednisolone (1–1.5 mg/kg) or IV methylprednisolone 1 g daily for 3 days (pulse therapy)—severe disease with major organ involvement
Mycophenolate mofetil	Titrating the dose from 500 mg twice daily to 1–1.5 g twice daily with weekly increases (0.3–3 g)
Cyclophosphamide	50–200 mg
Methotrexate	7.5–20 mg/week
Azathioprine	2–3 mg/kg (75–200 mg)
IV immunoglobulin	400 mg/kg/day over 5 days
Cyclosporine	For nonrenal lupus—2.5–5 mg/kg
Biologicals	Rituximab, belimumab, tocilizumab, abatacept, sifalimumab, and rontalizumab

Table 40.5 Emergencies: Specific management aspects

Skin	*Lupus erythematosus (LE)–specific lesions*: Photoprotection, topical steroids, antimalarials *LE nonspecific lesions*: *Bullous lesions*: Dapsone alone/combination with prednisolone *Vascular involvement*: Glucocorticoids, cyclophosphamide, plasmapheresis, other immunosuppressives Immunoglobulins and rituximab in refractory cases *Urticaria*: Dapsone, antihistaminics *Urticarial vasculitis*: Indomethacin, antihistamines, moderate to high doses of oral steroids (>40 mg/day), dapsone, colchicine, and hydroxychloroquine
Antiphospholipid syndrome	*Treat and prevent further thrombosis*: Anticoagulants (low molecular weight heparin, warfarin, acetylsalicylic acid) *Settle the cytokine storm*: High-dose steroid, hydroxychloroquine *Reduce the antiphospholipid antibody burden*: Plasmapheresis, IV immunoglobulin (IVIg), eliminating the potential infectious factors *Recalcitrant cases*: Rituximab
Hematologic	*Severe neutropenia*: Granulocyte colony-stimulating factor *Low lymphocytic count*: Prophylactic therapy for infections *Severe thrombocytopenia*: Pulse corticosteroids, IVIg or rituximab *Autoimmune hemolytic anemia (AIHA)*: Pulse glucocorticoids *Refractory AIHA*: Rituximab or splenectomy *Thrombotic thrombocytopenic purpura*: Plasmapheresis or plasma exchange, IV cyclophosphamide, rituximab
Renal	Pulse IV cyclophosphamide Maintenance with mycophenolate mofetil or azathioprine
Gastrointestinal	IV methylprednisolone pulse therapy
Pulmonary	Treatment of infections Methylprednisolone pulse therapy Pulmonary hypertension d/t thromboembolic disease: Surgical embolectomy or thrombolytic agent or heparin
Cardiovascular	IV methylprednisolone pulse therapy Cyclophosphamide pulse
Neuropsychiatric	SLE myelitis: IV methylprednisolone pulse therapy f/b high-dose oral corticosteroids Rituximab
Rheumatologic	*Mild disease*: Low-dose prednisone, nonsteroidal anti-inflammatory drugs *Moderate to severe disease*: High-dose glucocorticoids, often in combination with immunosuppressant (azathioprine, methotrexate)
Neonatal and childhood	*Neonatal LE*: Sun avoidance, low-potency topical steroids, rarely antimalarials in case of persistent skin lesions Early recognition of cardiac problems, permanent pacemaker Oral steroids or antimalarials: First 16 weeks of pregnancy Dexamethasone: If heart block detected early *Childhood LE*: Management similar to adult LE
Pregnancy	*Hydroxychloroquin* continued in pregnancy *For disease flares*: Short courses of high doses steroids and/or IV pulse methylprednisolone *Maintenance*: Azathioprine, calcineurin inhibitors, IVIg, plasmapheresis *Obstetrics antiphospholipid syndrome*: • Low-dose aspirin before conception • Combine low molecular weight heparin (LMWH) after conception and maintain it throughout the pregnancy • Switch to full-dose LMWH with hydroxychloroquine and low prednisone dose when necessary
Medication-related adverse effects	Prompt recognition of adverse events and specific management

systemic manifestations, including renal, skin, blood, and joint involvement [56,57]. Besides lupus flares, there is a higher risk of complicated pregnancies, regardless of whether or not SLE is active. Active lupus nephritis and APS-related outcomes including preeclampsia, preterm birth, intrauterine growth retardation, and fetal loss can occur [58].

Emergencies due to medications used in lupus erythematosus

SLE patients are often on immunosuppressive medications for a prolonged period and hence can present in the ED with clinical manifestations of adverse effects. Invasive infections occurring due to immunosuppression have a poor prognostic outcome in SLE emergencies. The adverse effects can occur due to prolonged or high-dose corticosteroids, disease-modifying antirheumatic drugs, or other immunosuppressives (Table 40.2).

INVESTIGATIONS

Laboratory investigations, imaging studies, serological tests, and biopsies are required when evaluating a case of SLE [6,31]. Evaluation for antibodies and tissue biopsies are useful for confirming the diagnosis when SLE is considered as a differential diagnosis in certain emergency clinical settings; however, these tests are not helpful for evaluating complications in LE. Various investigations in LE and their relevance are outlined in Table 40.3.

MANAGEMENT

General measures for SLE patients include avoidance of sun exposure, use of broad-spectrum sunscreen, topical therapy with steroids/calcineurin inhibitors for skin lesions, and oral nonsteroidal anti-inflammatory drugs (NSAIDS) for joint pain [6,28,31]. Systemic agents include antimalarials, corticosteroids, azathioprine, cyclophosphamide, methotrexate, mycophenolate mofetil, IVIg, cyclosporine, rituximab, and other biologicals (Table 40.4). Specific management of emergencies in various clinical scenarios has been summarized in Table 40.5.

CONCLUSION

SLE, a multisystem disorder, is characterized by organ inflammation and immunological abnormalities. Even though skin, joints, and vasculature are most commonly affected, renal, cardiac, pulmonary, and neurological involvement may occur, with increased mortality. APS and SLE in special populations (pregnancy and children) may show varied clinical presentations and need to be dealt with accordingly. Hence, it is important to recognize clinical variations and prognostic parameters in SLE and thereby provide better care in a risk-based approach for SLE patients in emergencies.

KEY POINTS

- SLE can manifest with various emergencies involving kidney, heart, lungs and central nervous system.
- Certain cutaneous features of lupus erythematosus act as markers for systemic involvement thus leading to early diagnosis of complications if these cutaneous features are diagnosed.
- Antiphospholipid syndrome in association can also be diagnosed by early cutaneous features.

REFERENCES

1. Ferucci ED et al. Prevalence and incidence of systemic lupus erythematosus in a population-based registry of American Indian and Alaska Native People, 2007–2009. *Arthritis Rheum* 2014;66:2494–502.
2. Lim SS, Drenkard C. Epidemiology of systemic lupus erythematosus: Capturing the butterfly. *Curr Rheumatol Rep* 2008;10:265–72.
3. Lim SS, Bayakly AR, Helmick CG, Gordon C, Easley K, Drenkard C. The incidence and prevalence of systemic lupus erythematosus, 2002–2004: The Georgia Lupus Registry. *Arthritis Rheum* 2014;66(2):357–68.
4. Gilliam JN, Sontheimer RD. Distinctive cutaneous subsets in the spectrum of lupus erythematosus. *J Am Acad Dermatol* 1981;4(4):471–5.
5. Yell JA, Mbuagbaw J, Burge SM. Cutaneous manifestations of systemic lupus erythematosus. *Br J Dermatol* 1996;135(3):355–62.
6. Goodfield MJ, Dutz J, McCourt C. Lupus erythematosus. In: Griffiths CEM, Barker J, Bleiker T, Chalmers R, Creamer D (Eds), *Rook's Textbook of Dermatology*. 9th ed. Oxford, UK: Wiley Blackwell; 2016:51.14–37.
7. Cojocaru M, Cojocaru IM, Silosi I, Vrabie CD. Manifestations of systemic lupus erythematosus. *Mædica* 2011;6(4):330–6.
8. Mok CC, Lau CS. Pathogenesis of systemic lupus erythematosus. *J Clin Pathol* 2003;56(7):481–90.
9. Choi J, Kim ST, Craft J. The pathogenesis of systemic lupus erythematosus—An update. *Curr Opin Immunol* 2012;24(6):651–7.
10. Costner MI, Sontheimer RD. Lupus erythematosus. In: Goldsmith L, Katz S, Gilchrest B, Paller A, Leffell D, Wolff K (Eds), *Fitzpatrick's Dermatology in General Medicine*. 8th ed. New York: McGraw-Hill; 2012, Chapter 155.
11. Petri M et al. Derivation and validation of Systemic Lupus International Collaborating Clinics (SLICC) classification criteria for systemic lupus erythematosus. *Arthritis Rheum* 2012;64:2677–86.

12. Chen C, Chen G, Zhu C, Lu X, Ye S, Yang C. Severe systemic lupus erythematosus in emergency department: A retrospective single-center study from China. *Clin Rheumatol* 2011;30:1463–9.

13. Monga B, Ghosh S, Jain VK. Toxic epidermal necrolysis-like rash of lupus: A dermatologist's dilemma. *Indian J Dermatol* 2014;59:401–2.

14. Aggarwal K, Jain V K, Dayal S. Lupus erythematosus profundus. *Indian J Dermatol Venereol Leprol* 2002;68:352–3.

15. Barbosa WS et al. Bullous systemic lupus erythematosus: Differential diagnosis with dermatitis herpetiformis. *An Bras Dermatol* 2011;86(4 Suppl. 1):S92–5.

16. Gamba G et al. Purpura fulminans as clinical manifestation of atypical SLE with antiphospholipid antibodies: A case report. *Haematologica* 1991;76(5):426–8.

17. Spadoni M et al. Chronic autoimmune urticaria as the first manifestation of juvenile systemic lupus erythematosus. *Lupus* 2011;20(7):763–6.

18. Habibagahi Z, Ruzbeh J, Yarmohammadi V, Kamali M, Rastegar MH. Refractory angioedema in a patient with systemic lupus erythematosus. *Iranian Dokkyo J Med Sci* 2015;40(4):372–5.

19. Pai VV, Naveen KN, Athanikar SB, Dinesh US, Reshme P, Divyashree RA. Subacute cutaneous lupus erythematosus presenting as erythroderma. *Indian J Dermatol* 2014;59:634.

20. Safwan H, Sake E, Russell B, Jasin HE. Systemic lupus erythematosus and calciphylaxis. *J Rheumatol* 2004;31:1851–3.

21. Aliaga LG et al. Calciphylaxis in a patient with systemic lupus erythematosus without renal insufficiency or hyperparathyroidism. *Lupus* 2012;21(3):329–31.

22. Kim MS et al. Calcinosis cutis in systemic lupus erythematosus: A case report and review of the published work. *J Dermatol* 2010;37(9):815–8.

23. Gunasekera NS et al. Intralesional sodium thiosulfate treatment for calcinosis cutis in the setting of lupus panniculitis. *JAMA Dermatol* 2017 1;153(9):944–5.

24. González-Moreno J et al. Pyoderma gangrenosum and systemic lupus erythematosus: A report of five cases and review of the literature. *Lupus* 2015;24(2):130–7.

25. Lederhandler M et al. Leg ulcers in systemic lupus erythematosus associated with underlying dystrophic calcinosis and bone infarcts in the absence of antiphospholipid antibodies. *JAAD Case Rep* 2016;2(2):164–7.

26. Ruffatti A et al. Treatment strategies and pregnancy outcomes in antiphospholipid syndrome patients with thrombosis and triple antiphospholipid positivity. A European multicentre retrospective study. *Thromb Haemost* 2014;112(4):727–35.

27. Nayer A, Ortega LM. Catastrophic antiphospholipid syndrome: A clinical review. *J Nephropathol* 2014;3(1):9–17.

28. Michelle P. Life-threatening complications of systemic lupus erythematosus. In: Khamashta MA, Ramos-Casals M (Eds), *Autoimmune Diseases: Acute and Complex Situations*. New York: Springer; 2011:9–17.

29. Bertsias GK et al. Joint European League Against Rheumatism and European Renal Association European Dialysis and Transplant Association (EULAR/ERA-EDTA) recommendations for the management of adult and paediatric lupus nephritis. *Ann Rheum Dis* 2012;71(11):1771–82.

30. Dhingra S, Qureshi R, Abdellatif A, Gaber LW, Truong LD. Tubulointerstitial nephritis in systemic lupus erythematosus: Innocent bystander or ominous presage. *Histol Histopathol* 2014;29(5):553–65.

31. Vymetal J et al. Emergency situations in rheumatology with a focus on systemic autoimmune diseases. *Biomed Pap Med Fac Univ Palacky Olomouc Czech Repub* 2016;160(1):20–9.

32. Hughson MD, Nadasdy T, McCarty GA, Sholer C, Min KW, Silva F. Renal thrombotic microangiopathy in patients with systemic lupus erythematosus and the antiphospholipid syndrome. *Am J Kidney Dis* 1992;20(2):150–8.

33. Horak P, Ciferska H, Krajsova B. Organ manifestation of rheumatic diseases. In: Pavelka K, Vencovsky J, Horak P, Šenolt L, Mann H, Štěpan J (Eds), *Rheumatology*. Prague: Maxdorf-Jessenius; 2012:106–37.

34. Martinez-Martinez MU, Abud-Mendoza C. Diffuse alveolar hemorrhage in patients with systemic lupus erythematosus. Clinical manifestations, treatment, and prognosis. *Reumatol Clin* 2014;10(4):248–53.

35. Martinez-Taboada VM, Blanco R, Armona J, Fernandez-Sueiro JL, Rodriguez-Valverde V. Acute reversible hypoxemia in systemic lupus erythematosus: A new syndrome or an index of disease activity? *Lupus* 1995;4(4):259–62.

36. Abramson SB, Dobro J, Eberle MA, Benton M, Reibman J, Epstein H, Rapoport DM, Belmont HM, Goldring RM. Acute reversible hypoxemia in systemic lupus erythematosus. *Ann Intern Med* 1991;114(11):941–7.

37. Galve E, Candell-Riera J, Pigrau C, Permanyer-Miralda G, Garcia-Del-Castillo H, Soler-Soler J. Prevalence, morphologic types, and evolution of cardiac valvular disease in systemic lupus erythematosus. *N Engl J Med* 1988;319(13):817–23.

38. Khan RM, Namas R, Parikh S, Rubin B. Lupus. Embolic stroke as the initial manifestation of systemic lupus erythematosus. *Case Rep Rheumatol* 2015;24(8):885–8.

39. Doria A, Iaccarino L, Sarzi-Puttini P, Atzeni F, Turriel M, Petri M. Cardiac involvement in systemic lupus erythematosus. *Lupus* 2005;14(9):683–6.

40. Moder KG, Miller TD, Tazelaar HD. Cardiac involvement in systemic lupus erythematosus. *Mayo Clin Proc* 1999;74(3):275–84.

41. Salmon JE, Roman MJ. Accelerated atherosclerosis in systemic lupus erythematosus: Implications for patient management. *Curr Opin Rheumatol* 2001;13:341–4.

42. Smrzova A, Horak P, Skacelova M, Zurek M, Frysakova L, Vymetal J, Vaverkova H. Cardiovascular events in patients with systemic lupus erythematosus. *Cor Vasa [Serial on the Internet]* 2014;56:e145–52.

43. Brey RL et al. Neuropsychiatric syndromes in lupus: Prevalence using standardized definitions. *Neurology* 2002;58(8):1214–20.

44. Koskenmies S, Vaarala O, Widen E, Kere J, Palosuo T, Julkunen H. The association of antibodies to cardiolipin, beta 2-glycoprotein I, prothrombin, and oxidized low-density lipoprotein with thrombosis in 292 patients with familial and sporadic systemic lupus erythematosus. *Scand J Rheumatol* 2004;33(4):246–52.

45. Cimaz R, Meroni PL, Shoenfeld Y. Epilepsy as part of systemic lupus erythematosus and systemic antiphospholipid syndrome (Hughes syndrome). *Lupus* 2006;15(4):191–7.

46. Bertsias GK et al. EULAR recommendations for the management of systemic lupus erythematosus with neuropsychiatric manifestations: Report of a task force of the EULAR standing committee for clinical affairs. *Ann Rheum Dis* 2010;69(12):2074–82.

47. Wolfe F et al. Fibromyalgia, systemic lupus erythematosus (SLE) and the evaluation of SLE activity. *J Rheumatol* 2009;36(1):82–8.

48. Rinsho N, Kaishi MG. Neonatal lupus erythematosus. *Lupus* 2017;40(2):124–30.

49. Bhatt TA, Fatani HA, Mimesh S. Congenital lupus erythematosus. *Indian J Dermatol* 2011;56:734–6.

50. Yousef-Yengej FA, van Royen-Kerkhof A, Derksen RHWM, Fritsch-Stork RDE. The development of offspring from mothers with systemic lupus erythematosus. A systematic review. *Autoimmun Rev* 2017;16(7):701–11.

51. Bundhun PK, Kumari A, Huang F. Differences in clinical features observed between childhood-onset versus adult-onset systemic lupus erythematosus: A systematic review and meta-analysis. *Medicine (Baltim)* 2017;96(37):e80–6.

52. Thakur N, Chandra J, Dhingra B, Singh V. Pediatric lupus: Varied haematological picture and presentation. *Indian J Hematol Blood Transfus* 2015;31(1):68–70.

53. Gültekingil-Keser A, Ertuğrul İ, Tekşam Ö, Konuşkan B, Özkutlu S, Özen S. Unusual presentations of childhood systemic lupus erythematosus to emergency department. *Pediatr Emerg Care* 2016;16(7):701–11.

54. Petri M, Howard D, Repke J. Frequency of lupus flare in pregnancy. The Hopkins Lupus Pregnancy Center experience. *Arthritis Rheum* 1991;34(12):1538–45.

55. Molad Y et al. Maternal and fetal outcome of lupus pregnancy: A prospective study of 29 pregnancies. *Lupus* 2005;14(2):145–51.

56. Clowse ME, Magder LS, Witter F, Petri M. The impact of increased lupus activity on obstetric outcomes. *Arthritis Rheum* 2005;52(2):514–21.

57. Gluhovschi C, Gluhovschi G, Petrica L, Velciov S, Gluhovschi A. Pregnancy associated with systemic lupus erythematosus: Immune tolerance in pregnancy and its deficiency in systemic lupus erythematosus—An immunological dilemma. *J Immunol Res* 2015;2015:241547.

58. Stojan G, Baer AN. Flares of systemic lupus erythematosus during pregnancy and the puerperium: Prevention, diagnosis and management. *Expert Rev Clin Immunol* 2012;5:439–53.

41

Scleroderma and associated complications

YASMEEN JABEEN BHAT AND SAFIYA BASHIR

INTRODUCTION

Scleroderma refers to a rare connective tissue disorder characterized by sclerosis of the skin and subcutaneous tissue along with variable visceral involvement. Broadly scleroderma is classified into two categories: *systemic sclerosis* which encompasses cutaneous sclerosis and visceral involvement and *localized scleroderma or morphea* in which disease is mainly limited to the skin and underlying tissues. Systemic sclerosis is associated with multiple systemic complications and can present as emergencies. This chapter highlights the manifestations, complications, and management of systemic sclerosis.

SYSTEMIC SCLEROSIS

Introduction

Systemic sclerosis is a complex autoimmune disease presenting with a multitude of clinical manifestations. Autoimmunity along with vasculopathy and fibrosis are the basis for the protean manifestations of this chronic disease. The disease is quite heterogeneous in its clinical presentation, progressing with time and therapeutic response. Systemic sclerosis is presumably the autoimmune rheumatic disease with the highest disease-related morbidity and mortality and an impaired quality of life [1].

Epidemiology

Systemic sclerosis is a rare disease with a substantial female predominance with female-to-male ratio of 3–6:1 [2]. The disease most commonly affects the young and middle-aged adults. The peak incidence of the disease is in the fourth and fifth decades. Approximately 85% of cases develop in individuals aged 20–60 years. Epidemiological studies suggest that systemic sclerosis is more common in African Americans than in Caucasians and occurs at a younger age and is more severe in this population [3,4].

Etiopathogenesis

The etiopathogenesis of systemic sclerosis is poorly understood. Various genetic and environmental factors are implicated in the etiology of the disease. It is widely believed that certain environmental factors such as drugs, infection, and toxins may trigger skin disease in genetically predisposed individuals. A strong human leukocyte antigen (HLA) association particularly with DRB1 and DQB1 has been demonstrated.

GENETIC FACTORS

The incidence of this disease in families with a history of systemic sclerosis is 1.5%–1.7% [4]. Siblings of patients with systemic sclerosis have a 15- to 19-fold risk of developing the disease, whereas the risk is 13- to 15-fold in first-degree relatives [5–7]. A major role of the HLA region in systemic sclerosis and in determining the autoantibodies and clinical features has been confirmed.

A number of gene alleles have been linked to disease susceptibility and clinical features, which include transforming growth factor-β (TGF-β), monocyte chemoattractant protein-1 (MCP-1), interleukin-1a (IL-1a), tumor necrosis factor-α (TNF-α), connective tissue growth factor (CTGF), fibrillin-1, interferon regulatory factor-5 (IRF-5), signal transducer, and activator-4 [8]. The association of HLA B8 with severe cases [9], and the presence of raised DR2, DR5, and anticentromere antibodies with mild cases of systemic sclerosis have also been determined. HLA-DRB1*11–DQB1*0301 haplotypes have been associated with antitopoisomerase I positivity, whereas HLA-DRB1*01–DQB1*0501 haplotypes are more common in anticentromere antibodies (ACA) positive patients [10].

Multiple susceptibility loci for systemic sclerosis have also been identified at non-HLA regions such as *STAT4, TNFSF4, CD247,* and *MIF* [11].

ENVIRONMENTAL FACTORS

The development of systemic sclerosis has been associated with silica exposure, use of chlorinated solvents, aromatic solvents, trichloroethylene, and ketones [12]. In addition, infections and vaccinations have preceded the development of systemic sclerosis in some cases [13]. Drugs such as anorexigens, pentazocine, and bromocriptine have been implicated in the etiology of systemic sclerosis [3].

MICROCHIMERISM

Fetomaternal and maternofetal microchimerisms have also been proposed as mechanisms triggering autoimmunity in systemic sclerosis and other autoimmune diseases. A graft versus host disease type of response could be initiated by microchimerisms with microchimeric cells acting as effectors or targets of an immune response [14,15].

The etiopathogenesis of systemic sclerosis is summarized in Figure 41.1.

Pathogenesis

The key early process in the pathogenesis of systemic sclerosis involves endothelial cell damage particularly involving the arterioles [16]. Various mechanisms suggested for the endothelial cell damage include viral agents, especially human cytomegalovirus, cytotoxic T cells,

antibody-dependent cellular toxicity, antiendothelial cell antibodies, and ischemic reperfusion injury [17,18].

Endothelial cell injury leads to overproduction of growth factors, cytokines, and other mediators of hyperplasia and hypertrophy including endothelin-1(ET-1), connective tissue growth factor, and transforming growth factor (TGF) β in addition to matrix-modulating proteins like matrix metalloproteinases (MMPs) [19,20].

ET-1 appears to play a significantly important role in the pathogenesis of systemic sclerosis by activating adhesion molecule expression, which in turn is important in regulating the inflammatory response. ET-1 has a major role in vasoconstriction and is an important mediator in extracellular matrix (ECM) deposition and remodeling [21].

It is likely that both innate and adaptive immunity are altered in systemic sclerosis and both share a role in the pathogenesis of systemic sclerosis. T cells induce fibrosis and vasculopathy through cell-cell contact and production of profibrotic cytokines. B cells further contribute to vasculopathy and fibrosis by production of cytokines and antibodies, which in turn activate endothelial cells and fibroblasts to a profibrotic phenotype [22].

Diagnostic criteria

Presently the most widely accepted classification criteria for systemic sclerosis is the Joint Committee of American College of Rheumatology (ACR) and European League Against Rheumatism (EULAR) criteria, which removed the limitations of the previous ACR criteria (Table 41.1) [23,24].

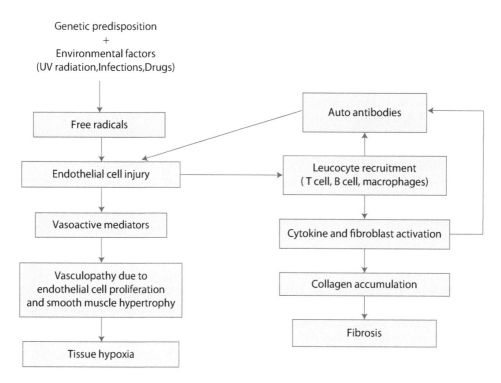

Figure 41.1 Etiopathogenesis of systemic sclerosis.

Table 41.1 Classification criteria by Joint Committee of the American College of Rheumatology and European League Against Rheumatism (EULAR) (2013)

Item	Subitem	Score
Skin thickening of the fingers of both hands extending proximal to the metacarpophalangeal joints (sufficient criterion)		9
Skin thickening of the fingers (only count the highest score)	Puffy fingers	2
	Sclerodactyly of the fingers (distal to the metacarpophalangeal joints but proximal to the proximal interphalangeal joints)	4
Fingertip lesions	Digital tip ulcers	2
	Fingertip pitting scars	3
Telangiectasias		2
Abnormal nail fold capillaries		2
Pulmonary arterial hypertension and/or interstitial lung disease	Pulmonary arterial hypertension/interstitial lung disease	2
Raynaud phenomenon		3
Systemic sclerosis–related autoantibodies	Anticentromere	1
	Antitopoisomerase I (Anti-ScL-70)	1
	Anti-RNA polymerase III	1

Note: The total score is determined by adding the maximum score in each category; patients with total score of ≥9 are classified as having definite systemic sclerosis.

Clinical features

The disease can have varied clinical presentations with vascular damage and fibrosis underlying most of them. The disease may present in various forms:

- Diffuse systemic sclerosis (dSSc)
- Limited systemic sclerosis (lSSc)
- Transitory form (dSSC/lSSc)
- Systemic sclerosis sine scleroderma
- Malignant scleroderma

The principal forms of systemic sclerosis include:

- Diffuse systemic sclerosis
- Limited systemic sclerosis

The characteristic features of these two forms are given in Table 41.2.

The disease involves the skin as well as internal organs. The presenting symptoms depend on the affected organs in addition to skin disease [1,25].

CUTANEOUS INVOLVEMENT

Cutaneous involvement in systemic sclerosis has three phases:

- The edematous phase, which is characterized by puffiness and swelling and decreased flexibility of joints and tendons.
- The indurative phase in which the skin appears shiny, is thickened, and is bound down (Figure 41.2). Pruritus may be seen in early stages of the disease.
- The atrophic phase in which atrophic changes are more apparent over the bony prominences. The dermis may soften and the thickness of skin may return to normal during this phase (Figure 41.3).

Table 41.2 Characteristic features of systemic sclerosis

Type of systemic sclerosis	Characteristic features
Limited systemic sclerosis	• Skin fibrosis involving the face and extremities distal to the elbows and knees • Atrophic changes over lips, alae nasi • Raynaud phenomenon precedes the skin sclerosis by a long period of time • Gastrointestinal involvement is common • Late pulmonary involvement, mainly in the form of pulmonary hypertension • Anticentromere antibodies seen in 70%–80% of patients
Diffuse systemic sclerosis	• Skin fibrosis involving proximal limbs and trunk as well • Short history of Raynaud phenomenon • Pulmonary, renal, and cardiac involvement more common • Rapid onset and progression • Nail fold capillary dilatation and capillary destruction • Antitopoisomerase I (ScL-70) antibodies positive in approximately 30% of patients

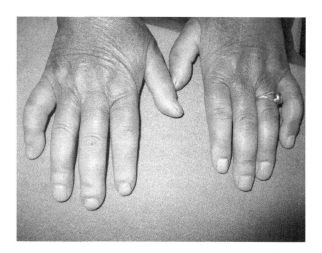

Figure 41.2 Indurated phase of systemic sclerosis with erythema of proximal part of fingers and pallor of tips.

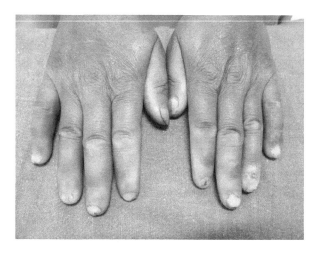

Figure 41.3 Atrophic phase of systemic sclerosis with sclerodactyly.

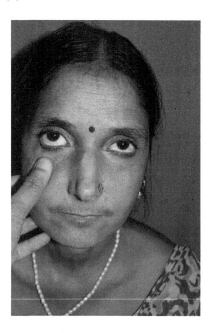

Figure 41.4 Ingram sign.

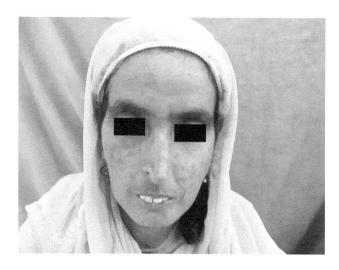

Figure 41.5 Mask face with pursing of lips and mat telangiectasia on face.

Skin thickening or fibrosis occurs in nearly all patients with systemic sclerosis. Skin fibrosis may reflect as facial amimia, inability to retract the lower eyelids in patients with progressive disease (Ingram sign) (Figure 41.4), reduced mouth aperture, and sclerosis of the frenulum. Radial furrowing around the mouth may also be seen. Atrophy of nasal alae leads to pinched appearance of the nose. This facial involvement leads to the typical mauskopf appearance (Figure 41.5).

Measurement of skin thickness can be used as a surrogate marker of disease severity and subsequent mortality [26]. Modified Rodnan score is the most widely accepted and validated method of measurement of skin thickness [27]. Skin thickening and tethering are measured for 17 body sites as shown in Table 41.3, and each site is given a score of 0 (normal skin), 1 (possible thickening), 2 (definite thickening but mobile skin), or 3 (thickened and fixed skin), depending on the degree of involvement, making up a maximum score of 51. Initial and follow-up scores are valuable in disease assessment.

Table 41.3 Modified Rodnan score

Site	Maximum score		
	Right		Left
Upper arm	3		3
Forearm	3		3
Hand	3		3
Fingers	3		3
Thigh	3		3
Leg	3		3
Foot	3		3
	21		21
Face		3	
Chest		3	
Abdomen		3	
Subtotal		9	
Total score		51	

Painful digital ulcers and pitted scars (Figure 41.6) are commonly seen due to local ischemia and vascular insufficiency. Digital ulcers may be complicated by secondary bacterial infections leading to gangrene, atrophy, and autoamputation (Figure 41.7) [27]. Pigmentary changes of the skin are seen in the form of localized hyperpigmentation, diffuse hyperpigmentation, or dyspigmentation (salt and pepper appearance) characterized by vitiligo-like depigmentation with perifollicular pigmentary retention [28]. Other cutaneous changes include telangiectasias, nail fold capillary alterations (dilated loops at the nail bed and distended venules) (Figure 41.8a–c), and subcutaneous calcinosis occurring mainly in periarticular tissues (Figure 41.9).

RAYNAUD PHENOMENON

This occurs in nearly 95% of systemic sclerosis patients and usually precedes other signs of the disease. Long-standing Raynaud phenomenon in patients with systemic sclerosis may lead to the disappearance of the peaked contour on fingertips (Mizutani sign).

NONCUTANEOUS MANIFESTATIONS AND COMPLICATIONS

Pulmonary involvement

Interstitial lung disease (ILD) and pulmonary arterial hypertension (PAH) are the two primary pulmonary manifestations of systemic sclerosis, though other manifestations like pleuritis, pleural effusion, and aspiration may also occur in a fraction of affected patients [29]. Some degree of parenchymal involvement is seen in most patients with systemic sclerosis. Diffuse cutaneous systemic sclerosis has a strong association with ILD, especially in patients with a positive anti-Scl-70 antibody [30]. ILD is the leading cause of morbidity and mortality due to systemic sclerosis [31]. Pulmonary parenchymal involvement does not appear to be related to the extent and severity of cutaneous involvement

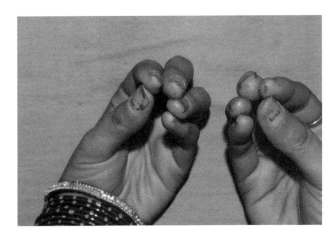

Figure 41.6 Digital pitted scars and ulcers.

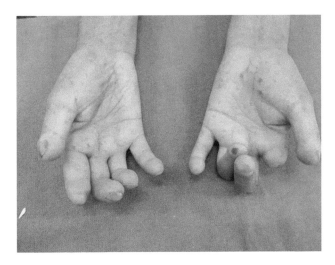

Figure 41.7 Sclerodactyly, fingertip ulcers, and autoamputation in systemic sclerosis.

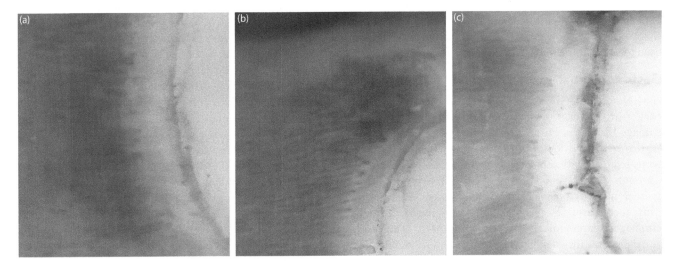

Figure 41.8 Nail fold capillaroscopy in (a) early changes with few enlarged capillaries; (b) active disease with frequently enlarged capillaries and frequent hemorrhages; and (c) late changes with irregular enlargement, severe loss of capillaries, and avascular areas.

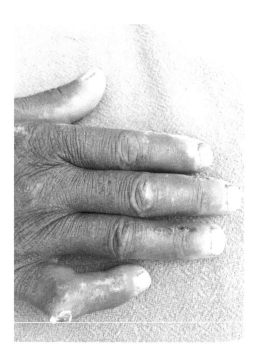

Figure 41.9 Fingertip ulcers, depigmentation, and calcinosis.

[32]. Auscultation of lung bases reveals the typical bilateral inspiratory and expiratory crackles ("Velcro" crackles).

The signs and symptoms of ILD are often preceded by changes in the pulmonary function tests that reveal a restrictive ventilatory defect [33]. A decrease in diffusing capacity of the lung for carbon monoxide (DLCO) is probably the earliest indicator of ILD in systemic sclerosis [34]. High-resolution computed tomography (HRCT) changes like subpleural infiltrates, interstitial reticular infiltrates, and subpleural honeycombing suggest ILD in systemic sclerosis (Figure 41.10).

PAH usually presents with dyspnea on exertion and is seen more commonly in association with limited cutaneous systemic sclerosis. Accentuation of a second component of heart sound (S2) and signs of heart failure are seen, and echocardiogram along with cardiac catheterization can be used to confirm the diagnosis.

Gastrointestinal involvement

Gastrointestinal (GI) involvement in systemic sclerosis occurs in the form of motility dysfunction and mucosal damage that occurs in different segments of the GI tract. GI involvement is found in 75%–90% of patients with systemic sclerosis with esophageal involvement being the most common [35,36]. Abnormalities of esophageal motility may present with dysphagia or gastroesophageal reflux with consequent erosive esophagitis, Barrett esophagus, or rarely esophageal carcinoma [37]. Food stasis may result from gastric dysmotility. Esophageal and gastric telangiectasias ("watermelon stomach") may lead to GI hemorrhage. Severe intestinal involvement can result in pseudo-obstruction syndrome with resultant bacterial overgrowth and malabsorption. Volvulus of the small intestine and involvement

of the colon leading to constipation and colonic diverticula may sometimes be seen [38].

Musculoskeletal involvement

Nearly 40%–80% of patients with systemic sclerosis present with musculoskeletal complaints. Joint involvement in the form of generalized inflammatory arthralgias is seen in 46%–97% of patients with systemic sclerosis [39]. Rheumatoid factor positivity is seen in up to 30% of patients with systemic sclerosis [40]. Joint involvement may be a predictor of poor outcome in the form of severe organ damage [4]. Synovitis and tendon friction rubs usually associated with the diffuse cutaneous form may be indicative of rapid progression of cutaneous disease and an early onset of kidney disease [41,42]. Acro-osteolysis characterized by bony resorption of terminal digits is seen in up to 20% of patients [43]. Myopathy, which is often mild in nature, presents with proximal muscle weakness and minimal or slightly increased creatine kinase levels.

Cardiac manifestations

Cardiac involvement in systemic sclerosis may be "primary" in the form of myocardial fibrosis (pathognomonic "mosaic" or "patchy" distribution), fibrosis of the conduction system, and pericardial involvement (acute or chronic pericarditis, constrictive pericarditis) or may be secondary to PAH, ILD, or renal pathology [44,45]. Cardiac involvement usually manifests as diastolic or less commonly systolic dysfunction (symptomatic or asymptomatic). In addition, atrial and ventricular arrhythmias may occur [44].

Renal involvement

Renal involvement is uncommon in systemic sclerosis and is more frequently associated with diffuse cutaneous systemic sclerosis than with the limited forms [46]. *Scleroderma renal crisis* is a potentially life-threatening complication of systemic sclerosis that occurs in 10%–15% of patients with diffuse cutaneous systemic sclerosis and only 1%–2% of limited cutaneous systemic sclerosis patients [47,48]. Scleroderma renal crisis almost invariably occurs in early, rapidly progressive diffuse systemic sclerosis. It manifests as an abrupt rise in blood pressure over days or weeks, rapidly progressing to renal failure. Use of corticosteroids or cyclosporine and the presence of anti-RNA polymerase III antibodies may precipitate scleroderma renal crisis [49,50]. Apart from scleroderma renal crisis, some less severe complications due to reduced renal blood flow and decreased glomerular filtration rate (GFR) may occur. Unusual renal complications like glomerulonephritis and renal vasculitis may be seen in the setting of antineutrophil cytoplasmic antibody reactivity [51].

Neurological involvement

Neurological involvement in systemic sclerosis may occur in the form of compressive neuropathies like carpal tunnel syndrome, trigeminal neuralgia, motor and sensory neuropathy, headache, epilepsy, and cognitive disorders. Anxiety and depressive symptoms are commonly seen.

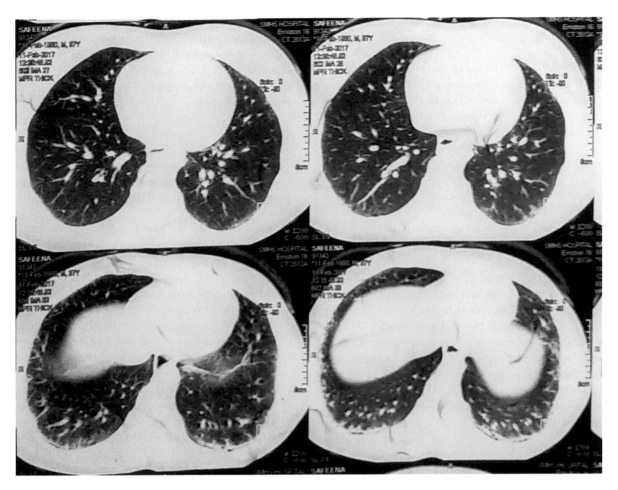

Figure 41.10 High-resolution computed tomography chest of 19-year-old female showing subpleural areas of honeycombing in posterobasal segments of bilateral lower lobes with tiny nodules in superior segment of left lower lobe.

SCLERODERMA SINE SCLERODERMA

This is a rare condition and is probably a form of limited cutaneous systemic sclerosis, as all clinical and laboratory features are similar to the classical form except for the skin fibrosis and thickening, a lower frequency of telangiectasias, digital ulcers, antitopoisomerase I and anti-RNA polymerase III antibodies.

Diagnosis

Early identification of systemic sclerosis patients is of prime importance to prevent progression to severe organ involvement. Diagnosis is based on the clinical as well as laboratory features.

Differential diagnosis

Systemic sclerosis needs to be differentiated from several conditions that present with clinical features resembling systemic sclerosis (Table 41.4).

Investigations

Hematological studies: These often reveal anemia of chronic disease or iron deficiency anemia due to chronic GI hemorrhage. Other hematological parameters are usually normal, although cases of autoimmune hemolytic anemia and neutropenia associated with systemic sclerosis have been reported [52].

Biomarkers: Antinuclear antibodies are detected in up to 90% of cases of systemic sclerosis [23]. Anticentromere antibodies (ACA) are seen in nearly 70% of patients with limited cutaneous disease [53]. Anti-ScL-70 (antitopoisomerase I) antibodies are more likely to be associated with diffuse

Table 41.4 Differential diagnosis of systemic sclerosis

- Generalized morphea
- Nephrogenic systemic fibrosis
- Eosinophilic fasciitis
- Eosinophilia-myalgia syndrome
- Chronic graft versus host disease
- Scleromyxedema
- Scleredema
- Porphyria cutanea tarda
- Drug-induced scleroderma
- Environmental exposure to organic solvents, petroleum distillate, contaminants of L-tryptophan, adulterated cooking oil, and use of vibratory tools

Table 41.5 Other autoantibodies in systemic sclerosis

Autoantibodies	Associations
Anti-U1RNP	Mixed connective tissue disease
Anti-Th/Tho antibodies	Pulmonary arterial hypertension
Antifibrillarin/U3 ribonucleoprotein antibodies	Limited cutaneous systemic sclerosis
	Scleroderma renal crisis
	Muscle involvement
	Increased risk of pulmonary arterial hypertension
	Digital ulcers
	Pericarditis
	Lower gastrointestinal involvement

systemic sclerosis and indicate a poor prognosis with a higher rate of internal organ involvement.

The sensitivity of these tests is however quite low, being 30% and 40%, respectively, for ACA and anti-ScL-70 antibodies. Anti-RNA polymerase III antibodies are commonly associated with diffuse cutaneous systemic sclerosis and are predictive of scleroderma renal crisis or development of malignancy in systemic sclerosis [54,55]. Other autoantibodies that may be uncommonly found in systemic sclerosis are given in Table 41.5.

SPECIFIC TESTS

Evaluation of pulmonary complaints with chest radiography, pulmonary function tests, or HRCT of the chest may be needed. Similarly systemic sclerosis patients with cardiac symptoms may require evaluation using electrocardiogram, echocardiogram, or cardiac catheterization. Rarely endomyocardial biopsy may be warranted. Endoscopy, colonoscopy, or rectal manometry may be needed to rule out any GI involvement. Renal involvement can be ruled out by simple renal function tests and 24-hour urinary protein estimation. Patients with Raynaud phenomenon will require nail fold capillaroscopy. Durometry and optical coherence tomography (OCT) can be used to measure skin thickness.

SKIN BIOPSY

A skin biopsy is generally not needed for diagnosis except in the event of diagnostic doubt with other scleroderma-like disorders (nephrogenic systemic fibrosis, eosinophilic fasciitis, scleromyxedema, etc.). It can also be used as an outcome measure where skin biopsies obtained before and after treatment can be compared by determining the hyalinized collagen score and myofibroblast score [56,57].

Histopathology of the skin in systemic sclerosis shows an abnormal accumulation of extracellular matrix constituents. An early cellular stage and a late fibrotic stage can be appreciated on histopathological examination. In the early stage, thick collagen bundles in the reticular dermis along with a perivascular lymphohistiocytic inflammatory infiltrate that can extend to the deeper tissues is seen. Overlying epidermis is often atrophic and thin. The inflammatory infiltrate tends to decrease over time due to increasing vascularity. The fibrotic stage depicts more of sclerosis with closely packed collagen bundles and atrophic or absent sweat glands. The fat cells may then also be replaced by collagen.

Treatment

The treatment of systemic sclerosis is based on the *organ-targeted therapy* in which specific treatment options are utilized depending on the specific organ involvement.

RAYNAUD PHENOMENON

The various drugs recommended for the treatment of systemic sclerosis–associated Raynaud phenomenon include

- *Dihydropyridine-type calcium channel blockers (CCBs)*: These tend to decrease the severity as well as frequency of ischemic attacks in systemic sclerosis–associated Raynaud phenomenon [58–60] and should be considered as the first-line therapy for the same. Among the dihydropyridine-type CCBs, oral nifedipine (30–60 mg/day) is the drug mostly preferred for the treatment of Raynaud phenomenon. Other CCBs like nicardipine, amlodipine, and diltiazem have also been used in the treatment of Raynaud phenomenon.
- *Phosphodiesterase-5 (PDE-5) inhibitors*: PDE-5 inhibitors (sildenafil, tadalafil, verdanafil) also tend to decrease the frequency, severity, and duration of attacks in systemic sclerosis–associated Raynaud phenomenon and may be used in patients who do not show satisfactory improvement with the use of CCBs or those who tend to have more severe disease [61–63].
- *Prostanoids*: IV Iloprost (0.5–2 µg/kg/min) for 3–5 days and repeated every 6–8 weeks is quite helpful in reducing the frequency and severity of attacks in refractory cases [64–66].
- *Fluoxetine*: Fluoxetine may be comparable or even superior to nifedipine in treatment of systemic sclerosis–associated Raynaud phenomenon [67]. *Fluoxetine* in a dose of 20 mg/day orally may be considered in patients who show intolerance or poor response to vasodilators.
- α1-*adrenergic receptor antagonists*: Prazosin (1–3 mg/day) may be moderately effective in treating Raynaud phenomenon [68].
- *ACE inhibitors*: Losartan (50 mg/day) has been found to be efficacious in decreasing the severity and frequency of attacks of Raynaud phenomenon [69].

DIGITAL ULCERS

- *Prostanoids*: Prostanoids like IV iloprost or oral treprostinil have been shown to reduce the number of digital ulcers in comparison with placebo [70]. Other prostanoids like epoprostenol and beraprost may improve digital ulceration in systemic sclerosis patients.

- *PDE-5 inhibitors*: Sildenafil (50 mg twice daily) or tadalafil (20 mg on alternate days) have shown beneficial effects in the healing of digital ulcers in systemic sclerosis [71].
- *Bosentan*: It is a dual-receptor antagonist that does not appear to be effective in the healing of active digital ulcers but has been used to prevent recurrences in patients with multiple digital ulcers [72].

Other drugs that have been used in the treatment of both Raynaud phenomenon and digital ulcers with variable results include aspirin, dipyridamole, pentoxifylline, and topical nitroglycerin.

In addition to these pharmacological treatments, exclusion of aggravating factors like smoking, exposure of hands to cold, and use of vasoconstrictor drugs helps in improving the outcome. In recalcitrant cases, sympathetic blocks (stellate ganglion block and lumbar sympathetic block) and surgical sympathectomy can be performed [73].

SKIN DISEASE

D-penicillamine has been shown to improve skin disease at a low dose of 125 mg every other day. Methotrexate in a dose of 10–15 mg/week has been shown to improve skin scores in early diffuse systemic sclerosis [74]. Other immunosuppressants such as cyclophosphamide, mycophenolate mofetil, cyclosporine, tacrolimus, and azathioprine have also shown benefits in patients with systemic sclerosis [75,76].

Rituximab and tocilizumab have also shown efficacy in improving skin disease in some patients. Antifibrotic agents, such as tyrosine kinase inhibitors (imatinib, nintedanib, nilotinib), by blocking the TGF-β and PDGF signaling pathways improve skin fibrosis in systemic sclerosis. In patients with rapidly deteriorating skin disease, IV immunoglobulins may have a role [77]. Hematopoietic stem cell transplant may also have a role.

SYSTEMIC SCLEROSIS–RELATED GI DISEASE

Proton pump inhibitors (PPIs) are the first-line treatment for systemic sclerosis–related gastroesophageal reflux and for prevention of esophageal ulcers and strictures [78]. In refractory cases of gastroesophageal reflux disease, a twice daily PPI or dual therapy with H2 blockers may be needed. In addition, prokinetic drugs like metoclopramide, octreotide, and domperidone may improve esophageal dysmotility [79]. Treatment with antibiotics such as metronidazole, rifaximin, neomycin, or doxycycline might improve small intestinal bacterial overgrowth. Intestinal microbiome may improve with the use of pre- and probiotics [80].

SYSTEMIC SCLEROSIS–RELATED PULMONARY INVOLVEMENT

Pulmonary arterial hypertension

Endothelin-receptor antagonists (bosentan, ambrisentan, macitentan, sitaxsentan) have been recommended as the initial therapy in systemic sclerosis–related PAH. In addition, phosphodiesterase inhibitors (sildenafil, tadalafil) [81] and Riociguat (soluble guanylate cyclase stimulator) [82] have been shown to improve exercise capacity and halt clinical progression in PAH. Prostacyclin analogues (epoprostenol, treprostinil) are best reserved for severe therapy-resistant PAH.

Interstitial lung disease: Cyclophosphamide in combination with high-dose corticosteroids is effective in early stages [83]. Tyrosine kinase inhibitors such as imatinib offer a promising future option [84]. Hematopoietic stem cell transplant and lung transplant may be considered in rapidly progressive and end-stage lung disease, respectively.

Scleroderma renal crisis

Prompt initiation of treatment with ACE inhibitors may significantly improve the outcome in scleroderma renal crisis [85]. Other antihypertensives such as angiotensin receptor blockers (ARBs) and calcium channel blockers (CCBs) can also be used. In addition, low-dose prostacyclin infusion may be beneficial in controlling blood pressure and in improving renal perfusion.

Systemic sclerosis–related cardiac complications

Pericarditis and myocarditis both respond to low-dose steroids. Massive pericardial effusion may require pericardiocentesis.

CONCLUSION

Scleroderma is a heterogenous disease varying in clinical presentation, antibody profile, and outcome. Biological markers are useful in defining the phenotype and prognosis in scleroderma patients. Despite recent advances and progress in management, the treatment of scleroderma still remains a challenge. Targeted therapies that are currently being investigated offer hope for the future.

KEY POINTS

- Widespread vascular injury and progressive fibrosis form the basis of the protean manifestations of scleroderma.
- Morphea is distinguished from systemic sclerosis by the lack of sclerodactyly, Raynaud phenomenon, and nail fold capillary changes.
- The gold standard for measuring skin thickness in systemic sclerosis is the modified Rodnan skin score (mRSS). More extensive skin involvement coincides with poor prognosis.
- Screening strategies aimed at early identification of systemic sclerosis–related systemic complications are the key to improved disease outcome.

REFERENCES

1. Almeida C, Almeida I, Vasconcelos C. Quality of life in systemic sclerosis. *Autoimmun Rev* 2015;14:1087–96.

2. Pakozdi A, Nihtyanova S, Moinzadeh P, Ong VH, Black CM, Denton CP. Clinical and serological hallmarks of systemic sclerosis overlap syndromes. *J Rheumatol* 2011;38(11):2406–9.

3. Chifflot H, Fautrel B, Sordet C, Chatelus E, Sibilia J. Incidence and prevalence of systemic sclerosis: A systematic literature review. *Semin Arthritis Rheum* 2008;37(4):223–35.

4. Reveille JD. Ethnicity and race and systemic sclerosis: How it affects susceptibility, severity, antibody genetics, and clinical manifestations. *Curr Rheumatol Rep* 2003;5(2):160–7.

5. Luo Y, Wang Y, Wang Q, Xiao R, Lu Q. Systemic sclerosis: Genetics and epigenetics. *J Autoimmun* 2013;41:161–7.

6. Arnett FC, Cho M, Chatterjee S, Aguilar MB, Reveille JD, Mayes MD. Familial occurrence frequencies and relative risks for systemic sclerosis (scleroderma) in three United States cohorts. *Arthritis Rheum* 2001;44(6):1359–62.

7. Broen JC, Coenen MJ, Radstake TR. Genetics of systemic sclerosis: An update. *Curr Rheumatol Rep* 2012;14:11–21.

8. Balbir-Gurman A, Braun-Moscovici Y. Scleroderma—New aspects in pathogenesis and treatment, best practice and research. *Clin Rheumatol* 2012;26:13–24.

9. Goodfield MJ, Jones SK, Veale DJ. The Connective Tissue Diseases. In: Burns T, Breathnach S, Cox N, Griffiths C (Eds), *Rook's Textbook of Dermatology*. 8th ed. Edinburgh: Wiley Blackwell; 2010;51:87–109.

10. Allanore Y, Dieude P, Boileau C. Genetic background of systemic sclerosis: Autoimmune genes take centre stage. *Rheumatology* 2010;49:203–10.

11. Jin J, Chou C, Lima M, Zhou D, Zhou X. Systemic sclerosis is a complex disease associated mainly with immune regulatory and inflammatory genes. *Open Rheumatol J* 2014;8:29–42.

12. Marie I. Systemic sclerosis and occupational exposure: Towards an extension of legal recognition as occupational disorder in 2014? *Rev Médecine Interne Fondée Par Société Natl Francaise Médecine Interne* 2014;35:631–5.

13. Marie I et al. Prospective study to evaluate the association between systemic sclerosis and occupational exposure and review of the literature. *Autoimmun Rev* 2014;13:151–6.

14. Nelson JL. Microchimerism and scleroderma. *Curr Rheumatol Rep* 1999;1(1):15–21.

15. Prescott RJ, Freemont AJ, Jones CJ, Hoyland J, Fielding P. Sequential dermal microvascular and perivascular changes changes in the development of scleroderma. *J Pathol* 1992;166(3):255–63.

16. Kahaleh B. Vascular disease in scleroderma: Mechanisms of vascular injury. *Rheum Dis Clin North Am* 2008;34(1):57–71.

17. Kahaleh B, Meyer O, Scorza R. Assessment of vascular involvement. *Clin Exp Rheumatol* 2003;21(3 Suppl. 29):S9–14.

18. Newby AC. Matrix metalloproteinases regulate migration, proliferation, and death of vascular smooth muscle cells by degrading matrix and non-matrix substrates. *Cardiovasc Res* 2006;69:614–24.

19. Nagase H, Visse R, Murphy G. Structure and function of matrix metalloproteinases and TIMPs. *Cardiovasc Res* 2006;69:562–73.

20. Distler O, Abraham D. How does endothelial cell injury start? The role of endothelin in systemic sclerosis. *Arthritis Res Ther* 2007;9(Suppl. 2):S2.

21. Sakkas L, Platsoucas C D. T cells and B cells in systemic sclerosis. *Curr Rheumatol Rev* 2010;6(4):276–82.

22. Giacomelli R, Cipriani P, Fulminis A, Nelson JL, Matucci-Cerinic M. Gamma/delta T cells in placenta and skin: Their different functions may support the paradigm of microchimerism in systemic sclerosis. *Clin Exp Rheumatol* 2004;22(3 Suppl. 33):S28–30.

23. Preliminary criteria for the classification of systemic sclerosis/scleroderma. Subcommittee for Scleroderma Criteria of the American Rheumatism Association Diagnostic and Therapeutic Criteria Committee. *Arthritis Rheum* 1980;23:581–90.

24. Van den Hoogen F et al. 2013. Classification criteria for systemic sclerosis: An American College of Rheumatology/European League Against Rheumatism collaborative initiative. *Ann Rheum Dis* 2013;72:1747–55.

25. Clements PJ et al. Skin thickness score as a predictor and correlate of outcome in systemic sclerosis: High-dose versus low-dose penicillamine trial. *Arthritis Rheum* 2000;43(11):2445–54.

26. Clements PJ et al. Skin thickness score in systemic sclerosis: An assessment of interobserver variability in 3 independent studies. *J Rheumatol* 1993;20:1892–6.

27. Ingraham KM, Steen VD. Morbidity of digital tip ulcers in scleroderma. *Arthritis Rheum* 2006;54(9):78.

28. Rai VM, Balachandran C. Pseudovitiligo in systemic sclerosis. *Dermatol Online J* 2005;10:41.

29. Owens GR, Follansbee WP. Cardiopulmonary manifestations of systemic sclerosis. *Chest* 1987;91:118–27.

30. Walker UA et al. Clinical risk assessment of organ manifestations in systemic sclerosis: A report from the EULAR Scleroderma Trials and Research group database. *Ann Rheum Dis* 2007;66:754–63.

31. Steen VD, Medsger TA. Changes in causes of death in systemic sclerosis, 1972–2002. *Ann Rheum Dis* 2007;66:940–4.

32. Morelli S et al. Relationship between cutaneous and pulmonary involvement in systemic sclerosis. *J Rheumatol* 1997;24:81–5.

33. Nihtyanova SI et al. Prediction of pulmonary complications and long-term survival in systemic sclerosis. *Arthritis Rheumatol* 2014;66:1625–35.

34. Wells AU, Rubens MB, du Bois RM, Hansell DM. Serial CT in fibrosingalveolitis: Prognostic significance of the initial pattern. *AJR Am J Roentgenol* 1993;161:1159–65.

35. Ellen CE. Esophageal disease in scleroderma. *J Clin Gastroenterol* 2006;40:796–875.

36. Szamosi S, Szekanecz Z, Szucs G. Gastrointestinal manifestations in Hungarian scleroderma patients. *Rheumatol Int* 2006;26:1120–4.

37. Marie I. Gastrointestinal involvement in systemic sclerosis. *Presse Med* 2006;35:1952–65.

38. Robinson JC, Teitelbaum SL. Stercoral ulceration and perforation of the sclerodermatous colon: Report of two cases and review of the literature. *Dis Colon Rectum* 1974;17:622–32.

39. Lóránd V, Czirják L, Minier T. Musculoskeletal involvement in systemic sclerosis. *Presse Med* 2014;43:e315–328.

40. Horimoto AM, Costa IP. Overlap between systemic sclerosis and rheumatoid arthritis: A distinct clinical entity? *Rev Bras Reumatol* 2016;56:287–98.

41. Elhai M et al. Ultrasonographic hand features in systemic sclerosis and correlates with clinical, biologic, and radiographic findings. *Arthritis Care Res* 2012;64:1244–9.

42. Avouac J et al. Joint and tendon involvement predict disease progression in systemic sclerosis: A EUSTAR prospective study. *Ann Rheum Dis* 2016;75:103–9.

43. Avouac J et al. Radiological hand involvement in systemic sclerosis. *Ann Rheum Dis* 2006;65:1088–92.

44. Varga J, Denton CP, Wigley FM. *Scleroderma*. New York: Springer; 2012:361–371;373–95.

45. Dinser R, Frerix M, Meier FM, Klingel K, Rolf A. Endocardial and myocardial involvement in systemic sclerosis—Is there a relevant inflammatory component? *Joint Bone Spine* 2013;80:320–3.

46. Minier T et al. Preliminary analysis of the very early diagnosis of systemic sclerosis (VEDOSS) EUSTAR multicentre study: Evidence for puffy fingers as a pivotal sign for suspicion of systemic sclerosis. *Ann Rheum Dis* 2014;73:2087–93.

47. Penn H et al. Scleroderma renal crisis: Patient characteristics and long-term outcomes. *Q J Med* 2007;100:485–94.

48. Teixeira L et al. Mortality and risk factors of scleroderma renal crisis: A French retrospective study of 50 patients. *Ann Rheum Dis* 2008;67:110–6.

49. DeMarco PJ et al. Predictors and outcomes of scleroderma renal crisis: The high-dose versus low-dose D-penicillamine in early diffuse systemic sclerosis trial. *Arthritis Rheum* 2002;46:2983–9.

50. Steen VD, Medsger TA Jr. Case-control study of corticosteroids and other drugs that either precipitate or protect from the development of scleroderma renal crisis. *Arthritis Rheum* 1998;41:1613–9.

51. Kamen DL, Wigley FM, Brown AN. Antineutrophil cytoplasmic antibody-positive crescentic glomerulonephritis in scleroderma—A different kind of renal crisis. *J Rheumatol* 2006;33:1886–8.

52. Sumithran E. Progressive systemic sclerosis and autoimmune haemolytic anaemia. *Postgrad Med J* 1976;52:173–6.

53. Sobanski V et al. Prevalence of anti-RNA polymerase III antibodies in systemic sclerosis: New data from a French cohort and a systematic review and meta-analysis: Prevalence of anti-RNAP III in SSc. *Arthritis Rheumatol* 2014;66:407–17.

54. Hesselstrand R, Scheja A, Wuttge D. Scleroderma renal crisis in a Swedish systemic sclerosis cohort: Survival, renal outcome, and RNA polymerase III antibodies as a risk factor. *Scand J Rheumatol* 2012;41:39–43.

55. Nikpour M et al. Prevalence, correlates and clinical usefulness of antibodies to RNA polymerase III in systemic sclerosis: A cross-sectional analysis of data from an Australian cohort. *Arthritis Res Ther* 2011;13:R211.

56. Smith V, Van Praet JT, Vandooren B, Van der Cruyssen B, Naeyaert JM, Decuman S, Elewaut D, De Keyser F. Rituximab in diffuse cutaneous systemic sclerosis: An open-label clinical and histopathological study. *Ann Rheum Dis* 2010;69:193–7.

57. Nash RA et al. High-dose immunosuppressive therapy and autologous hematopoietic cell transplantation for severe systemic sclerosis: Long-term follow-up of the US multicenter pilot study. *Blood* 2007;110:1388–96.

58. Thompson AE et al. Calcium-channel blockers for Raynaud's phenomenon in systemic sclerosis. *Arthritis Rheum* 2001;44:1841–7.

59. Ettinger WH et al. Controlled double-blind trial of dazoxiben and nifedipine in the treatment of Raynaud's phenomenon. *Am J Med* 1984;77:451–6.

60. Kahan A et al. Calcium entry blocking agents in digital vasospasm (Raynaud's phenomenon). *Eur Heart J* 1983;4(Suppl. C):123–9.

61. Roustit M et al. Phosphodiesterase-5 inhibitors for the treatment of secondary Raynaud's phenomenon: Systematic review and meta-analysis of randomised trials. *Ann Rheum Dis* 2013;72:1696–9.

62. Herrick AL et al. Modified-release sildenafil reduces Raynaud's phenomenon attack frequency in limited cutaneous systemic sclerosis. *Arthritis Rheum* 2011;63:775–82.

63. Fries R et al. Sildenafil in the treatment of Raynaud's phenomenon resistant to vasodilatory therapy. *Circulation* 2005;112:2980–5.

64. Pope J et al. Iloprost and cisaprost for Raynaud's phenomenon in progressive systemic sclerosis. *Cochrane Database Syst Rev* 2000;(2):Cd000953.

65. McHugh NJ et al. Infusion of iloprost, a prostacyclin analogue, for treatment of Raynaud's phenomenon in systemic sclerosis. *Ann Rheum Dis* 1988;47:43–7.

66. Belch JJ et al. Oral iloprost as a treatment for Raynaud's syndrome: A double blind multicentre placebo controlled study. *Ann Rheum Dis* 1995;54:197–200.

67. Coleiro B et al. Treatment of Raynaud's phenomenon with the selective serotonin reuptake inhibitor fluoxetine. *Rheumatology (Oxf)* 2001;40:1038–43.

68. Pope J et al. Prazosin for Raynaud's phenomenon in progressive systemic sclerosis. *Cochrane Database Syst Rev* 2000;2:CD000956.

69. Dziadzio M et al. Losartan therapy for Raynaud's phenomenon and scleroderma: Clinical and biochemical findings in a fifteen week, randomized, parallel-group, controlled trial. *Arthritis Rheum* 1999;42:2646–55.

70. Wigley FM, Seibold JR, Wise RA, McCloskey DA, Dole WP. Intravenous iloprost treatment of Raynaud's phenomenon and ischemic ulcers secondary to systemic sclerosis. *J Rheumatol* 1992;19:1407–14.

71. Tingey T et al. Meta-analysis of healing and prevention of digital ulcers in systemic sclerosis. *Arthritis Care Res* 2013;65:1460–71.

72. Matucci-Cerinic M et al. Bosentan treatment of digital ulcers related to systemic sclerosis: Results from the RAPIDS-2 randomised, double-blind, placebo-controlled trial. *Ann Rheum Dis* 2011;70:32–8.

73. Wasserman A, Brahn E. Systemic sclerosis: Bilateral improvement of Raynaud's phenomenon with unilateral digital sympathectomy. *Semin Arthritis Rheum* 2010;40(2):137–46.

74. Pope JE et al. A randomized, controlled trial of methotrexate versus placebo in early diffuse scleroderma. *Arthritis Rheum* 2001;44:1351–8.

75. Tashkin DP et al. Cyclophosphamide versus placebo in scleroderma lung disease. *N Engl J Med* 2006;354:2655–66.

76. Morton SJ, Powell RJ. Cyclosporin and tacrolimus: Their use in routine clinical setting for scleroderma. *Rheumatology* 2000;39(8):865–9.

77. Desbois AC, Cacoub P. Systemic sclerosis: An update in 2016. *Autoimmun Rev* 2016;15(5):417–26.

78. Pakozdi A et al. Does long term therapy with lansoprazole slow progression of oesophageal involvement in systemic sclerosis? *Clin Exp Rheumatol* 2009;27(Suppl. 54):5–8.

79. Wollheim FA, Akesson A. Management of intestinal involvement in systemic sclerosis. *J Clin Rheumatol* 2007;13:116–8.

80. Bures J et al. Small intestinal bacterial overgrowth syndrome. *World J Gastroenterol* 2010;16:2978–90.

81. Galie N et al. Sildenafil citrate therapy for pulmonary arterial hypertension. *N Engl J Med* 2005;353:2148–57.

82. Ghofrani HA et al. Riociguat for the treatment of pulmonary arterial hypertension. *N Engl J Med* 2013;369:330–40.

83. Goldin J et al. Treatment of scleroderma-interstitial lung disease with cyclophosphamide is associated with less progressive fibrosis on serial thoracic high resolution CT scan than placebo: Findings from the scleroderma lung study. *Chest* 2009;136(5):1333–40.

84. Spiera RF et al. Imatinib mesylate (Gleevec) in the treatment of diffuse cutaneous systemic sclerosis: Results of a 1-year, phase IIa, single-arm, open-label clinical trial. *Ann Rheum Dis* 2011;70:1003–9.

85. Denton CP. Renal manifestations of systemic sclerosis—Clinical features and outcome assessment. *Rheumatology (Oxf)* 2008;47(Suppl. 5):v54–6.

42

Dermatomyositis and its associated complications

IFFAT HASSAN SHAH AND SANIYA AKHTAR

INTRODUCTION

Dermatomyositis (DM) is a rare, idiopathic, inflammatory disease in which the patients present with characteristic cutaneous findings with signs of muscle weakness and myopathy. It is one of three idiopathic inflammatory myopathies (IIMs) commonly encountered; the other two are polymyositis (PM) and inclusion body myositis. It primarily affects the skin and muscles, but widespread systemic involvement may be seen with affection of blood vessels, joints, esophagus, lungs, and less commonly, the heart [1,2].

EPIDEMIOLOGY

Dermatomyositis can affect both adults and children and can sometimes be associated with underlying malignancy in the form of carcinoma or lymphoma in adults. It affects women approximately two to three times more than men and has a bimodal distribution in the age of onset. In juvenile cases, it can occur between 5 and 15 years of age with girl-to-boy ratio of 5:1 [3], and can even occur in infancy [4]. In adult cases, onset is between 40 and 60 years of age with mean age of onset being later in men than in women [5]. No racial or geographical predilection is seen.

ETIOPATHOGENESIS

The exact cause of DM is not known; however, several genetic, immunological, infectious, and environmental factors have been implicated.

Genetics: An increased incidence has been linked to certain HLA types, such as HLA-B8 [6], HLA-DR3 [7], and HLA-B14 [8]; however, the disease is not known to occur in families.

Immunological: Immunological abnormalities are common in patients with DM, and they frequently present with several circulating autoantibodies including PM-1, Jo-1, PL-12, and in Japanese patients, KU. Also antibodies directed against specific myositis-related antigens, for example, p155 and p155/140 have been reported [9]. Childhood dermatomyositis appears to be a true autoimmune disorder with granular deposits of IgG, IgM, and C3, alone or in combination, being described in the walls of skeletal muscle and blood vessels [10].

Infections: Various infectious agents have been postulated to be responsible for the disease. In childhood cases, the symptoms may be preceded by an attack of respiratory or gastrointestinal infection. Viruses such as coxsackie B virus [11], parvovirus B19 [12], echovirus, human T-cell lymphotropic virus type 1, and HIV have been implicated. Also staphylococcal [13] and streptococcal [14] infections and toxoplasmosis [15] have been identified as triggering factors.

Drugs: Certain drugs have been associated with dermatomyositis-like skin changes. Drugs such as hydroxyurea [16], penicillamine [17], tamoxifen [18], TNF-α inhibitors [19], nonsteroidal anti-inflammatory drugs, lipid-lowering drugs (statins-gemfibrozil) [20] and the bacillus Calmette-Guérin (BCG) vaccine have been associated with dermatomyositis and polymyositis.

Malignancy: The association of malignancy occurs with adult and amyopathic dermatomyositis, but not with the juvenile form or with polymyositis. The incidence of carcinoma in association with dermatomyositis varies from 15% to 34% [21]. Dermatomyositis precedes the neoplasm in 40%, both conditions may occur together (26%), or the neoplasm may occur first (34%) [22]. Malignancies found in association with DM include tumors of the breast, lung, stomach, pancreas, female genital tract, colon, kidney, testis, and in some cases, lymphomas [23,24]. In the Chinese, nasopharyngeal carcinoma accounted for 75% of malignant disease [25]. Many myositis-related antigens are expressed by tumors that are antigenically different from the tissues of origin, possibly triggering an autoimmune response directed against muscle [26].

Infections and drugs may trigger activation of T and B cells, plasmacytoid dendritic cells, production of type I interferons, and complement-mediated endothelial cell damage resulting in vasculopathy. One mechanism proposes that the binding of antibodies to the endothelium of the endomysial capillaries leads to activation of the complement system with subsequent MAC (membrane attack complex) deposition that leads to endothelial swelling, capillary necrosis, perivascular inflammation, and muscle ischemia [27]. Another model suggests that endothelial cells and myofibers may be injured by the chronic intracellular overproduction of one or more interferon-α/β inducible proteins [28].

CLASSIFICATION

The most commonly used clinical classification of IIMs was proposed by Bohan and Peter [29,30]. Their classification system is given in Table 42.1. A revised classification of the IIMs (Table 42.2) that includes amyopathic forms of dermatomyositis, with muscle involvement no longer required for a definitive diagnosis, has been proposed [31]. Newer classifications have been proposed based on autoantibody subgroups [32] or on muscle histopathology [33].

CLINICAL FEATURES

Cutaneous involvement

The cutaneous manifestations of DM can occur before, shortly after, or at the same time as muscle weakness, but

Table 42.1 Clinical classification of idiopathic inflammatory myopathies proposed by Bohan and Peter

1. Primary idiopathic polymyositis (PM)
2. Primary idiopathic dermatomyositis (DM)
3. Juvenile DM
4. PM or DM with malignancy
5. PM or DM with associated collagen vascular diseases

Source: Bohan A, Peter JB. *N Engl J Med* 1975;292:344–7; Bohan A, Peter JB. *N Engl J Med* 1975;292:403–7.

Table 42.2 Revised classification system for the idiopathic inflammatory dermatomyopathies

1. Dermatomyositis
   a. Adult-onset
      i. Classic dermatomyositis (DM)
      ii. Classic DM with malignancy
      iii. Classic DM as part of an overlapping connective tissue disorder
      iv. Clinically amyopathic DM
         • Amyopathic DM
         • Hypomyopathic DM
   b. Juvenile-onset
      i. Classic DM
      ii. Clinically amyopathic DM
         • Amyopathic DM
         • Hypomyopathic DM
2. Polymyositis
      i. Isolated polymyositis
      ii. Polymyositis as part of an overlapping connective tissue disorder
      iii. Polymyositis associated with internal malignancy
3. Inclusion body myositis

Source: Sontheimer RD. *Curr Opin Rheumatol* 1999;11:475–82.

a proportion of patients with characteristic skin findings may never develop clinical or laboratory signs of myositis, a condition known as *amyopathic dermatomyositis*. Some patients with typical features of muscle involvement show little or no evidence of skin involvement; the condition is then known as *polymyositis* [34]. The classical cutaneous manifestations of the disease are shown in Table 42.3 [35].

Heliotrope rash is a characteristic sign of DM which consists of confluent violaceous macular erythema of the upper eyelids, often with associated edema and telangiectasia. It can extend to the cheeks and sometimes over the nasal bridge, forehead, lateral face, and ears, and can also involve the nasolabial folds (Figure 42.1a and b) [36].

The hallmark sign of DM is *Gottron papules* which primarily consist of erythematous to violaceous papules and plaques over the extensor surfaces of the knuckles and

Table 42.3 Classical cutaneous manifestations of the disease

- Heliotrope rash
- Gottron sign
- Gottron papules
- V-sign
- Shawl sign
- Skin ulcers
- Vasculitis
- Flagellate erythema
- Mechanic's hand
- Nail fold changes

Source: Jinnin M. *Brain Nerve* 2013;65(11):1283–90.

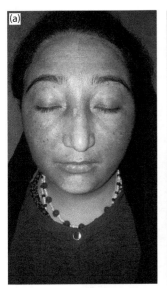
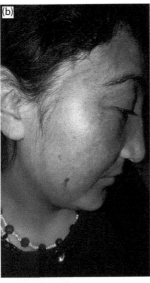

Figure 42.1 **(a)** A patient of dermatomyositis with heliotrope rash and extension of erythema over both cheeks. **(b)** Same patient showing extension of the erythema over lateral part of the face.

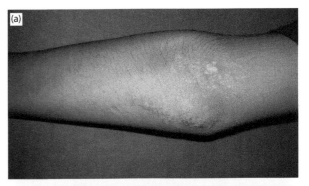
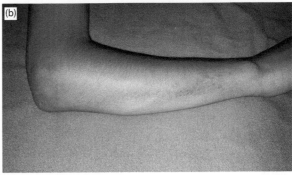

Figure 42.3 **(a)** Presence of erythematous macules and papules (Gottron sign) over the right elbow in a case of dermatomyositis. **(b)** Same patient showing extension of the lesions to the ulnar aspect of the right forearm.

interphalangeal joints of the fingers (Figure 42.2). These lesions may have accompanying scale, and can sometimes develop ulcerations; active lesions tend to resolve with dyspigmentation, atrophy, and scarring.

Gottron sign refers to erythematous macules and patches overlying the elbows and sometimes extending to the forearms (Figure 42.3a and b) and/or knees (Figure 42.4), and these are less specific findings for DM [37].

Confluent macular erythema over the sun-exposed upper anterior chest can also be seen, which is called the *V sign* (Figure 42.5). *Shawl sign* (Figure 42.6) refers to erythema over the upper back, posterior neck, and shoulders, sometimes with extension to the lateral arms.

Erythema when present over the lateral aspect of the thighs is known as the *Holster sign*.

Patients may develop *mechanics hands* (Figure 42.7) in which they present with rough, cracked hands with hyperkeratosis, fissuring, and linear hyperpigmentation of radial and palmar surfaces of the fingers.

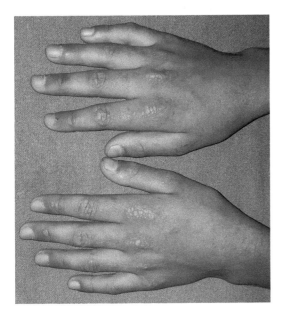

Figure 42.2 Presence of Gottron papules over extensor surfaces of the knuckles and interphalangeal joints of the fingers in a case of dermatomyositis.

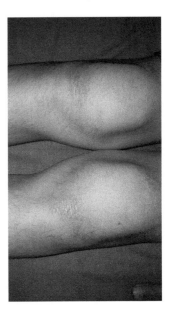

Figure 42.4 Gottron sign overlying both knees in a case of dermatomyositis.

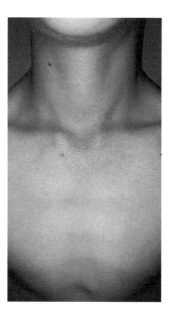

Figure 42.5 Classical "V sign" seen over the sun-exposed upper anterior chest.

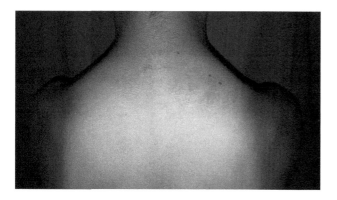

Figure 42.6 "Shawl sign" seen over the upper back in a case of dermatomyositis.

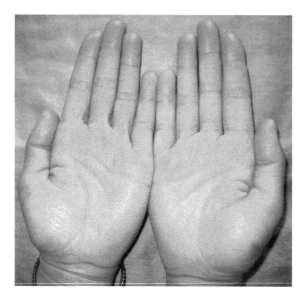

Figure 42.7 Mechanic's hands in a patient with dermatomyositis.

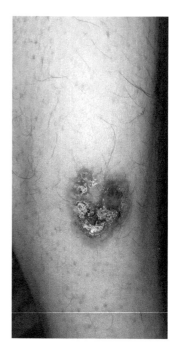

Figure 42.8 A patient of dermatomyositis showing an ulcerated plaque on shin.

Vasculopathic lesions of DM include livedo reticularis, ulceration (Figure 42.8), gingival, and periungual telangiectasia.

Calcinosis (Figure 42.9) involving the skin, subcutaneous tissue, fascia, or muscle seen in areas of potential trauma or inflammation is often a late complication, seen more often in juvenile than in adult cases [36].

Some patients may develop red, firm, tender areas of *panniculitis* that may ulcerate or break down to form sinuses. Some patients may present with *flagellate erythema* with linear, violaceous, itchy, and edematous streaks on the trunk occurring in association with excoriations

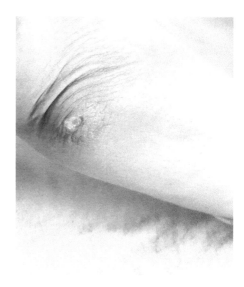

Figure 42.9 A patient with dermatomyositis showing calcinosis near elbow joint.

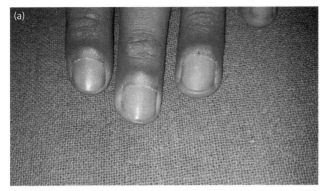

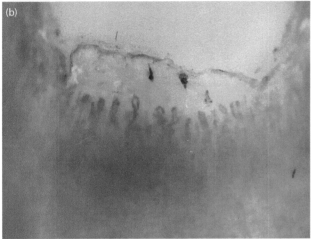

Figure 42.10 (a) Nail fold changes seen in a patient of dermatomyositis with dilated, irregular capillary loops as appreciated with the naked eye. (b) Magnified view of the nail fold capillaries of the same patient showing dilated, irregular, and tortuous capillary loops.

from pruritus [37]. In chronic disease, the patients may present with *poikiloderma* and focal or diffuse areas of alopecia.

Nail fold changes are also noted in patients of DM and act as a clinical clue to the diagnosis (Figure 42.10a). The capillary loops of the nail folds may be dilated, irregular, and tortuous, and easily visible with or without a lens, or by capillaroscopy (Figure 42.10b). The degree of telangiectasias and vessel drop-out reflects ongoing disease activity, particularly in the skin [38].

Other rare skin findings include the following:

- Cutaneous mucinosis
- Follicular hyperkeratosis
- Hyperpigmentation
- Ichthyosis
- White plaques on the buccal mucosa
- Cutaneous vasculitis
- Flagellate erythema
- Diffuse subcutaneous edema
- Vesiculobullous or erosive lesions
- Exfoliative erythroderma

Muscle involvement

Muscle weakness in DM is insidious in onset and gradually worsens over weeks to months. Initial symptoms are variable and may include a feeling of malaise, difficulty in going up stairs or rising from a chair, or difficulty in raising the arms high enough to comb the hair. The initial presentation of muscle involvement is typically symmetric and proximal, with distal muscle weakness occurring late in the course of the disease. Examination for muscle disease in dermatomyositis may demonstrate the following:

- Quadriparesis involving proximal musculature
- Difficulty rising from a seated or supine position without support
- Extensor muscles often more affected than the flexor muscles
- Neck flexor muscle weakness

Distal muscle strength, sensation, and tendon reflexes are maintained (unless the patient has severely weak and atrophic muscle). With more severe disease, patients can develop dysphagia, dysphonia, and weakness in the muscles of respiration. Such symptoms need to be tackled as an emergency as patients can develop respiratory failure that can even be fatal.

Other organ involvement

Lung involvement in DM can be in the form of interstitial lung disease (ILD), pulmonary fibrosis, and pulmonary hypertension. It has been estimated that 35%–40% of patients with either polymyositis or dermatomyositis will suffer from ILD during the course of their illness [39]. Patients present with subjective dyspnea on exertion with nonproductive cough and hypoxemia. Myocarditis, myocardial fibrosis, disorders of conduction, and cardiac failure have been reported in approximately one-third of cases [40]. Esophageal disease in DM patients most commonly presents with dysphagia to solids and liquids due to loss of pharyngoesophageal muscle tone. Other signs of pharyngoesophageal involvement include nasal speech, hoarseness, nasal regurgitation, and aspiration pneumonia.

DIAGNOSIS

Among the connective tissue disorders, dermatomyositis can be confused with systemic sclerosis, systemic lupus erythematosus (SLE), and mixed connective tissue disease (MCTD). True lupus erythematosus and scleroderma may be present in the setting of an overlap syndrome. The papulosquamous lesions on the knees and elbows can be misdiagnosed as psoriasis. Airborne or allergic contact dermatitis or photo-aggravated dermatoses can mimic the heliotrope rash of DM. Poikiloderma in DM can be confused with cutaneous T-cell lymphoma. In cases of juvenile DM, atopic dermatitis is an important differential diagnosis.

Table 42.4 Bohan and Peter criteria for diagnosis of polymyositis/dermatomyositis (PM/DM)

- Proximal muscle weakness: Usually symmetrical
- Elevated serum muscle enzymes
- Myopathic changes on electromyography
- Muscle biopsy findings typical of PM or DM
- Typical rash of DM (a distinguishing feature between DM and PM)

Source: Greenberg SA. *Curr Rheumatol Rep* 2010;12:198–203; Bohan A, Peter JB. *N Engl J Med* 1975;292:344–7.

Note: Definite diagnosis of DM requires four criteria (including rash), whereas definite diagnosis of PM requires four criteria (without rash).
Probable disease comprises three criteria (including rash) for DM and three criteria (without rash) for PM.
Possible disease requires two criteria (including rash) for DM and two criteria (without rash) for PM.

Bohan and Peter criteria proposed in 1975 (Table 42.4) are the most widely used criteria for diagnosis of polymyositis and dermatomyositis [29,30]. The workup includes muscle and skin biopsy, selected laboratory tests, and diagnostic imaging (Table 42.5).

Table 42.5 Workup of patients with suspected polymyositis/dermatomyositis (PM/DM)

Pathology
- Skin biopsy
- Muscle biopsy

Laboratory studies
Muscle enzymes
- Creatine kinase (CK)
- Aldolase
- Lactic dehydrogenase (LDH)
- Aspartate aminotransferase (AST)

Myositis-specific antibodies (MSAs)
- Antinuclear antibody (ANA)
- Anti-Mi-2 antibodies
- Anti-Jo-1 antibodies
- Anti-p155/140 antibodies
- Anti-SRP antibodies
- Anti-NXP-2 antibodies
- Anti-CADM140 antibodies

Imaging studies
- Magnetic resonance imaging
- Ultrasonography
- Electromyography
- Esophageal manometry
- Chest radiography
- Chest computed tomography scan (with pulmonary function studies with diffusion capacity)
- Echocardiogram
- Electrocardiogram
- Colonoscopy to screen for underlying malignancy
- Transvaginal ultrasonography in females for malignancy screening
- Papanicolaou smear and mammography in women for malignancy screening
- CEA, PSA, CA-125, and CA-19-9 for malignancy screening

Histopathology

Skin biopsy: The typical histopathologic findings in DM skin include epidermal basal cell vacuolar degeneration, apoptosis of epidermal basal and suprabasal cells often with epidermal atrophy, and increased dermal mucin deposition [41]. A cell-poor interface dermatitis composed of plasmacytoid dendritic cells at the dermal-epidermal junction is also characteristic. On direct immunofluorescence, IgM, IgG, and C3 may be found at the dermal-epidermal junction in 50% of cases [42]. In early stages the histopathological findings resemble subacute LE while in later stages the changes are similar to scleroderma. Mucin deposits commonly occur in the dermis, and mucin in an otherwise nonspecific skin biopsy is suggestive of dermatomyositis [43].

Muscle biopsy: Muscle biopsy is done from a muscle that is clinically weak or shows abnormality on magnetic resonance imaging (MRI) scanning. The typical histopathologic findings of DM in muscle include perifascicular atrophy, endothelial cell swelling, vessel wall membrane attack complex (MAC) deposition, capillary necrosis, infarcts, major histocompatibility complex (MHC) I upregulation, and the presence of an inflammatory infiltrate consisting of T and B lymphocytes, macrophages, and plasma cells [44]. The histopathological findings depend on the stage of the disease with atrophy and sclerosis seen in the late stages.

Laboratory studies

Muscle enzymes are often raised in patients of dermatomyositis. The most sensitive/specific enzyme abnormality is elevated creatine kinase (CK) and aldolase. Other tests like lactate dehydrogenase (LDH) and aspartate aminotransferase (AST) may also yield abnormal results as these are released once muscle damage occurs. In the amyopathic variant of the disease, the muscle enzymes may be in normal range [45].

Rarely, urine creatinine levels may be elevated in some patients with normal serum CK levels. Myoglobin released by damaged muscles can be detected in the serum of patients with mild muscle disease. However, its detection in urine is a cause for concern as severe myoglobinuria can result in acute renal failure [46]. This is another setting where PM/DM can present as an acute dermatological emergency.

Myositis-specific antibodies (MSAs) occur in about 30% of all patients with dermatomyositis or polymyositis.

A positive antinuclear antibody (ANA) finding is common in patients with dermatomyositis, but not diagnostic. Antibodies against Mi-2 (a nuclear helicase protein) are highly specific for dermatomyositis, but sensitivity is low. Seen in both adult DM (15%) and juvenile DM (<10%), its presence indicates a better prognosis.

Anti-Jo-1 antibodies, directed against histidyl transfer RNA (t-RNA) synthetase, are seen in up to 20% of cases of adult dermatomyositis. They are associated with the antisynthetase syndrome that comprises fever, arthritis, pulmonary involvement (interstitial lung disease), Raynaud phenomenon, and mechanic's hands.

Anti-p155/140 antibodies are highly specific for DM and are seen in cancer-associated adult DM. They are characterized by severe cutaneous disease in both adult and juvenile population and with markedly increased risk of malignancy. Many other MSAs also exist [47–49].

Imaging studies

MRI (Figure 42.11a and b) of muscles is routinely prescribed as it is useful in selecting the muscle for biopsy and also in assessing the presence of an inflammatory myopathy in patients without weakness. MRI may be the most sensitive test for muscle disease, but it is more expensive [45]. *Ultrasonography* of the muscles is less expensive and can also be useful in determining the appropriate site for muscle biopsy, but it is not as sensitive. *Electromyography* (EMG) is a sensitive but nonspecific test that helps in detecting muscle inflammation and damage (Figure 42.12). It is less helpful in patients with polymyositis because there is overlap with other myopathies [50].

For evaluation of esophageal dysmotility, barium swallow and esophageal manometry can be done in selected cases. In cases with suspected lung involvement, chest radiography and CT scan with pulmonary function studies can be helpful. Electrocardiogram (ECG) and in symptomatic cases echocardiogram can be done.

In adult patients with dermatomyositis, assessment for malignancy should be performed upon initial diagnosis and repeated at least annually for 3 years as the risk of malignancy increases with age. Table 42.5 summarizes the investigations to be done in a case of suspected dermatomyositis and in some specific conditions for malignancy screening.

The Dermatomyositis Skin Severity Index (DSSI) [51] and the updated Cutaneous Dermatomyositis Disease Area and Severity Index (CDASI) [52] are valid instruments to determine the severity of cutaneous disease and also to monitor the treatment response.

EMERGENCIES IN DERMATOMYOSITIS

In patients of dermatomyositis, the reasons for intensive care unit (ICU) admission are infection, especially pneumonia or acute exacerbation of IIM alone. During acute exacerbation, patients can end up in rapid progressive interstitial lung disease (RP-ILD), which is the most common problem encountered. Acute respiratory failure (ARF) is the most common type of organ failure. Cardiac failure is the other main contributor. Mortality is quite high when it comes to acute exacerbations and organ damage. Factors associated with increased ICU mortality include a diagnosis of DM (including CADM), a high APACHE II score, coexistence of infection or IIM exacerbation, the presence of ARF or shock, a decreased PaO_2/FiO_2 ratio, and a low lymphocyte count at the time of ICU admission.

TREATMENT

Dermatomyositis is a difficult condition to treat. Table 42.6 summarizes the treatment strategy in patients with DM. Rest may be advised in the acute fulminant stages and in cases presenting as erythroderma. Physical therapy for muscle symptoms can also be beneficial. Photoprotection and application of sunscreens can be helpful in management of the cutaneous disease. Making the patient aware of the disease and explaining the prognosis is important for better compliance to treatment.

Systemic corticosteroids are the mainstay of treatment. Prednisolone is started in relatively high doses initially (1 mg/kg/day) depending on the severity of the disease. The steroid dose should gradually be reduced as the patient improves clinically and the muscle enzymes become normal. It is possible to reduce the dose to half of the starting dose by 6–8 months of treatment initiation in most cases. However, a maintenance dosage of 5–15 mg/day may be required for many months, or even years [53]. Prevention of osteoporosis and monitoring of potential side effects of long-term steroids is equally important in the management of these patients. Weakness arising from corticosteroid myopathy may be difficult to distinguish from disease exacerbation. In corticosteroid-induced myopathy, the serum enzymes are normal, but the 24-hour urinary creatine excretion is raised. Another cause of weakness in dermatomyositis may be hypokalemia arising as a result of corticosteroid therapy where regular electrolyte monitoring may be helpful. Recovery on reduction of dosage takes up to 4 months [53].

Patients not showing improvement on daily steroid therapy or having a severe disease may need IV methylprednisolone pulse (1 g for 3 successive days) or the addition of a steroid-sparing drug.

Steroid-sparing drugs are started in patients who do not respond to prednisolone treatment or relapse while on tapering dose of steroids. Also these drugs are started with steroids from the beginning in patients with severe disease or life-threatening complications. They are also started from the outset in patients who cannot tolerate high-dose steroids or have active contraindications for steroid therapy [54]. Among steroid-sparing drugs, important ones are methotrexate, azathioprine, mycophenolate mofetil, and IV immunoglobulin (IVIg).

Methotrexate (MTX) is started at a dose of 7.5 mg weekly that is increased by 2.5 mg increments to reach a dose of

(a)

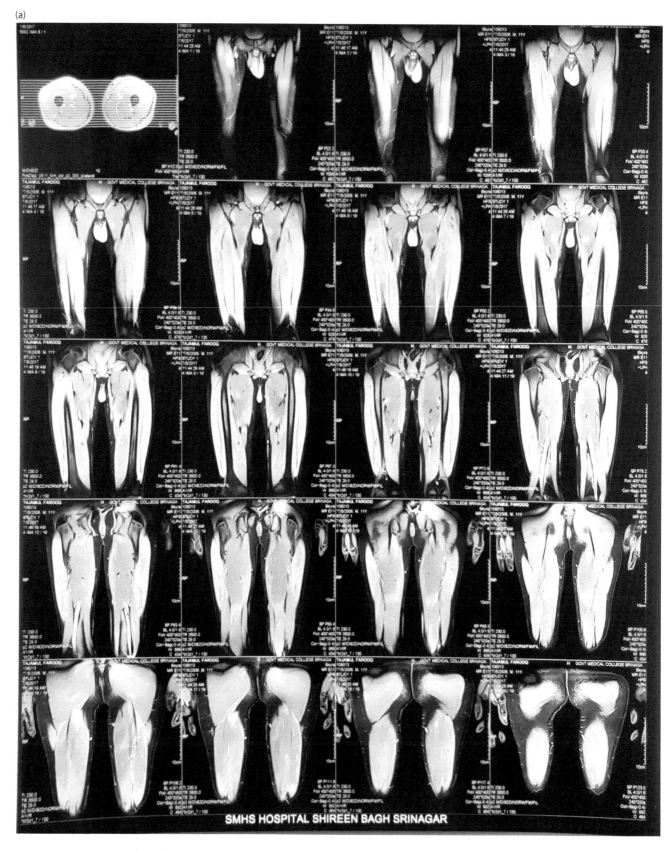

Figure 42.11 **(a)** T2-weighted magnetic resonance imaging (MRI) in inversion recovery coronal sections of a case of dermatomyositis showing high signal intensity in the lateral compartment of the thigh muscles.

(Continued)

(b)

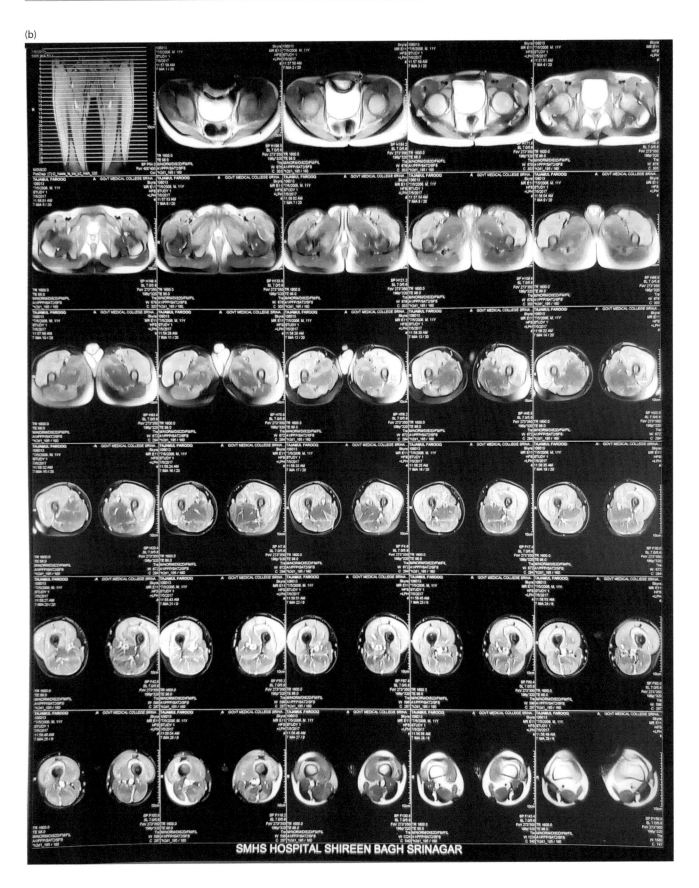

Figure 42.11 (Continued) **(b)** T2-weighted MRI images in fat-suppressing axial sections of a case of dermatomyositis showing high signal intensity in the lateral compartment of the thigh muscles.

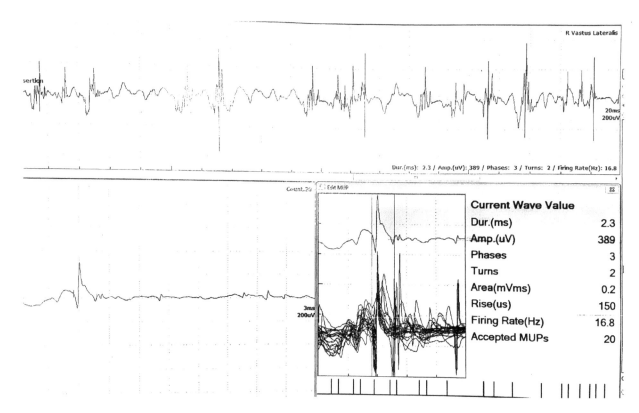

Figure 42.12 Electromyogram of a case of dermatomyositis showing small-amplitude, brief duration potentials in vastus lateralis muscle of thigh on motor unit action potential analysis.

25 mg weekly. If there is no improvement after 1 month of 25 mg weekly of oral MTX, some experts switch to weekly subcutaneous MTX and increase the dose by 5 mg every week up to 60 mg weekly [55]. MTX can rarely induce

Table 42.6 Treatment strategy of patients with dermatomyositis

---

Supportive therapy

Corticosteroids—mainstay of treatment (pulsed IV methylprednisolone in case of severe disease)

Steroid-sparing agents
- Methotrexate
- Azathioprine
- Mycophenolate mofetil
- Intravenous immunoglobulin

Alternative treatment options
- Ciclosporin
- Tacrolimus
- Chlorambucil
- Fludarabine
- Cyclophosphamide

Biologicals
- Infliximab
- Etanercept
- Rituximab

---

pneumonitis and should be used with caution in patients with ILD or Jo-1 antibodies.

Azathioprine is an antimetabolite that is started at an initial dose is 25–50 mg daily; with increment of 25 mg/week to reach a dose of 2–3 mg/kg body weight. It has a delayed onset of response that begins in 4–8 months and peaks at 1–2 years [56]. It is important to check thiopurine methyltransferase (TPMT) levels before initiating treatment.

Mycophenolate mofetil (MMF) is initiated at a dose of 500 mg twice daily and increased by 500 mg weekly to a dose of 2–3 gram/day. Patients with anti-synthetase syndrome especially ILD may respond favorably to MMF [56].

Intravenous immunoglobulin (IVIg) can be used as a disease-modifying and steroid-sparing agent in DM especially in patients with severe esophageal dysfunction. High-dose (2 g/kg body weight) IVIg is given over 2 or 5 days once a month up to 3–6 months [57]. Renal function needs to be monitored due to the risk of IVIg-induced renal failure [58].

Alternative treatment options that have been tried include ciclosporin (3–5 mg/kg/day) [59], tacrolimus [60], chlorambucil [61], and fludarabine [62]. Monthly cyclophosphamide (0.5–1.0 g/m^2) pulses have also been tried, especially in pulmonary disease [63]. Ciclosporin, tacrolimus, and cyclophosphamide have been found effective in treating PM/DM with associated ILD.

Among *biologicals*, tumor necrosis factor alpha (TNF-α) blockers like infliximab and etanercept have been tried and have demonstrated steroid-sparing effects [64]. Recent trials

Table 42.7 Treatment strategy in specific clinical situations encountered in dermatomyositis (DM)

For cutaneous lesions
- Suncreens
- Topical steroids
- Topical tacrolimus
- Hydroxychloroquine
- Low-dose methotrexate
- Mycophenolate mofetil
- IVIg
- Thalidomide
- Dapsone

For juvenile DM
- Systemic corticosteroids; oral prednisone in a dose of 2 mg/kg up to a maximum of 60 mg daily
- MTX (main steroid-sparing agent)
- Azathioprine
- Cyclosporine
- Tacrolimus
- IVIg
- Rituximab

For calcinosis cutis
- Surgical excision
- Diltiazem
- Low-dose warfarin
- Bisphosphonates
- Probenecid
- Aluminum hydroxide
- Electric shock wave lithotripsy

KEY POINTS

- Dermatomyositis is a disease with characteristic cutaneous symptoms and muscle weakness.
- Amyopathic dermatomyositis is recognized as a distinct entity where only cutaneous disease is seen.
- Many implicating factors have been identified in the etiopathogenesis of the disease with adult cases being associated with malignancy in some cases where thorough investigations are helpful in identifying the cause.
- For proper evaluation of the disease, history and examination need to be combined with various laboratory investigations and imaging modalities.
- Corticosteroids are the mainstay of treatment along with various steroid-sparing agents used according to the disease presentation and severity.

PROGNOSIS

The prognosis is variable. About 5% of patients have a fulminant progressive course with eventual death. Risk factors for a poorer prognosis in patients with dermatomyositis include the following:

- An associated malignancy
- Cardiac, pulmonary, or esophageal involvement
- Older age (i.e., older than 60 years)

CONCLUSION

To conclude, dermatomyositis is a disease with varied presentations. Patients can present with mild cutaneous symptoms only or can end up with erythroderma or respiratory failure or severe myopathy. Proper knowledge of the disease and a high amount of suspicion in atypical cases is very important for prompt diagnosis. Workup of the patients should include detailed history and examination coupled with laboratory investigations and imaging studies. Management of the disease is prolonged and difficult, especially for the cutaneous lesions that are refractory to treatment. An extensive search for underlying malignancy is crucial in adult cases of PM and DM to rule out any sinister cause for the symptoms.

have found rituximab as an effective treatment option in resistant IIM, especially in association with antisynthetase syndrome, which can be associated with life-threatening ILD [65,66].

Emerging therapies include anakinra, alemtuzumab, belimumab, and sifalimumab [56].

For the treatment of *skin disease*, topical steroids and tacrolimus have been used [67]. Hydroxychloroquine has been used to treat cutaneous manifestations in DM and juvenile DM (JDM) and is given at a dose of 200 mg twice daily [68]. Methotrexate can also be beneficial in the management of skin disease.

In cases of JDM, the treatment strategy is similar to the one used for adults, except that an initial prednisone dose of 2 mg/kg is used up to a maximum of 60 mg daily. MTX is the main steroid-sparing agent, with others being azathioprine, cyclosporine, and tacrolimus. MMF is not used routinely in children. IVIg and rituximab are efficacious and safe for refractory cases [56].

Calcinosis cutis is a troublesome complication of severe DM with poor response to treatment, although spontaneous improvement can occur. Diltiazem has been used successfully [69]. Surgical excision is another option. Table 42.7 summarizes the treatment strategy in specific situations seen in DM.

REFERENCES

1. Callen JP. Dermatomyositis. *Lancet* 2000;355(9197):53–7.
2. Callen JP, Wortmann RL. Dermatomyositis. *Clin Dermatol* 2006;24(5):363–73.
3. Symmons DPM, Sills JA, Davis SM. The incidence of juvenile dermatomyositis: Results from a nationwide study. *Br J Rheumatol* 1995;34:732–6.

4. Carlisle JW, Good RA. Dermatomyositis in childhood: Report of studies on several cases and review of the literature. *Lancet* 1959;79:266–73.

5. Degos R, Civatte J, Belaich S, Delarue A. The prognosis of adult dermatomyositis. *Trans St John's Hosp Dermatol Soc Lond* 1971;57:98–104.

6. Friedman JM et al. Immunogenetic studies of juvenile dermatomyositis. *Tissue Antigens* 1983;21:45–9.

7. Song MS, Farber D, Bitton A, Jass J, Singer M, Karpati G. Dermatomyositis associated with celiac disease: Response to a gluten-free diet. *Can J Gastroenterol* 2006;20:433–5.

8. Machulla HK, Stein J, Gautsch A, Langner J, Schaller HG, Reichert S. HLA-A, B, Cw, DRB1, DRB3/4/5, DQB1 in German patients suffering from rapidly progressive periodontitis (RPP) and adult periodontitis (AP). *J Clin Periodontol* 2002;29:573–9.

9. Benveniste O, Dubourg O, Herson S. New classifications and pathophysiology of the inflammatory myopathies. *Rev Med Interne* 2007;28:603–12.

10. Whitaker JN, Engel WK. Vascular deposits of immunoglobulin and complement in idiopathic inflammatory myopathy. *N Engl J Med* 1972;286:333–8.

11. Christensen ML, Pachman LM, Schneiderman R, Patel DC, Friedman JM. Prevalence of Coxsackie B virus antibodies in patients with juvenile dermatomyositis. *Arthritis Rheum* 1986;11:1365–70.

12. Crowson AN, Magro CM, Dawood MR. A causal role for parvovirus B19 infection in adult dermatomyositis and other autoimmune syndromes. *J Cutan Pathol* 2000;27:505–15.

13. Lane S, Doherty M, Powell RJ. Dermatomyositis following chronic staphylococcal joint sepsis. *Ann Rheum Dis* 1990;49:405–6.

14. Martini A et al. Recurrent juvenile dermatomyositis and cutaneous necrotizing arteritis with molecular mimicry between streptococcal type 5 m protein and human skeletal myosin. *J Pediatr* 1992;121:739–42.

15. Harland CC, Marsden JR, Vernon SA, Allen BR. Dermatomyositis responding to treatment of associated toxoplasmosis. *Br J Dermatol* 1991;125:76–8.

16. Daoud MS, Gibson LE, Pittelkow MR. Hydroxyurea dermopathy: A unique lichenoid eruption complicating long-term therapy with hydroxyurea. *J Am Acad Dermatol* 1997;36:178–82.

17. Doyle DR, McCurley TL, Sergent JS. Fatal polymyositis in d-penicillamine treated rheumatoid arthritis. *Ann Intern Med* 1983;98:327–30.

18. Harris AL, Smith IE, Snaith M. Tamoxifen-induced tumour regression associated with dermatomyositis. *BMJ* 1982;284:1674–5.

19. Flendrie M, Vissers WH, Creemers MC, de Jong EM, van de Kerkhof PC, van Riel PL. Dermatological conditions during TNF-alpha-blocking therapy in patients with rheumatoid arthritis: A prospective study. *Arthritis Res Ther* 2005;7:666–76.

20. Noël B. Lupus erythematosus and other autoimmune diseases related to statin therapy: A systematic review. *J Eur Acad Dermatol Venereol* 2007;21(1):17–24.

21. Callen JP, Hyla JF, Bole GG, Kay DR. The relationship of dermatomyositis and polymyositis to internal malignancy. *Arch Dermatol* 1980;116:295–8.

22. Callen JP. The value of malignancy evaluation in patients with dermatomyositis. *J Am Acad Dermatol* 1982;6:253–9.

23. Hill CL et al. Frequency of specific cancer types in dermatomyositis and polymyositis: A population-based study. *Lancet* 2001;357:96–100.

24. Barnes BE, Mawr B. Dermatomyositis and malignancy. A review of the literature. *Ann Intern Med* 1976;84:68–76.

25. Wong KQ. Dermatomyositis: A clinical investigation of 23 cases in Hong Kong. *Br J Dermatol* 1969;81:544–7.

26. Stockton D, Doherty VR, Brewster DH. Risk of cancer in patients with dermatomyositis or polymyositis, and follow-up implications: A Scottish population based cohort study. *Br J Cancer* 2001;6:41–5.

27. Greenberg SA, Amato AA. Uncertainties in the pathogenesis of adult dermatomyositis. *Curr Opin Neurol* 2004;17:359–64.

28. Greenberg SA. Dermatomyositis and type 1 interferons. *Curr Rheumatol Rep* 2010;12:198–203.

29. Bohan A, Peter JB. Polymyositis and dermatomyositis (first of two parts). *N Engl J Med* 1975;292:344–7.

30. Bohan A, Peter JB. Polymyositis and dermatomyositis (second of two parts). *N Engl J Med* 1975;292:403–7.

31. Sontheimer RD. Cutaneous features of classical dermatomyositis and amyopathic dermatomyositis. *Curr Opin Rheumatol* 1999;11:475–82.

32. Miller FW. New approaches to the assessment and treatment of the idiopathic inflammatory myopathies. *Ann Rheum Dis* 2012;71(2):82–5.

33. Pestronk A. Acquired immune and inflammatory myopathies: Pathologic classification. *Curr Opin Rheumatol* 2011;23:595–604.

34. Bohan A, Peter JB, Bowman RL, Pearson CM. A computer-assisted analysis of 153 patients with polymyositis and dermatomyositis. *Medicine* 1977;56:255–86.

35. Jinnin M. Myositis and the skin: Cutaneous manifestations of dermatomyositis. *Brain Nerve* 2013;65(11):1283–90.

36. Marvi U, Chung L, Fiorentino DF. Clinical presentation and evaluation of dermatomyositis. *Indian J Dermatol* 2012;57:375–81.

37. Sontheimer RD. Dermatomyositis: An overview of recent progress with emphasis on dermatologic aspects. *Dermatol Clin* 2002;20:387–408.

38. Smith RL, Sundberg J, Shamiyah E, Dyer A, Pachman LM. Skin involvement in juvenile dermatomyositis is associated with loss of end row nailfold capillary loops. *J Rheumatol* 2004;31:1644–9.

39. Fathi M, Lundberg IE, Tornling G. Pulmonary complications of polymyositis and dermatomyositis. *Semin Respir Crit Care Med* 2007;28:451–8.

40. Haupt HM, Hutchins GM. The heart and cardiac conduction system in polymyositis–dermatomyositis. *Am J Cardiol* 1982;50:998–1006.

41. Costner MI, Jacobe H. Dermatopathology of connective tissue diseases. *Adv Dermatol* 2000;16:323–59.

42. Vaughan-Jones SA, Bhogal BS, Black MM. Direct immunofluorescence findings in dermatomyositis. *Br J Dermatol* 1995;133(45):55.

43. Janis JF, Winkelmann RK. Histopathology of the skin in dermatomyositis. *Arch Dermatol* 1968;97:40–50.

44. Dalakas MC. Muscle biopsy findings in inflammatory myopathies. *Rheum Dis Clin North Am* 2002;28:779–98.

45. Stonecipher MR, Jorizzo JL, Monu J, Walker F, Sutej PG. Dermatomyositis with normal muscle enzyme concentrations. A single-blind study of the diagnostic value of magnetic resonance imaging and ultrasound. *Arch Dermatol* 1994;130:1294–9.

46. Jorizzo JL, Vleugels RA. Dermatomyositis. In: Bolognia JL, Jorizzo JL, Schaffer JV (Eds), *Dermatology*. 3rd ed. China: Elsevier Saunders; 2012:1(3):638.

47. Valenzuela A, Chung L, Casciola-Rosen L, Fiorentino D. Identification of clinical features and autoantibodies associated with calcinosis in dermatomyositis. *JAMA Dermatol* 2014;150(7):724–9.

48. Sato S et al. RNA helicase encoded by melanoma differentiation-associated gene 5 is a major autoantigen in patients with clinically amyopathic dermatomyositis: Association with rapidly progressive interstitial lung disease. *Arthritis Rheum* 2009;60(7):2193–200.

49. Sato S et al. Autoantibodies to a 140-kd polypeptide, CADM-140, in Japanese patients with clinically amyopathic dermatomyositis. *Arthritis Rheum* 2005;52(5):1571–6.

50. Bromberg MB, Albers JW. Electromyography in idiopathic myositis. *Mt Sinai J Med* 1988;55:459–64.

51. Carroll CL, Lang W, Snively B, Feldman SR, Callen J, Jorizzo JL. Development and validation of the Dermatomyositis Skin and Severity Index. *Br J Dermatol* 2008;158:345–50.

52. Yassaee M et al. Modification of the cutaneous Dermatomyositis Disease Area and Severity Index, an outcome instrument. *Br J Dermatol* 2010;162:669–73.

53. Goodfield MJD, Jones SK, Veale DJ. The Connective Tissue Diseases. In: Burns T, Breathnach S, Cox N, Griffiths C (Eds), *Rook's Textbook of Dermatology*. Edinburgh: Wiley-Blackwell; 2010;3(8):51.129.

54. Amato AA, Griggs RC. Treatment of idiopathic inflammatory myopathies. *Curr Opin Neurol* 2003;16(5):569–75.

55. Amato AA, Barohn RJ. Evaluation and treatment of inflammatory myopathies. *J Neurol Neurosurg Psychiatry* 2009;80(10):1060–8.

56. Malik A, Hayat G, Kalia JS, Guzman MA. Idiopathic inflammatory myopathies: Clinical approach and management. *Front Neurol* 2016;7(64):1–19.

57. Dalakas MC II et al. A controlled trial of high-dose intravenous immune globulin infusions as treatment for dermatomyositis. *N Engl J Med* 1993;329:993–2000.

58. Dalakas MC. Mechanism of action of intravenous immunoglobulin and therapeutic considerations in the treatment of autoimmune neurologic diseases. *Neurology* 1998;51(6):S2–8.

59. Casato M, Bonomo L, Caccavo D, Giorgi A. Clinical effects of cyclosporin in dermatomyositis. *Clin Exp Dermatol* 1990;15:121–3.

60. Oddis CV, Sciurba FC, Elmagd KA, Starzl TE. Tacrolimus in refractory polymyositis with interstitial lung disease. *Lancet* 1999;353:1211–7.

61. Sinoway PA, Callen JP. Chlorambucil: An effective corticosteroid-sparing agent for patients with recalcitrant dermatomyositis. *Arthritis Rheum* 1993;36:319–24.

62. Adams EM et al. A pilot study: Use of fludarabine for refractory dermatomyositis and polymyositis, and examination of end-point measures. *J Rheumatol* 1999;26:352–60.

63. Riley P, Maillard SM, Wedderburn LR, Woo P, Murray KJ, Pilkington CA. Intravenous cyclophosphamide pulse therapy in juvenile dermatomyositis. A review of efficacy and safety. *Rheumatology (Oxf)* 2004;43:491–6.

64. Amato A. A randomized, pilot trial of etanercept in dermatomyositis. *Ann Neurol* 2011;70(3):427–36.

65. Nalotto L et al. Rituximab in refractory idiopathic inflammatory myopathies and antisynthetase syndrome: Personal experience and review of the literature. *Immunol Res* 2013;56(2–3):362–70.

66. Limaye V, Hissaria P, Liew CL, Koszyka B. Efficacy of rituximab in refractory antisynthetase syndrome. *Intern Med J* 2012;42(3):4–7.

67. Yoshimasu T, Ohtani T, Sakamoto T, Oshima A, Furukawa F. Topical FK506 (tacrolimus) therapy for facial erythematous lesions of cutaneous lupus erythematosus and dermatomyositis. *Eur J Dermatol* 2002;12(1):50–2.

68. Woo TY, Callen JP, Voorhees JJ, Bickers DR, Hanno R, Hawkins C. Cutaneous lesions of dermatomyositis are improved by hydroxychloroquine. *J Am Acad Dermatol* 1984;10:592–600.

69. Palmieri GM et al. Treatment of calcinosis with diltiazem. *Arthritis Rheum* 1995;38:1646–54.

43

Sjögren syndrome and mixed connective tissue disease

VISHAL GUPTA AND NIDHI KAELEY

INTRODUCTION

Sjögren syndrome is a chronic autoimmune disease characterized by the triad of dry skin (xerosis), dry eyes (keratoconjunctivitis sicca), and dry mouth (xerostomia). It is termed *primary* when it occurs alone, and *secondary* when associated with other autoimmune connective tissue disorders such as rheumatoid arthritis, systemic lupus erythematosus, systemic sclerosis, and primary biliary cirrhosis. The prevalence of primary Sjögren syndrome varies widely, depending on the classification criteria used. A large population-based study in Norway estimated its point-prevalence as 0.44% and 0.22% using the European and the revised criteria, respectively [1,2]. Females are affected roughly nine times more frequently than men. It has two age peaks: the first peak occurs after menarche at around 20–30 years of age, and the second peak occurs in the 50s [3,4].

CLINICAL FEATURES

Sjögren syndrome primarily affects exocrine glands, mainly lacrimal and salivary glands. Extraglandular organ system involvement can include skin, joints, heart, lungs, gastrointestinal tract, kidney, nervous system, and hematological system.

Cutaneous manifestations

Cutaneous features of Sjögren syndrome include xerosis, Raynaud phenomenon, cutaneous vasculitis, and annular erythema (Table 43.1). Xerosis of skin is the most common cutaneous finding in patients with Sjögren syndrome, occurring in 23%–67% patients [5,6]. Dry skin is prone to itching, and chronic scratching can lead to lichenification (Figure 43.1). Initially thought to be due to reduced sweating because of lymphocytic infiltration of the eccrine glands, xerosis in Sjögren syndrome is now believed to occur as a result of alterations in the stratum corneum layer [7]. Cutaneous vasculitis is reported in about 10%–30% patients, and usually affects the small-caliber vessels presenting as palpable purpura or urticarial lesions. Medium vessel involvement is infrequent and is often associated with cryoglobulinemia [8,9]. Annular erythema of Sjögren syndrome favors head and neck, and morphologically resembles the annular papulosquamous skin lesions in subacute cutaneous lupus erythematosus. Its histopathology shows perivascular and periappendigeal lymphocytic infiltrate, while lacking the interface changes of lupus erythematosus. It has been mostly reported in Japanese cohorts and is more common in patients with antibodies against SS-A/SS-B [10–12]. Other skin findings can include vitiligo, lichen planus, cutaneous amyloidosis, livedo reticularis, and erythema nodosum [4,5]. Patients with secondary Sjögren syndrome can have additional manifestations depending on the associated autoimmune disease.

Extracutaneous manifestations

Patients have dry eyes and dry mouth as a result of lymphocytic infiltration in the lacrimal and salivary glands, respectively (Table 43.1). Salivary gland enlargement occurs in 30%–50% of patients. Parotid and submandibular glands

Table 43.1 Mucocutaneous features of Sjögren syndrome

Mucocutaneous manifestation	Presentation	Management
Dry skin	Dry, scaly skin predominantly affecting lower legs Pruritus, burning sensation Chronic scratching can lead to lichenification	Liberal emollients Antihistamines
Xerophthalmia	Foreign-body sensation or grittiness Absence of tears Blurred vision	Artificial tears/lubricant eye drops Do not rub eyes frequently Moist cotton balls over eyes while sleeping Cyclosporine eye drops (0.05%) Hydroxychloroquine sulfate
Xerostomia	Dry mouth Altered taste Burning sensation in mouth Dry, fissured tongue	Frequent mouth rinsing with water Salivary gland message to promote salivary flow Dental hygiene, chlorhexidine rinses, topical fluoride treatments, oral antifungal prophylaxis Cholinergics: cevimeline, pilocarpine
Vaginal dryness	Vaginal itching Dyspareunia	Emollients
Cutaneous vasculitis	Crops of palpable purpura on lower extremities, buttocks Urticarial vasculitis	Nonsteroidal anti-inflammatory drugs Dapsone Colchicine Corticosteroids Other immunosuppressives: azathioprine, cyclosporine, cyclophosphamide
Raynaud phenomenon	Episodic bluish discoloration of finger tips, triggered by cold exposure	Cold protection Calcium channel blockers: nifedipine
Annular erythema	Erythema multiforme-like Erythema annularecentrifugum-like Seen in Asians, typically Japanese	Topic steroids, tacrolimus Hydroxychloroquine Low-dose oral steroids

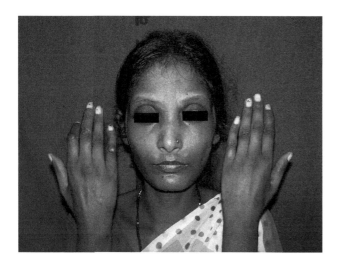

Figure 43.1 Lichenification and hyperpigmentation on dorsum of hand.

are commonly affected [13]. About half of the patients with Sjögren syndrome have musculoskeletal symptoms such as fatigue, myalgias, and arthralgias; arthritis being infrequent. Lungs can be involved in 10%–20% patients, in the form of small airway disease (bronchiolitis) and interstitial lung disease [14]. Renal involvement most commonly occurs as chronic tubulointerstitial nephritis, while glomerular involvement is associated with poor prognosis. An important renal involvement of Sjögren syndrome is distal renal tubular acidosis, which occurs in about 30% of patients with Sjögren syndrome. It can lead to symptomatic hypokalemia, which can present as sudden-onset quadriparesis, and can rarely cause respiratory arrest. Its diagnosis can be confirmed by documenting hypokalemia and hyperchloremic metabolic acidosis. Potassium supplementation should be started immediately with careful monitoring [15,16].

Risk of lymphoma in Sjögren syndrome

Patients with Sjögren syndrome with vasculitic manifestations are more likely to develop non-Hodgkin lymphoma, as compared to patients without vasculitis. The 10-year risk of developing lymphoma has been documented to be 4% in patients with cutaneous vasculitis and/or low C4 levels [17,18]. Apart from vasculitis and hypocomplementemia, the presence of persistent salivary gland enlargement, lymphadenopathy, cryoglobulinemia, glomerulonephritis, and lymphopenia also increase the risk of lymphoma [19,20]. Persistent salivary gland swelling, commonly affecting the parotid gland, or a hard, nodular unilateral salivary gland swelling should raise the suspicion of lymphoma in a patient with Sjögren syndrome.

COMPLICATIONS RELATED TO CUTANEOUS INVOLVEMENT

Cutaneous vasculitis is a marker of more severe disease. Apart from the risk of lymphoma, patients with Sjögren syndrome who develop vasculitis are also more likely to have systemic involvement such as arthritis, peripheral neuropathy, Raynaud phenomenon, and glomerulonephritis. Waldenstrom macroglobulinemia is a relatively common vasculitic manifestation of primary Sjögren syndrome. It presents as palpable purpura, polyclonal hypergammaglobulinemia, and elevated titers of rheumatoid factor and anti-SS-A/SS-B autoantibodies. Though itself benign, it is associated with sensory peripheral neuropathy [5].

Cryoglobulinemic vasculitis

In a study of 52 patients with Sjögren syndrome, cryoglobulinemia accounted for leukocytoclastic vasculitis in 30% of cases. Cryoglobulinemia can be associated with life-threatening systemic vasculitis, such as affecting the kidneys, gastrointestinal, and central nervous system [9]. Skin findings include palpable purpura that can become necrotic and ulcerate, erythematous papules, ecchymoses, dermal nodules, urticarial lesions, livedo reticularis, and digital gangrene [21].

Digital gangrene

Digital gangrene may develop as a complication of cryoglobulinemic vasculitis or Raynaud phenomenon. Another cause of digital gangrene in Sjögren syndrome can be the occurrence of antiphospholipid antibody syndrome, especially those with an overlap with systemic lupus erythematosus [22].

Xerosis-related complications

Patients with xerophthalmia often develop blepharitis either due to staphylococcal infection or due to frequent rubbing of the eyelids. A more serious but less frequent complication is corneal ulceration and perforation. Due to reduced salivary secretions, patients with xerostomia are at risk of developing dental caries. Oral candidiasis and angular cheilitis can also develop due to poor oral hygiene. Salivary glands can become swollen and are prone to recurrent attacks of bacterial infections, due to impaired salivary flow [4,5,23].

DIAGNOSIS

Several classification criteria have been proposed for the diagnosis of primary Sjögren syndrome. The criteria proposed by the American-European Consensus Group and the Sjögren International Collaborative Clinical Alliance have been the

Table 43.2 American College of Rheumatology/European League Against Rheumatism classification criteria for primary Sjögren syndrome

Item	Score
Labial salivary gland with focal lymphocytic sialadenitis, and focus score of >1 foci/mm²	3
Anti SS-A/Ro positive	3
Ocular staining score >5 (or van Bijesterveld score >4) in at least one eye	1
Schirmer test <5 mm/5 minutes in at least one eye (Figure 43.2)	1
Unstimulated whole salivary flow rate <0.1 mL/min	1

Note: Diagnosis of primary Sjögren syndrome can be made if an individual meets the inclusion criteria (symptomatic ocular or oral dryness), does not have any of the exclusion criteria (history of head/neck radiation, active hepatitis C infection, AIDS, sarcoidosis, amyloidosis, graft versus host disease, IgG4-related disease), and has a score of ≥4 on summation of criteria as mentioned previously.

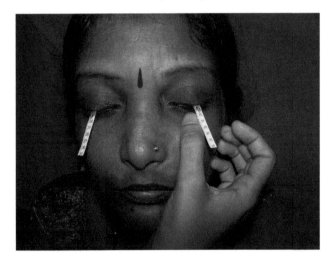

Figure 43.2 Schirmer test showing decreased tearing.

most widely used [24]. Recently, the American College of Rheumatology and European League Against Rheumatism collaborated to update the diagnostic criteria for Sjögren syndrome [25]. Diagnosis of Sjögren syndrome requires a score of >4 on summation of items (Table 43.2) [25].

TREATMENT

Currently, there is no one treatment that can take care of all of the manifestations of Sjögren syndrome or that can modify its natural course. Treatment is directed toward the affected system. Treatment strategies for different cutaneous manifestations are summarized in Table 43.1 [4,5]. Drawing from the experience from other rheumatic diseases, hydroxychloroquine is often used for fatigue, muscle, and joint pains. For more severe internal organ involvement, systemic corticosteroids and steroid-sparing agents such as methotrexate, azathioprine, and cyclophosphamide are used [26]. TNF-α blockers such as infliximab and etanercept have also been tried for the treatment of sicca symptoms with variable results [27,28].

MIXED CONNECTIVE TISSUE DISEASE

Introduction

Mixed connective tissue disease (MCTD) was first described by Sharp et al. as a clinically and serologically distinct entity in 1972 [29]. Patients exhibit clinical features overlapping with those of systemic lupus erythematous, systemic sclerosis, and polymyositis, and have high titers of anti-U1RNP (ribonucleoprotein) antibody. However, there is controversy whether MCTD exists as a distinct clinical entity or is merely an overlap of clinical features of different connective tissue diseases. As a subset of patients with MCTD develops features consistent with classic systemic lupus or scleroderma over time, some researchers believe that it represents an early nonspecific phase of an evolving connective tissue disease (often referred to as *undifferentiated connective tissue disease*) [30–32]. MCTD is the least common of all the connective tissue disorders. A population-based study in Norway estimated its point-prevalence as 3.8 per 100,000 adults and the annual incidence rate as 2.1 per million. Females are affected more frequently than males (female-to-male ratios range from 3.3:1 to 16:1) [33–35]. Most patients are affected in their second or third decades of life. MCTD can have a juvenile onset in 7%–23% patients [36].

Clinical features

MCTD affects several organ systems. Early in the course of the disease, it has cutaneous-predominant findings along with nonspecific constitutional symptoms such as easy fatigability, myalgias, and arthralgias.

CUTANEOUS MANIFESTATIONS

Common cutaneous features include Raynaud phenomenon, periungual telangiectasias, acrosclerosis or sclerodactyly, swollen inflamed digits ("sausage fingers"), and symmetrically swollen hands ("puffy hands"). Raynaud phenomenon is the earliest skin manifestation and is present in almost all patients. Patients can develop painful digital ulcers, and even digital infarcts/gangrene in severe cases. Acute lupus-like features such as photosensitivity and malar rash can develop during disease flares [33–38]. Patients with MCTD often develop glandular features of Sjögren syndrome such as dry eyes and dry mouth (*sicca complex*) [39]. There may be well-defined sclerodermoid (unlike the diffuse binding down of skin in systemic sclerosis) or poikilodermatous (areas of mottled or reticulate dyspigmentation, telangiectasias, atrophy) lesions on the upper trunk and proximal limbs; however, other dermatomyositis-specific changes are usually absent. Oral ulcers and nasal septal perforation have also been described.

EXTRACUTANEOUS MANIFESTATIONS

Arthritis is a common feature of MCTD, seen in about 60% patients. Usually, it is nonerosive but occasionally erosions and an arthritis mutilans-like picture may develop [40]. Most patients develop an inflammatory myopathy during the course of their disease; however, it is rarely present at the onset of the disease.

Pulmonary involvement may occur in the form of interstitial lung disease (20%–65%), pleural effusion (50%), pulmonary hypertension (10%–45%), and pleurisy (20%). Pulmonary hypertension is thought to develop independent of interstitial lung disease and is a major cause of death in MCTD [41,42].

Symptomatic cardiac involvement occurs in 30% of patients. Pericarditis is the most common manifestation of cardiac involvement, although endocardium (conduction abnormalities) and myocardium can also be involved [43].

Other organ system involvement is milder and less common and includes esophageal dysmotility, trigeminal neuralgia, glomerulonephritis, and cytopenias. Notably, patients have less severe neurological and renal involvement as compared to systemic lupus erythematosus [33,44,45].

Complications related to cutaneous involvement

DIGITAL GANGRENE

Patients with MCTD can develop digital gangrene as a complication of Raynaud phenomenon. Medium vessel vasculitis or antiphospholipid antibody syndrome can also occur in the setting of MCTD [46,47], which can lead to digital gangrene.

LIVEDOID VASCULOPATHY

Livedoid vasculopathy presents as small punched-out painful ulcers on the lower legs, with peripheral retiform purpura, which heal with characteristic porcelain-white stellate scars (atrophie blanche) [48–52]. Sometimes, upper limbs may also be affected. Livedoid vasculopathic ulcers in a patient with MCTD can also occur as a part of coexistent antiphospholipid antibody syndrome.

CUTANEOUS VASCULITIS

Small vessel leukocytoclastic vasculitis and urticarial vasculitis (urticarial lesions with a purpuric hue) can occur in MCTD [53]. Multiple large painful leg ulcers have also been reported as a manifestation of cutaneous vasculitis in MCTD [54].

Table 43.3 Alarcon-Segova criteria for the diagnosis of mixed connective tissue disease

Serological criteria	Anti-RNP antibodies with a titer of >1:1,600
Clinical criteria	Raynaud phenomenon
	Acrosclerosis
	Swollen hands
	Synovitis
	Myositis

Note: Diagnosis of mixed connective tissue disease requires the presence of the serological criteria and at least three clinical criteria, one of which must include synovitis or myositis.

CALCINOSIS CUTIS

Dystrophic calcification in the skin has been described in patients with MCTD, which can present as whitish-yellowish hard deep-seated nodules and/or plaques [55]. The overlying skin can ulcerate with discharge of chalky white material. The ulcers are painful and are difficult to heal. The diagnosis can be confirmed by visualizing the soft-tissue calcification on radiography [56].

DIAGNOSIS

The presence of antibodies to U1RNP is a *sine qua non* for the diagnosis of MCTD. Because the overlapping clinical features of systemic lupus erythematosus, systemic sclerosis, and polymyositis/dermatomyositis occur sequentially, several years may elapse before the diagnosis of MCTD is suspected. Various criteria have been proposed for diagnosis of MCTD [57]. The Alarcon-Segova criteria have been regularly used (Table 43.3) [58]. As a practical rule, MCTD should be suspected in a patient presenting with Raynaud phenomenon, swollen hands, elevated anti-U1RNP antibodies, and at least two of the following: arthritis, myositis, leukopenia, esophageal dysmotility, pleuritis, pericarditis, interstitial lung disease, or pulmonary artery hypertension [33].

TREATMENT

Treatment of MCTD depends on the symptoms and organs affected. Calcium channel blockers such as nifedipine (20–60 mg/day) are the first-line agents for Raynaud phenomenon. Hydroxychloroquine is often used for musculoskeletal pains, while internal organ involvement is treated with systemic corticosteroids and other immunosuppressives such as methotrexate, azathioprine, cyclosporine, cyclophosphamide, and mycophenolate mofetil. Other options in refractory cases may include plasmapheresis and stem cell transplantation. Pulmonary artery hypertension requires treatment with endothelin receptor antagonists (bosentan, ambrisentan), phosphodiesterase-5 inhibitors (sildenafil, tadalafil), and/or prostacyclins [33].

KEY POINTS

- Sjögren syndrome is a chronic autoimmune disease characterized by xerosis, keratoconjunctivitis sicca and xerostomia.
- Sjögren syndrome primarily affects mainly lacrimal and salivary glands. Extraglandular organ system involvement can include skin, joints, heart, lungs, gastrointestinal tract, kidney, nervous system, and hematological system.
- Patients with Sjögren syndrome with vasculitic manifestations are more likely to develop non-Hodgkin lymphoma, as compared to patients without vasculitis.
- Patients exhibiting clinical features overlapping with those of systemic lupus erythematous, systemic sclerosis, and polymyositis, and have high titers of anti-U1RNP antibody are classified as having MCTD.

REFERENCES

1. Haugen AJ et al. Estimation of the prevalence of primary Sjögren's syndrome in two age-different community-based populations using two sets of classification criteria: The Hordaland Health Study. *Scand J Rheumatol* 2008;37(1):30–4.
2. Bowman SJ, Ibrahim GH, Holmes G, Hamburger J, Ainsworth JR. Estimating the prevalence among Caucasian women of primary Sjögren's syndrome in two general practices in Birmingham, UK. *Scand J Rheumatol* 2004;33(1):39–43.
3. Cimaz R et al. Primary Sjögren syndrome in the paediatric age: A multicentre survey. *Eur J Pediatr* 2003;162(10):661–5.
4. Fox RI, Liu AY. Sjögren's syndrome in dermatology. *Clin Dermatol* 2006;24(5):393–413.
5. Kittridge A, Routhouska SB, Korman NJ. Dermatologic manifestations of Sjögren syndrome. *J Cutan Med Surg* 2011;15(1):8–14.
6. Roguedas AM, Misery L, Sassolas B, Le Masson G, Pennec YL, Youinou P. Cutaneous manifestations of primary Sjögren's syndrome are underestimated. *Clin Exp Rheumatol* 2004;22(5):632–6.
7. Bernacchi E et al. Xerosis in primary Sjögren syndrome: Immunohistochemical and functional investigations. *J Dermatol Sci* 2005;39(1):53–5.
8. Bernacchi E et al. Sjögren's syndrome: A retrospective review of the cutaneous features of 93 patients by the Italian Group of Immunodermatology. *Clin Exp Rheumatol* 2004;22(1):55–62.
9. Ramos-Casals M et al. Cutaneous vasculitis in primary Sjögren syndrome: Classification and

clinical significance of 52 patients. *Medicine (Baltim)* 2004;83(2):96–106.

10. Katayama I, Teramoto N, Arai H, Nishioka K, Nishiyama S. Annular erythema. A comparative study of Sjögren syndrome with subacute cutaneous lupus erythematosus. *Int J Dermatol* 1991;30(9):635–9.

11. Katayama I, Yamamoto T, Otoyama K, Matsunaga T, Nishioka K. Clinical and immunological analysis of annular erythema associated with Sjögren syndrome. *Dermatol Basel Switz* 1994;189(Suppl 1):14–7.

12. Brito-Zerón P et al. Annular erythema in primary Sjögren syndrome: Description of 43 non-Asian cases. *Lupus* 2014;23(2):166–75.

13. Daniels TE, Fox PC. Salivary and oral components of Sjögren's syndrome. *Rheum Dis Clin North Am* 1992;18(3):571–89.

14. Kreider M, Highland K. Pulmonary involvement in Sjögren syndrome. *Semin Respir Crit Care Med* 2014;35(2):255–64.

15. Slobodin G, Hussein A, Rozenbaum M, Rosner I. The emergency room in systemic rheumatic diseases. *Emerg Med J EMJ* 2006;23(9):667–71.

16. Soy M, Pamuk ON, Gerenli M, Celik Y. A primary Sjögren's syndrome patient with distal renal tubular acidosis, who presented with symptoms of hypokalemic periodic paralysis: Report of a case study and review of the literature. *Rheumatol Int* 2005;26(1):86–9.

17. Ioannidis JPA, Vassiliou VA, Moutsopoulos HM. Long-term risk of mortality and lymphoproliferative disease and predictive classification of primary Sjögren's syndrome. *Arthritis Rheum* 2002;46(3):741–7.

18. Skopouli FN, Dafni U, Ioannidis JP, Moutsopoulos HM. Clinical evolution, and morbidity and mortality of primary Sjögren's syndrome. *Semin Arthritis Rheum* 2000;29(5):296–304.

19. Voulgarelis M, Tzioufas AG, Moutsopoulos HM. Mortality in Sjögren's syndrome. *Clin Exp Rheumatol* 2008;26(5 Suppl. 51):S66–71.

20. Papageorgiou A et al. Predicting the outcome of Sjögren syndrome-associated non-Hodgkin's lymphoma patients. *PLOS ONE* 2015;10(2):e0116189.

21. Ferri C, Mascia MT. Cryoglobulinemic vasculitis. *Curr Opin Rheumatol* 2006;18(1):54–63.

22. Cervera R et al. Antiphospholipid syndrome: Clinical and immunologic manifestations and patterns of disease expression in a cohort of 1,000 patients. *Arthritis Rheum* 2002;46(4):1019–27.

23. Connolly MK. Sjogern's syndrome. *Semin Cutan Med Surg* 2001;20(1):46–52.

24. Franceschini F, Cavazzana I, Andreoli L, Tincani A. The 2016 classification criteria for primary Sjögren syndrome: What's new? *BMC Med* 2017;15.

25. Shiboski CH et al. 2016 American College of Rheumatology/European League Against Rheumatism classification criteria for primary Sjögren's syndrome: A consensus and data-driven methodology involving three international patient cohorts. *Ann Rheum Dis* 2017;76(1):9–16.

26. Saraux A, Pers J-O, Devauchelle-Pensec V. Treatment of primary Sjögren syndrome. *Nat Rev Rheumatol* 2016;12(8):456–71.

27. Betül Türkoğlu E, Tuna S, Alan S, İhsan Arman M, Tuna Y, Ünal M. Effect of systemic infliximab therapy in patients with Sjögren's syndrome. *Turk J Ophthalmol* 2015;45(4):138–41.

28. Sankar V et al. Etanercept in Sjögren's syndrome: A twelve-week randomized, double-blind, placebo-controlled pilot clinical trial. *Arthritis Rheum* 2004;50(7):2240–5.

29. Sharp GC, Irvin WS, Tan EM, Gould RG, Holman HR. Mixed connective tissue disease: An apparently distinct rheumatic disease syndrome associated with a specific antibody to an extractable nuclear antigen (ENA). *Am J Med* 1972;52(2):148–59.

30. Cappelli S et al. "To be or not to be," ten years after: Evidence for mixed connective tissue disease as a distinct entity. *Semin Arthritis Rheum* 2012;41(4):589–98.

31. Aringer M, Steiner G, Smolen JS. Does mixed connective tissue disease exist? Yes. *Rheum Dis Clin North Am* 2005;31(3):411–20, v.

32. Swanton J, Isenberg D. Mixed connective tissue disease: Still crazy after all these years. *Rheum Dis Clin North Am* 2005;31(3):421–36, v.

33. Gunnarsson R, Hetlevik SO, Lilleby V, Molberg Ø. Mixed connective tissue disease. *Best Pract Res Clin Rheumatol* 2016;30(1):95–111.

34. Gunnarsson R, Molberg O, Gilboe I-M, Gran JT, PAHNOR1 Study Group. The prevalence and incidence of mixed connective tissue disease: A national multicentre survey of Norwegian patients. *Ann Rheum Dis* 2011;70(6):1047–51.

35. Nakae K et al. A nationwide epidemiological survey on diffuse collagen diseases: Estimation of prevalence rate in Japan. In: Kasukawa R, Sharp G (Eds), *Mixed Connective Tissue Disease and Anti-Nuclear Antibodies*. Amsterdam: Excerpta Medica; 1987:9.

36. Kotajima L, Aotsuka S, Sumiya M, Yokohari R, Tojo T, Kasukawa R. Clinical features of patients with juvenile onset mixed connective tissue disease: Analysis of data collected in a nationwide collaborative study in Japan. *J Rheumatol* 1996;23(6):1088–94.

37. Venables PJW. Mixed connective tissue disease. *Lupus* 2006;15(3):132–7.

38. Sen S et al. Cutaneous manifestations of mixed connective tissue disease: Study from a tertiary care hospital in Eastern India. *Indian J Dermatol* 2014;59(1):35–40.

39. Setty YN, Pittman CB, Mahale AS, Greidinger EL, Hoffman RW. Sicca symptoms and anti-SSA/Ro antibodies are common in mixed connective tissue disease. *J Rheumatol* 2002;29(3):487–9.

40. Bennett RM, O'Connell DJ. The arthritis of mixed connective tissue disease. *Ann Rheum Dis* 1978;37(5):397–403.

41. Wigley FM, Lima JAC, Mayes M, McLain D, Chapin JL, Ward-Able C. The prevalence of undiagnosed pulmonary arterial hypertension in subjects with connective tissue disease at the secondary health care level of community-based rheumatologists (the UNCOVER study). *Arthritis Rheum* 2005;52(7):2125–32.

42. Kozuka T et al. Pulmonary involvement in mixed connective tissue disease: High-resolution CT findings in 41 patients. *J Thorac Imaging* 2001;16(2):94–8.

43. Ungprasert P et al. Cardiac involvement in mixed connective tissue disease: A systematic review. *Int J Cardiol* 2014;171(3):326–30.

44. Kitridou RC, Akmal M, Turkel SB, Ehresmann GR, Quismorio FP, Massry SG. Renal involvement in mixed connective tissue disease: A longitudinal clinicopathologic study. *Semin Arthritis Rheum* 1986;16(2):135–45.

45. Bennett RM. Mixed connective tissue disease and overlap syndromes. In: Harris ED et al. (Eds), *Textbook of Rheumatology*. 7th ed. Philadelphia: WB Saunders; 2004:1241.

46. Kameda T et al. A case of catastrophic antiphospholipid syndrome, which presented an acute interstitial pneumonia-like image on chest CT scan. *Mod Rheumatol* 2015;25(1):150–3.

47. Komatireddy GR, Wang GS, Sharp GC, Hoffman RW. Antiphospholipid antibodies among anti-U1-70 kDa autoantibody positive patients with mixed connective tissue disease. *J Rheumatol* 1997;24(2):319–22.

48. Oh YB et al. Mixed connective tissue disease associated with skin defects of livedoid vasculitis. *Clin Rheumatol* 2000;19(5):381–4.

49. Lee JM, Kim I-H. Case series of recalcitrant livedoid vasculopathy treated with rivaroxaban. *Clin Exp Dermatol* 2016;41(5):559–61.

50. Weishaupt C et al. Anticoagulation with rivaroxaban for livedoid vasculopathy (RILIVA): A multicentre, single-arm, open-label, phase 2a, proof-of-concept trial. *Lancet Haematol* 2016;3(2):e72–79.

51. Bennett DD, Ohanian M, Cable CT. Rituximab in severe skin diseases: Target, disease, and dose. *Clin Pharmacol Adv Appl* 2010;2:135–41.

52. Zeni P, Finger E, Scheinberg MA. Successful use of rituximab in a patient with recalcitrant livedoid vasculopathy. *Ann Rheum Dis* 2008;67(7):1055–6.

53. Calistru AM, Lisboa C, Cruz MJ, Delgado L, Poças L, Azevedo F. Hypocomplementemic urticarial vasculitis in mixed connective tissue disease. *Dermatol Online J* 2010;16(12):8.

54. Rozin AP et al. Large leg ulcers due to autoimmune diseases. *Med Sci Monit Int Med J Exp Clin Res* 2011;17(1):CS1–7.

55. Goolamali SI, Gordon P, Salisbury J, Creamer D. Subcutaneous calcification presenting in a patient with mixed connective tissue disease and cutaneous polyarteritis nodosa. *Clin Exp Dermatol* 2009;34(5):e141–144.

56. Reiter N, El-Shabrawi L, Leinweber B, Berghold A, Aberer E. Calcinosis cutis: Part II. Treatment options. *J Am Acad Dermatol* 2011;65(1):15–22, quiz 23–24.

57. Alarcón-Segovia D, Cardiel MH. Comparison between 3 diagnostic criteria for mixed connective tissue disease. Study of 593 patients. *J Rheumatol* 1989;16(3):328–34.

58. Alarcon-Segovia D, Villarreal M. Classification and diagnostic criteria for mixed connective tissue disease. In: Kasukawa R, Sharp GC (Eds), *Mixed Connective Tissue Disease and Anti-Nuclear Antibodies*. Amsterdam: Elsevier Science Publishers (Biomedical Division); 1987: 33e40.

PART 11

Systemic Emergencies Presenting with Dermatological Signs

G. K. SINGH

44

Dermatological manifestations of renal failure

G. K. SINGH AND N. S. BENIWAL

INTRODUCTION

Chronic kidney disease is defined as either kidney damage or decreased kidney function (decreased glomerular filtration rate [GFR]) for 3 or more months. The National Kidney Foundation defines kidney failure as either (a) GFR less than 15 mL/min per 1.73 m^2, which is accompanied in most cases by signs and symptoms of uremia, or (b) a need to start kidney replacement therapy (dialysis or transplantation). Kidney failure is not synonymous with end-stage renal disease (ESRD) [1]. Chronic kidney disease is a universal public health problem. The data from the United States show a rising trend of incidence and prevalence. The number of persons with kidney failure who are treated with dialysis and transplantation has increased from 340,000 in 1999 to 651,000 in 2010 [2].

CUTANEOUS MANIFESTATIONS

Acute renal failure does not cause any skin changes. Chronic kidney failure is the persistent accumulation of toxic metabolic products that have failed to clear from the body system producing varied forms of skin conditions. Dermatological manifestations of chronic renal failure are not uncommon in clinical practice. In a study by Pico et al., all of the patients with CRF had one or more skin manifestations [3]. Chronic renal failure (CRF), irrespective of its cause, often produces specific skin changes that can develop long before failure manifests clinically. Few of the cutaneous problems pose serious impacts on the quality of life of patients. Characteristic dermatological manifestations usually seen in CRF are highlighted in the following section.

CLASSIFICATION OF CUTANEOUS MANIFESTATIONS

Traditionally, cutaneous problems in CRF are divided into two categories: nonspecific and specific cutaneous disorders. Nonspecific disorders include xerosis (Figure 44.1), pigmentary disorders, pruritus, and half-and-half nail. Specific disorders include acquired perforating dermatosis, calciphylaxis, bullous dermatoses, and nephrogenic fibrosing dermopathy [4].

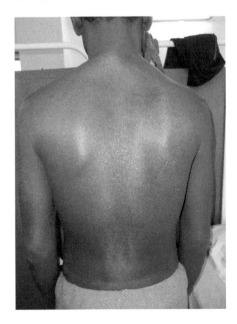

Figure 44.1 A case of xerosis. Generalized fine scaling and dryness of the body are seen in patient of chronic kidney disease.

There are many underlying disease conditions that may lead to ESRD; they may have distinct cutaneous signs by themselves. Similarly, patients with uremia and patients undergoing renal transplant will have unique cutaneous signs. Thus, more scientifically, dermatological manifestations of CRF can also be classified into three broad categories:

1. Dermatological manifestations of diseases associated with the development of ESRD
2. Dermatological manifestations of uremia
3. Dermatological disorders associated with renal transplantation

DERMATOLOGICAL MANIFESTATIONS OF DISEASES ASSOCIATED WITH END-STAGE RENAL DISEASE

There are many underlying diseases that can ultimately lead to ESRD. They are depicted in Table 44.1 along with their dermatological manifestations [4–8]. It is electrolyte imbalance, accumulation of uremic substances, and comorbid diseases that are commonly implicated in the pathogenesis of the cutaneous manifestations of ESRD.

DERMATOLOGICAL MANIFESTATIONS OF UREMIA

State-of-the-art dialysis and renal transplantation cannot substitute for a natural healthy kidney in terms of clearing toxic substances and performing other essential metabolic functions of the kidney. Most patients with ESRD develop significant metabolic abnormalities that are directly related to the loss of kidney function, e.g., metabolic acidosis, anemia, alteration in calcium-phosphate homeostasis, hyperparathyroidism, hyperlipidemia, and glucose intolerance. In the long run, uremic patients develop dermatological manifestations including xerosis, pruritus, pigmentary alteration, half-and-half nails, alopecia, uremic frost, porphyria cutanea tarda, and arterial steal syndrome [4,5,6]. Nonspecific dermatological manifestations, their clinical pictures, and their management are described in brief in Table 44.2. Specific dermatological manifestations of uremia are described in the following sections.

Acquired perforating dermatosis

This comprises a heterogeneous group of dermatoses characterized by transepidermal elimination of dermal

Table 44.1 Systemic diseases causing end-stage renal disease with their renal involvement and dermatological manifestations

Underlying systemic disease	Renal disease	Dermatological manifestations
Diabetes mellitus [9]	Diabetic nephropathy	Diabetic dermopathy, necrobiosis lipoidica, acanthosis nigricans, eruptive xanthoma, Kyrle disease, scleredema, cutaneous changes of pruritus such as excoriation
Systemic lupus erythematosus (SLE) [10,11]	Glomerulonephritis, nephrotic syndrome	Mucosal ulcers, photosensitivity, malar rash, discoid rash, hair loss, purpuric lesions, vasculitic lesions, skin lesions of chronic cutaneous lupus and subacute cutaneous lupus, tumid lupus, SLE-associated neutrophilic skin lesions
Henoch–Schönlein purpura [4,5]	Vasculitis, glomerulonephritis	Palpable purpura
Wegener granulomatosis [12,13]	Vasculitis, glomerulonephritis	Palpable purpura, subcutaneous nodules, ulcers
Polyarteritis nodosa [14]	Vasculitis, glomerulonephritis	Palpable purpura, subcutaneous nodules, ulcers
Subacute bacterial endocarditis	Renal emboli, glomerulonephritis	Purpura, petechiae
Cholesterol emboli [15]	Renal emboli	Petechiae, livedo reticularis, blue toes
Hepatitis C virus [16,17]	Glomerulonephritis	Purpura, lichen planus, porphyria cutanea tarda, cutaneous polyarteritis nodosa, necrolytic acral erythema, sclerodermatous plaques
Human immunodeficiency virus (HIV) [18]	HIV-associated nephropathy	Eosinophilic folliculitis, oral hairy leukoplakia, bacillary angiomatosis, Kaposi sarcoma
Systemic sclerosis [19]	Malignant hypertension	Diffuse scleroderma
Amyloidosis [20]	Nephritic syndrome	Purpura, macroglossia
Fabry disease [6]	Nephritic syndrome	Angiokeratoma
Nail-patella syndrome [6,7]	Renal tubular defects	Absent or displaced patella, absent or pitted nails
Tuberous sclerosis [4]	Renal hamartomas, renal cell carcinoma	Adenoma sebaceum, ash leaf macule, shagreen patch, periungual fibromas

Table 44.2 Common nonspecific dermatological manifestations in uremia with their pathogenesis, clinical presentation, and management

Dermatological manifestations	Pathogenesis	Clinical features	Management
Xerosis [6–8]	• Alteration in corneocyte maturation due to uremic condition • Decrease in water content in the epidermis, decrease in sweat volume, atrophy of sebaceous glands, i.e., hypervitamin-A-like state	• In 50%–92% of the dialysis population • Generalized dryness, fine scaling, fissuring, more predominantly involving limbs (Figure 44.1)	Routine use of emollients
Pruritus [6–8,21,22]	• Not fully understood • Proposed causes are xerosis, decreased transepidermal elimination of pruritogenic factors, hyperparathyroidism, hypercalcemia, hyperphosphatemia, elevated histamine levels, increased dermal mast cell proliferation, uremic sensory neuropathy, middle molecule theory (unidentified pruritogenic substances)	• 50%–90% of patients with ESRD • Independent of sex, age, race • May be associated with excoriations, prurigo nodularis, and lichen simplex chronicus • May frequently affect the patient's sleep pattern and psychologic well-being	• Emollients • Augmentation of dialysis efficacy • Normalization of serum calcium and phosphate levels, and parathyroidectomy • Ultraviolet (UV) B phototherapy probably is the most effective • Naloxone and naltrexone • Miscellaneous: cholestyramine and activated charcoal
Pigmentary changes [6–8]	• Lack of erythropoietin causes anemia • Brown pigmentation due to hemosiderin deposition due to iron overload from excessive transfusions • Blackish pigmentation due to increase in melanin production because of increase in ß-melanocyte stimulating hormone	• 25%–70% of the dialysis population • Pallor • Brown to slate-gray discoloration • Brownish hyperpigmentation	Correct anemia for pallor by erythropoietin • Effective dialysis • Photoprotection
Half-and-half nails [6,7,23,24]	Exact mechanism is unknown; one hypothesis is that there is an increased tissue concentration of melanocyte-stimulating hormone	• Characterized by a dark distal band that occupies 20%–60% of the nail bed and by a white proximal band • Not pathognomonic for renal failure • 40% of patients on dialysis	Disappear several months after successful renal transplantation
Alopecia [4,6,7]	Due to chronic telogen effluvium or underlying systemic disease like SLE	• Chronic hair loss leading to diffuse alopecia, thinning of hair, lack of hair lustre	• Treat the underlying disease • Supplement with iron, calcium, vitamins

structures. The perforating disorders seen in ESRD, known as acquired perforating dermatosis (APD), are both clinically and histologically similar to the primary perforating dermatoses [9]. Onset of APD is usually seen after dialysis treatment has started. The prevalence in dialysis patients is between 2% and 11% [25–27].

Usually, patients present with moderate to severe, firm, dome-shaped papules or nodules with a central keratotic plug distributed on the extensor aspects of the extremities, gluteal areas, and trunk (Figure 44.2). Koebnerization is common. Spontaneous resolution may occur in a few cases [9,25–28].

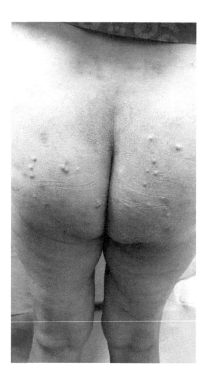

Figure 44.2 A case of acquired perforating disorder.

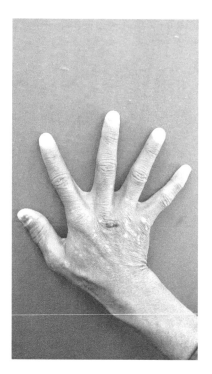

Figure 44.3 A case of porphyria cutanea tarda in a patient of end-stage renal disease.

To date, there is no single effective therapy. Topical mid-potent steroid or potent steroid, steroid with salicylic acid, and retinoid can be tried. Oral antihistamines, retinoid, allopurinol, doxycycline, and minocycline can be given. Other therapies include narrow-band ultraviolet B (UVB), photodynamic therapy, and cryotherapy [25,27,29].

Uremic frost

This is rarely seen nowadays, especially with aggressive management of chronic kidney disease. It is a result of a very high level of blood urea nitrogen (usually >250–300 mg/dL), which leads to the concentration of urea in sweat, which once evaporated results in the deposition of urea crystals on the skin. Clinically seen as fine white-to-yellow crystals that dissolve readily when challenged by a drop of water, it is present commonly on the beard or on other parts of the face, neck, and trunk [4,5].

Porphyria cutanea tarda

Failed kidneys lead to the accumulation of photosensitive metabolites in the skin that, on exposure to ultraviolet light, cause skin fragility and vesiculation. Porphyria cutanea tarda (PCT) is due to deficiency or dysfunction of uropor-phyrinogen-decarboxylase (URO-D). Porphyrins may form complexes with high molecular weight proteins, which are poorly dialyzed by conventional methods. Patients of PCT present with tense vesicles/bullae, erosions, and crusts distributed on the face, extensor surface of the forearms, and dorsal hands (Figure 44.3). Lesions typically heal with atro-phic scarring and milial cysts [4,5,30,31].

Unlike hemodialysis (HD), PCT is uncommonly seen with peritoneal dialysis (PD), most probably because PD achieves more effective clearance of larger metabolites. Increased serum levels of iron and ferritin, increased uri-nary uroporphyrin excretion, and increased levels of plasma uroporphyrin are typical of PCT [30].

Patients of PCT should strictly avoid triggers, like sun exposure, alcohol, and hepatotoxic medications. Applying sunscreen and decreasing iron overload are required for symptomatic management. Small volume phlebotomy (50–100 mL once or twice weekly) that stimulates erythropoi-esis, desferrioxamine to decrease hepatic iron stores, and high-flux membrane hemodialysis can induce remission within several months [31].

Metastatic calcification

Altered calcium/phosphate metabolism in patients of ESRD results in elevated serum levels of calcium, which leads to deposition of calcium salts in the cutaneous and/or subcu-taneous tissues. It can also affect blood vessels and viscera. Clinically it presents as calcinosis cutis or calcific uremic arteriolopathy [32].

CALCINOSIS CUTIS

Patients present with firm white papules/plaques and nod-ules that are most commonly distributed in the periarticu-lar areas and fingertips (Figure 44.4). Periarticular lesions are normally asymptomatic, but lesions on the fingertips are usually painful. A whitish discharge can be seen from these lesions. It is a benign nodular calcification, without tissue

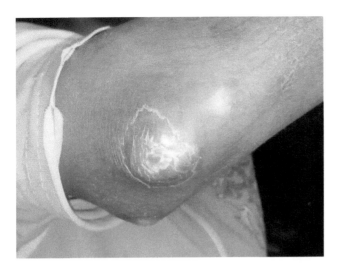

Figure 44.4 A case of calcinosis cutis.

necrosis. Hyperphosphatemia is typical and is secondary to diminished renal clearance of phosphate and inadequate clearance by dialysis. The number and size of lesions correlate with the serum phosphate level. Dietary phosphate restriction, phosphate binders, and parathyroidectomy, if necessary in patients with elevated iPTH levels, may help lower serum phosphate levels. Lesions tend to regress after the hyperphosphatemia resolves [32–35].

CALCIFIC UREMIC ARTERIOLOPATHY

Calcific uremic arteriolopathy (CUA), also known as calciphylaxis, is a rare and potentially life-threatening condition characterized by thrombosis of calcified small and medium-sized arteries and arterioles as well as fibrosis, involving most commonly the dermis and subcutaneous fat [32,36–41]. It has an estimated incidence of 1% and prevalence of 1%–4% in the ESRD population. CUA has a mortality rate of 60%–80%. Death is most commonly secondary to sepsis and organ failure [32]. Metabolic factors, systemic inflammation, oxidative stress, and endothelial injury along with certain triggers have been implicated. Apart from local trauma, other etiological factors include hypoalbuminemia, therapy with calcium salts, vitamin D supplements, erythropoiesis-stimulating agents, warfarin, iron supplements, liver disease, and systemic corticosteroids. Independent risk factors include female sex, Caucasian ethnicity, and obesity (body mass index: 30 kg/m²) [36–38].

Clinically, these lesions present as excruciatingly painful subcutaneous nodules with violaceous mottling, similar to livedo reticularis. These lesions can ulcerate and form eschar as a result of ischemic necrosis (Figure 44.5). They tend to develop over areas that have more subcutaneous fat such as the abdomen, thigh, breast, hip, and shoulder [32,36].

The pathognomonic histological findings of CUA have been described as medial calcification of small arteries and arterioles up to 600 micrometer with intimal hyperplasia, inflammation, endovascular fibrosis, thrombosis, and tissue necrosis. Associated panniculitis can also be present. Close examination, multiple tissue sections, and von Kossa

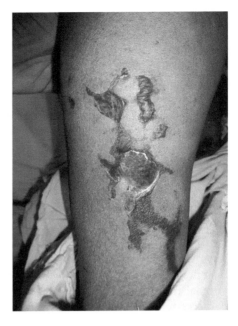

Figure 44.5 A case of calciphylaxis in a patient of end-stage renal disease.

staining, highlighting the calcium deposits, may be required for an accurate diagnosis [36,39].

Patients may present with hypercalcemia, hyperphosphatemia, elevated calcium-phosphate products, and elevated parathyroid hormone (PTH) levels. Bone scintigraphy may be helpful in making the diagnosis as well as in monitoring the treatment.

Treatment of CUA requires a multidisciplinary approach involving avoidance of risk factors/triggers, wound management, antibiotics for infections, and correction of biochemical abnormalities [36,40]. Serum electrolyte levels should be, where possible, maintained at target per National Kidney Foundation guidelines [42].

Lowering the calcium concentration in the dialysate to 1.0–1.5 mEq/L as can be tolerated and intensifying dialysis to four to six times per week; parathyroidectomy if medical management fails; bisphosphonates, both IV and oral preparations, are other treatment options. Sodium thiosulfate, a dialyzable calcium chelator, and hyperbaric oxygen therapy are other modalities available [36,40–42].

Nephrogenic systemic fibrosis

Nephrogenic systemic fibrosis (NSF) is a scleroderma-like disorder caused by exposure to gadolinium-based contrast agents (GBCAs), which are used in diagnostic imaging in the setting of renal failure [43,44]. The rapid development and symmetrical NSF lesions and the proliferation of dermal spindle cells typically seen on biopsy specimens support the pathogenic role of circulating fibroblast in NSF [45]. The initial presentation is severely painful, symmetric erythema and edema that evolve into sclerodermatous and erythematous induration of the skin with firm plaques and nodules, commonly distributed symmetrically on the lower extremities and less often on the arms and trunk. There may be associated hyper- or hypopigmentation of the skin and contracture of adjacent joints, especially of the hands [43,45].

Histological features show dermal fibrosis with thickened collagen bundles, proliferation of dermal spindle cells, increased stromal mucin, and minimal inflammatory infiltrate. The epidermis is usually unaffected, and patients may have abnormal calcification in the dermis and subcutaneous tissue. Fibrosis can extend through the fascia and into the skeletal muscle [43].

Avoiding linear and ionic GBCAs in patients with a GFR of 30 mL/min or less, avoiding high-dose GBCA, and early dialysis after GBCA exposure are some recommendations to prevent NSF [43]. Spontaneous improvement of NSF has been reported in a few cases of acute kidney injury (AKI) [43,45]. Improving renal function seems to slow NSF progression and may improve the signs and symptoms of disease. Post renal transplant, the majority of cases of NSF have had successful outcomes. Treatments with limited benefit include oral corticosteroids, UVA phototherapy, plasmapheresis, sirolimus, high-dose IVIg, methotrexate, pentoxifylline, and extracorporeal photopheresis. Imatinib mesylate and alefacept have been tried with improvement in the disease [43–45].

Arterial steal syndrome

The arterial steal syndrome or dialysis-associated steal syndrome is a rare but quite morbid complication of the vascular access meant for hemodialysis. If proximal shunting of blood is significant, it may lead to distal ischemia. The arteriovenous connection causes a reversal of blood flow through the distal arteries due to a low-pressure system. It presents as pain and numbness. Prolonged ischemia may result in digital gangrene, peripheral neuropathy, or cutaneous atrophy. Patients of peripheral vascular disease and diabetes mellitus are at higher risk for this complication [46].

DERMATOLOGICAL MANIFESTATIONS ASSOCIATED WITH RENAL TRANSPLANTATION

Dermatological signs visible in patients who have undergone renal transplants are either due to adverse effects of immunosuppressive drugs or the immune-compromised state created by the drugs. Almost 50%–100% of renal transplant recipients (RTRs) have transplant-related dermatological manifestations. However, other factors, such as duration following transplantation, geographic region, skin type, and climate, greatly modify the clinical disorders associated with renal transplantation [47].

Adverse effects of corticosteroids include moon facies, buffalo hump, striae distensae, cutaneous atrophy, and telangiectasias (Figure 44.6). These changes may resolve or improve when the corticosteroid dose is reduced, although these cutaneous changes may continue, as steroids are usually used long term.

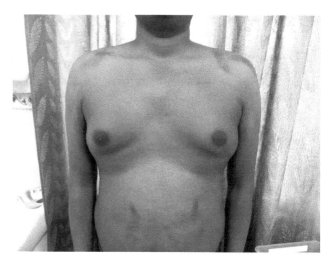

Figure 44.6 Features of Cushing disease.

Adverse effects of cyclosporine include gingival hyperplasia and hypertrichosis. These tend to occur early in the course and improve with time.

Other dermatological features include acne, folliculitis, keratosis pilaris, epidermal cysts, and sebaceous gland hyperplasia.

Immunocompromised state causing infections

Patients are at higher risk for developing opportunistic infections during the first 6 months after transplantation because of the use of higher doses of immunosuppressive agents. The following infections can be seen following renal transplant:

- *Viral infections*: Herpes simplex, varicella-zoster infection, Epstein-Barr virus infection, human papilloma virus causing warts
- *Bacterial infections*: *Staphylococcus aureus*, *Bartonella henselae*, *Mycobacterium tuberculosis*, and atypical mycobacterial
- *Fungal infections*: Superficial mycoses (e.g., dermatophytes, *Pityrosporum* species, candidiasis) and deep fungal infections (e.g., *Aspergillus*, *Cryptococcus*, *Nocardia*, *Rhizopus* species)
- *Parasitic infection*: Scabies. Pityriasis versicolor has been shown to be the most common fungal infection and occurs in 18%–48% of renal transplant recipients [48,49]

Malignancy

The incidence of malignancies proportionately increases with duration of immunosuppressant [50,51]. Incidence of nonmelanoma skin cancer is 20–40 times greater in RTRs than in the general population. The cumulative risk of cutaneous malignancy is 10%–30% at 5 years, 10%–44% at 10 years, and 30%–40% at 20 years. Most malignancies occur on sun-exposed areas and usually are found on the head, neck, and upper extremities. Multiple malignancies are a common occurrence in post-renal-transplant patients, e.g., nonmelanoma skin cancer (squamous cell carcinoma, basal cell carcinoma); Kaposi sarcoma, melanoma; and other malignancies (malignant fibrous histiocytomas, atypical fibroxanthomas, and dermatofibrosarcoma protuberans, Merkel cell carcinoma).

Miscellaneous conditions

Miscellaenous conditions include transfusion-associated graft versus host disease, actinic keratosis, and porokeratosis.

CONCLUSION

Understanding dermatological manifestations of renal failure and chronic kidney disease not only gives clues in the early diagnosis of the disease but also helps in monitoring the cases. On several occasions patients develop skin conditions purely because of administration of new treatment. Knowledge of these dermatological manifestations helps in better understanding the diseases and their management.

KEY POINTS

- Cutaneous manifestations of chronic renal failure form the bulk of these manifestations.
- Nonspecific manifestations include xerosis pigmentary disorders, pruritus, and half-and-half nail.
- Specific disorders include acquired perforating dermatosis, calciphylaxis, bullous dermatoses, and nephrogenic fibrosing dermopathy.
- Features of uremic include xerosis, pruritus, pigmentary alteration, half-and-half nails, alopecia, uremic frost, porphyria cutanea tarda, and arterial steal syndrome.

REFERENCES

1. Levey AS et al. National Kidney Foundation practice guidelines for chronic kidney disease: Evaluation, classification, and stratification. *Ann Intern Med* 2003;139:137–47.
2. United States Renal Data System. Excerpts from the 2000 U.S. Renal Data System Annual Data Report: Atlas of End-Stage Renal Disease in the United States. *Am J Kidney Dis* 2000;36:S1–279.
3. Pico MR, Lugo-Somolinos A, Sanchez JL, Burgos-Calderon R. Cutaneous alterations in patients with chronic renal failure. *Int J Dermatol* 1992;31:860–3.
4. Galperin TA, Cronin AJ, Leslie KS. Cutaneous manifestations of ESRD. *Clin J Am Soc Nephrol* 2014;9(1):201–18.
5. Goldman L, Schafer AI. Chronic kidney disease. In: *Goldman's Cecil Medicine, Expert Consult Premium Edition*. 24th ed. Philadelphia: Elsevier Saunders; 2012.
6. Kurban MS, Boueiz A, Kibbi AG. Cutaneous manifestations of chronic kidney disease. *Clin Dermatol* 2008;26:255–64.
7. US Renal Data System (USRDS). *2015 Annual Data Report: Atlas of Chronic Kidney Disease and End-Stage Renal Disease in the United States*. Bethesda, MD: National Institutes of Health, National Institute of Diabetes and Digestive and Kidney Diseases; 2007. Available at http://www.usrds.org/adr.aspx. Accessed: August 11, 2017.
8. Markova A et al. Diagnosis of common dermopathies in dialysis patients: A review and update. *Semin Dial* 2012;25:408–18.
9. Farrell AM. Acquired perforating dermatosis in renal and diabetic patients. *Lancet* 1997;349(9056):895–6.
10. Tebbe B, Mansmann U, Wollina U, et al. Markers in cutaneous lupus erythematosus indicating systemic involvement. A multicenter study on 296 patients. *Acta Derm Venereol* 1997;77(4):305–8.
11. Lopez-Longo FJ, Monteagudo I, Gonzalez CM, Grau R, Carreño L. Systemic lupus erythematosus: Clinical expression and anti-Ro/SS—A response in patients with and without lesions of subacute cutaneous lupus erythematosus. *Lupus* 1997;6(1):32–9.
12. Walsh JS, Gross DJ. Wegener's granulomatosis involving the skin. *Cutis* 1999;64(3):183–6.
13. Francès C et al. Wegener's granulomatosis. Dermatological manifestations in 75 cases with clinicopathologic correlation. *Arch Dermatol* 1994;130(7):861–7.
14. Sharma A, Sharma K. Hepatotropic viral infection associated systemic vasculitides-hepatitis B virus associated polyarteritis nodosa and hepatitis C virus associated cryoglobulinemic vasculitis. *J Clin Exp Hepatol* 2013;3(3):204–12.
15. Fine MJ, Kapoor W, Falanga V. Cholesterol crystal embolization: A review of 221 cases in the English literature. *Angiology* 1987;38(10):769–84.
16. Daghestani L, Pomeroy C. Renal manifestations of hepatitis C infection. *Am J Med* 1999;106(3):347–54.
17. Chuang TY, Brashear R, Lewis C. Porphyria cutanea tarda and hepatitis C virus: A case-control study and meta-analysis of the literature. *J Am Acad Dermatol* 1999;41(1):31–6.
18. Szczech LA et al. The clinical epidemiology and course of the spectrum of renal diseases associated with HIV infection. *Kidney Int* 2004;66(3):1145–52.
19. Steen VD. Clinical manifestations of systemic sclerosis. *Semin Cutan Med Surg* 1998;17(1):48–54.

20. Noël LH, Zingraff J, Bardin T, Atienza C, Kuntz D, Drüeke T. Tissue distribution of dialysis amyloidosis. *Clin Nephrol* 1987;27(4):175–8.

21. Murphy M, Carmichael AJ. Renal itch. *Clin Exp Dermatol* 2000;25:103–6.

22. Lugon JR. Uremic pruritus: A review. *Hemodial Int* 2005;9:180–8.

23. Lindsay PG. The half-and-half nail. *J Lab Clin Med* 1965;66:892–7.

24. Leyden JJ, Wood MG. The "half-and-half nail": A uremic onychopathy. *Arch Dermatol* 1972;105(4):591–2.

25. Hong SB, Park J-H, Ihm C-G, Kim N-I. Acquired perforating dermatosis in patients with chronic renal failure and diabetes mellitus. *J Korean Med Sci* 2004;19:283–8.

26. Morton CA, Henderson IS, Jones MC, Lowe JG. Acquired perforating dermatosis in a British dialysis population. *Br J Dermatol* 1996;135:671–7.

27. Hari Kumar KV, Prajapati J, Pavan G, Parthasarathy A, Jha R, Modi KD. Acquired perforating dermatoses in patients with diabetic kidney disease on hemodialysis. *Hemodial Int* 2010;14:73–7.

28. Saray Y, Seçkin D, Bilezikçi B. Acquired perforating dermatosis: Clinicopathological features in twenty-two cases. *J Eur Acad Dermatol Venereol* 2006;20:679–88.

29. Weng C-H, Hu C-C, Ueng S-H, Yu C-C, Hui C-Y, Lin J-L, Yang C-W, Hung C-C, Hsu C-W, Yen T-H. Predictors of acquired perforating dermatosis in uremic patients on hemodialysis: A case-control study. *Scientific World J* 2012:158075.

30. Ryali ME, Whittier WL. Bullous skin lesions in a patient undergoingchronic hemodialysis. *Semin Dial* 2010;23:83–7.

31. Balwani M, Desnick RJ. The porphyrias: Advances in diagnosis and treatment. *Blood* 2012;120:4496–504.

32. Zhou Q, Neubauer J, Kern JS, Grotz W, Walz G, Huber TB. Calciphylaxis. *Lancet* 2014;383(9922):1067.

33. Reiter N, El-Shabrawi L, Leinweber B, Berghold A, Aberer E. Calcinosis cutis: Part I. Diagnostic pathway. *J Am Acad Dermatol* 2011;65:1–12.

34. Saliba W, El-Haddad B. Secondary hyperparathyroidism: Pathophysiology and treatment. *J Am Board Fam Med* 2009;22:574–81.

35. Martin KJ, González EA. Prevention and control of phosphate retention/hyperphosphatemia in CKD-MBD: What is normal, when to start, and how to treat? *Clin J Am Soc Nephrol* 2011;6:440–6.

36. Daudén E, Oñate M-J. Calciphylaxis. *Dermatol Clin* 2008;26:557–68.

37. Weenig RH, Sewell LD, Davis MDP, McCarthy JT, Pittelkow MR. Calciphylaxis: Natural history, risk factor analysis, and outcome. *J Am Acad Dermatol* 2007;56:569–79.

38. Fine A, Zacharias J. Calciphylaxis is usually non-ulcerating: Risk factors, outcome and therapy. *Kidney Int* 2002;61:2210–7.

39. Hayashi M, Takamatsu I, Kanno Y, Yoshida T, Abe T, Sato Y; Japanese Calciphylaxis Study Group. A case-control study of calciphylaxis in Japanese end-stage renal disease patients. *Nephrol Dial Transplant* 2012;27:1580–4.

40. Vedvyas C, Winterfield LS, Vleugels RA. Calciphylaxis: A systematic review of existing and emerging therapies. *J Am Acad Dermatol* 2012;67:e253–60.

41. Baldwin C, Farah M, Leung M, Taylor P, Werb R, Kiaii M, Levin A. Multi-intervention management of calciphylaxis: A report of 7 cases. *Am J Kidney Dis* 2011;58:988–91.

42. National Kidney Foundation. K/DOQI clinical practice guidelines for bone metabolism and disease in chronic kidney disease. *Am J Kidney Dis* 2003;42(Suppl 3):S1–201.

43. Zou Z, Zhang HL, Roditi GH, Leiner T, Kucharczyk W, Prince MR. Nephrogenic systemic fibrosis: Review of 370 biopsy-confirmed cases. *JACC Cardiovasc Imaging* 2004;4:1206–16.

44. Elmholdt TR, Pedersen M, Jørgensen B, Søndergaard K, Jensen JD, Ramsing M, Olesen AB. Nephrogenic systemic fibrosis is found only among gadolinium-exposed patients with renal insufficiency: A case-control study from Denmark. *Br J Dermatol* 2011;165:828–36.

45. Introcaso CE, Hivnor C, Cowper S, Werth VP. Nephrogenic fibrosing dermopathy/nephrogenic systemic fibrosis: A case series of nine patients and review of the literature. *Int J Dermatol* 2007;46:447–52.

46. Berman SS et al. Distal revascularization-interval ligation for limb salvage and maintenance of dialysis access in ischemic steal syndrome. *J Vasc Surg* 1997;26(3):393–4.

47. Bottomley MJ, Harden PN. Update on the long-term complications of renal transplantation. *Br Med Bull* 2013;106:117–34.

48. Karuthu S, Blumberg EA. Common infections in kidney transplant recipients. *Clin J Am Soc Nephrol* 2012;7:2058–70.

49. Hogewoning AA et al. Skin infections in renal transplant recipients. *Clin Transplant* 2001;15:32–8.

50. Zwald FO, Brown M. Skin cancer in solid organ transplant recipients: Advances in therapy and management: Part I. Epidemiology of skin cancer in solid organ transplant recipients. *J Am Acad Dermatol* 2011;65:253–61.

51. Laing ME et al. Malignant melanoma in renal transplant recipients. *Br J Dermatol* 2006;155:857.

45

Dermatological manifestations of serious gastrointestinal disorders

G. K. SINGH AND KUNAL GHOSH

INTRODUCTION

As skin is the largest organ of the body, it is known to behave as the "mirror of the body"; subtle cutaneous signs such as icterus, acanthosis, pigmentation, or telangiectasia may give clues to further evaluation of underlying serious gastrointestinal (GI) disorders. The skin can provide significant clues to screen, investigate, diagnose, and formulate management protocols with the help of a GI physician or specialist in internal medicine. These cutaneous manifestations are highly varied, diverse, and can include specific or nonspecific changes [1,2,3]. There are myriad of skin presentations as there are GI diseases; however, for the sake of understanding, dermatological manifestations of GI disorders are described under the following broad headings:

1. Dermatological manifestations of disorders of pharynx, esophagus, and stomach
2. Dermatological manifestations of disorders of intestinal involvement
3. Dermatological manifestations of liver and pancreas disorders
4. Dermatological manifestations of miscellaneous gastrointestinal disorders

DERMATOLOGIC MANIFESTATIONS OF DISORDERS AFFECTING PHARYNX, ESOPHAGUS, AND STOMACH

Systemic sclerosis (scleroderma)

Systemic sclerosis (SSc) causes fibrotic changes not only in the skin but also in the GI tract. The GI tract is the most commonly involved internal organ in SSc. Gastric reflux disease and dysphagia are the two most common GI tract (GIT) symptoms. However, SSc can also cause abdominal distension, obstruction, and features of malabsorption in the long run [4]. In limited systemic sclerosis (LSSc), also known as CREST syndrome (calcinosis, Raynaud phenomenon, esophageal dysmotility, sclerodactyly, telangiectasia), there is esophageal abnormality consisting of decreased and disordered peristalsis [5].

Plummer–Vinson syndrome (Patterson–Brown–Kelly syndrome)

Plummer–Vinson syndrome or sideropenic dysphagia is a rare disease characterized by long-standing intermittent dysphagia, esophageal webs, and iron deficiency anemia. Cutaneous features include atrophic glossitis, angular

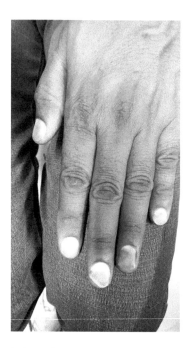

Figure 45.1 Koilonychia.

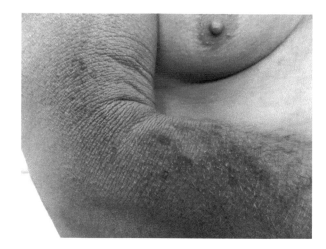

Figure 45.2 Acanthosis nigricans.

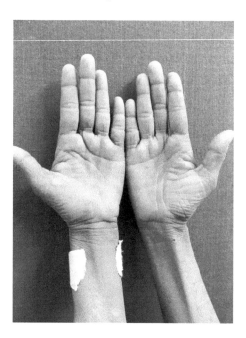

Figure 45.3 Tripe palms.

stomatitis, and koilonychias (Figure 45.1). This is associated with increased risk of squamous cell carcinoma of the esophagus and pharynx. Evaluation of iron deficiency anemia and cineradiography for esophageal webs gives clues to diagnosis. Treatment primarily aims at correcting iron deficiency anemia, which provides prompt resolution of dysphagia. Mechanical dilatation of esophagus and regular follow-up are essential to keep the patient symptom free [6].

Blistering disorders

Mechanobullous disorders and immunobullous disorders present primarily with skin symptoms but may also have systemic involvement. GIT involvement in the form of gastric and esophageal erosions and ulcerations can lead to scarring and stenosis. In epidermolysis bullosa (EB) simplex, children may develop constipation and gastroesophageal reflux, while in junctional epidermolysis bullosa there is chance of failure to thrive and protein-losing enteropathy, and in dystrophic EB there may be constipation [7]. In the long run, patients may develop malabsorption and its associated features on the skin.

Acanthosis nigricans

Acanthosis nigricans (AN) is poorly defined, brown-black, velvety hyperpigmentation predominantly involving the nape of the neck, axillae, forehead, navel, and groin regions. It is a common dermatological finding in obesity and runs in families. However, it may be associated with various systemic conditions including GIT manifestations [8]. The malignancies associated with acanthosis nigricans include adenocarcinoma (85% of cases), of which gastric carcinoma is the most common at 60%. Tripe palm (prominent acanthosis nigricans of palms) can be a first sign of underlying cancer,

especially gastric carcinoma or lung carcinoma [9]. Patients of adenocarcinoma of the stomach with acanthosis and tripe palm are shown in Figures 45.2 and 45.3, respectively. Any patients with rapidly progressive AN lesions, extensive involvement, and weight loss should be screened for diabetes and internal malignancies [10]. Malignant acanthosis nigricans will resolve if the causative tumor is removed.

Acrokeratosis neoplastica (Bazex syndrome)

There are psoriasis-like skin lesions in this syndrome, which most often involves distal extremities but can also occur on the nose and helices of the ears. Acrokeratosis neoplastica is highly associated with malignancy, particularly squamous cell carcinoma of the upper digestive tract. It precedes the detection of malignancy in 65%–70% of cases. So, detailed history, clinical examination, and workup may give an early clue to an internal malignancy [11].

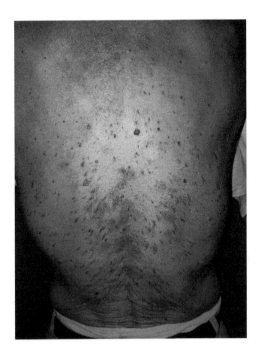

Figure 45.4 Sign of Lesar Trélat.

Seborrheic keratosis

Seborrheic keratosis is characterized by rough, well-demarcated, verrucous plaques with a "stuck-on" appearance. They are commonly seen in elderly people. Rapid development of multiple such lesions might be associated with GI adenocarcinomas. This sign is popularly known as the sign of Leser-Trélat (Figure 45.4) [12]. This sign has been controversial because age is a confounding factor for these cutaneous lesions as well as malignancies. But it gives an early clue in younger patients, who develop rapid increase in the size and number of such lesions or have other features of GIT involvement. Similar to acanthosis nigricans, patients presenting with the sign of Leser-Trélat have a poor prognosis [13,14].

Sister Mary Joseph nodule

The name of this condition originates from the historic observation by Sister Mary Joseph Dempsey, who was the surgical assistant to William J. Mayo. It is characterized by a palpable firm but mobile nodule bulging into the umbilicus and is a manifestation of cutaneous metastasis of internal malignancy. Approximately 90% of these malignancies are adenocarcinomas, with gastric or ovarian being the most commonly discovered primary site. Even carcinoma from the colon and the pancreas can metastasize to the umbilicus [15].

Hereditary hemorrhagic telangiectasia (Osler–Weber–Rendu Syndrome)

This is a rare autosomal dominant disorder characterized by abnormal blood vessel dilatation in skin and mucosae as well as liver, lungs, and brain. The most common and often cardinal clinical presentation is epistaxis. Dermatologic

examination reveals multiple small-sized, sharply demarcated telangiectasias on the face, lips, palate, tongue, ears, chest, or extremities. Diagnosis can be suspected on clinical presentation of recurrent epistaxis, telangiectasia, arteriovenous malformation, visceral lesions, and positive family history. Elevated levels of γ-glutamyltransferase (GGT) or alkaline phosphatase can aid in diagnosis, which can further be confirmed by computed tomography scan or color Doppler [16].

DERMATOLOGIC MANIFESTATIONS OF INTESTINAL DISORDERS

Dermatitis herpetiformis as manifestation of celiac disease

Celiac disease is an autoimmune, gluten-dependent enteropathy, manifesting in genetically predisposed individuals. The disease shows a strong human leukocyte antigen (HLA) association: more than 90% of patients express the HLADQ ($\alpha 1*501,\beta 1*02$) heterodimer, i.e., HLA-DQ2, and almost all the remainder have HLA-DQ8 [2,3].

The clinical manifestations of celiac disease are caused by the inability to absorb gluten from the diet. Patients develop weight loss, diarrhea, bloating, and steatorrhea. In the long run it causes malabsorption, eventually leading to iron or folate-deficient anemia. The most common skin manifestation is dermatitis herpetiformis. Other skin diseases that have been described in the context of celiac disease include aphthous stomatitis, urticaria, hereditary angioedema, cutaneous vasculitis, erythema nodosum, and erythema elevatum diutinum [17,18].

Dermatitis herpetiformis (DH) presents with an extremely pruritic rash with microvesicles or excoriation marks on extensor aspects of the body. There is characteristic granular deposition of IgA within the dermal papillae on direct immunofluorescence. Patients may have elevated serum IgA antibodies against transglutaminase 2 and 3. All patients with DH have demonstrable pathologic changes of celiac disease on small intestinal biopsy, while 20% of patients with DH have a clinically overt celiac disorder [17].

For diagnosis, a high index of suspicion is required, which can be subsequently confirmed by serological tests for antigliadin, tissue transglutaminase, and antiendomysial antibodies. Intestinal biopsies and upper GI endoscopy further aid in diagnosis. Management includes adoption of a gluten-free diet, with avoidance of foods such as wheat, barley, and rye. Therapy with dapsone or sulfapyridine results in a dramatic improvement in both GI and dermatologic symptoms; a prompt improvement following therapy can also confirm the diagnosis [19].

Henoch–Schönlein purpura

Henoch–Schönlein purpura (HSP), which is also known as anaphylactoid purpura or IgA vasculitis, is a small vessel vasculitis that manifests clinically as palpable purpura, arthralgia, abdominal pain, and renal involvement (hematuria, proteinuria, or glomerulonephritis). It generally occurs in early childhood, but it also can present in late adulthood. Most HSP patients respond well to systemic corticosteroids [20].

Inflammatory bowel disease

Crohn disease (CD) and ulcerative colitis (UC) are two principal types of inflammatory bowel disease (IBD). There are distinct differences between these two types of IBD: UC is restricted to the colon, whereas CD can involve the entire GIT; UC is associated with HLA-B27 and smoking, while CD is not; CD is TH1 mediated, while UC is a TH2-mediated disease [2,3,21]. Dermatologic involvement in IBD can be grouped into four categories as depicted in Table 45.1. Direct involvement of skin and mucosa are common in CD, whereas these are rare in UC. The most commonly

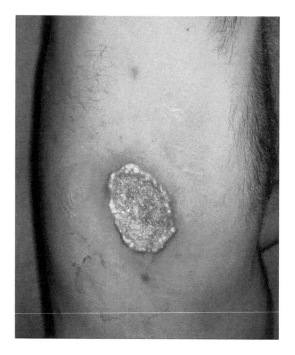

Figure 45.5 Pyoderma gangrenosum.

associated skin lesions are erythema nodosum and pyoderma gangrenosum (Figure 45.5), which also are markers of disease activity (more seen in UC). Oral aphthous ulcers are more common in CD [21].

Bowel-associated dermatosis arthritis syndrome

Also known as bowel bypass syndrome, BADAS has been linked with IBD, diverticulitis, and gastrectomy. BADAS patients present with flu-like symptoms, polyarthralgia, myalgia, and cutaneous lesions. Skin lesions usually start with erythematous macules evolving into papulopustular lesions predominantly affecting the upper chest and extremities [2,3,21].

Whipple disease

Whipple disease, caused by bacterium *Tropheryma whipplei*, is a rare systemic disorder primarily involving the small intestine. The most common cutaneous sign is diffuse hyperpigmentation in photo-exposed areas. Erythroderma, purpura, vasculitis, panniculitis, and urticaria can be other cutaneous manifestations although they are very rare. Affected patients may have abdominal pain, diarrhea, and malabsorption in the advanced stage. Neurological, ophthalmic, cardiac, or pleural involvement has also been seen in advanced disease [22]. Diagnosis can further be confirmed by demonstration of periodic acid-Schiff (PAS) positive particles in duodenal endoscopy biopsy, by immunohistochemistry, or polymerase chain reaction [23]. An appropriate antibiotic such as penicillin, tetracycline, or cotrimoxazole for 1–2 years can alleviate the disease process.

Table 45.1 Cutaneous manifestations of inflammatory bowel disease

Specific lesions (reflect direct skin involvement, found only in Crohn disease [CD])	1. Direct skin and mucosal involvement • Anal tags, perianal abscesses, fissures, fistula (perianal and abdominal), watering-can perineum • Oral lesions: aphthous ulcers, granulomatous infiltrates, angular cheilitis 2. Cutaneous CD at distant site having histological picture of CD
Reactive lesions (seen in both CD and ulcerative colitis [UC])	Erythema nodosum, pyoderma gangrenosum, Sweet syndrome, pyodermatitis–pyostomatitis vegetans, cutaneous polyarteritis nodosa, leukocytoclastic vasculitis, thrombosis, oral aphthous ulcers
Associated lesions	Psoriasis, epidermolysis bullosa acquisita, hidradenitis suppurativa, erythema multiforme, vitiligo, lichen planus, secondary amyloidosis, linear IgA disease, urticaria, bowel-associated dermatosis arthritis syndrome
Complications or treatment related	Anti-TNF inhibitor induced psoriasis, immunosuppressant-induced cancer, acrodermatitis enteropathica

Source: Shah KR et al. *J Am Acad Dermatol* 2013;68:189.e1–21, quiz 210; Thrash B et al. *J Am Acad Dermatol* 2013;68:211. e1–33; quiz 244–6.

Intestinal polyposis

Hereditary conditions account for about 15% of colorectal cancers worldwide. There are multiple disorders having hereditary GI cancers with cutaneous manifestations. This includes familial adenomatous polyposis (FAP), hereditary nonpolyposis colon cancer (Muir-Torre; Lynch syndrome), Peutz-Jeghers syndrome (PJS), juvenile polyposis syndrome (JPS), Cowden syndrome, Bannayan-Riley-Ruvalcaba syndrome, and Cronkhite-Canada syndrome (CCS) [1]. Distinct skin manifestations of these syndromes give clues to the underlying disease and therefore have important roles in prompt diagnosis. Few details regarding their etiology, cutaneous manifestations, and GI features are summarized in Table 45.2.

Hypertrichosis lanuginosa

Acquired hypertrichosis lanuginosa, which consists of abnormal and excessive growth of fine lanugo hair, can be associated with an underlying malignancy, especially colorectal cancer (Figure 45.6). This condition may regress with removal of the tumor [28].

DERMATOLOGIC MANIFESTATIONS OF LIVER AND PANCREAS DISORDERS

Dermatological manifestations related to the hepatobiliary system and pancreas are not uncommon in a routine clinical setting. These disorders are usually associated with a constellation of specific or nonspecific mucocutaneous signs. Acute damage to the liver is most often due to viral hepatitis, alcohol, or hepatotoxic drugs. Initial cutaneous signs may be absent or just may be jaundice. In most cases, only pruritus with marks of excoriation can be early features of obstructive jaundice. Hepatitis B virus (HBV) and hepatitis C virus (HCV) are two important viruses that can have acute as well as chronic liver damage. These viruses themselves have been associated with

Table 45.2 Hereditary gastrointestinal cancers with their etiology and cutaneous manifestations

Syndrome	Inheritance pattern, gene involved, chromosome location	Cutaneous manifestations	Gastrointestinal (GI) involvement	Malignancies associated
Peutz-Jeghers syndrome [24]	AD, *STK11* (a tumor suppressor), 19p13.3	Pigmented macules involving oral mucosa, perioral area, face, and tongue	Hamartomatous polyps throughout GI tract, predominantly involving small intestine	Possibly increased incidence of GI neoplasia
Muir-Torre syndrome [25]	AD, DNA mismatch repair (MMR) genes	Sebaceous neoplasia and multiple keratoacanthoma	• Colonic polyposis in only approximately half the cases • Possibility of various GI malignancies	Multiple low grade visceral cancers possible, for instance, lymphomas, genitourinary tract
Gardner syndrome/ Familial adenomatous polyposis (FAP) [26]	AD, *APC*, 5q21-q22	Epidermoid cysts, lipomas, fibromas, desmoid tumors, pilomatricomas	Widespread colorectal polyps	Adenocarcinoma colon is dreaded complication
Cowden syndrome (GS) (Multiple hamartoma syndrome) [27]	AD, *PTEN*, 10q23.31	Multiple periorbital or perioral papules (trichelemmomas) Cobblestoning of oral mucosa	Polyps throughout GI tract	Can be associated with fibrocystic disease of breast and thyroid tumors
Bannayan-Riley-Ruvalcaba syndrome	Overlapping to genitourinary system	Vascular malformations, lipomatosis, speckled lentigines of the penis and vulva, facial acanthosis nigricans–like lesions, and multiple acrochordons	Polyps throughout GI tract	Unlike CS is not associated with an increased risk of malignancy, being *PTEN* associated disease require regular GI screening of cancers
Cronkhite-Canada syndrome	Not understood, however associated with few autoimmune disease	Nail dystrophy, alopecia, onycholysis, onychomadesis, diffuse macular hyperpigmentation	Diarrhea, significant weight loss, and abdominal pain	Transformation into malignancies reported

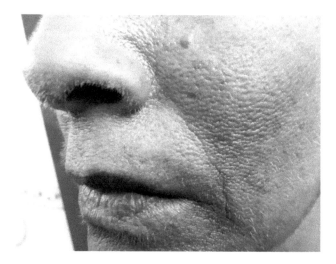

Figure 45.6 Hypertrichosis lanuginose.

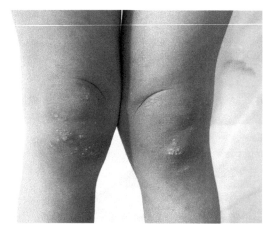

Figure 45.7 Gianotti-Crosti syndrome with grouped papules on extensor aspect of both knees.

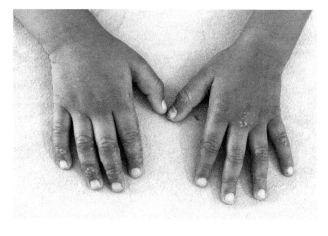

Figure 45.8 Gianotti-Crosti syndrome manifesting as grouped papules on dorsum of hands.

dermatoses such as urticaria, erythema multiforme, Gianotti-Crosti syndrome (Figures 45.7 and 45.8) [30], mixed cryoglobulinemia, lichen planus, and dermatomyositis [2,3,29,20]. Liver cell failure can lead to a constellation of signs such as icterus; spider nevus; other telangiectasias; dilated abdominal wall veins (caput medusa); palmar erythema; parotidomegaly; Terry nails (white nail bed); Muehrcke nails (transverse white bands); sparse axillary, pubic, and pectoral hair; gynecomastia; and striae distensae.

Hemochromatosis

Hemochromatosis, which is also known as *Bronze diabetes*, is a disorder of iron overload leading to iron deposition in multiple body organs, including the liver, pancreas, and skin. Classically it is described as a triad of liver cirrhosis, diabetes, and bronze skin pigmentation. Hepatomegaly is the most common GI finding. Pigmentation of skin is a metallic gray or bronze-brown color that is generally diffuse, but it may be prominent in areas of scars or on the face, neck, extensors of upper extremities, and genitalia. Other important cutaneous signs may be skin atrophy, ichthyosis, partial hair loss (most often in the pubic region), and koilonychia [31]. Clinically there may be features of liver cell failure; however, even in advanced stages there is no derangement in liver enzymes. Cirrhosis followed by hepatocellular carcinoma is a long-term complication when left untreated. Phlebotomy and chelating agents are available therapies [32].

Porphyria cutanea tarda

Porphyria cutanea tarda (PCT) is the most common subtype of porphyria occurring in adults. Decreased activity of the enzyme uroporphyrinogen decarboxylase (UROD), the fifth enzyme in the heme biosynthetic pathway, is the cause of PCT. Skin findings include photosensitivity, skin fragility, poikiloderma, facial hypertrichosis, blistering, and scarring with milia formation predominantly in sun-exposed areas. There are many aggravating factors including HCV infection, alcohol, estrogen, iron, hemochromatosis, etc. [33,34]. Management involves removal of possible triggers (alcohol, estrogen, iron deficiency) along with chloroquine, hydroxychloroquine, and phlebotomy. Skin care should be emphasized with a liberal application of sunscreen and moisturizers [2,3].

Lichen planus

Lichen planus, which is an idiopathic inflammatory condition, has been linked to various hepatic ailments. HBV, HCV, and primary biliary cirrhosis have been associated with increased incidence of lichen planus [2,3,35].

Pancreatitis

Purpura, bruising, and jaundice may occur in patients with acute pancreatitis, but none of these are specific for pancreatitis. The tracking of hemorrhagic fluid in interfascial defect produces purpura or bruise. Classically Grey Turner sign manifests as bruise in the left flank due to left-sided acute pancreatitis. However, there are many sites of retroperitoneal hemorrhage, such as splenic rupture, ectopic pregnancy, metastatic tumor, or aortic aneurysm, that may mimic acute pancreatitis. Patients of pancreatitis may also have dermatological signs related to their etiological conditions, e.g., alcohol abuse, hepatic cirrhosis, or xanthomas due to hypertriglyceridemia [36].

Trousseau syndrome

Trousseau syndrome or Trousseau sign of malignancy consists of migratory thrombophlebitis of superficial veins that can be an early sign of gastric or pancreatic cancer. Migratory thrombophlebitis presents as inflamed, erythematous, tender subcutaneous nodules migrating across the upper trunk and extremities. Trousseau syndrome usually resolves with management of the underlying malignancy [36,37].

Necrolytic migratory erythema

This is the cutaneous manifestation of the glucagonoma syndrome, which results from a glucagon-secreting α-cell tumor of the pancreas. It presents as annular patches of erythema that forms vesicles or bullae which over a period get eroded and crusted. All stages of lesions, from patches, to vesicles, to crusts, may be seen synchronously. The lesions can be pruritic or painful and are commonly distributed over the perioral region, lower abdomen, buttocks, groin, and lower legs. Apart from elevated serum glucagon levels, the clinical spectrum also includes diarrhea, weight loss, weakness, thrombosis, and psychiatric disturbances [38].

DERMATOLOGIC MANIFESTATIONS OF MISCELLANEOUS GASTROINTESTINAL DISORDERS

Long-term involvement of the GIT can lead to malabsorption of many essential nutrients, vitamins, and minerals that are vital for the body's function. Scurvy, pellagra, and acrodermatitis enteropathica are known diseases that occur due

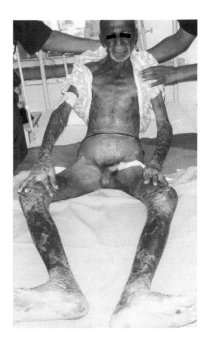

Figure 45.9 Pellagra.

to deficiencies of ascorbic acid, niacin, and zinc, respectively. These disorders have distinct cutaneous features. Perifollicular hyperkeratotic papules, corkscrew hairs, petechiae, ecchymosis, splinter hemorrhages of the nails, bleeding of the gingiva, poor wound healing, and alopecia are characteristic cutaneous signs of scurvy [39]. Photosensitive dermatitis, perineal lesions, and thick hyperpigmented skin over bony prominences are characteristic cutaneous lesions of pellagra (Figure 45.9). However, it is better known by the 4D's, i.e., diarrhea, dermatitis, dementia, and death, usually presenting sequentially in that order [40]. In acrodermatitis enteropathica, cutaneous lesions start as erythematous scaly patches and plaques similar to eczema, but progress to develop erosions and crusts mainly affecting perioral and perianal areas [41]. Patients also

Table 45.3 Rare genetic gastrointestinal (GI) disorders having features of GI bleed with their cutaneous manifestations

Disorder	Cutaneous manifestations	GI findings	Other important features
Pseudoxanthoma elasticum	Yellow papules arranged in linear/reticulate pattern (plucked chicken appearance) involving neck, intertriginous regions	Upper and lower GI bleed	Hypertension, uterine hemorrhage, angioid streaks in eyes
Blue rubber bleb nevus syndrome	Soft bluish subcutaneous venous malformation	GI hemangioma, GI bleed	Other vascular malformation like central nervous system (CNS), lungs
Ehlers–Danlos Syndrome	Hyperelastic fragile skin; frequent bruising	GI bleed due to arterial rupture or intestinal perforation	Hyperextensibility of joints, acrogeric facies
Malignant atrophic papulosis (Degos disease)	Pale red papules with central necrosis in early phase, whereas atrophic ivory scars in later stage	Similar lesions in GI mucosa GI hemorrhage that may be life threatening	Abdominal pain, melena and vomiting; pleuritis, pericarditis, CNS involvement

have diarrhea and hair loss. These conditions show dramatic improvement after supplementing the required deficiencies.

There are many rare, genetic conditions like *elasticum*, blue rubber bleb nevus syndrome, Ehlers–Danlos syndrome, Dowling Degos, etc., which manifest as bleeding from the GIT. They also have distinct cutaneous features [42–45]. There are other important systemic features that help in establishing the diagnosis. The summary of such conditions is presented in Table 45.3.

SKIN MANIFESTATIONS OF STOMAS

At many occasions, various GI disorders require formation and maintenance of stomas, e.g., IBD, bowel obstruction, and bowel cancer. While managing stomas, a treating physician can encounter many complications including dermatological ones, e.g., (1) contact dermatitis: irritant as well as allergic which may be due to adhesive plaster, dressing materials, or leakage from the bag; (2) secondary infections, maceration, erosions, and pressure necrosis; (3) pyoderma gangrenosum: common in Crohn disease; and (4) Koebnerization leading to psoriasis and lichen planus [46].

CONCLUSION

There are numerous specific as well as nonspecific cutaneous signs of GI involvement. However, a high index of suspicion and sound knowledge of cutaneous manifestations of GIT can help in prompt diagnosis and planning of subsequent therapies. An interdisciplinary approach is essential to establish the diagnosis, and thorough management can alleviate most of these manifestations.

KEY POINTS

- Systemic sclerosis, blistering disorders and Plummer–Vinson syndromes affect esophagus and can be diagnosed by cutaneous features.
- Bazex syndrome and Lesar Trélat sign are paraneoplastic manifestations.
- Various disorders with intestinal involvement like coeliac sprue, inflammatory bowel disease, whipple's disease and intestinal polyposis can be diagnosed by their cutaneous features.

REFERENCES

1. Rahvar M, Kerstetter J. Cutaneous manifestations of gastrointestinal disease. *J Gastrointest Oncol* 2016;7:44–54.
2. Shah KR et al. Cutaneous manifestations of gastrointestinal disease: Part I. *J Am Acad Dermatol* 2013;68:189.e1–21; quiz 210.
3. Thrash B et al. Cutaneous manifestations of gastrointestinal disease: Part II. *J Am Acad Dermatol* 2013;68:211.e1–33; quiz 244–6.
4. Tian XP, Zhang X. Gastrointestinal complications of systemic sclerosis. *World J Gastroenterol* 2013;19(41):7062–8.
5. Gilliland BC. Systemic sclerosis. In: Braunwald E et al. (Eds), *Harrison's Principles of Internal Medicine*. 14th ed. New York: McGraw-Hill; 1998:1888–95.
6. Hoffman RM, Jaffe PE. Plummer-Vinson syndrome. A case report and literature review. *Arch Intern Med* 1995;155(18):2008–11.
7. Freeman EB et al. Gastrointestinal complications of epidermolysis bullosa in children. *Br J Dermatol* 2008;158(6):1308–14.
8. Singh GK, Sen D, Mulajkar DS, Suresh M. Acanthosis nigricans associated with transitional cell carcinoma of urinary bladder. *Indian J Dermatol* 2011;56:722–5.
9. Cohen PR, Grossman ME, Almeida L, Kurzrock R. Tripe palms and malignancy. *J Clin Oncol* 1989;7(5):669–78.
10. Longshore SJ, Taylor JS, Kennedy A, Nurko S. Malignant acanthosis nigricans and endometrioid adenocarcinoma of the parametrium: The search for malignancy. *J Am Acad Dermatol* 2003;49(3):541–3.
11. Ljubenovic MS, Ljubenovic DB, Binic II, Jankovic AS, Jovanovic DL. Acrokeratosis paraneoplastica (Bazex syndrome). *Indian J Dermatol Venereol Leprol* 2009;75(3):329.
12. Kleyn CE, Lai-Cheong JE, Bell HK. Cutaneous manifestations of internal malignancy: Diagnosis and management. *Am J Clin Dermatol* 2006;7(2):71–84.
13. Ginarte M, Sánchez-Aguilar D, Toribio J. Sign of Leser-Trélat associated with adenocarcinoma of the rectum. *Eur J Dermatol* 2001;11(3):251–3.
14. Schwartz RA, Burgess GH. Florid cutaneous papillomatosis. *Arch Dermatol* 1978;114(12):1803–6.
15. Powell FC, Cooper AJ, Massa MC, Goellner JR, Su WP. Sister Mary Joseph's nodule: A clinical and histologic study. *J Am Acad Dermatol* 1984;10(4):610–5.
16. Haitjema T et al. Hereditary hemorrhagic telangiectasia (Osler-Weber-Rendu disease): New insights in pathogenesis, complications, and treatment. *Arch Intern Med* 1996;156(7):714–9.
17. Abenavoli L et al. Cutaneous manifestations in celiac disease. *World J Gastroenterol* 2006;12:843–52.
18. Reunala T. Dermatitis herpetiformis: Coeliac disease of the skin. *Ann Med* 1998;30(5):416–8.
19. Hull CM et al. Elevation of IgA anti-epidermal transglutaminase antibodies in dermatitis herpetiformis. *Br J Dermatol* 2008;159(1):120–4.
20. Kraft DM, Mckee D, Scott C. Henoch-Schönlein purpura: A review. *Am Fam Physician* 1998;58(2):405–8, 411.
21. Huang BL, Chandra S, Shih DQ. Skin manifestations of inflammatory bowel disease. *Front Physiol* 2012;3:13.
22. Fenollar F, Lagier JC, Raoult D. *Tropheryma whipplei* and Whipple's disease. *J Infect* 2014;69(2):103–12.

23. Gunther U et al. Gastrointestinal diagnosis of classical Whipple disease: Clinical, endoscopic, and histopathologic features in 191 patients. *Medicine (Baltimore)* 2015;94(15):e714.

24. Boardman LA et al. Increased risk for cancer in patients with the Peutz-Jeghers syndrome. *Ann Intern Med* 1998;128(11):896–9.

25. Esche C et al. Muir-Torre syndrome: Clinical features and molecular genetic analysis. *Br J Dermatol* 1997;136(6):913–7.

26. Perniciaro C. Gardner's syndrome. *Dermatol Clin* 1995;13(1):51–6.

27. Allbritton J, Simmons-O'Brien E, Hutcheons D, Whitmore SE. Cronkhite-Canada syndrome: Report of two cases, biopsy findings in the associated alopecia, and a new treatment option. *Cutis* 1998;61(4):229–32.

28. Slee PH, van der Waal RI, Schagen van Leeuwen JH, Tupker RA, Timmer R, Seldenrijk CA, van Steensel MA. Paraneoplastic hypertrichosis lanuginosa acquisita: Uncommon or overlooked? *Br J Dermatol* 2007;157(6):1087–92.

29. Ghosn SH, Kibbi AG. Cutaneous manifestations of liver diseases. *Clin Dermatol* 2008;26:274–82.

30. Karakaş M et al. Gianotti-Crosti syndrome in a child following hepatitis B virus vaccination. *J Dermatol* 2007;34:117–20.

31. Yen AW, Fancher TL, Bowlus CL. Revisiting hereditary hemochromatosis: Current concepts and progress. *Am J Med* 2006;119(5):391–9.

32. Chevrant-Breton J, Simon M, Bourel M, Ferrand B. Cutaneous manifestations of idiopathic hemochromatosis. Study of 100 cases. *Arch Dermatol* 1977;113(2):161–5.

33. Herrero C et al. Is hepatitis C virus infection a trigger of porphyria cutanea tarda? *Lancet* 1993;341(8848):788–9.

34. Tsukazaki N, Watanabe M, Irifune H. Porphyria cutanea tarda and hepatitis C virus infection. *Br J Dermatol* 1998;138(6):1015–7.

35. Powell FC, Rogers RS3rd, Dickson ER. Primary biliary cirrhosis and lichen planus. *J Am Acad Dermatol* 1983;9(4):540–5.

36. Lankisch PG et al. Skin signs in acute pancreatitis: Frequency and implications for prognosis. *J Intern Med* 2009;265:299–301.

37. Varki A. Trousseau's syndrome: Multiple definitions and multiple mechanisms. *Blood* 2007;110(6):1723–9.

38. van Beek AP, de Haas ER, van Vloten WA, Lips CJ, Roijers JF, Canninga-van Dijk MR. The glucagonoma syndrome and necrolytic migratory erythema: A clinical review. *Eur J Endocrinol* 2004;151(5):531–7.

39. Hampl JS, Taylor CA, Johnston CS. Vitamin C deficiency and depletion in the United States: The Third National Health and Nutrition Examination Survey, 1988 to 1994. *Am J Public Health* 2004;94:870–5.

40. Hegyi J, Schwartz RA, Hegyi V. Pellagra: Dermatitis, dementia, and diarrhea. *Int J Dermatol* 2004;43(1):1–5.

41. Maverakis E et al. Acrodermatitis enteropathica and an overview of zinc metabolism. *J Am Acad Dermatol* 2007;56(1):116–24.

42. Finger RP et al. Pseudoxanthoma elasticum: Genetics, clinical manifestations and therapeutic approaches. *Surv Ophthalmol* 2009;54(2):272–85.

43. Oksüzoglu BC, Oksüzoglu G, Cakir U, Bayir T, Esen M. Blue rubber bleb nevus syndrome. *Am J Gastroenterol* 1996;91(4):780–2.

44. Castori M et al. Spectrum of mucocutaneous manifestations in 277 patients with joint hypermobility syndrome/Ehlers-Danlos syndrome, hypermobility type. *Am J Med Genet C Semin Med Genet* 2015;169C(1):43–53.

45. Bhagwat PV, Tophakhane RS, Shashikumar BM, Noronha TM, Naidu V. Three cases of Dowling Degos disease in two families. *Indian J Dermatol Venereol Leprol* 2009;75(4):398–400.

46. Duchesne JC, Wang Y, Weintraub SL, Boyle M, Hunt JP. Stoma complications: A multivariate analysis. *Am Surg* 2002;68:961–6.

46

Dermatological manifestations of cardiovascular emergencies

ASEEM SHARMA, O. BIBY CHACKO, AND MADHULIKA MHATRE

INTRODUCTION

Cardiovascular diseases comprise a significantly common set of pathologies, often linked to a grave prognosis. As with other organ systems, they often affect the integumentary system, either as part of the primary pathogenetic mechanism, or an association, or even a sequela. Good knowledge of the same, a high index of suspicion, and prompt diagnosis of the cutaneous lesions may act as a premonition of underlying and ongoing cardiovascular disease.

The manifestations can be classified as general signs of cardiac disease, signs specific to certain conditions and systemic diseases affecting both systems. Treatment of the cardiovascular condition results in remission of the cutaneous signs.

GENERAL CUTANEOUS SIGNS OF CARDIOVASCULAR DISEASE

Edema

Fluid excess in the interstitium causes edema. Peripheral edema is hallmark of cardiovascular disease [1,2]. The dependent areas, viz., the distal lower extremities, the back, and the face (in bedridden patients), are involved initially and can progress to involve the proximal parts as well. A plethora of conditions like right and left heart failure, pulmonary hypertension, myocardial infarction, congenital heart disease, valvular dysfunction, or cardiomyopathies may result in peripheral edema.

MANAGEMENT PEARLS

- Rest for the dependent/affected area, e.g., limb elevation for the extremities
- Reduction in salt intake
- Compression-elastic stockings
- Diuretics in the early stages only
- Angiotensin dopamine converting enzyme inhibitors have definitive role in persistent edema

Cyanosis

Cyanosis occurs as a result of decreased oxygen perfusion or increased desaturated, deoxygenated blood. It is of two types: central and peripheral. Central cyanosis is a marker of congenital heart disease (cyanotic), while peripheral cyanosis may be seen in low-output cardiac failure as a consequence of low blood flow. Treatment of the underlying cause generally corrects this particular sign.

Clubbing

This is defined as a bulbous appearance of the distal curvature of the nail plate, rendering it spongy on palpation. The normal angle between the nail and cuticle becomes convex and clublike. Though classically linked with pulmonary disease, it has been seen in conjunction with endocarditis (of various etiologies) as well as congenital heart disease.

Corneal arcus

A grayish-white lipid deposition involving the periphery (arc) of the cornea is seen mostly in males, especially in the elderly, and with long-standing alcohol abuse. The presence of corneal arcus correlates with cholesterol levels and age, and premature development may indicate familial hypercholesterolemia. Furthermore, studies have suggested that corneal arcus is associated with the presence of atherosclerosis and coronary artery disease [3].

Mitral facies

Associated with mitral stenosis, the mitral facies comprises mild cyanosis of the lips, cheeks, and malar prominences, often with an erythematous or violaceous hue. It results from slight arterial hypoxia owing to pulmonary fibrosis secondary to persistently low cardiac output [4].

Acanthosis nigricans

Acanthosis nigricans (AN) and overlying acrochordons develop as a result of hyperinsulinemia subsequent to persistent hyperglycemia owing to an increase in insulin-like growth factor-1 (IGF-1). Acanthosis, alone, presenting over the face, has been delineated as a marker of metabolic syndrome, aptly termed *facial metabolic melanosis*. The coexistence of acrochordons (skin tags) and acanthosis is also slated to be a marker of the same. Although not a primary marker of emergency, per se, AN has been included in the preview of this chapter, on account of its strong association with syndrome X or metabolic syndrome, which has emerged as the leading cause for ischemic heart disease and sudden cardiac death [5].

MANAGEMENT PEARLS

- Correction of deranged metabolic parameters
- Oral biguanides
- Oral retinoids
- Myoinositol, D-chiro-inositol, α-lipoic acid
- Topical retinoids, keratolytics
- Dermabrasion, erbium:yttrium-aluminum-garnet (Er:YAG) laser ablation [5]

Xanthelasma palpebrarum and others

A special mention is being made of xanthelasma palpebrarum that, even though it is thought of as a marker of dyslipidemia and familial hypercholesterolemia, in more than half of the cases, it is not considered a significant marker for cardiovascular disease. The same goes for eruptive xanthomas and premature canities [6].

SPECIFIC CUTANEOUS MANIFESTATIONS OF CERTAIN CARDIOVASCULAR DISEASES

Stated in the following sections are cardiac diseases and their "specific" cutaneous manifestations.

Diagonal earlobe crease

Synonymous with Frank sign, this association of a diagonal crease over the earlobe (lobule) with coronary artery disease was first reported in 1973 [1]. In a few studies, it has been delineated as an independent marker of coronary artery disease, conferring increased risk of acute myocardial infarction and death secondary to cardiovascular morbidity and mortality

[2]. Significant evidence exists that a systemic microvascular pathology causes end-artery occlusion in the earlobe and heart, confirmed by histologic evidence of small artery arteriosclerosis, generalized elastin loss, and tearing of elastic fibers in the subcutaneous tissue, conferring the anatomical aberration [2].

Infective endocarditis

This is mainly a result of endocardial microbial proliferation. The infection most frequently involves the heart valves, both native and prosthetic, but may also occur on the ventricular septum and on intracardiac devices *in situ*. The characteristic lesion is vegetation, an admixture of platelets, fibrin, and microbe colonies, which adhere to the valves of the heart.

Endocarditis, left untreated, is fatal in an acute setting due to hematogenous spread of microbes and imminent sepsis, whereas in subacute endocarditis, structural damage to the heart valves ensues, resulting in emboli or aneurysms [7].

CUTANEOUS MANIFESTATIONS

These occur as a result of septic emboli and immunological reactions generated by chronic bacterial infection. They include the following:

- *Splinter hemorrhages*: Splinter hemorrhages are subungual, linear, dark-red streaks seen most commonly in the nail bed.
- *Roth spots*: Roth spots are oval to ellipsoid hemorrhages with a clear, pale center seen over the retina.
- *Osler nodes*: Osler nodes are small, tender nodules that develop on the finger or toe pads and persist for a few hours to days.
- *Janeway lesions*: Janeway lesions are polysized hemorrhagic nodules occurring on the palms and soles.
- *Peripheral digital emboli*: Peripheral arterial septic emboli from valvular bacterial endocarditis are also seen. These may result in digital infarcts.

Treatment includes prolonged, bactericidal antibiotics to target the avascular vegetations. Antibiotic selection depends on the susceptibility of the particular organism involved. Surgical management is indicated in cases of cardiac failure secondary to valvular insufficiency, refractory infection due to a surgically removable focus, and life-threatening embolization [8–11].

Acute rheumatic fever

Acute rheumatic fever (ARF) is postinfectious sequela of a group A β-hemolytic streptococcal (GABHS) pharyngitis. In most cases, appropriate preemptive antibiotic treatment of streptococcal pharyngitis prevents ARF [7].

ARF is mediated by an autoimmune response, wherein antibodies directed against group A streptococcal antigens cross-react to similar antigens in human tissue. Symptoms manifest as fever accompanied by migratory polyarthritis, Sydenham's chorea, rash, subcutaneous nodules, and pancarditis.

CUTANEOUS MANIFESTATIONS

a. *Erythema marginatum*: It is one of the first signs to appear and the last to disappear [8,9]. It appears as a nonpruritic, transient, blanching, erythematous plaque with an annular serpiginous margin that involves the trunk and the proximal extremities, while classically sparing the face. It progresses along with central clearing.

b. *Subcutaneous nodules*: They appear after the first weeks of the illness and are persistent for a month. The nodules are small, firm, and painless and most commonly affect the tendons or bony surfaces, particularly the elbows and knees.

Treatment of rheumatic fever is composed of anti-inflammatory agents, namely acetylsalicylic acid, for symptomatic relief of fever and arthritis. The use of corticosteroids is controversial. A 10-day course of oral penicillin V (Phenoxymethyl penicillin) is used for eradication of streptococcal pharyngitis [10]. For prevention of recurrences, continuous antibiotic prophylaxis is started immediately after resolution of the acute episode with parenteral penicillin [12]. Furthermore, patients with valve damage are at risk for bacterial heart infections when undergoing dental procedures and, in these circumstances, require an additional short course of antibiotic prophylaxis other than penicillin [13].

Cholesterol embolization syndrome

Synonymous with atheroembolism, this is a multisystem disease resulting from the disruption of cholesterol crystals from atheromatous plaques over the aorta and other arteries. This fragmented atheromatous material subsequently occludes smaller arteries, hampering tissue and organ perfusion. It occurs spontaneously, following cardiovascular manipulation, and rarely after overzealous thrombolysis [14,15].

CUTANEOUS MANIFESTATIONS

- *Livedo reticularis*: An erythematous to livid-blue, mottled, net, or lace-like discoloration is the classic finding. Other findings include ulceration, cyanosis, purpura, necrosis, gangrene, and painful nodules. Most cases involve the lower extremities and are often symmetrical and bilateral. Treatment of the primary condition (after ruling out vasculitis) causes improvement [14].
- *Hollenhurst plaques*: Evidence of cholesterol emboli in the retinal arteries may be observed on ophthalmologic examination. This is a significant diagnostic clue.
- *Blue-toe syndrome*: Vascular occlusion in the digits, and progression to digital necrosis and gangrene may develop [15].

Treatment involves appropriate supportive care and limb amputation, where indicated. In cases of an identifiable and accessible embolic source, surgical treatment may be used. The use of statins may be considered for their lipid-lowering properties as well as their effect in plaque stabilization. Corticosteroids, rheologics like pentoxifylline, cilostazol, rutoside, calcium dobesilate and flavonoids, and endothelial antagonist iloprost have also been reported to be of therapeutic value [16,17].

Sarcoidosis

This is a multisystem, autoimmune disease, affecting the lungs and skin commonly; cardiac involvement is seen in one-third of patients, and more often than not, it is heralded by cutaneous manifestations that could be specific or nonspecific.

The difference between these is histological, with specific lesions showing the classical noncaseating or "naked" granulomas, and their absence in the latter. Erythema nodosum, or painful erythematous nodules, primarily over the lower limbs, is the hallmark specific lesion. Other specific lesions include lupus pernio, ulcerative, ichthyosiform, Boeck scar and angiolupoid variants, along with classic types, viz., macular, papular, nodular, plaque, annular, lichenoid, verrucous, and psoriasiform lesions.

Lupus pernio, presenting as erythematous to violaceous, often disfiguring plaques over the malar region of the face, specifically signals extracutaneous involvement [18].

Aortic insufficiency

Synonymous with *aortic regurgitation* (AR), it is defined as the regurgitation of blood to the left ventricle from the aorta, during diastole, owing to valve dysfunction, or incompetence. The etiological agents can be grouped into the following:

Primary: Congenital, rheumatic, endocarditis (sequelae), autoimmune disease, trauma, degenerative disease

Secondary: Aortic root dilatation, aorto-annular pathology, postsurgery, senile ectasia, and uncontrolled hypertension [19]

Based on the previously mentioned information, AI can be classified as primary or secondary, and acute or chronic. In developing countries, rheumatic heart disease commonly occurs secondarily to bacterial endocarditis, whereas in first-world countries, the common etiology is localized to aortic root disease. Needless to say, acute disease is associated with mortality, and chronic AR leads to significant morbidity.

CUTANEOUS MANIFESTATIONS

All the signs mentioned, hereinafter, are synchronous with the pulse rate, and are resultant of chronic AR. They can be attributed to a change in the peripheral dynamic, rather than the regurgitant jet into the left ventricle. Due to chronic AR, the systemic arteriolar resistance decreases, thereby increasing the velocity of the flow, and a higher cardiac output, which results in bounding and collapsing peripheral pulsations. They are all clinical markers of aortic regurgitation and resolve with treatment of the same. They are as follows [20]:

Quincke sign: Visible pulsation of the nail bed capillaries, causing pallor (blanching) and erythema (flushing) of the same

De Musset sign: A rhythmic bobbing and nodding of the head

Lighthouse sign: Alternating flushing and blanching of the forehead

Muller sign: Uvular pulsation

Landolfi sign: Alternating dilation and constriction of the pupils

Becker sign: Visible pulsation of retinal arteries (ophthalmoscopic finding)

Ashrafian sign: Pulsatile pseudo-proptosis [19,20]

MANAGEMENT

Patients with mild or moderate AR can usually be managed conservatively, with inotropic agents and calcium channel blockers, unless valvular surgery is indicated for correction of concomitant lesions, such as a markedly dilated aortic root, whereas in severe AR, left ventricular (LV) dysfunction or pronounced LV enlargement are considered as indications for surgery. The role of angiotensin-converting enzyme inhibitors remains to be studied [21].

MULTIORGAN SYSTEM DISEASES AFFECTING BOTH SKIN AND THE HEART

This chapter would be incomplete without the mention of systemic diseases affecting both the integumentary and cardiovascular systems. In this section, the authors aim to tabulate certain such conditions with their common cutaneous and cardiac manifestations, briefly.

Disease	Cutaneous manifestations	Cardiac features
Genetic [22]		
Neurofibromatosis-1 (Von Recklinghausen disease)	Café-au-lait macules (CALMs) Neurofibromas Freckling (flexural, palmoplantar)	Coronary artery disease Hypertension Pulmonary stenosis Pulmonary hypertension
Costello syndrome	Skin laxity Papillomatosis Alopecia Acanthosis nigricans	Cardiomyopathies Cardiac arrhythmias (supraventricular tachycardia, most common)
Noonan syndrome	Lymphedema Cutis verticis gyrata	Fallot tetralogy Atrioventricular septal defects Cardiomyopathies
LEOPARD syndrome	Café-noir spots Lentiginosis	Pulmonary stenosis Cardiomyopathies Electrocardiogram anomalies
Cardiofaciocutaneous syndrome	Keratosis pilaris—all variants Palmoplantar keratoderma Multiple melanocytic nevi	Pulmonary stenosis Cardiomyopathies Atrial septal defects
Carney complex "NAME"	Multiple nevi Ephelides	Atrial myxomas
Carney complex "LAMB"	Lentiginosis Blue nevi Mucocutaneous myxomas	Atrial myxoma
Pseudoxanthoma elasticum	Yellow, waxy flexural papules Skin laxity	Mitral valve prolapse Cardiomyopathies Myocardial infarction Renovascular hypertension Aortic aneurysm
Marfan syndrome	Generalized striae Elastosis perforans serpiginosa Lipoatrophy	Aortic dissection Aortic regurgitation Mitral valvular dysfunction
Ehlers–Danlos	Skin fragility, hyperelasticity Atrophic scarring Ecchymoses Elastosis perforans serpiginosa	Aortic root dilatation Tricuspid regurgitation Aortic dissection
Cutis laxa	Dermatochalasia Inelastic skin	Aortic dilatation Aortic aneurysm Right heart failure

(Continued)

Disease	Cutaneous manifestations	Cardiac features
Homocystinuria	Livedo reticularis	Atherosclerosis
	Malar rash	Coronary artery disease
	Dyspigmentation	Vascular thrombosis
	Nail dystrophy	
	Alopecia	
	Superficial thrombophlebitis	
Hutchinson-Gilford progeria	Premature aging	Premature atherosclerosis
	Wrinkling	Cardiovascular and cerebrovascular accidents
	Alopecia	
	Premature canities	Left ventricular hypertrophy
Naxos disease	Palmoplantar keratoderma (PPK)—diffuse	Arrhythmogenic right ventricular cardiomyopathy
	Woolly hair	
Carvajal syndrome	PPK—striate	Left-sided cardiomyopathy
	Skin fragility	
	Clubbing	
Connective Tissue Disease [23]		
Systemic lupus erythematosus (SLE)	Malar rash	Pericarditis
	Discoid lupus erythematosus	Libman-Sach endocarditis
	Photosensitivity	Pericardial effusion
	Livedo reticularis	Valvular heart disease
	Oral ulceration	Myocardial infarction
	Nail fold capillary changes	
	Alopecia—"lupus hair"	
Scleroderma—limited cutaneous	Raynaud phenomenon	Pulmonary arterial hypertension
	Sclerodactyly	
	Calcinosis cutis	
	Trophic ulcers	
	Telangiectasia	
Diffuse scleroderma	Symmetric skin sclerosis and fibrosis	Arrythmias
	Hidebound skin	Pericarditis
	Pseudo-vitiligo	Cardiomyopathy
	Raynaud phenomenon	Congestive cardiac failure
		Angina pectoris
Relapsing polychondritis	Auricular chondritis	Aorto-arteritis
	Saddle-nose deformity	Complete heart block
	Vasculitis	Aortic aneurysms
	Panniculitis	
Behçet disease	Orogenital aphthosis	Pericarditis
	Vasculitis	Myocarditis
	Acneiform eruptions	Coronary artery aneurysm
	Livedo reticularis	Aortic insufficiency
	Superficial thrombophlebitis	
Miscellaneous [23]		
Amyloidosis—full spectrum of disease	Macular amyloidosis	Congestive heart failure
	Lichen amyloidosis	Arrhythmias
	Pinch purpuras	Atrial fibrillation
		Anteroseptal infarction
Carcinoid syndrome	Cutaneous flushing	Valvular heart disease
	Telangiectasias	Tricuspid regurgitation
	Facial edema	Pulmonary stenosis
Malignant atrophic papulosis (Degos disease)	White atrophic papules with a telangiectatic rim	Cardiopulmonary syndrome
		Pericarditis
Hemochromatosis	Gray-brown mucocutaneous hyperpigmentation	Cardiomegaly
	Ichthyosis	Arrhythmias
	Alopecia	Myocardial infarction
	Koilonychia	Congestive cardiac failure

(Continued)

Disease	Cutaneous manifestations	Cardiac features
Kawasaki disease	Acral erythema, edema, and desquamation Polymorphous exanthema Strawberry tongue Conjunctival and pharyngeal congestion	Coronary arteritis Coronary artery aneurysm

CONCLUSION

Skin has been touted, since evermore, as a mirror of the internal homeostatic milieu. It has proven to be a worthy marker of grave systemic disease, especially of cardiovascular origin. In fact, it may be the only manifestation, thus signaling an impending, underlying disease at an early stage, which could change the outcome of the same. A high index of suspicion should always be kept while examining the integumentary system.

KEY POINTS

- Serious cardiac conditions can have cutaneous manifestations which helps early diagnosis, e.g., Diagonal Earlobe crease.
- Infective endocarditis, acute rheumatic fever and cholesterol embolization syndromes have characteristic cutaneous features by which they can be diagnosed.
- Certain multisystem diseases have associated cutaneous and cardiac features by which they can be diagnosed, e.g., Hemochromatosis, Carney's complex and Marfan's syndrome.

REFERENCES

1. Frank ST. Aural sign of coronary artery disease. *N Engl J Med* 1973;289:327–8.
2. Miric D et al. Dermatological indicators of coronary risk: A case-control study. *Int J Cardiol* 1998;67:251–5.
3. Chambless LE et al. The association of corneal arcus with coronary disease and cardiovascular mortality in the lipid research clinics mortality follow-up study. *Am J Public Health* 1990;80:1200–4.
4. Armstrong GP. Mitral stenosis. *Merck Manual* 2016;2:34–6.
5. Hess PL et al. The metabolic syndrome and risk of sudden cardiac death: The atherosclerosis risk in communities study. *J Am Heart Assoc* 2017;5:61–73.
6. Panda S et al. Facial acanthosis nigricans: A morphological marker of metabolic syndrome. *Ind J Dermatol* 2017;62(6):591–7.
7. Dwivedi S, Jhamb R. Cutaneous markers of coronary artery disease. *World J Cardiol* 2010;2(9):252–69.
8. Moreillon P, Yok-Ai Q. Infective endocarditis. *Lancet* 2004;363:139–49.
9. Li JS et al. Proposed modifications to the Duke criteria for the diagnosis of infective endocarditis. *Clin Infect Dis* 2000;30:633–8.
10. Larbalestier RI et al. Acute bacterial endocarditis: Optimizing surgical results. *Circulation* 1992;86:II 68–74.
11. Van de Rijn I, Zabriskie JB, McCarty M. Group A streptococcal antigens cross-reactive with myocardium: Purification of heart-reactive antibody and isolation and characterization of the streptococcal antigen. *J Exp Med* 1977;146:579–99.
12. Special Writing Group of the Committee on Rheumatic Fever. Guidelines for the diagnosis of acute rheumatic fever: Jones criteria, 1992 update. *JAMA* 1992;268:2069–73.
13. American Academy of Pediatrics. Group A streptococcal infections. In: Pickering LK (Ed), *Report of the Committee on Infectious Diseases*. Itasca, IL: American Academy of Pediatrics; 2003:573–83.
14. Fine MJ, Kapoor W, Falanga V. Cholesterol crystal embolization: A review of 221 cases in the English literature. *Angiology* 1987;38:769–84.
15. Fukumoto Y et al. The incidence and risk factors of cholesterol embolization syndrome, a complication of cardiac catheterization: A prospective study. *J Am Coll Cardiol* 2003;42:211–6.
16. Mann SJ, Sos TA. Treatment of atheroembolism with corticosteroids. *Am J Hypertens* 2001;14:831–4.
17. Elinav E, Chajek-Shaul T, Stern M. Improvement in cholesterol emboli syndrome after iloprost therapy. *BMJ* 2002;324:268–9.
18. Doughan AR, Williams BR. Cardiac sarcoidosis. *Heart* 2006;92(2):282–8.
19. Carabello BA. Vasodilators in aortic regurgitation—What is the evidence of their effectiveness? *N Engl J Med* 2005;35(3):1400–2.
20. Klodas E et al. Optimizing timing of surgical correction in patients with severe aortic regurgitation: Role of symptoms. *J Am Col Cardiol* 1997;30:746–52.
21. Chaliki HP et al. Outcomes after aortic valve replacement in patients with severe aortic regurgitation and markedly reduced left ventricular function. *Circulation* 2002;10(6):2687–93.
22. O'Neill JL, Narahari S, Sane DC, Yosipovitch G. Cardiac manifestations of cutaneous disorders. *J Am Acad Dermatol* 2013;68(1):156–66.
23. McDonnell JK. Cardiac disease and skin. *Dermatol Clin* 2002;20(4):503–11.

47

Dermatological manifestations of pulmonary and neurological emergencies

JATINDER SINGH AND RAJAN SINGH GREWAL

INTRODUCTION

Skin, being the largest single organ of the body, is affected in various systemic illnesses. Many medical emergencies primarily involving the lungs or the neurological system can have cutaneous manifestations. Similarly, various dermatological emergencies or acute skin failure can affect the pulmonary and neurological systems. We provide an overview of both of these conditions in this chapter.

LUNGS AND SKIN

The respiratory system is closely related to skin, as both of these systems are the first ones to face external insult or pathogens. Various pulmonary disorders have characteristic cutaneous manifestations such as yellow nail syndrome, sarcoidosis, and certain vasculitis syndromes, whereas other general features like clubbing and cyanosis can be seen in many respiratory disorders. Similarly, many dermatoses are known to affect the lungs primarily or are complications. In the following text, we discuss how skin changes and lung disease together can present in an emergency. This will help both primary care physicians and intensivists to make quick diagnoses and manage cases prudently.

Skin changes in primary pulmonary emergencies

Cutaneous manifestations of respiratory emergencies commonly encountered in emergency departments or intensive care unit settings are as follows:

Fat embolism syndrome: It is characterized by a classical triad of respiratory distress, altered mental status, and thrombocytopenia, typically presenting within 72 hours of long bone or pelvic fracture. The classic cutaneous manifestation (seen in almost one-third to one-half of patients) is transient petechial eruptions involving upper portions of the body (i.e., upper chest, neck, axillae, conjunctivae) [1]. It results from occlusion and increased fragility of dermal capillaries [2]. The distribution corresponds to fat globules floating in the aortic arch getting embolized to its major branches [2].

Acute miliary tuberculosis: It is defined as hematogenous dissemination of *Mycobacterium tuberculosis* from an internal focus, mostly lung. It consists of 1%–3% of all tuberculosis (TB) cases and is particularly more common in immunocompromised patients. Cutaneous manifestations include multiple discrete bluish-red to skin-colored papules, pustules, and purpuric lesions, and uncommonly, umbilicated vesicles [3–7]. The vesicles may subsequently rupture into an ulcer followed by healing with atrophic scars with a brown halo by the end of the fourth week.

Severe pneumonia: Severe atypical pneumonia, especially that caused by mycoplasmal pneumonia, may present with myriad cutaneous manifestations in addition to respiratory symptoms. Classically erythema multiforme (EM) which presents as target lesions (bull's-eye) has been associated with *Mycoplasma*, especially in children. Various other lesions are associated with it, including erythema multiforme/Stevens-Johnson syndrome/toxic epidermal necrolysis (EM/SJS/TEN), anaphylactoid purpura, urticaria, erythema nodosum (tender erythematous nodules depicting septal panniculitis on shins), papular purpuric gloves and socks syndrome (PPGSS), mucositis, cutaneous vasculitis, subcorneal pustular dermatosis, and Sweet syndrome-like presentation [8].

Birt-Hogg-Dubé (BHD) syndrome: First described in 1977 by the Canadian physicians Birt, Hogg, and Dubé, it is a rare, genetic disorder with the propensity to develop benign skin tumors, lung cysts, and spontaneous pneumothorax. The overall prevalence of spontaneous pneumothorax in BHD varies from 28% to 36%, which can be particularly precipitated by air travel [9–11]. Cutaneous manifestations of BHD include fibrofolliculomas, trichodiscomas, acrochordons, and perifollicular fibromas, which look similar and are described as 2–4 mm skin-colored, smooth, dome-shaped papules that favor the face, neck, and trunk [12]. Cutaneous lesions typically appear in the third and fourth decades of life [13]. The lesions tend to increase in size with age, and males generally have larger and more numerous lesions compared to females [12,13].

Vascular disorders: These are multisystem disorders of unknown etiology that can affect almost any organ in the body. Some small-vessel vasculitides can affect both lungs and skin, occasionally presenting as a medical emergency.

Granulomatosis with polyangiitis or Wegener granulomatosis, which affects the respiratory system (upper and lower) primarily along with kidney and skin, can present with acute-onset epistaxis or hemoptysis. Cutaneous manifestations that are seen in 30%–45% of patients include, but are not limited to, palpable purpura, papules, nodules, plaques, necrotic ulcers especially on legs, oral ulcers, and gingival hyperplasia [14–16].

Similarly, eosinophilic granulomatosis with polyangiitis or Churg-Strauss syndrome can also present as an acute asthmatic attack with vasculitis lesions, urticaria, and reticulate erythema (livedo reticularis). As many as 70% of patients with Churg-Strauss syndrome have cutaneous manifestations. A variety of lesions may be seen, the most common of which are palpable purpura, subcutaneous nodules, urticarial rashes, and livedo reticularis [17].

Pulmonary arteriovenous malformations (PAVMs): Acute dyspnea, hemoptysis, or rarely hemothorax may be the initial presentation of PAVMs. In almost 70% of cases, PAVMs is associated with hereditary hemorrhagic telangiectasia (HHT), also termed Osler–Weber–Rendu syndrome, characterized by mucocutaneous macular telangiectasia with 1–3 mm of diameter that generally appear 10–30 years after epistaxis episodes (two-thirds of patients) [18]. Palms and fingers are the only sites affected in 71% of patients, whereas lips and tongue involvement are seen in 66% [18]. The mucosal lesions usually blanch on pressure and are highly vulnerable to spontaneous rupture and cause bleeding [19].

Anaphylaxis: This is a very common medical emergency worldwide that invariably presents with cutaneous flushing and urticaria in addition to dyspnea and hypotension.

Pulmonary involvement in dermatological emergencies

SJS/TEN complex: Both SJS and TEN are characterized by widespread necrosis of epidermal and mucous membrane mostly secondary to an offending drug. Mortality rates vary from 5% to above 30% depending on the extent of body surface area (BSA) involved [20]. Early pulmonary manifestations, seen in almost 25% of cases, presenting within 1–2 days of rash onset result from bronchial sloughing presenting as dyspnea, which may result in respiratory failure warranting mechanical ventilation [21]. Late features include development of pulmonary edema, bronchiolitis obliterans, infective pneumonitis, and lung atelectasis [21].

Erythroderma: Erythroderma or exfoliative dermatitis is characterized by diffuse erythema, and scaling involving more than 90% of BSA can be caused by a number of conditions including eczemas, psoriasis, drug reactions, lymphomas (cutaneous T-cell lymphoma and others), infections, and certain genodermatoses. High-output cardiac failure resulting in pulmonary edema can be seen in any erythroderma patient [22–24]. Pulmonary involvement closely mimicking pneumonia can be seen in Sézary syndrome or erythrodermic cutaneous T-cell lymphoma [25].

Drug reaction with eosinophilia and systemic symptoms (DRESS): Also called *drug hypersensitivity syndrome,* a potentially life-threatening acute drug reaction, it classically presents after 2–6 weeks of drug intake, resulting in diverse cutaneous manifestations, mostly exanthematous rash. Pulmonary involvement can cause acute interstitial pneumonitis, lymphocytic interstitial pneumonia, pleuritis, and acute respiratory distress syndrome. Minocycline is the most common drug associated with lung involvement [26].

NERVOUS SYSTEM AND SKIN

The skin and the neurological system share a common embryonic origin; thereby many genetic disorders affecting the skin also involve the neurological system, commonly referred to as neurocutaneous syndromes. Many of such genodermatoses, also called phakomatoses, in addition to a number of other acquired infective, inflammatory, or malignant conditions affecting the skin, can present with a neurological emergency such as stroke or seizure. In the following text we briefly discuss such scenarios.

Sturge-Weber syndrome (SWS): It is a congenital condition involving the brain, skin, and eye, characterized by a facial capillary malformation (port-wine stain [PWS]) in the distribution of ophthalmic division of the trigeminal nerve (forehead and/or eyelid) and very rarely maxillary and mandibular distribution of the facial region. Primary neurological symptoms of SWS include seizures, headaches, stroke-like episodes, hemiparesis, visual field deficits, and cognitive impairments. Risk of brain involvement is 8%–20% in unilateral PWS, whereas it increases to about 35% in bilateral extensive PWS [27,28]. Neurological symptoms generally start from infancy only, but onset in adulthood has also been reported [29–31]. Seizures occur in roughly 75% of patients with unilateral brain involvement, and 95% of patients with bilateral brain involvement [32,33].

Meningococcal meningitis: Caused by gram-negative diplococci *Neisseria meningitidis* generally presents with a nonspecific prodrome of fever, cough, coryza, and prostration which can rapidly go on to develop features of meningitis, i.e., severe headache, photophobia, vomiting, neck rigidity, and altered sensorium. Skin rash that initially starts as nonspecific exanthem can rapidly evolve into petechiae on limbs and trunk, which in turn can progress to large ecchymotic patches or peripheral gangrene within hours (purpura fulminans) [34,35].

Rocky Mountain spotted fever (spotted fever): It is the most common rickettsial illness caused by *Rickettsia rickettsii*. Because of its diverse clinical features, it is also known by the names of "wolf in sheep's clothing" and "the great imitator" of other diseases [36]. It classically presents with a prodrome of fever, headache, and myalgia followed by development of a rash on days 3–5 starting around the ankles and wrists. It starts as tiny erythematous macules evolving into papules, petechiae, ecchymoses, and rarely necrosis. It can spread to proximal limbs, perineum, and trunk, usually sparing the face. Central nervous system (CNS) involvement may cause confusion, lethargy, seizures, blindness, deafness, or coma.

Lyme disease: Lyme disease (LD) is a tick-borne illness caused by *Borrelia burgdorferi sensu stricto* [37]. Cutaneous manifestations are divided into early localized infection, early disseminated disease, and late infection. The rash is classically described as targetoid or bull's-eye appearance, with an area of erythema surrounded by central clearing, named as *erythema migrans* [38]. Early neurologic presentations typically include cranial neuritis, radiculitis, and meningitis. Rare neurological manifestations include Horner syndrome, pseudotumor cerebri, and transverse myelitis [39].

Viral exanthems: Practically any viral infection can result in aseptic meningitis.

Vascular disorders: Any multisystem disease involving cutaneous vasculature, i.e., vasculitides and vasculopathy, can involve the neurological system as well, presenting with cerebrovascular accident or stroke. Basically all the defects that give rise to anticoagulation (protein C deficiency, Coumadin necrosis, purpura fulminans, calciphylaxis), fibrinolytic disorders (antithrombin III deficiency, disseminated intravascular coagulation), platelet abnormalities (abnormal structure or function, heparin necrosis, drug-induced platelet dysfunction, cryoglobulinemia), antibodies to endothelial cells in connective tissue diseases (systemic lupus erythematosus, dermatomyositis, systemic sclerosis, relapsing polychondritis, Sjögren syndrome, Degos disease, lupus anticoagulant, thrombotic thrombocytopenic purpura, cholesterol emboli, septic emboli), and states of hyperviscosity (cryoglobulinemias, cryofibrinogenemias, cold agglutinins, hypergammaglobulinemia) may lead to both skin and neural involvement.

Behçet disease: Named after the Turkish dermatologist Hulusi Behçet, who described a triad of oral ulcers, genital ulcers, and ocular inflammation in 1937, it is a rare, chronic, autoinflammatory disorder of unknown origin. Oral aphthous ulcers seen in 98% of cases are considered a *sine qua non* feature of Behçet disease [40]. A typical ulcer is round with a sharp, erythematous, and elevated border, mostly 1–3 cm in diameter, but larger lesions can also occur. Neurological involvement is seen in 20%–40% of cases and includes parenchymal and nonparenchymal (i.e., cerebral venous thrombosis or arterial aneurism) lesions [41,42]. Parenchymal lesions or neuro-Behçet disease frequently presents as acute episodes/attacks of headache, meningitis/meningoencephalitis, hemiplegia, or cranial nerve palsies [43].

Intravascular malignant lymphomatosis: It may initially cause dizziness, confusion, and hemiparesis that precedes the development of a generalized telangiectasia [44].

Sneddon syndrome: A rare, progressive condition primarily affecting blood vessels characterized by livedo reticularis (mottled red-blue discoloration in net-like appearance) especially over the legs, and exacerbated by cold, and neurological abnormalities such as transient ischemic attacks (TIAs) (mini-strokes) and strokes, headache, and dizziness [45,46].

Pseudoxanthoma elasticum: It is an autosomal recessive connective tissue disease affecting skin, eyes, and vasculature. The characteristic skin changes include small yellowish papules on the nape and sides of the neck and in flexural areas such as the axillae, the antecubital fossae, and periumbilical, inguinal, and popliteal areas [47]. CNS involvement manifests as subarachnoid and intracerebral hemorrhages, bilateral carotid occlusion, and cerebral and multilacunar infarctions [48–51].

Fabry disease: It is an X-linked lysosomal storage disorder resulting in accumulation of globotriaosylceramide in multiple organs, resulting in severely reduced quality of life and premature death. Angiokeratoma, a characteristic skin rash of flat dark red to blue-colored lesions, is found primarily in the bathing trunk area and the mucosal membranes from adolescence. Cerebrovascular events, such as stroke or TIA, are frequent in Fabry disease, giving rise to paresis, ataxia, dysarthria, nausea, dizziness, and probably poststroke neuropathic pain. The stroke episodes start at a mean age of 29 years in males and slightly later in females; however, the prevalence of stroke or TIA is higher in female patients [52,53].

CONCLUSION

Lungs and CNS can be involved commonly in dermatological emergencies. Similarly, many neurological and pulmonary emergencies can have varied cutaneous manifestations. Knowledge of these features can help all specialists involved to manage these emergencies in a much better way.

KEY POINTS

- Pulmonary and neurological emergencies can have cutaneous manifestations, which help to diagnose them early and vice versa.
- Fat embolism syndrome, Birt Hogg Dube and acute miliary tuberculosis are examples of such pulmonary emergencies.
- SJS/TEN, erythroderma and DRESS are primary skin disorders can affect the lungs.
- Fabry's disease, Pseudoxanthoma elasticum, Sturge Weber syndrome are few conditions which can present as neurological emergencies and have specific cutaneous features.

REFERENCES

1. Kaplan RP, Grant JN, Kaufman AJ. Dermatologic features of the fat embolism syndrome. *Cutis* 1986;38:52–5.
2. Alho A. Fat embolism syndrome, etiology pathogenesis and treatment. *Acta Chir Scand Suppl* 1980;499:75–85.
3. Barbagallo J et al. Cutaneous tuberculosis: Diagnosis and treatment. *Am J Clin Dermatol* 2002;3:319–28.
4. Sethuraman G, Ramesh V, Raman M, Sharma V. Skin tuberculosis in children: Learning from India. *Dermatol Clin* 2008;26:285–94.
5. Tappeiner G, Wolff K. Tuberculosis and other mycobacterial infections. In: Fitzpatrick TB, Freedberg IM, Eisen AZ, Wolff K, Austen KF (Eds), *Dermatology in General Medicine*. 5th ed. New York: McGraw-Hill; 2003:1933–50.
6. Sehgal V, Wagh S. Cutaneous tuberculosis: Current concepts. *Int J Dermatol* 1990;28:355–62.
7. Sehgal V. Cutaneous tuberculosis. *Dermatol Clin* 1994;12:645–53.
8. Narita M. Classification of extrapulmonary manifestations due to *Mycoplasma pneumoniae* infection on the basis of possible pathogenesis. *Front Microbiol* 2016;7:23.
9. Toro JR et al. Lung cysts, spontaneous pneumothorax, and genetic associations in 89 families with Birt-Hogg-Dubé syndrome. *Am J Respir Crit Care Med* 2007;175:1044–53.
10. Toro JR et al. BHD mutations, clinical and molecular genetic investigations of Birt-Hogg-Dubé syndrome: A new series of 50 families and a review of published reports. *J Med Genet* 2008;45:321–31.
11. Houweling AC et al. Renal cancer and pneumothorax risk in Birt-Hogg-Dubé syndrome: An analysis of 115 FLCN mutation carriers from 35 BHD families. *Br J Cancer* 2011;105:1912–9.
12. Aivaz O, Berkman S, Middelton L, Linehan WM, DiGiovanna JJ, Cowen EW. Comedonal and cystic fibrofolliculomas in Birt-Hogg-Dubé syndrome. *JAMA Dermatol* 2015;151:770–4.
13. Schaffer JV, Gohara MA, McNiff JM, Aasi SZ, Dvoretzky I. Multiple facial angiofibromas: A cutaneous manifestation of Birt-Hogg-Dubé syndrome. *J Am Acad Dermatol* 2005;53(2 Suppl):S108–11.
14. Ferri F. Granulomatosis with polyangiitis (Wegener's granulomatosis). In: Ferri FF (Ed). *Ferri's Clinical Advisor*. Philadelphia: Elsevier; 2016:555–6.
15. Wolff K, Johnson R, Saavedra AP. Section 14: The skin in immune, autoimmune, and rheumatic disorders. In: *Fitzpatrick's Color Atlas and Synopsis of Clinical Dermatology*. 7th ed. New York: McGraw-Hill; 2013.
16. Avcin T, Singh-Grewal D, Silverman ED, Schneider R. Severe digital ischaemia in a child with Wegener's granulomatosis. *Scand J Rheumatol* 2007;36:78–80.
17. Schwartz RA, Churg J. Churg-Strauss syndrome. *Br J Dermatol* 1992;127:199–204.
18. Barbosa AB, Hans-Filho G, Vicari CFS, Medeiros MZ, Couto DV, Takita LC. Rendu-Osler-Weber syndrome: Dermatological approach. *An Bras Dermatol* 2015;90(3 Suppl 1):S226–8.
19. Khoja AM, Jalan RK, Jain DL, Kajale OV. Osler-Weber-Rendu disease: A rare cause of recurrent hemoptysis. *Lung India* 2016;33:313–6.
20. Borchers AT, Lee JL et al. Stevens-Johnson syndrome and toxic epidermal necrolysis. *Autoimmun Rev* 2008;7:598–605.
21. McIvor RA, Zaidi J, Peters WJ, Hyland RH. Acute and chronic respiratory complications of toxic epidermal necrolysis. *J Burn Care Rehabil* 1996;17:237–40.
22. Grant-Kels JM, Fedeles F, Rothe MJ. Exfoliative dermatitis. In: Goldsmith LA, Katz SI, Gilchrest BA, Paller AS, Leffell DJ, Wolff K (Eds), *Fitzpatrick's Dermatology in General Medicine*. 8th ed. New York: McGraw Hill Medical; 2012.
23. Sterry W, Steinhoff M. Erythroderma. In: Bolognia JL, Jorizzo JL, Schaffer JV (Eds) *Dermatology*. 3rd ed. Philadelphia: Elsevier Saunders; 2012:171–81.
24. Lancrajan C, Bumbacea R, Giurcaneanu C. Erythrodermic atopic dermatitis with late onset—Case presentation. *J Med Life* 2010;3:80–3.
25. Mukherjee R et al. Sézary syndrome with pulmonary involvement: A case report. *Int J Sci Report* 2016;2:168–71.
26. De A, Rajagopalan M, Sarda A, Das S, Biswas P. Drug reaction with eosinophilia and systemic symptoms: An update and review of recent literature. *Indian J Dermatol* 2018;63:30–40.
27. Enjolras O, Riche MC, Merland JJ. Facial port-wine stains and Sturge-Weber syndrome. *Pediatrics* 1985;76:48–51.

28. Tallman B et al. Location of port-wine stains and the likelihood of ophthalmic and/or central nervous system complications. *Pediatrics* 1991;87:323–7.

29. Comi AC. Presentation, diagnosis, pathophysiology, and treatment of the neurological features of Sturge-Weber syndrome. *Neurologist* 2011;17:179–84.

30. Traub R, Riley C, Horvath S. Teaching NeuroImages: Sturge-Weber syndrome presenting in a 58-year-old woman with seizures. *Neurology* 2010;75:e52.

31. Kumar KR et al. Transient changes on brain magnetic resonance imaging in a patient with Sturge-Weber syndrome presenting with hemiparesis. *Neurologist* 2009;15:351–4.

32. Bebin EM, Gomez MR. Prognosis in Sturge-Weber disease: Comparison of unihemispheric and bihemispheric involvement. *J Child Neurol* 1988;3:181–4.

33. Oakes WJ. The natural history of patients with the Sturge-Weber syndrome. *Pediatr Neurosurg* 1992;18:287–90.

34. Nadel S, Kroll JS. Diagnosis and management of meningococcal disease: The need for centralized care. *FEMS Microbiol Rev* 2007;31:71–83.

35. Meningitis Research Foundation 2010. Lessons from research for doctors in training.

36. Sexton DJ, Corey GR. Rocky Mountain "spotless" and "almost spotless" fever: A wolf in sheep's clothing. *Clin Infect Dis* 1992;15:439–48.

37. Borchers AT, Keen CL, Huntley AC, Gershwin ME. Lyme disease: A rigorous review of diagnostic criteria and treatment. *J Autoimmun* 2015;57:82–115.

38. Miraflor AP, Seidel GD, Perry AE, Castanedo-Tardan MP, Guill MA, Yan S. The many masks of cutaneous Lyme disease. *J Cutan Pathol* 2015;43:32–40.

39. Morrison C, Seifter A, Aucott JN. Unusual presentation of Lyme disease: Horner syndrome with negative serology. *J Am Board Fam Med* 2009;22:219–22.

40. International Study Group for Behçet's Disease. Criteria for diagnosis of Behçet's disease. *Lancet* 1990;335:1078–80.

41. Akman-Demir G, Serdaroglu P, Tasci B. Clinical patterns of neurological involvement in Behçet's disease: Evaluation of 200 patients, The Neuro-Behçet Study Group. *Brain* 1999;122:2171–82.

42. Wechsler B, Sbai A, Du-Boutin LT, Duhaut P, Dormont D, Piette JC. Neurological manifestations of Behçet's disease. *Rev Neurol (Paris)* 2002;158:926–33.

43. Greco A, Gallo A, Fusconi M, Marinelli C, Macri GF, de Vincentiis M. Bell's palsy and autoimmunity. *Autoimmun Rev* 2012;12:323–8.

44. Eto M et al. Intravascular malignant lymphomatosis: An autopsy case with generalized telangiectasia and various neurological manifestations. *Rinsho Shinkeigaku* 2001;41:107–12.

45. Sneddon Syndrome. National Organization for Rare Disorders (NORD). 2016.

46. Berlit P. Sneddon syndrome. *Orphanet* 2015 March.

47. Marconi B et al. Pseudoxanthoma elasticum and skin: Clinical manifestations, histopathology, pathomechanism, perspectives of treatment. *Intractable Rare Dis Res* 2015;4:113–22.

48. Dixon JM. Angioid streaks and pseudoxanthoma elasticum with aneurysm of internal carotid artery. *Am J Ophthalmol* 1951;34:1322–3.

49. Goto K. Involvement of central nervous system in pseudoxanthoma elasticum. *Fol Psychiatr Neurol* 1975;9:263–77.

50. McKusick VA. *Heritable Disorders of Connective Tissue.* St. Louis, MO: CV Mosby; 1966:286–322.

51. Messis CP, Budzilovich GN. Pseudoxanthoma elasticum: Report of an autopsied case with cerebral involvement. *Neurology (Minneap)* 1970;20:703–9.

52. Rolfs A et al. Prevalence of Fabry disease in patients with cryptogenic stroke: A prospective study. *Lancet* 2005;366:1794–6.

53. Mehta A et al. Fabry disease defined: Baseline clinical manifestations of 366 patients in the Fabry Outcome Survey. *Eur J Clin Invest* 2004;34:236–42.

48

Endocrine emergencies with skin manifestations

RAJESHWARI DABAS

INTRODUCTION

Endocrine diseases may result in a multitude of dermatological manifestations. Some of the endocrine disorders can present as life-threatening emergencies. Awareness of the skin markers of such conditions may facilitate prompt and early diagnosis, which in turn can be lifesaving. This chapter focuses on some of the endocrine emergencies with dermatological manifestations.

ADDISON DISEASE

Adrenal insufficiency was first described by Thomas Addison at London Guy's Hospital in 1855 [1]. It is defined as the failure of the adrenal cortex to produce sufficient amounts of steroid hormones. It is a potentially life-threatening condition because of the central role of glucocorticoid and mineralocorticoid hormones in the energy, salt, and fluid homeostasis. Primary adrenal insufficiency or Addison disease is due to the diseases affecting the adrenal cortex and is less frequent than secondary adrenal insufficiency (SAI), which is due to diseases of pituitary or hypothalamus secondarily affecting the adrenal gland.

Causes of Addison disease mainly include tuberculosis and autoimmune adrenal failure [2,3].

Pathogenesis

Addison disease is caused by reduced adrenal function and is characterized by low levels of both glucocorticoids and mineralocorticoids and high adrenocorticotrophic hormone (ACTH) levels, whereas SAI is caused by disordered function of the hypothalamus and pituitary gland and is characterized by a low cortisol production rate and a normal or low plasma ACTH concentration.

The cause of the hyperpigmentation in Addison disease, being debated, is likely due to increased stimulation of the MC1R (Melanocortin-1 receptor) on cutaneous melanocytes by the high circulating levels of ACTH and α-MSH [4].

Clinical features

Rate of onset and the severity of adrenal insufficiency dictate the clinical picture. Addisonian crisis (acute adrenal insufficiency or adrenal crisis) is an emergency manifesting as hypotension and acute circulatory failure. Other features include anorexia, nausea, vomiting, diarrhea, and occasionally, abdominal pain. Fever and hypoglycemia may occur.

Adrenal hemorrhage presents acutely with hypotension; pain in the abdomen, flanks, or lower chest; anorexia; and vomiting.

The skin markers can give a clue to the diagnosis. The most common cutaneous manifestation of Addison disease is hypermelanosis of skin and mucous membranes. It is the most obvious clinical feature that differentiates primary from secondary hypoadrenalism. The hyperpigmentation is generalized but is most prominent in sun-exposed areas (such as the face, neck, back of hands), palmar creases, pressure points, intertriginous areas, external genitalia, nail beds, oral mucosa, lips, and recent rather than old scars. Hyperpigmentation is present in as high as 94% of cases. Women may complain of loss of axillary and pubic hair and frequently have dry and itchy skin because of loss of adrenal androgen secretion. Vitiligo is found to be associated with autoimmune adrenal insufficiency. In SAI, there is only glucocorticoid insufficiency leading to hypotension and hyponatremia without acidosis and hyperkalemia. ACTH-mediated hyperpigmentation is not seen in SAI [5].

Investigations

The diagnosis of Addison disease is made by the short cosyntropin test. The cut-off level for adrenal failure is taken as cortisol level <500–550 nmol/L estimated 30–60 minutes after ACTH stimulation, that is, after IV or intramuscular (IM) administration of 250 μg of cosyntropin. After the diagnosis of Addison disease is made, imaging of the adrenals (contrast-enhanced computed tomography [CECT]) is done to exclude any hemorrhage, infiltration, and metastases. Other laboratory investigations show hyponatremia, hyperkalemia, and hyperchloremic metabolic acidosis [6].

Treatment

Treatment of Addison disease consists of replacing glucocorticoids (hydrocortisone 15–20 mg on awakening and 5–10 mg in evening) and mineralocorticoids (fludrocortisone 0.1 mg/day) in adults. During a minor febrile illness and stress, glucocorticoid dose is increased by two- to threefold for the few days of illness. When undergoing surgery or a major procedure, systemic corticosteroids are administered [5].

CUSHING SYNDROME

Cushing syndrome comprises the symptoms and signs associated with prolonged exposure to inappropriately elevated levels of free plasma glucocorticoids (both endogenous and exogenous). *Cushing syndrome* is used to describe all causes, whereas *Cushing disease* is reserved for pituitary-dependent causes.

Pathogenesis

The causes of Cushing syndrome can be classified as ACTH-dependent or ACTH-independent causes. ACTH-dependent causes include Cushing disease (pituitary-dependent), ectopic ACTH syndrome, or ectopic corticotropin-releasing hormone syndrome, macronodular adrenal hyperplasia, or iatrogenic (treatment with 1–24 ACTH). ACTH-independent causes include cortisol secreting adrenal adenoma and carcinoma, primary pigmented nodular adrenal hyperplasia and Carney syndrome, McCune-Albright syndrome, and iatrogenic (e.g., pharmacologic doses of prednisolone, dexamethasone). The end result is an increase in the cortisol levels [5].

Clinical features

The clinical features are moon facies (Figure 48.1), buffalo hump, centripetal obesity, gonadal dysfunction, psychiatric manifestations, osteoporosis and pathological fractures/fractures following minor trauma, proximal myopathy, and hypertension. Patients are prone to infections such as tuberculosis, fungal infections, bowel perforation, wound

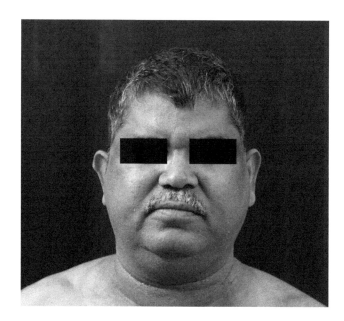

Figure 48.1 Moon facies.

infection, and poor wound healing. Adverse cardiovascular events are more common in such patients. There can be associated diabetes/glucose intolerance and increase in circulating cholesterol and triglycerides.

The skin findings include thinning of skin and easy bruisability. On examination, wrinkling of the skin on the dorsum of the hand may be seen, resulting in a "cigarette paper" appearance (Liddle sign). The plethoric appearance of the patient with Cushing syndrome is secondary to the thinning of the skin combined with loss of facial subcutaneous fat and is not caused by true polycythemia. Acne and papular lesions may occur over the face, chest, and back. The typical, almost pathognomonic, red-purple livid striae greater than 1 cm in width are most frequently found on the abdomen but may also be present on the upper thighs, breasts, and arms. They are very common in younger patients and less so in those older than 50 years of age. Skin pigmentation is rare in Cushing disease but common in the ectopic ACTH syndrome. It arises because of overstimulation of melanocyte receptors by ACTH and possibly proopiomelanocortin (POMC)-derived peptides. Vellus hypertrichosis on the face is common [7].

Investigations

Diagnostic confirmation of Cushing syndrome requires demonstration of excess cortisol. The tests recommended are overnight low-dose dexamethasone suppression test, 24-hour urinary free cortisol levels, or midnight salivary cortisol levels. The choice of imaging once biochemical tests are suggestive of Cushing includes magnetic resonance imaging (MRI) for pituitary and CECT of abdomen for adrenals [5].

Treatment

The primary treatment of Cushing syndrome is removal of the source of excess glucocorticoid. This is achieved by excision of the pituitary adenoma by transsphenoidal approach or by adrenalectomy in cases of adrenal tumors or adenomas. Pasireotide is the only drug approved for use in Cushing disease in those refractory to surgeries or in patients not suitable for surgery. It has high affinity for somatostatin receptor subtype 5, overexpressed by adenoma cells in the pituitary [8].

THYROID DYSFUNCTION

Hypothyroidism

Hypothyroidism is one of the most frequently encountered endocrinology disorders. The prevalence of hypothyroidism in India is 11%, compared with only 2% in the United Kingdom and 4%–6% in the United States [9].

Hypothyroidism can affect all organ systems, and the manifestations depend on the degree of hormone deficiency. A rare, life-threatening condition encountered in long-standing untreated hypothyroidism is myxedema coma. However, most patients are not in a coma, and hence, *myxedema crisis* may be the apt term. There is decompensation of various organs due to severe hypothyroidism. The clinical signs include altered mental status, hypothermia, bradycardia, hypoventilation, seizures, severe hypotension, and shock. There is usually a precipitating cause such as exposure to cold, infection, trauma, and certain drugs, and mortality remains high despite treatment [10].

PATHOGENESIS

Myxedema is the most classic dermatological finding associated with hypothyroidism. This is due to the loss of inhibitory effect of the thyroid hormones on the deposition of hyaluronates, fibronectin, and collagen by fibroblasts. The dermal deposition of mucopolysaccharides, namely, hyaluronic acid and chondroitin, causes the classic mucinous nonpitting edema termed as *myxedema*. This is most apparent in the skin and can occur in many organs.

CLINICAL FEATURES

Clinical features of hypothyroidism depend on the etiology, rapidity, and severity of deficiency of thyroid hormones. The skin is dry (hypofunctioning sebaceous and sweat glands), pale (reduced dermal perfusion and anemia), and scaly and rough (mucinous swelling of the dermis and hyperkeratosis of the stratum corneum). There is yellowish discoloration, especially of palms and soles (deposition of carotene due to slow/lack of conversion to vitamin A). Characteristic facial changes termed *myxedema facies* can be seen, which include a broad nose, thickened lips, puffy eyelids, and macroglossia. Hairs are dull, coarse, and brittle. Hair loss occurs in 50%, which is diffuse and involves the scalp, beard, genital hair, and lateral aspect of the eyebrows. Nails are also affected and become thin, brittle, and develop grooves, and their rate of growth is retarded. Wound healing is impaired. Other symptoms include cold intolerance, constipation, lethargy and fatigue, menstrual disturbances, hoarseness of voice, decreased sweating, weight gain, and hyporeflexia [11].

Hyperthyroidism

The terms *hyperthyroidism* and *thyrotoxicosis* are used interchangeably and refer to the classical or subtle manifestations of excessive quantities of thyroid hormones. The disproportionate amount of thyroid hormone leads to an accelerated metabolic state.

Thyroid storm, also called *accelerated hyperthyroidism*, is an extreme accentuation of thyrotoxicosis. It is an emergency that if not treated in a timely fashion carries a high mortality rate. The common precipitating factors are infection, trauma, or surgical emergencies. Other conditions include diabetic ketoacidosis, toxemia of pregnancy, or parturition. The clinical signs include hyperpyrexia; cardiovascular decompensation leading to tachycardia, atrial fibrillation, and congestive heart failure; gastrointestinal dysfunction; and central nervous system disturbance in the form of delirium, seizures, and coma [12].

CLINICAL FEATURES

Warm and moist skin is the most characteristic finding of hyperthyroidism. This is because of cutaneous vasodilatation and increased diaphoresis. Scalp hair becomes fine and fragile, and in 20%–40% of the patients diffuse hair loss occurs. A characteristic but rare finding is Plummer nails, onycholysis involving the fourth and fifth fingers. A rare form of skin involvement occurs in Graves disease, called *thyroid dermopathy*, and it occurs in less than 1% of cases. It is also called *pretibial myxedema* because most commonly it occurs as hyperpigmented, nonpitting induration of skin over the shins. This is a late manifestation and almost 99% of these patients will have Graves orbitopathy. There is compression of lymphatics in dermis resulting in nonpitting edema. Later in the course of disease, there is nodule and plaque formation. Rare sites of such lesions are the face, eyebrows, elbows, or dorsa of hands. The Graves triad consists of thyrotoxicosis and goiter, orbitopathy, and dermopathy. Thyroid acropachy (painful clubbing, soft tissue swelling, and periosteal bone changes) occurs due to hypermetabolic state leading to axial bone destruction. This is presumably due to increased osteoclast activity. Vitiligo is common in autoimmune thyroid disorders [13].

Other features of hyperthyroidism are unintentional weight loss, heat intolerance, increased sweating, increased appetite, palpitations, menstrual disturbances, fine tremors, presence of goiter, ophthalmopathy, tachycardia, atrial fibrillation, and high-output cardiac failure [12].

Investigations

The diagnosis of thyroid disease is confirmed by thyroid function tests. Screening is done with serum levels of TSH, and any abnormalities in TSH should be followed by measurements of serum free T4 and T3 and antithyroid antibodies.

Treatment

The mainstay of treatment for thyroid disease is to bring the thyroid function back to normal. The treatment of hypothyroidism is by replacement of thyroid hormone. The definite treatment of hyperthyroidism depends on the etiology, which includes antithyroid drugs, radioactive iodine, thyroid surgery, and medications for symptom control.

PARATHYROID DISORDERS

Hypoparathyroidism

Parathyroid hormone (PTH) is one of the major hormones that regulates serum calcium along with vitamin D. Hypoparathyroidism occurs when there is destruction of the parathyroid glands (autoimmune, surgical), abnormal parathyroid gland development, altered regulation of PTH production, or impaired PTH action. When PTH secretion is insufficient, hypocalcemia develops. Hypocalcemia varies from an asymptomatic biochemical abnormality to a life-threatening disorder, depending on the duration, severity, and rapidity of development.

CLINICAL FEATURES

The predominant clinical symptoms and signs of hypocalcemia are those of neuromuscular irritability, which include perioral paresthesias, tingling of the fingers and toes, and spontaneous or latent tetany. Tetany can be elicited by Chvostek sign (percussion of the facial nerve below the zygoma, resulting in ipsilateral contractions of the facial muscle) or Trousseau sign (carpal spasm elicited by inflation of a blood pressure cuff to 20 mm Hg above the patient's systolic pressure for 3 minutes). Electrocardiographic abnormalities in the form of prolonged QT interval, ventricular arrhythmias, laryngospasm, and seizures can also occur [14].

The dermatological manifestations include coarse brittle hair, alopecia, dry and rough skin, and nail abnormalities, such as discoloration, distal onycholysis, and transverse ridges [15].

TREATMENT

The treatment for hypoparathyroidism is supplementation with calcium and vitamin D. Patients with acute symptomatic hypocalcemia (calcium level less than 7.0 mg/dL) should be treated promptly with IV calcium, preferably calcium gluconate [13.14].

Hyperparathyroidism

Primary hyperparathyroidism results from an abnormal function of parathyroid gland. This in turn causes increased levels of PTH. The most common cause of primary hyperparathyroidism is an autonomous PTH secreting adenoma. Secondary hyperparathyroidism may arise from vitamin D deficiency or from disturbances of the calcium-phosphate balance, mainly in patients with chronic kidney disease.

Skin manifestations are rarely seen in hyperparathyroidism. Calcinosis cutis due to elevated calcium and phosphate levels may be present. Calciphylaxis is a rare but life-threatening condition that is commonly associated with secondary hyperparathyroidism in the setting of chronic renal failure [16]. It is characterized by vascular calcification and thrombosis. It clinically presents with severe painful skin lesions (livedo reticularis, reticulate purpura, violaceous plaques, or indurated nodules) that evolve into nonhealing ulcers covered with black eschar and finally lead to tissue gangrene. Both the trunk and extremities can be involved [17].

TREATMENT

For calciphylaxis, medical therapy includes bisphosphonates, sodium thiosulfate, antibiotics, hyperbaric oxygen, and aggressive wound care and débridement of necrotic tissue. Total or subtotal parathyroidectomy with autotransplantation may be of therapeutic benefit [17].

Diabetes mellitus

Diabetes mellitus is characterized by a state of relative or complete insulin deficiency. The two acute and life-threatening complications of diabetes are diabetic ketoacidosis (DKA) and hyperosmolar hyperglycemic syndrome (HHS), which require early diagnosis and aggressive management to optimize clinical outcomes.

DKA is due to absolute or profound relative deficiency of insulin, and patients present with hyperglycemia, ketonemia, and metabolic acidosis. HHS is characterized by a greater severity of plasma glucose elevation, marked increase of plasma osmolality, absent to mild ketosis, and altered mental status. In HHS, residual insulin secretion minimizes ketone body production but is not able to control hyperglycemia. Most patients with DKA have type 1 diabetes. Patients with advanced or severe type 2 diabetes can also be at risk during acute illnesses. HHS occurs almost exclusively in type 2 diabetes patients, who continue to demonstrate some degree of insulin secretion. Infection is a major precipitating factor for hyperglycemic emergencies [18].

Pathogenesis

Individuals with type 2 diabetes are more likely than those with type 1 diabetes to develop cutaneous manifestations. The skin changes in diabetes are due to metabolic changes, namely, hyperglycemia and hyperlipidemia, and may be a result of progressive damage to vascular, neurologic, or immune systems. Hyperglycemia leads to nonenzymatic glycosylation of various structural and regulatory proteins, including collagen, which in turn causes formation of advanced glycation end products (AGEs). Disorders such as diabetic thick skin and limited joint mobility are thought to result directly from accumulation of AGEs. Certain infections, such as necrotizing soft tissue infections, mucormycosis, pyodermas, and candidiasis, occur more frequently in patients with diabetes. Acanthosis nigricans is due to the action of insulin on the insulin-like growth factor-1 receptor that stimulates epidermal proliferation. The altered lipid metabolism is responsible for hypertriglyceridemia, which manifests as eruptive xanthomas. Nonhealing leg ulcers are due to macro- and microangiopathy and peripheral neuropathy [16].

Clinical features

In DKA, patients present with poor skin turgor, tachycardia, and hypotension. There may be a fruity odor to the breath due to ketosis as well as Kussmaul breathing. Patients with HHS can present with focal neurological signs, seizures, and coma. The dermatological manifestations might serve as an indicator of diabetes mellitus in such patients.

ACANTHOSIS NIGRICANS

Acanthosis nigricans (AN) is the most common manifestation and can predict hyperinsulinemia. It is also a prognostic indicator for developing type 2 diabetes. Heredity, obesity, endocrine disorders, certain drugs, and malignancy are also associated with AN [19].

ACROCHORDONS

Acrochordons or skin tags are soft, pedunculated lesions most commonly located on the eyelids, neck, axillae, and groin. The relationship between hyperinsulinemia and skin tags has been well established. Treatment is usually cosmetic or in cases where it causes irritation. They can be removed by excision, cryotherapy with liquid nitrogen, or electrodessication [20].

DIABETIC DERMOPATHY

Diabetic dermopathy, also called shin spots or pigmented pretibial patches, presents as multiple, asymptomatic, oval, dull red papules or plaques predominantly on the pretibial skin, but they can also occur on the forearms, thighs, and lateral malleoli. As it is asymptomatic, no treatment is required.

ERUPTIVE XANTHOMA

Eruptive xanthoma (EX) presents on the buttocks, elbows, and knees as sudden onset of crops of yellow papules with an erythematous base. It is rare and occurs more often in patients with poorly controlled type 2 diabetes with hyperlipidemia. People with EX are at higher risk of early coronary artery disease and pancreatitis due to hypertriglyceridemia. Treatment is with diet modification and systemic medications to lower the triglycerides.

RUBEOSIS FACEI

Rubeosis facei is a microangiopathic complication of diabetes. If present, other microangiopathic complications such as retinopathy should be looked for. It presents as flushing on the face (Figure 48.2). This condition is seen in 3%–5% of people with diabetes. No treatment is required. Strict glycemic control can improve the appearance and prevent complications of microangiopathy in other organ systems as well.

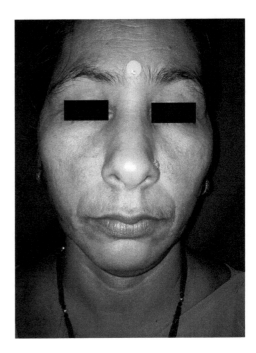

Figure 48.2 Rubeosis facei.

NECROBIOSIS LIPOIDICA

Necrobiosis lipoidica (NL) appears in 0.3%–1.6% of diabetic patients. Although the exact cause of NL is not known, it is suggested that an antibody-mediated vasculitis with secondary collagen degeneration is the main cause of this disorder. It is stated that approximately 75% of patients with NL have or will develop diabetes. Therefore, it is also called *necrobiosis lipodica diabeticorum*. The lesions begin as small, firm, erythematous papules that enlarge radially to form indurated, annular plaques with a yellowish atrophic center, prominent superficial telangiectasia, and a slightly elevated erythematous-violaceous margin. The lesions are most commonly distributed bilaterally on the lower extremities, particularly the pretibial areas, but may occur on the face, trunk, and upper extremities as well. Various treatment modalities have been tried, and the response is generally disappointing. The treatment modalities include topical and intralesional steroids, tacrolimus, PUVA, and other immunosuppressive drugs [19].

LIMITED JOINT MOBILITY

Limited joint mobility (LJM), or diabetic cheiroarthropathy, presents with mildly restricted extension of the metacarpophalangeal and interphalangeal joints that generally begins with involvement of the fifth digit and then progresses to involve all fingers. It is characterized by the "prayer sign." It is caused by thickening of periarticular connective tissue causing stiffness [13].

SCLEREDEMA DIABETICORUM

Scleredema diabeticorum is characterized by ill-defined, painless induration of the skin, most commonly on the neck and upper back. It is mainly seen in type 2 diabetes associated with obesity [20].

BULLOSIS DIABETICORUM

Bullosis diabeticorum occurs in people with long-standing type 1 diabetes mellitus. The exact etiology is still not known. It presents with painless bullae with clear, sterile fluid on a noninflamed base. The onset is spontaneous and affects the dorsa and the sides of the legs and feet; the lesions resolve in 2–5 weeks.

DIABETIC ULCERS

Foot ulcers are a major problem for patients with diabetes, occurring in 15%–25% of diabetic patients. Peripheral neuropathy, trauma, and pressure play important roles in the development of such ulcers. There is initially callus formation over the bony prominences of the feet, usually on the first and/or second metatarsophalangeal joints followed by necrosis of tissue which forms the ulcer. They can extend and cause soft tissue infection and osteomyelitis. Treatment for neuropathic diabetic ulcers includes wound débridement and protective dressings along with offloading measures [4].

Other conditions that may be seen in patients with diabetes include granuloma annulare, vitiligo, generalized pruritus, and acquired perforating dermatosis.

Investigations

A fasting plasma glucose value of $\geq$126 mg/dL or random plasma glucose value of $\geq$200 mg/dL confirms the diagnosis of diabetes. Hemoglobin A1c is used in conjunction with fasting plasma glucose for the diagnosis of diabetes mellitus.

Treatment

The treatment of diabetes includes lifestyle modification and oral hypoglycemic agents or insulin.

GLUCAGONOMA

Glucagonoma is a rare neuroendocrine tumor that originates from the α-2 cells of the pancreas. Approximately 80% of tumors occur sporadically, with the remainder associated with the MEN1 (multiple endocrine neoplasia type 1) syndrome. About 75% of glucagonomas are malignant and have metastasized by the time of diagnosis.

Clinical features

A hallmark of this syndrome is necrolytic migratory erythema. It presents as a painful migratory rash with a predilection for intertriginous areas, especially the anogenital region, perioral area, and distal part of the extremities. It starts as erythematous plaques with occasional bullae, which erode rapidly and form crust. These lesions coalesce into large geographic areas. This rash eventually resolves to reappear again. Patients with glucagonomas may have weight loss, abdominal pain, diabetes, stomatitis, glossitis, cheilitis, nail dystrophy,

thromboembolic events, anemia, and neuropsychiatric symptoms. The triad of hyperglucagonemia, necrolytic migratory erythema, and a pancreatic tumor is seen in some cases.

Investigations

There is elevation of elevated serum glucagon, usually well over 1000 pg/mL (normal range 50–150 pg/mL). There may be associated hyperglycemia, normochromic normocytic anemia, low serum levels of amino acids, total protein, albumin, cholesterol, and zinc. Somatostatin receptor scintigraphy is positive in approximately 95% of patients with glucagonoma.

Treatment

For patients with glucagonoma, symptomatic relief is provided by resection of the tumor.

If tumor metastasis has occurred, the long-acting somatostatin analogue, octreotide, is given to decrease the glucagon levels. Supplementation with zinc, amino acids, and essential fatty acids appears to be beneficial in some cases [21].

PHEOCHROMOCYTOMA

Pheochromocytoma is a potentially life-threatening catecholamine-secreting endocrine neoplasm of the adrenal medulla. Although it can occur anywhere along the sympathetic chain, 85%–90% are discovered within the adrenal gland. Traditional teachings regarding pheochromocytoma include the Rule of 10s: 10% bilateral, 10% malignant (higher in familial cases), 10% extra-adrenal (most commonly in the sympathetic chain in the thorax, abdomen, and pelvis), and 10% familial (now estimated to be as high as 24%) [22].

Clinical features

It clinically presents with paroxysmal "spells" of headache, palpitations, diaphoresis, and severe hypertension. Other features include arrhythmias, acute coronary syndrome, cardiomyopathy, heart failure, acute respiratory distress syndrome, diabetes mellitus, hypertensive retinopathy, tremors, seizures, and hemiplegia. Skin manifestations include hyperhidrosis, paroxysmal facial pallor, Raynaud phenomenon, and livedo reticularis.

Investigations

Biochemical tests include 24-hour collection of urinary metanephrines and vanillylmandelic acid and plasma metanephrines. Imaging modalities include CT, MRI, and scintigraphy scans.

Treatment

The treatment of choice for pheochromocytoma is complete surgical resection [22].

CARCINOID SYNDROME

Carcinoid syndrome is a paraneoplastic syndrome comprising the signs and symptoms that occur secondary to carcinoid tumors. Carcinoid tumors are derived from neuroendocrine cells and most commonly involve the lungs and gastrointestinal tract. They can also originate from the thymus, ovaries, testes, heart, and middle ear.

Clinical features

The features of the classic carcinoid syndrome are flushing, diarrhea, right-sided heart failure, and sometimes bronchial constriction. Other features include weight loss, sweating, and pellagra-like skin lesions. Flushes may be spontaneous or may be precipitated by stress, infection, alcohol, spicy foods, or certain drugs. The pathophysiology of flushing in the carcinoid syndrome is not yet elucidated. Serotonin, tachykinins, like neuropeptide K and substance P, kallikrein, bradykinins, and histamine have all been implicated to be mediators of the flushes.

Investigations

The most specific test is a measurement of 24-hour urinary excretion of 5-hydroxyindoleacetic acid (5-HIAA), a degradation product of serotonin. Serum chromogranin A (CgA) is another biochemical test commonly used for the diagnosis of carcinoid. CgA is a more sensitive marker than urinary 5-HIAA in detecting carcinoid tumors, but because CgA is released and secreted from various types of neuroendocrine tumors, the specificity is lower. Imaging modalities include CT, MRI, and octreotide scintigraphy scans.

Treatment

Avoiding stress, both psychological and physical, as well as substances such as alcohol, spicy foods, and medications that precipitate a flushing reaction might be sufficient in early cases. Medical treatment with somatostatin analogues (octreotide and lanreotide) has proven extremely efficacious for symptomatic relief. In metastatic carcinoid, interferon-α and chemotherapy can be used. Because most tumors in patients with the carcinoid syndrome are malignant at the time of clinical presentation, surgical cure is seldom obtained. Resection of local disease or regional nodular metastatic disease can cure some patients. However, even if radical surgery cannot be performed, debulking procedures and bypass should always be considered [23].

CONCLUSION

Endocrine diseases may result in a myriad of skin manifestations that might be helpful in arriving at a diagnosis in emergency situations. Awareness of these cutaneous signs may result in early diagnosis and prompt management that, at times, can even be lifesaving.

KEY POINTS

- Addisonian crisis is an emergency manifesting as hypotension and acute circulatory failure. Hypermelanosis of skin and mucous membranes is clue to its diagnosis.
- Thinning of skin and easy bruisability are features of Cushing's disease.
- Pretibial myxedema in thyrotoxicosis, necrobiosis lipoidica in diabetes and necrolytic migratory erythema in glucagonoma are characteristic cutaneous features.

REFERENCES

1. Addison T. On the constitutional and local effects of disease of the suprarenal capsule. In: *A Collection of the Published Writings of the Late Thomas Addison MD*. London: New Sydenham Society; 1868.
2. Husebye ES et al. Consensus statement on the diagnosis, treatment and follow-up of patients with primary adrenal insufficiency. *J Intern Med* 2014;275:104–15.
3. Agarwal G, Bhatia E, Pandey R, Jain SK. Clinical profile and prognosis of Addison's disease in India. *Natl Med J India* 2001;14:23–5.
4. Barthel A, Willenberg HS, Gruber M, Bornstein SR. Adrenal insufficiency. In: Jameson L, De Groot LJ, de Kretser DM, Giudice LC, Grossman AB, Melmed S, Potts JT, Jr., Weir GC (Eds), *Endocrinology Adult and Pediatric*. Vol 2. 7th ed. Philadelphia: Elsevier; 2016:1763–74.
5. Stewart PM, Newell-Price JDC. The adrenal cortex. In: Melmed S, Polonsky KS, Larsen PR, Kronenberg HM (Eds), *Williams Textbook of Endocrinology*. 13th ed. Philadelphia: Elsevier; 2016:490–555.
6. Arlt W. Disorders of adrenal cortex. In: Kasper DL, Fauci AS, Hauser SL, Longo DL, Jameson JL, Loscalzo J (Eds), *Harrison's Principles of Internal Medicine*. 19th ed. New York: McGraw-Hill; 2015:2309–29.
7. Paus R. The skin and endocrine disorders. In: Griffiths CEM, Barker J, Bleiker T, Chalmers R, Creamer D (Eds), *Rook's Textbook of Dermatology*. Vol. 4. 9th ed. Chichester, West Sussex: Wiley Blackwell; 2016:149.1–149.23.
8. McKeage K. Pasireotide: A review of its use in Cushing's disease. *Drugs* 2013;73:563–74.
9. Bagcchi S. Hypothyroidism in India: More to be done. *Lancet Diabetes Endocrinol* 2014;2:778.
10. Dubbs SB, Spangler R. Hypothyroidism. *Emerg Med Clin North Am* 2014;32:303–17.
11. Brent GA, Weetman AP. Hypothyroidism and thyroiditis. In: Melmed S, Polonsky KS, Larsen

PR, Kronenberg HM (Eds), *Williams Textbook of Endocrinology*. 13th ed. Philadelphia: Elsevier; 2016:416–48.

12. Devereaux D, Tewelde SZ. Hyperthyroidism and thyrotoxicosis. *Emerg Med Clin N Am* 2014;277–92.

13. Jabbour SA. Cutaneous manifestations of endocrine disorders: A guide for dermatologists. *Am J Clin Dermatol* 2003;4:315–31.

14. Bringhurst FR, Marie B, Demay MB, Kronenberg HM. Hormones and disorders of mineral metabolism. In: Melmed S, Polonsky KS, Larsen PR, Kronenberg HM (Eds), *Williams Textbook of Endocrinology*. 13th ed. Philadelphia: Elsevier; 2016:1254–322.

15. Demirkesen C. Skin manifestations of endocrine diseases. *Turk Patoloji Derg* 2015;31:145–54.

16. Kalus AA, Chien AJ, Olerud JE. Diabetes mellitus and other endocrine diseases. In: Goldsmith LA, Katz SI, Gilchrest BA, Paller AS, Leffell DJ, Wolff K (Eds), *Fitzpatrick's Dermatology in General Medicine*. Vol. 2. 8th ed. New York: McGraw-Hill; 2012:1840–68.

17. Nigwekar SU et al. Calciphylaxis: Risk factors, diagnosis, and treatment. *Am J Kidney Dis* 2015;66:133–46.

18. Corwell B, Knight B, Olivieri L, Willis GC. Current diagnosis and treatment of hyperglycemic emergencies. *Emerg Med Clin N Am* 2014;32:437–52.

19. Murphy-Chutorian B, Han G, Cohen SR. Dermatologic manifestations of diabetes mellitus. *Endocrinol Metab Clin North Am* 2013;42:869–98.

20. Bourke J. Skin disorders in diabetes mellitus. In: Griffiths CEM, Barker J, Bleiker T, Chalmers R, Creamer D (Eds), *Rook's Textbook of Dermatology*. Vol. 2. 9th ed. Edinburgh: Wiley Blackwell; 2016:64.1–7.

21. Shi W, Liao W, Mei X, Xiao Q, Zeng Y, Zhou Q. Necrolytic migratory erythema associated with glucagonoma syndrome. *J Clin Oncol* 2010;28:e329–31.

22. Young WF, Jr. Endocrine hypertension. In: Melmed S, Polonsky KS, Larsen PR, Kronenberg HM (Eds), *Williams Textbook of Endocrinology*. 13th ed. Philadelphia: Elsevier; 2016:556–88.

23. Öberg K. Neuroendocrine gastrointestinal and lung tumors (carcinoid tumors), the carcinoid syndrome and related disorders. In: Melmed S, Polonsky KS, Larsen PR, Kronenberg HM (Eds), *Williams Textbook of Endocrinology*. 13th ed. Philadelphia: Elsevier; 2016:1833–53.

49

Skin manifestations of poisoning

NILENDU SARMA AND SUSHILA HANSDA

INTRODUCTION

Poisoning is a harmful condition due to exposure to some chemicals. It may be acute and chronic. Poisoning can affect one or a few individuals or even may affect the masses. Numerous chemicals have the potential to cause harm to human beings, such as natural gases (as in the gas leak in China in 2003 that killed many) and toxic gases (release of carbon monoxide, hydrogen sulfide, and methylisocyanate in Bhopal in 1984 that caused many deaths), and methanol. However, only a few important chemicals are discussed in this chapter with particular attention to the dermatological effects of such poisoning.

ARSENICOSIS

Arsenic is a known carcinogen (group 1 human carcinogen, as classified by the U.S. Environmental Protection Agency), and a genotoxic molecule [1]. In the present era, it has proved to be the prime cause of one of the deadliest disasters mankind has ever witnessed, killing millions of people through drinking the (ground) water and possibly many other foods grown in the fields with contaminated water.

Arsenic is a heavy metal that is widely spread in nature in its various environmental sources, such as soil and water. Arsenic is a colorless, odorless, tasteless agent that makes it a suitable choice for a poison that is easily incorporated with food or drink [1–3]. A significant population of the world, especially the Asian countries such as Bangladesh, India, and China [4], are battling the deleterious effects of arsenic from groundwater contamination, in the form of various respiratory, hepatobiliary, neurological, and vascular system abnormalities along with characteristic cutaneous features that are possibly mediated via the damage caused to epidermal stem cells [5].

Source

Arsenic exposure in humans may be through inhalation, ingestion, or absorption via skin. However, the main source of human toxicity is through contaminated groundwater. The discovery that arsenic exposure can occur through food and crops grown in fields with high arsenic content in the groundwater is really worrisome. Other possible sources are pesticides, paints, smelting, semiconductors, and transistors. Arsenic toxicity has been repeatedly reported following use of traditional ayurvedic and homeopathic medicines. Moreover, the concentration of arsenic in these products is much above the level found in groundwater. Some organic sources are seafood and algae, etc.

Pathogenesis

Arsenic has the ability to bind various molecular side chains of different enzymes required for normal physiological function. The trivalent and pentavalent forms are responsible for human toxicity. The trivalent form of arsenic (As^{3+}) binds to the sulfhydryl group of keratin present in skin, hair, nail, and mucosae, and thus it gets deposited in these sites. The pentavalent form binds to the tissue by replacing phosphate. Arsenic induces premalignant and malignant dermatological lesions, nondermatological health effects, and cancers in humans through various known and unknown complex mechanisms [6–9].

Clinical features

ACUTE POISONING

Acute poisoning results from accidental ingestion, suicidal attempts, or when arsenic is used as a homicidal agent. The lethal doses of acute ingested inorganic arsenic compounds range from 120 to 200 mg, but toxicity can appear with a dose range of 5–50 mg [10]. Gastrointestinal, cardiovascular, neurological, and renal systems are principally affected in acute poisoning. Gastrointestinal (GI) symptoms such as acute abdominal pain, vomiting, diarrhea, and excess salivation are the usual presenting symptoms. There is a typical garlic-like odor of the breath and perspiration. Arsenic causes severe irritation and transudation of fluid in the GI mucosa leading to bloody diarrhea. Death from arsenic is generally caused by circulatory collapse associated with intense gastroenteritis. Other manifestations are hemoglobinuria, disseminated intravascular coagulation, pulmonary edema, cardiomyopathy, encephalopathy, and renal failure. Arsenic also causes peripheral neuropathy that may present as ascending weakness like that of Guillain-Barré syndrome.

Diagnosis

Complete blood count done in such cases may show microcytic hypochromic anemia and at times, acute hemolytic anemia. Serum electrolyte levels are usually abnormal because of severe diarrhea. The normal blood arsenic concentration is between 2 and 23 µg/L [11]. But in case of acute poisoning, the serum level is usually more than 50 µg/L. A 24-hour urine collection for total arsenic excretion can be diagnostic, and a level >50 mcg is suggestive of high arsenic exposure. Consumption of seafood within the last 3 days and high presence of organic arsenic from nutritional sources can give false positivity.

Treatment

Following acute poisoning, supportive treatment is needed first. Gastric lavage may be done in early presentation. Bowel irrigation with polyethylene glycol may be effective to prevent GI tract absorption of arsenic. Various chelation therapies that may be tried are Dimercaprol (British anti-Lewisite [BAL]), Succimer (dimercaptosuccinic acid [DMSA]), and Dimaval (dimercaptopropane sulfonate [DMPS]). Chelation therapy should be started as early as possible to get the desired effects.

Follow-up may be required for months after acute poisoning, as peripheral neuropathy can occur as a long-term sequelae.

CHRONIC ARSENICOSIS

The World Health Organization (WHO) has defined chronic arsenicosis as a "chronic health condition arising from prolonged ingestion (not less than 6 months) of arsenic above a safe dose, usually manifested by characteristic skin lesions, with or without involvement of internal organs" [12].

Manifestation of chronic arsenicosis

CUTANEOUS MANIFESTATIONS

Cutaneous features are the earliest and most common manifestation of chronic arsenicosis. These may range from pigmentary changes of various types and hyperkeratosis to cutaneous malignancy [5,13–17].

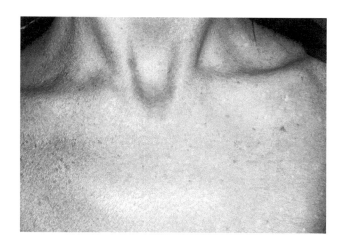

Figure 49.1 Raindrop pigmentation of arsenicosis.

Figure 49.2 Spotty depigmentation.

PIGMENTARY CHANGES

Diffuse hyperpigmentation mostly over the trunk, patchy pigmentation with prominence over skin folds, and fine freckles of spotted pigmentary changes are also seen, known as *raindrop pigmentation* (Figure 49.1) [13–15]. Besides hyperpigmentation, macular areas of depigmentation sometimes appear on normal skin or hyperpigmented skin known as *leukomelanosis* (Figure 49.2). Pigmentary changes may not be limited to skin only but may also manifest as diffuse or discrete pigmentation in buccal mucosa and transverse white bands in finger- or toenails known as Mees lines (Figure 49.3).

HYPERKERATOSIS

Another characteristic feature of chronic arsenicosis is hyperkeratosis of palms and soles (Figures 49.4 and 49.5). Hyperkeratosis may be graded as mild where there are minute wart-like papules (<2 mm), moderate form with raised wart-like thickening (2–5 mm), and severe with large (>5 mm) discrete or confluent elevations and even fissuring. Arsenical keratosis is more marked in areas subjected

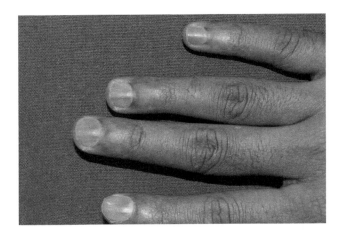

Figure 49.3 Mees lines.

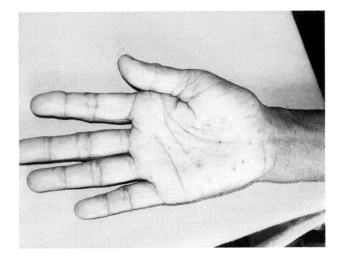

Figure 49.4 Characteristic palmar lesions.

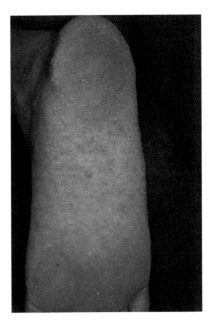

Figure 49.5 Characteristic plantar lesions.

to trauma and friction. Sometimes it may also be seen over the dorsum of extremities and trunk [5]. Apart from the classical keratotic papules, diffuse palmoplantar thickening and fissuring may sometimes be seen.

MALIGNANCY

Malignant change may occur in skin, lung, bladder, kidney, prostate, liver, and uterus, but skin is considered the most sensitive site for arsenic-induced malignancies [13,18–20].

Bowen disease, basal cell carcinoma (BCC), and squamous cell carcinoma (SCC) are commonly encountered [21], with rare reports of Merkel cell carcinoma [22]. Arsenic-related BCC are multiple in number and found in covered parts as well [23–25].

GASTROINTESTINAL SYMPTOMS

Apart from nausea, anorexia, constipation, and diarrhea, other serious manifestations are hepatomegaly and portal hypertension. Histopathological examination of the liver mostly shows noncirrhotic portal fibrosis [26].

CARDIOVASCULAR

Chronic arsenic toxicity can result in a form of peripheral vascular disease named Blackfoot disease [27]. Clinically it presents as coldness of extremities (usually in the feet), decreased peripheral pulses, pain, and intermittent claudication, progressing to gangrene and spontaneous amputation [28]. Underlying histopathology often shows arteriosclerosis obliterans and thromboangiitis obliterans, particularly affecting small vessels [29]. Other than peripheral vascular disease hypertension [30], ischemic heart disease can also occur [31].

NERVOUS SYSTEM

Peripheral neuropathy (sensory > motor) manifesting as paresthesias, pain, weakness, and atrophy of the affected limb further impairs the quality of life of patients with chronic arsenic toxicity [5,32].

OTHER SYSTEMS

Some other reported symptoms are chronic cough, bronchitis, anemia, leukopenia, and thrombocytopenia. Arsenic exposure during pregnancy is associated with adverse pregnancy outcomes such as spontaneous abortions, stillbirths, and preterm births [5].

Diagnosis

The maximum permissible limit of arsenic in drinking water was provisionally reduced by the WHO in 1993 from 0.05 mg/L to 0.01 mg/L [33], but India still considers 0.05 mg/L as standard, because of a lack of adequate testing facilities for lower concentrations [33]. Measurement of 24-hour urinary arsenic level can be a good indicator of recent arsenic exposure as it is principally excreted via the kidneys [34,35]. Normal levels are <50 µg/L. Normal concentrations of arsenic in hair and nails are up to 1 and 1.5 mg/kg, respectively [13]. It takes about 100 days after

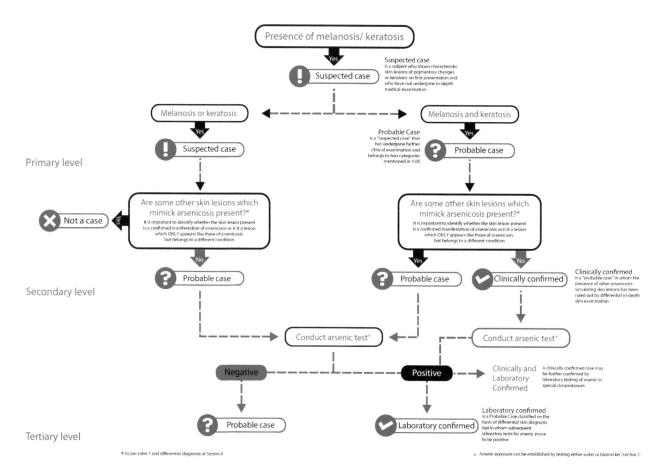

Flowchart 49.1 Alogorithmic approach for case definition and diagnosis of arsenicosis. (From Caussy D [Ed]. *A Field Guide for Detection, Management and Surveillance of Arsenicosis Cases.* New Delhi: World Health Organization, Regional Office of South-East Asia; 2005.)

exposure for arsenic to be detected at the tips of nails [36]. Arsenic has a very short half-life in blood, so blood arsenic level is not of much help in chronic poisoning.

Histology

Histological examination of the keratotic lesions reveals hyperkeratosis with or without parakeratosis, acanthosis, and enlargement of the rete ridges [37,38]. In some cases there may be basal cell pigmentation, dysplasia, and malignant changes [37]. Bowen disease, BCC, and SCC show usual characteristic features.

The WHO's regional office of Southeast Asia has come up with an algorithmic approach to diagnose arsenicosis with locally available resources (Flowchart 49.1) [14].

Treatment

GENERAL MEASURES

Once features of chronic arsenicosis are detected, the possible source should then be avoided. The method for removing arsenic content from water and making it operational at mass level are yet to be developed, so finding an arsenic-free water source would be of primary concern. Some proposed

options are deep wells, traditionally dug wells, and rainwater harvesting.

SPECIFIC MEASURES

Cutaneous lesions

Hyperkeratosis of the palm and sole can be treated by local application of 5%–10% salicylic acid and 10%–20% urea-based ointment and emollients. Retinoids are suitable choices for severe arsenical keratosis which has malignant potential [39,40]. Lesions of Bowen disease, BCC, and SCC need to be treated by surgical excision and close follow-up.

Treatment of systemic symptoms

GI symptoms such as dyspepsia and constipation can be controlled by H_2 receptor blockers and prokinetic drugs. More serious problems such as portal hypertension may require sclerotherapy or banding. Distressing peripheral neuropathy is often difficult to manage, but a tricyclic antidepressant can be helpful in some.

Peripheral vascular disease eventually ends up in gangrene requiring amputation, but pentoxifylline and calcium channel blockers can be tried with some benefit in the initial stage.

Chelation therapy

Various available chelating agents for arsenic toxicity are DMSA (dimercaptosuccinic acid), DMPS (dimercaptopropane succinate), and d-penicillamine [41–43]. DMPS has shown good results in some studies by increasing urinary excretion of arsenic.

Others

Free radicals play an important role in arsenic-induced toxicity. This prompts the use of agents such as vitamin C, vitamin E [44], polyphenols, and extracts of green and black tea [45] as antioxidants in ameliorating the symptoms of arsenic toxicity.

SILVER POISONING

Silver is a naturally occurring metallic compound that is amply found in nature [46]. The National Institute for Occupational Safety and Health (NIOSH) established a Recommended Exposure Limit (REL) of 0.01 mg/m^3 for both soluble silver compounds and silver metal dust. The WHO has set up limits up to 0.1 mg/L for drinking water levels and total lifetime oral intake of 10 g for no observable adverse effect.

Source

Exposure to silver can occur through ingestion or inhalation or by direct impregnation into the skin.

OCCUPATIONAL

Silver is widely used in various industrial works such as mining; manufacturing of mirrors, batteries, and jewelery; photography; etc. [47]. Exposure may be localized through direct skin contact, or it may be generalized by inhalation of fumes containing silver particles.

MEDICINAL

Traditionally, silver compounds and colloidal silver proteins because of their antimicrobial, caustic, astringent, and hemostatic properties have been used in the treatment of ophthalmia neonatorum, syphilis, GI disorders, oral ulcers, warts, and for bladder irrigation. Various cough syrups, eye drops, nasal sprays [48], and herbal dietary supplements [49] also contained a certain amount of silver. But now this has declined because of the availability of safer options. Currently the most common use of silver preparations as a medicinal agent is for burns as silver sulfadiazine cream. Medical devices such as prosthetic implants, splints, catheters, heart valves, stents, bone cement, and dental fillings are other possible sources [48,50].

COSMETICS AND OTHERS

Certain cosmetics such as eyelash dye [51] and silver earrings [52] can be a potential source of exposure. Mouth fresheners [53] and sweets sometimes have silver coatings on them.

ACCIDENTAL

There are reports of accidental exposure to silver through contaminated water during hemodialysis [54] and patients with psychiatric illness chewing photographic films [55].

Acute toxicity

Large doses of inorganic silver salts such as silver nitrate if ingested have a corrosive effect on the GI tract leading to abdominal pain, vomiting, and diarrhea. Respiratory tract irritation occurs if inhaled. Severe toxicity may progress to decreased blood pressure, depressed respiration, convulsions, and shock [47], although these corrosive effects are likely to be due to the nitrate in the compound rather than to the silver itself [47]. Organic silver compounds, such as colloidal silver, are less toxic but may have effects like pleural edema, hemolysis, and coma if consumed in large doses [49].

Chronic toxicity

Long-term exposure to silver and its compounds results in a distinctive condition known as argyria. It may be localized or generalized depending on the exposure type. Generalized argyria is a manifestation of long-term systemic absorption of silver affecting the skin, eyes, mucosa, nails, and internal organs such as the spleen and liver. But systemic symptoms and carcinogenicity are rare even after prolonged exposure. There is a typical blue-gray pigmentation with a bit of a shiny tinge with accentuation over the sun-exposed site. The pigmentation appears gradually over years and is often mistaken by the patient as tanning in the beginning. After absorption, silver binds to tissue proteins and is converted to metallic silver in the presence of light, which then further oxidizes to form silver sulfide and silver selenide, which are responsible for the blackish discoloration.

Differential diagnosis

Argyria is mimicked by metabolic disorders such as Addison disease, hemochromatosis, methemoglobinemia, Wilson disease, idiopathic dermatoses like erythema dyschromicum perstans, and lichen planus pigmentosus [50]. Other possible conditions that pose diagnostic difficulties are chronic exposure to drugs like minocycline, clofazimine, antimalarials, amiodarone, and chlorpromazine. Chronic exposure to heavy metals such as gold, mercury, and lead can also lead to similar skin pigmentation [56].

Histopathology

Histopathological examination reveals deposition of fine brown-black granules in the basement membrane of the eccrine gland [57], blood vessel walls, elastic fibers of the papillary dermis, and less frequently in the connective tissue sheaths surrounding pilosebaceous units, perineural tissues, and arrector pili muscles. When the deposit is inconspicuous under light microscopy, dark-field microscopy may help where the granules are seen as brightly refractile particles [58].

Management

Once evolved, the pigmentation in argyria is usually persistent, but identifying the source may help to prevent further progression. Sunscreen prevents additional pigmentary darkening. Hydroquinone and dermabrasion have been tried without much effect. Laser treatment with Q-switched 1064-nm neodymium:yttrium-aluminum-garnet (Nd:YAG) has shown better outcome in some [59].

LEAD

Lead is a heavy metal that is ubiquitous in nature though it does not have any physiological role in the human body. Lead and its various salts such as lead acetate, lead carbonate, lead chromate, and lead trioxide (component of vermillion [sindur]) all produce toxicity in humans if exposed to a significant amount.

Source

OCCUPATIONAL

Lead is an important material in industries such as battery, glass, paint, plastics, rubber, printing, and piping. Exposure occurs by inhaling dust and fumes during processing.

ENVIRONMENTAL

Water supplies through lead pipes and food storage cans where lead solder is used can cause toxicity in the long run. Lead exposure of children from lead paint is an important cause of childhood lead poisoning. With the gaining popularity of ayurvedic medicines, a considerable number of cases with lead toxicity are being reported following their consumption [60–62].

Acute poisoning

Acute lead poisoning, though not so frequent as chronic, can occur following occupational exposure [63], suicidal attempts [64], and accidental ingestion in psychiatric patients [65].

Acute poisoning is characterized by abdominal pain, diarrhea, vomiting, hemolytic anemia, hepatitis, and neurologic dysfunction in the form of paraesthesia. In severe cases there may be renal failure and cerebral edema. Lead prevents the incorporation of iron into the protoporphyrin molecule by interfering with the enzyme ferrochelatase. So free erythropoietic porphyrin level (EFP) could be an indicator of lead toxicity, especially helping to distinguish between acute and chronic poisoning where both blood lead level and EFP will be elevated but in acute EFP will not be elevated.

TREATMENT

In case of acute poisoning, gastric lavage with 1% solution of sodium or magnesium sulfate is given initially along with continuous supportive treatment according to the presenting symptoms. Oral chelation therapy with D-penicillamine and succimer and parenteral chelation with calcium disodium EDTA and BAL can be given.

Chronic poisoning

Chronic poisoning occurs with long-term exposure to various forms of lead in occupational fields and through food, water, cosmetics, hair dye, paints, and toys in the case of children, etc.

Both systemic as well as cutaneous symptoms may occur. There is anemia (due to impaired heme synthesis and hemolysis), colicky abdominal pain (lead colic), constipation or diarrhea, neuromuscular symptoms, myalgias, arthralgias, wrist drop (lead palsy), peripheral neuritis, hypertension, and menstrual disturbances in females. Central nervous system (CNS) symptoms, which are more common in children, occur in the form of irritability, sleeplessness, memory disturbances, convulsions, encephalopathy, etc. Over time, lead nephropathy may progress to chronic kidney disease.

CUTANEOUS FEATURES

There is prominent cutaneous pallor particularly over the face known as lead hue. Stippled blue lines over the gums are also seen and are known as lead lines or Burtonian lines, which are often difficult to demonstrate in case of good oral hygiene and should be differentiated from venous congestion of gums, cyanosis, and bismuth and other metallic deposits.

LABORATORY FINDINGS

There is anemia, reticulocytosis, and basophilic stippling of erythrocytes. In case of adults <10 µg/dL is considered to be a normal blood lead level, but in children adverse effects are seen even with levels below 10 µg/dL [66]. Under normal circumstances, a very small amount of lead (0.04–0.08 mg in 24 hours) is excreted via urine. In case of increased exposure, levels are usually >0.1 mg in 24 hours.

Treatment

Avoidance of the source of exposure is of utmost importance. Chelation therapy is indicated even in asymptomatic children with blood lead level >45 µg/dL. Dimercaprol or BAL, calcium disodium ethylene diamine tetra-acetic acid (CaNa2EDTA), D-penicillamine, and Meso-2,3-dimercaptosuccinic acid (DMSA), named succimer, are approved for the treatment of acute and chronic lead poisoning [67]. Thiamine in combination with CaNa2 EDTA, vitamins C and E, and garlic all have shown some efficacy in reducing lead-induced oxidative stress [68–70].

MERCURY TOXICITY

Mercury belongs to the heavy metal group and exists in several forms, such as elemental mercury, inorganic mercury which includes the mercuric or mercurous salts, and organic mercury. Effects on humans vary according to the form and routes of exposure.

Sources

OCCUPATIONAL

Industries for manufacturing batteries, thermometers, barometers, photography, jewelery, etc., use mercury during their processing. Mercury is also used in fungicides and pesticides in farming.

ENVIRONMENTAL

Human exposure to organic mercury is principally through consumption of seafood. Industrial mercury waste flowing into the water adds to the intake [71].

OTHERS

Significant mercury exposure can occur following prolonged intake of some ayurvedic medicines as mercury is one of the most widely used heavy metals for drug preparation in ayurveda [72,73]. Mercury concentrations often exceeding the recommended values have been found in skin lightening creams [74,75].

Exposure to mercury can occur through inhalation, ingestion, injection, or by direct skin contact.

Toxicity

Toxic manifestation of mercury on humans varies according to the form of this metal, such as metallic, organic, or inorganic.

METALLIC MERCURY

Exposure to metallic mercury is mostly occupational by inhalation of mercury vapor. Symptoms range from shortness of breath to bronchiolitis, pneumonitis, and pulmonary edema, ultimately terminating into severe respiratory failure and death. The CNS is also affected significantly, producing symptoms like tremor, decreased performance, mercurial erethism, etc. [76]. Elemental mercury is not usually absorbed by healthy GI mucosa but ulcerative gingivitis, loose teeth, and excess salivation may be seen in some.

INORGANIC MERCURY

Inorganic mercury is readily absorbed by GI mucosa and leads to severe gastroenteritis, excessive salivation, oral ulceration, and gingival bleeding. Excessive fluid loss may precipitate into shock and acute tubular necrosis [77].

ORGANIC MERCURY

Exposure to organic mercury through ingestion causes GI symptoms, but it is less corrosive than inorganic mercury. Long-term hazardous effects occur in the CNS, such as neuropsychiatric disturbances, neuropathy, and even visual loss. Seafood and many traditional medicinal preparations can be possible sources.

Cutaneous manifestations

Skin contact with mercury can have local side effects such as erythema, formation of indurated plaque, ulceration, etc. [78]. Cutaneous mercury granulomas have been reported following accidental injury from mercury [79,80]. Oral lichen planus following dental amalgam filling containing mercury is a well-established entity supported by positive patch test [81]. Allergic contact dermatitis to mercury can occur by both topical as well as systemic exposure [82]. Individuals previously sensitized by small doses of mercury can later develop a form of systemic contact dermatitis known as baboon syndrome [83]. Acrodynia thought to be a hypersensitivity reaction to mercury primarily occurs in infants and children [84], characterized by pinkish discoloration of hands and feet with severe pain and pruritus [85]. There may be blotchy erythema over the trunk as well. Other symptoms such as gingivitis, loosening of teeth, dyspnea, and reduced urine output may also occur [86,87].

DIAGNOSIS

Exposure to mercury can be suspected from measuring levels in blood, urine, hair, and nail. Normal blood mercury concentration is usually between 10 and 20 µg/L [88,89]. Long-term mercury exposure can be best assessed by its levels in hair and nail, which persist even after exposure has ceased. Under normal circumstances, hair mercury level is <10 mg/kg. In case of poisoning it may go up to 200–800 mg/kg [90].

Treatment

Treatment includes avoiding the source of exposure, supportive therapy for acute symptoms, and chelation therapy. After securing provision for ventilatory support and fluid management, all contaminated clothing should be removed and skin should be cleansed thoroughly to prevent further absorption of mercury via skin. Gastric lavage is avoided in inorganic mercury poisoning because of its corrosive action but is preferred in organic poisoning. Activated charcoal and bowel irrigation with polyethylene glycol may be helpful. Oral therapy with D-penicillamine may be used for inorganic and metallic mercury toxicity, but DMSA that can be given either orally or through IV has been found to be a better choice [91]. Other chelating agents are DMPS and BAL. Plasmapheresis may be tried when conventional hemodialysis is unable to remove protein-bound mercury [91].

KEY POINTS

- Poisoning is due to exposure to some chemicals and cutaneous clues may be helpful in diagnosis.
- Features of arsenicosis include pigmentary changes, hyperkeratosis and cutaneous malignancies.
- Argyria has typical blue-gray pigmentation with accentuation over sun-exposed sites.
- Lead poisoning is characterized by stippled blue lines over the gums known as lead lines or Burtonian lines.
- Treatment includes avoiding the source of exposure, supportive therapy for acute symptoms, and chelation therapy.

REFERENCES

1. Fowler's solution. Drugstore museum. http://drugstoremuseum.com/sections/level_info2.php?level_id=145d%22vel=2%20 (Accessed April 2, 2008).
2. Anonymous Arsenic. Victoria King discovers the history of the infamous element. *History Magazine*. http://www.history-magazine.com/arsenic.html (Accessed April 2, 2008).
3. Waxman S, Anderson KC. History of the development of arsenic derivatives in cancer therapy. *Oncologist* 2001;6:3–10.
4. Mukherjee A et al. Arsenic contamination in groundwater: A global perspective with emphasis on the Asian scenario. *J Health Popul Nutr* 2006;24:142–63.
5. Sarma N. Arsenicosis—Indian Perspective. In: Ghosh S, Sarma N, De D (Eds), *Recent Advances in Dermatology*. Vol. 3. New Delhi: Jaypee Brothers Medical Publishers; 2014:134–53.
6. De Chaudhuri S et al. Genetic variants associated with arsenic susceptibility: Study of purine nucleoside phosphorylase, arsenic (+3) methyltransferase, and glutathione S-transferase omega genes. *Environ Health Perspect* 2008;116(4):501–5.
7. Chatterjee D, Bhattacharjee P, Sau TJ, Das JK, Sarma N. Arsenic exposure through drinking water leads to senescence and alteration of telomere length in humans: A case-control study in West Bengal, India. *Mol Carcinog* 2015;54(9):800–9.
8. Banerjee M et al. DNA repair deficiency leads to susceptibility to develop arsenic-induced premalignant skin lesions. *Int J Cancer* 2008;123:283–7.
9. Chatterjee D et al. Role of microRNAs in senescence and its contribution to peripheral neuropathy in the arsenic exposed population of West Bengal, India. *Environ Pollut* 2018;233:596–603.
10. Gossel TA, Bricker JD. *Principles of Clinical Toxicology*. 3rd ed. New York: Raven Press; 1994:184–5.
11. Jolliffe DM, Budd AJ, Gwilt DJ. Massive acute arsenic poisoning. *Anesthesia* 1991;46:288–90.
12. Arsenicosis Case-Detection, Management and Surveillance. Report of a Regional Consultation. New Delhi: WHO Regional Office for South-East Asia; June 2003.
13. Sarma N. Skin manifestations of chronic arsenicosis. In: States JC (Ed), *Arsenic: Exposure Sources, Health Risks, and Mechanisms of Toxicity*. New York: John Wiley & Sons; 2016:127–36.
14. Caussy D (Ed). *A Field Guide for Detection, Management and Surveillance of Arsenicosis Cases*. New Delhi: World Health Organization, Regional Office of South-East Asia; 2005.
15. Tay CH. Cutaneous manifestations of arsenic poisoning due to certain Chinese herbal medicine. *Australas J Dermatol* 1974;15:121–31.
16. Saha KC. Chronic arsenical dermatoses from tubewell water in West Bengal during 1983–1987. *Ind J Dermatol* 1995;40:1–12.
17. Saha KC. Diagnosis of arsenicosis. *J Environ Sci Health A Tox Hazard Subst Environ Eng* 2003;38:255–72.
18. Peer review of EPA's research plan for arsenic in drinking water. Draft report. Ad-hoc subcommittee on arsenic research, board of scientific counselors (BOSC), office of research and development. US EPA (US Environmental Protection Agency) Washington, DC, U.S. Environmental Protection Agency. 1997.
19. Paul S et al. Arsenic-induced toxicity and carcinogenicity: A two-wave cross-sectional study in arsenicosis individuals in West Bengal, India. *J Expo Sci Environ Epidemiol* 2013;23(2):156–62.
20. Das N et al. Arsenic exposure through drinking water increases the risk of liver and cardiovascular diseases in the population of West Bengal, India. *BMC Public Health* 2012;12:639.
21. Yusra Ahmad BA. The largest mass poisoning in recorded history. *International Health* 2004;82:57–8.
22. Lien HC, Tsai TF, Lee YY, Hsiao CH. Merkel cell carcinoma and chronic arsenicism. *J Am Acad Dermatol* 1999;41:641–3.
23. Castren K, Ranki A, Welsh JA, Vähäkangas KH. Infrequent p53 mutations in arsenic-related skin lesions. *Oncol Res* 1998;10:475–82.
24. Lee CH et al. Effects and interactions of low doses of arsenic and UVB on keratinocyte apoptosis. *Chem Res Toxicol* 2004;17:1199–205.
25. Yu HS, Lee CH, Jee SH, Ho CK, Guo YL. Environmental and occupational skin diseases in Taiwan. *J Dermatol* 2001;28:628–31.
26. Mazumder DN. Effect of chronic intake of arsenic-contaminated water on liver. *Toxicol Appl Pharmacol* 2005;206:169–75.

27. Chang CC, Ho SC, Tsai SS, Yang CY. Ischemic heart disease mortality reduction in an arseniasis-endemic area in southwestern Taiwan after a switch in the tap-water supply system. *J Toxicol Environ Health* 2004;67:1353–61.

28. Tseng CH. An overview on peripheral vascular disease in blackfoot disease—Hyperendemic villages in Taiwan. *Angiology* 2002;53:529–37.

29. Yeh S, How SW. A pathological study on the blackfoot disease in Taiwan. *Reports Inst Pathol Natl Taiwan Univ* 1963;14:25–73.

30. Chen CJ et al. Increased prevalence of hypertension and long-term arsenic exposure. *Hypertension* 1995;25:53–60.

31. Chen CJ, Chiou HY, Chiang MH, Lin LJ, Tai TY. Dose-response relation between ischemic heart disease and mortality and long-term arsenic exposure. *Arterioscler Thromb Vasc Biol* 1996;16:504–10.

32. Mukherjee SC et al. Neuropathy in arsenic toxicity from groundwater arsenic contamination in West Bengal, India. *J Environ Sci Health A Tox Hazard Subst Environ Eng* 2003;38:165–83.

33. Smedley PL, Kinniburgh DG. Source and behaviour of arsenic in natural waters. http://www.who.int/entity/water_sanitation_health/dwq/arsenicun1.pdf

34. Buchet JP, Lauwerys R, Roels H. Comparison of the urinary excretion of arsenic metabolites after a single oral dose of sodium arsenite, monomethylarsonate or dimethylarsenate in man. *Int Arch Occup Environ Health* 1981;48:71–9.

35. Vahter M. Species differences in the metabolism of arsenic compounds. *Appl Organomet Chem* 1994;8:175–82.

36. Pounds CA, Pearson EF, Turner TD. Arsenic in fingernails. *J Forensic Sci Soc J* 1979;19:165–74.

37. Sikder MS, Rahman MH, Maidul AZ, Khan MS, Rahman MM. Study on the histopathology of chronic Arsenicosis. *J Pakistan Assoc Derma* 2004;14:205–9.

38. Yeh S. Skin cancer in chronic arsenicism. *Hum Pathol* 1973;4:469–85.

39. Thiaprasit M. Chronic cutaneous arsenism treated with aromatic retinoid. *J Med Assoc Thailand* 1984;67:93–100.

40. Miller WH. The emerging role of retinoids and retinoic acid metabolism blocking agents in the treatment of cancer. *Cancer* 1998;83:1471–82.

41. GuhaMazumder DN et al. Randomized placebo-controlled trial of 2.3- dimercapto-l-propanesulfonate (DMPS) in therapy of chronic arsenicosis due to drinking arsenic-contaminated water. *J Toxicol Clin Toxicol* 2001;39:665–74.

42. Shum S, Whitehead J, Vanghn LS, Shum RN, Hale T. Chelation of organo arsenate with dimercaptosuccinic acid (DMSA). *Vet Human Toxicol* 1995;37:239–42.

43. Guha MDN et al. Randomized placebo-controlled trial of 2,3-dimercaptosuccinic acid in therapy of chronic arsenicosis due to drinking arsenic-contaminated subsoil water. *J Toxicol Clin Toxicol* 1998;36:683–90.

44. Khandker S, Dey RK, Maidul Islam AZ, Ahmad SA, Mahmud IA. Arsenic-safe drinking water and antioxidants for the management of arsenicosis patients. *Bangladesh J Pharmacol* 2006;1:42–50.

45. Sinha D, Dey S, Bhattacharya RK, Roy M. In vitro mitigation of arsenic toxicity by tea polyphenols in human lymphocytes. *J Environ Pathol Toxicol Oncol* 2007;26:207–20.

46. Brandt D, Park B, Hoang M, Jacobe HT. Argyria secondary to ingestion of homemade silver solution. *J Am Acad Dermatol* 2005;53:S105–7.

47. Drake PL, Hazelwood KJ. Exposure-related health effects of silver and silver compounds: A review. *Ann Occup Hyg* 2005;49:575–85.

48. Lansdown AB. Silver in health care: Antimicrobial effects and safety in use. *Curr Probl Dermatol* 2006;33:17–34.

49. Wadhera A, Fung M. Systemic argyria associated with ingestion of colloidal silver. *Dermatol Online J* 2005;11:12.

50. Lansdown AB. A pharmacological and toxicological profile of silver as an antimicrobial agent in medical devices. *Adv Pharmacol Sci* 2010;2010:910686.

51. Weiler HH, Lemp MA, Zeavin BH, Suarez AF. Argyria of the cornea due to self-administration of eyelash dye. *Ann Ophthalmol* 1982;14:822–3.

52. Sugden P, Azad S, Erdmann M. Argyria caused by an earring. *Br J Plast Surg* 2001;54:252–3.

53. Shimamoto Y, Shimamoto H. Systemic argyria secondary to breath freshener "Jintan Silver Pills." *Hiroshima J Med Sci* 1987;36:245–7.

54. Sue YM, Lee JY, Wang MC, Lin TK, Sung JM, Huang JJ. Generalized argyria in two chronic hemodialysis patients. *Am J Kidney Dis* 2001;37:1048–51.

55. Plack W, Bellizzi R. Generalized argyria secondary to chewing photographic film. Report of a case. *Oral Surg Oral Med Oral Pathol* 1980;49:504–6.

56. Kubba A, Kubba R, Batrani M, Pal T. Argyria an unrecognized cause of cutaneous pigmentation in Indian patients: A case series and review of the literature. *Indian J Dermatol Venereol Leprol* 2013;79:805–11.

57. Hill W, Montgomery H. Argyria, with special reference to the cutaneous histopathology. *Arch Dermatol* 1941;44:588.

58. Jonas L, Bloch C, Zimmermann R, Stadie V, Gross GE, Schäd SG. Detection of silver sulfide deposits in the skin of patients with argyria after long-term use of silver-containing drugs. *Ultrastruct Pathol* 2007;31:379–84.

59. Hovenic W, Golda N. Treatment of argyria using the quality-switched 1,064-nm neodymium-doped yttrium aluminum garnet laser: Efficacy and persistence of results at 1-year follow-up. *Dermatol Surg* 2012;38:2031–4.

60. Centers for Disease Control and Prevention (CDC). Lead poisoning associated with Ayurvedic medications—Five states, 2000–2003. *Morb Mortal Wkly Rep* 2004;53:582–4.

61. Breeher L, Gerr F, Fuortes L. A case report of adult lead toxicity following use of Ayurvedic herbal medication. *J Occup Med Toxicol* 2013;8:26.

62. Raviraja A et al. Three cases of lead toxicity associated with consumption of Ayurvedic medicines. *Indian J Clin Biochem* 2010;25:326–9.

63. Ogawa M, Nakajima Y, Kubota R, Endo Y. Two cases of acute lead poisoning due to occupational exposure to lead. *Clin Toxicol (Phila)* 2008;46:332–5.

64. Nortier JW, Sangster B, van Kestern RG. Acute lead poisoning with hemolysis and liver toxicity after ingestion of red lead. *Vet Hum Toxicol* 1980;22:145–7.

65. Vance MV, Curry SC, Bradley JM, Kunkel DB, Gerkin RD, Bond GR. Acute lead poisoning in nursing home and psychiatric patients from the ingestion of lead-based ceramic glazes. *Arch Intern Med* 1990;150:2085–92.

66. Chandran L, Cataldo R. Lead poisoning: Basics and new developments. *Pediatr Rev* 2010;31:399–405.

67. Wang C et al. Effect of ascorbic acid and thiamine supplementation at different concentrations on lead toxicity in liver. *Ann Occup Hyg* 2007;51(6):563–9.

68. Sajitha GR et al. Garlic oil and vitamin E prevent the adverse effects of lead acetate and ethanol separately as well as in combination in the drinking water of rats. *Indian J Clin Biochem* 2010;25(3):280–8.

69. Kianoush S et al. Comparison of therapeutic effects of garlic and d-penicillamine in patients with chronic occupational lead poisoning. *Basic Clin Pharmacol Toxicol* 2012;110:476–81.

70. Environmental Health Department, Ministry of the Environment, Minimata Disease: The History and Measures, Ministry of the Environment, Government of Japan, Tokyo, Japan, 2002.

71. Karamanou M, Kyriakis K, Tsoucalas G, Androutsos G. Hallmarks in history of syphilis therapeutics. *Infez Med* 2013;21:317–9.

72. The Ayurvedic Formulary of India, Part-1, Edn-1, Ministry of Health and Family Planning, Government of India. 1978. pp. 141–219.

73. Dadzie OE, Petit A. Skin bleaching: Highlighting the misuse of cutaneous depigmenting agents. *J Eur Acad Dermatol Venereol* 2009;23:741–50.

74. Boyd AS, Seger D, Vannucci S, Langley M, Abraham JL, King LE. Mercury exposure and cutaneous disease. *J Am Acad Dermatol* 2000;43:81–90.

75. Hua MS, Huang CC, Yang WJ. Chronic elemental mercury intoxication: Neuropsychological follow-up case study. *Brain Inj* 1995;10:377–84.

76. Bates N. Metallic and inorganic mercury poisoning. *Emerg Nurse* 2003;11:25–31.

77. Jun JB, Min PK, Kim DW, Chung SL, Lee KH. Cutaneous nodular reaction to oral mercury. *J Am Acad Dermatol* 1997;37:131–3.

78. George A, Kwatra KS, Chandra S. Cutaneous mercury granuloma following accidental occupational exposure. *Indian J Dermatol Venereol Leprol* 2015;81:57–9.

79. Risher JF. *Elemental Mercury and Inorganic Mercury Compounds: Human Health Aspects.* Geneva: World Health Organization; 2003.

80. Sandra A, Srinivas CR, Pai S, Pai K. Oral lichen planus caused by dental amalgam. *Indian J Dermatol Venereol Leprol* 1996;62:127–8.

81. Dantzig PI. A new cutaneous sign of mercury poisoning? *J Am Acad Dermatol* 2003;49:1109, 1nn111.

82. Wen L, Yin J, Ma D-L, Lanier B. Baboon syndrome induced by mercury—First case report in China. *Contact Dermatitis* 2007;56:356–7.

83. Warkany J. Acrodynia: Postmortem of a disease. *Am J Dis Child* 1966;112:146–56.

84. Shandley K, Austin DW. Ancestry of pink disease (infantile acrodynia) identified as a risk factor for autism spectrum disorders. *J Toxicol Environ Health* 2011;74:1185–94.

85. AbréuVélez AM et al. Detection of mercury and other undetermined materials in skin biopsies of endemic pemphigus foliaceus. *Am J Dermatopathol* 2003;25:384–91.

86. Robledo MA. Chronic methyl mercury poisoning may trigger endemic pemphigus foliaceus "fogoselvagem." *Med Hypotheses* 2012;78:60–6.

87. Klaassen CD. *Casarett and Doull's Toxicology: The Basic Science of Poisons.* New York: McGraw-Hill; 2007.

88. "3rd National report on human exposure to environmental chemicals," Tech. Rep., Centers for Disease Control and Prevention, 2005.

89. Alhibshi EA. Subclinical neurotoxicity of mercury: A behavioural, molecular mechanisms and therapeutic perspective. *Res J Pharm Biol Chem Sci* 2012;3:34–42.

90. Katzung BG, Masters SB, Trevor AJ. *Basic and Clinical Pharmacology.* New York: McGraw-Hill; 2009.

91. Nenov VD, Marinov P, Sabeva J, Nenov DS. Current applications of plasmapheresis in clinical toxicology. *Nephrol Dial Transplant* 2003;5:v56–8.

PART 12

Psoriasis and Related Conditions

BIJU VASUDEVAN

50

Pustular psoriasis

SANTANU BANERJEE AND NEERJA SARASWAT

INTRODUCTION

Pustular psoriasis can present in two main forms: localized and generalized. The generalized pustular form can manifest as a dermatological emergency and is associated with life-threatening complications. Generalized pustular psoriasis is described here.

GENERALIZED PUSTULAR PSORIASIS

Introduction

Generalized pustular psoriasis (GPP) is one of the most severe forms of psoriasis and is characterized by uncontrolled, widespread severe generalized eruptions with many systemic complications. The dermatologist should start aggressive and the most effective treatment at the earliest to save patients from succumbing to sepsis, acute renal failure, congestive cardiac failure (CCF), and acute respiratory distress syndrome (ARDS).

Epidemiology

Annual incidence and prevalence are very low at 0.64–1.76 per million, with Japan having the maximum prevalence at 7.46 per million. The peak age of incidence is about 40–59 years of age with women outnumbering men in the ratio of 2:1. Inflammatory polyarthritis and metabolic syndrome is commonly associated with GPP [1].

Etiopathogenesis

A variety of factors have been proposed to trigger or aggravate acute GPP. The most common factors are briefly discussed as follows:

- *Infections*: Both bacterial and viral infections are known to precipitate acute GPP, most importantly, infections such as dental and upper respiratory tract infections,

otitis media, and group A streptococcal and staphylococcal infections. The proposed mechanism is the bacterial superantigen, which triggers the T-cell-mediated autoimmune reaction resulting in the development of pustular psoriasis. Antistreptolysin antibodies are reported to be positive in cases of acute GPP, providing an important association between the two [1].
- *Psychological stress*
- *Pregnancy*
- *Hypocalcemia*
- *Drugs*
  - Withdrawal of systemic steroids—acute withdrawal of systemic corticosteroids results in acute inflammatory process leading to acute GPP
  - Overuse of topical steroids
  - Withdrawal of cyclosporine
  - Terbinafine, propranolol, bupropion, lithium, phenylbutazone, salicylates, potassium iodide
- *Genetic*: Mutation in IL-1 and IL-36 receptor antagonistic genes (IL-36RN) leads to unopposed activity of proinflammatory signaling pathways, namely, the nuclear factor κ-light-chain-enhancer of activated B cells (NF-κB) and mitogen-activated protein kinase (MAP kinase) pathway. IL-6 and its receptor complex have gained attention due to their role in the pathogenesis of pustular psoriasis. This complex expresses gp130, activates JAK/STAT kinase pathway, leading to increased nuclear gene expression. Downstream effects of IL-6 are synthesis of acute phase reactants, maturation of B cells, differentiation of T cells, augmentation of Th17 cell development, neutrophil maturation, enhanced migration of neutrophils, and release of proinflammatory cytokines like IL-23 and IL-17, which further promote Th17 positive feedback loop. In addition, neutrophil-derived elastase is a potent IL-36 activating enzyme implicated in the pathogenesis of pustular psoriasis.

- Sometimes pustular dermatitis is part of systemic inflammatory syndromes.
- Deficiency of interleukin-1 receptor antagonist (DIRA) and deficiency of IL-36 receptor antagonist (DITRA).

IL36RN MUTATIONS: IMPORTANCE IN PATHOGENESIS AND TREATMENT

Evidence suggests that some cases of GPP may actually represent a new genetic auto-inflammatory disease based on mutations in the *IL36RN* gene, which encodes the IL-36 receptor antagonist. This disease is known as the deficiency of interleukin-36-receptor antagonist (DITRA).

Patients with *IL36RN* mutations upregulate IL-1, in response to IL-36 stimulation. Case reports documenting successful treatment of GPP in patients with *IL36RN* mutations with Anakinra, an IL-1 receptor antagonist, support the importance of this pathway.

The beneficial effects of TNF-inhibiting drugs and anti-IL-23/IL-17 antibodies for GPP appear independent of the presence of the *IL36RN* mutation. Whether agents targeting *IL36RN* or IL-1 will be more effective and/or safer for patients with the mutation remains to be determined [2].

Clinical features

PATIENTS AT RISK

- Patients on offending drugs as presented later in the chapter
- Pregnant patients
- Psoriasis patients with hypoparathyroidism and hypocalcemia
- Patients with HLA-B27 and HLA-Cw along with genetic mutations—*IL36RN* mutations

VARIANTS

1. Acute generalized pustular psoriasis (von Zumbusch)
   There are two main groups of patients.
   The acute variant (also known as generalized pustular psoriasis of von Zumbusch) is characterized by the sudden onset of generalized pustular formation, where pustules are sterile (Figure 50.1). There is accompanied widespread erythema and inflammation (Figure 50.2). Pustules expand and coalesce to form lakes of pus. Acute pustulation is associated with pain and is generally accompanied by fever, malaise, and anorexia. This acute phase resolves in 2–3 days only to be followed by repeated waves of inflammation and postulation (Figure 50.3). Erythema and pustulation can involve flexural areas of the body, the genital region, and web spaces of fingers. Nails may be thickened or separated by subungual lakes of pus. There can be involvement of mucous membranes in the form of geographic tongue, redness, scaling of lips, and ulceration of tongue and mouth. Systemic complications like hepatitis, pulmonary and renal dysfunction, and sepsis in addition to arthritis can also occur. Laboratory abnormalities, such as leukocytosis, elevated erythrocyte sedimentation

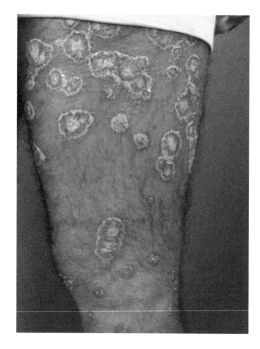

Figure 50.1 Appearance of multiple pustules.

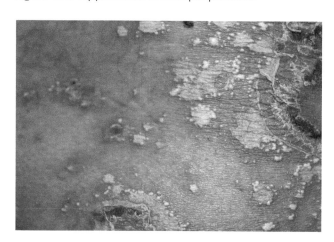

Figure 50.2 Extensive erythema and postulation.

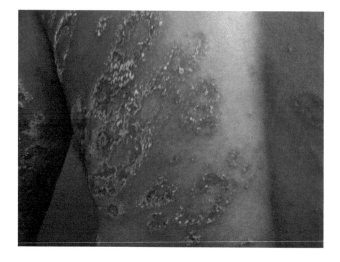

Figure 50.3 Waves of inflammation (erythema and pustulation).

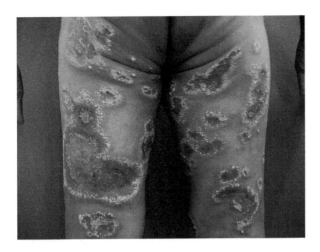

Figure 50.4 Annular generalized pustular psoriasis.

rate, hypocalcemia and other electrolyte abnormalities, hypoalbuminemia, reduced creatinine clearance, elevated urates, and elevated liver enzymes are common.

GPP may also present as a less acute disorder in which patients develop widespread annular or figurate erythematous plaques with peripheral pustules and scale (generalized annular pustular psoriasis) (Figure 50.4). Pain and fever may accompany these cutaneous manifestations.

Diagnostic criteria for acute GPP are as given in Table 50.1.

2. Impetigo herpetiformis

Described by Hebra in 1872, the disease generally has its onset in the last trimester in pregnancy or the first week of puerperium.

The rash is generally flexural in onset, with minute pustules arising symmetrically in acutely inflamed skin. Further progression leads to grouping of pustules extending centrifugally with drying in the center and either healing with reddish-brown pigmentation or progressing into widespread plaques. The tongue, buccal

Table 50.1 Diagnostic criteria for generalized pustular psoriasis

1. Multiple sterile pustules on erythematous skin
2. Systemic symptoms such as fever and malaise
3. The presence of histopathologically confirmed spongiform pustules
4. One or more of the following laboratory test alterations:
   a. Leukocytosis with left shift
   b. Elevated erythrocyte sedimentation rate
   c. Elevated C-reactive protein
   d. High antistreptolysin O antibody levels
   e. Elevation of IgG or IgA
   f. Hypoproteinemia
   g. Hypocalcemia, or recurrence of any of the aforementioned clinical and histologic findings

Source: Umezawa Y et al. *Arch Dermatol Res* 2003;295(Suppl.): S43–54.

mucosa, and even the esophagus may be involved, with circinate or erosive lesions following the appearance of short-lived pustules. Potential triggers for the development of pustular psoriasis of pregnancy include increased progesterone in the last trimester of pregnancy, hypocalcemia, and reduced elafin levels. Other associations are hormonal contraception, stress, seasonal variation, bacterial infections, and certain medications.

The disease is characterized by severe systemic symptoms; death may occur due to cardiac or renal failure. Severe fever, delirium, diarrhea, vomiting, and tetany have been described. The fetus can also be affected due to risk of placental insufficiency leading to stillbirth, premature rupture of membrane, preterm labor, intrauterine growth retardation, and neonatal death or fetal abnormalities.

Characteristically, the disease recurs in subsequent pregnancies. Recurrence has been described in up to nine pregnancies, and on subsequent use of oral contraceptives.

3. Infantile and juvenile generalized pustular psoriasis

Pustular psoriasis is rare in this age group, accounting for 1% of severe psoriasis cases. Over 25% of children affected are in their first year of life. The majority of children are aged 2–10 years at onset. The symptoms are mild with spontaneous remission in infancy. The majority have a past history of seborrheic dermatitis, napkin dermatitis, or sudden-onset napkin psoriasis is obtained. They may manifest as long-standing localized pustular psoriasis of the neck or evolve into more serious forms with constitutional symptoms as in the form of von Zumbusch pattern, but annular and circinate forms are more common in this age group. There is a history of recurrence, as in adults.

Differential diagnosis in pustular psoriasis

Although the diagnosis of GPP can be easily made clinically based on the classical picture discussed in presentation, many conditions can closely simulate signs and symptoms of pustular psoriasis, including pemphigus foliaceus, IgA pemphigus (subcorneal pustular dermatosis type or intraepidermal neutrophilic type), pustular miliaria, pustular erythema multiforme, generalized pustular drug eruptions, generalized pustular bacterid, extensive folliculitis, impetigo contagiosa, candidiasis, dermatitis herpetiformis, gram-negative septicemia, infected generalized atopic dermatitis and/or seborrheic dermatitis, acute generalized exanthematous pustulosis (AGEP), and necrolytic migratory erythema. In such conditions it is always prudent to carry out a biopsy, where the presence of intraepidermal spongiform pustules virtually rules out other possibilities.

Complications

- Renal failure—hypovolemia, oligemia
- Hypoalbuminemia—sudden loss of plasma proteins
- Hypocalcemia and tetany

- Decreased absorption of drugs
- Abnormal liver function test
- Cholestatic jaundice—neutrophilic cholangitis
- ARDS—psoriasis-associated aseptic pneumonitis
- Secondary staphylococcal infection
- Hair loss—telogen effluvium
- Amyloidosis

Management of generalized pustular psoriasis

1. *Triaging patient of GPP for hospitalization and investigate simultaneously*

   Due to the high risk of mortality and sudden deterioration of status, it is important to triage out patients who require immediate hospitalization. Simultaneously the patient needs to be investigated thoroughly. Complete blood count (CBC) with absolute lymphocyte counts may reveal absolute lymphopenia; erythrocyte sedimentation rate (ESR) may be raised; liver function tests with enzymes, renal function tests, and urinalysis may be deranged; Tzanck smear from the pustule; bacterial culture; and histopathology should be sent immediately. Histopathology of GPP is identical to that of psoriasis vulgaris, exhibiting parakeratosis, elongated rete ridges, mononuclear infiltrate in superficial dermis, and neutrophil aggregate in epidermis forming spongiform pustules of Kogoj. The treatment is usually governed by the extent of involvement and severity of disease with acitretin, cyclosporine, methotrexate, and infliximab remaining as first lines of therapy. Patients who have systemic symptoms of fever, chills, dyspnea, altered sensorium, and elderly patients with comorbidities such as cardiac, renal, endocrine, and immunodeficient problems will need immediate hospitalization.

2. *Identify and discontinue the causative drug (in drug-induced cases)*

   The withdrawal or administration of a variety of drugs has been linked to GPP as previously discussed. Systemic glucocorticoid withdrawal is a commonly cited contributor, and maintaining the glucocorticoid dose until disease control is achieved with other therapies and then tapering the systemic glucocorticoid with continuation of alternate therapy are advised.

3. *Supportive care*

   Recurrences are common in GPP. Thus, long-term treatment often is required to minimize recurrences of disease. Supportive skin care measures may help to soothe skin symptoms in patients with GPP. Use of moisturizers, wet wraps, and/or oatmeal baths can be beneficial in patients with this disease.

4. *Manage extracutaneous complications*

   Extracutaneous complications such as sepsis or internal organ dysfunction, acute respiratory distress syndrome, hepatic and renal failure, and cholestasis should be actively managed. Patients should be adequately investigated for any organ dysfunction. Routine

Table 50.2 First-line therapy in generalized pustular psoriasis in adults

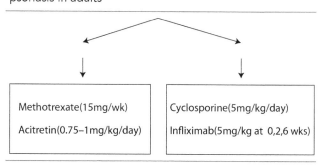

| Methotrexate(15mg/wk) | Cyclosporine(5mg/kg/day) |
| Acitretin(0.75–1mg/kg/day) | Infliximab(5mg/kg at 0,2,6 wks) |

blood count, C-reactive protein, renal and hepatic function, electrolyte levels, albumin, and chest x-ray should be done. Patient should be adequately managed with appropriate antibiotics, electrolytes, and hydration. Oral corticosteroids should be initiated if ARDS is suspected.

5. *Specific therapy*

   Medical treatment options for GPP consist of systemic therapies, topical therapies, and phototherapy [3]. We typically use systemic treatment for the initial management of adults with GPP because phototherapy tends to have a delayed onset of action and topical therapies are impractical for the treatment of widespread disease. Adult GPP (first-line therapy) is as given in Table 50.2.

PATIENTS WITH RELATIVELY STABLE DISEASE

Acitretin

Retinoids are the first line of therapy in a patient with GPP with a relatively stable disease, unless the patient is pregnant or planning pregnancy in the near future. The recommended daily dose is 0.75 mg to 1 mg/kg/day, with patients responding typically within a week of therapy with a maintenance dose of 0.125–0.25 mg/kg/day for several months to prevent recurrences [4].

When added with cyclosporine, it enhances the efficacy and rapidity of onset of action. When compared with other modalities of treatment, acitretin was found to be effective in 84% patients as compared to methotrexate (76%), cyclosporine (71%), and psoralen plus ultraviolet A (PUVA) (46%).

At such high doses, patients may develop serious side effects of pseudotumor cerebri and acute hypertriglyceridemia causing pancreatitis. There are minor, reversible, dose-dependent side effects including hair loss, periungual fibroma, xerosis, cheilitis, dry mucous membranes, hypertriglyceridemia, hair loss, liver function test abnormalities, bone changes, and visual changes which usually resolve when the dose of acitretin is reduced.

There is some evidence to suggest that isotretinoin, which is not considered effective for chronic plaque psoriasis, may be of benefit in GPP.

Methotrexate

This is a valid treatment alternative to acitretin for control of GPP in a patient with a relatively stable disease. It takes about

2 weeks to produce significant effect and is usually given in the dose of 15 mg/week to a maximum of 25 mg/week. The main limiting factor is the possibility of acute catastrophic side effects of pancytopenia, fulminant hepatitis, and pneumonitis [5]. Due to this drawback, a test dose of methotrexate for 1 week delays adequate treatment favoring cyclosporine, acitretin, and infliximab as first-line treatment.

PATIENTS WITH SEVERE ACUTE DISEASE

Cyclosporin

Cyclosporin is one of the most useful agents for rapidly bringing the intensity of generalized inflammation under control, and in some studies it is recommended as the first drug of choice in a patient with acute and severe disease. It is mandatory to use the drug in its maximum dermatological dose of 5 mg/kg/day in two to three divided doses. The onset of action is fairly rapid, as early as 2 weeks, with subsequent tapering of 0.5 mg/kg recommended every 2 weeks.

It is mandatory not to discontinue or decrease the dose of cyclosporine prematurely as intense inflammation has momentum. Therefore, it should be tapered over a period of 2–3 months. Few studies have suggested that if the patient is not controlled with 5 mg/kg/day, the dosage can be increased, which carries the advantage of suppressing the ongoing inflammation and reducing sepsis. Whenever cyclosporine is used in higher doses it is mandatory for the patient to be well hydrated to prevent renal hypoperfusion. Potential adverse effects of cyclosporine include hypertension, renal toxicity, and increased risk for infections and malignancy. Laboratory tests as well as blood pressure should be monitored closely during therapy.

Infliximab

A number of small case series have proven the efficiency of infliximab in the rapid control of GPP; hence, it has also been considered as first-line therapy among the biologicals [6]. The fast onset of infliximab has been evident in the time required to achieve clearance of pustules; pustules cleared in a median of 2 days (range 1–8 days). The dosing of infliximab followed in GPP is as in psoriasis 5 mg/kg at weeks 0, 2, and 6 and thereafter every 6–8 weeks. Alternatively, the patient can be put on other first-line therapies once the acute disease is controlled. Proper pretreatment screening for latent tuberculosis and hepatitis is mandatory.

Potential adverse effects of infliximab include infusion reactions and increased risk for infection, malignancy, heart failure, and demyelinating disease.

ADULT GENERALIZED PUSTULAR PSORIASIS (SECOND-LINE THERAPY)

The second-line therapy is as given in Table 50.3.

Patients who do not respond to or cannot tolerate first-line therapies for GPP may benefit from other approaches to therapy, such as IL-17 inhibitors, photochemotherapy, newer biologics (tumor necrosis factor-alpha [TNF-α] inhibitors), and combination therapy.

Table 50.3 Second-line therapy in adult generalized pustular psoriasis (GPP)

Adult GPP Second line
Adalimumab
Etanercept
Secukinumab
Ixekizumab
Brodalumab
PUVA
Topical corticosteroids
Topical calcipotrieine
Topical tacrolimus

Phototherapy

In an uncontrolled prospective study of eight patients with acute GPP, oral PUVA photochemotherapy (four times weekly) was associated with complete clearing of GPP in all patients within a mean of 13.5 ± 10 treatment sessions. Maintenance therapy (twice weekly PUVA treatments tapered to discontinuation if tolerated) was given upon complete remission, and seven patients remained in complete remission during follow-up periods of up to 1.5 years. The frequent clinic visits required for PUVA photochemotherapy make this a less favorable treatment option for some patients.

Combination therapy

Several case reports demonstrate efficacy when two or more classes of therapeutic agents are used in combination to treat recalcitrant GPP. Examples include methotrexate and cyclosporine, infliximab and methotrexate, infliximab and acitretin, adalimumab and acitretin, adalimumab and methotrexate, and acitretin and PUVA photochemotherapy.

Other therapies

Although systemic glucocorticoid therapy can lead to rapid improvement in GPP, the treatment must be used with caution because systemic glucocorticoids are implicated as potential inciting factors for GPP. In addition, there is concern for the serious side effects from long-term glucocorticoid therapy. Thus, we do not typically use systemic glucocorticoids in the treatment of GPP. In the event that systemic glucocorticoid treatment is given to obtain initial control of GPP, we suggest also initiating a second therapy in an attempt to reduce the likelihood of a disease flare during tapering and discontinuation of the systemic glucocorticoid. However, evidence to support this approach is lacking.

Several case reports document the successful use of granulocyte and monocyte apheresis for the treatment of refractory GPP. Other treatments that have been reported to be effective for GPP in case reports include anakinra, ustekinumab, canakinumab, mycophenolate mofetil, oral zinc, and dapsone. In addition, the onset or worsening of pustular psoriasis following ustekinumab treatment has been reported.

Table 50.4 Summary of treatment of adult generalized pustular psoriasis

Systemic therapy: Based on severity of disease, disease acuity, and contraindications to specific therapy

Slowly progressive/stable disease—Acitretin, methotrexate

Acute, severe, rapidly progressive—Cyclosporine, infliximab

No response to above therapies—Anti-IL-17 agents, combination therapy

Topical therapy as adjunct: Especially in persistent, recalcitrant lesions

Topical therapy—Corticosteroids, vitamin D analogues, tacrolimus

Phototherapy—Maintenance therapy

Topical therapy

Topical therapy acts as good adjunctive cooling procedure until the effects of systemic therapy kick in. Evidence suggests application of topical triamcinolone ointment with application of wet wraps, other topical steroids, topical calcipotriene, and tacrolimus, and some benefit does occur [7]. Topical corticosteroids are the topical agents we use most frequently in patients for whom corticosteroids are not the precipitating factor for the episode of GPP.

The key points in treatment of adult GPP are summarized in Table 50.4.

MANAGEMENT IN CHILDREN

> **Childhood GPP:**
> **First line**
> Acitretin (<1 mg/kg per day)
> Cyclosporine (1 to 3 mg/kg per day)
> Methotrexate (0.2 to 0.4 mg/kg per week)
> Etanercept (0.4 mg/kg per day)
>
> **Childhood GPP:**
> **Second line**
> Adalimumab
> Infliximab
> UVB phototherapy

The first-line internal therapy for GPP in children includes the following:

- Acitretin (<1 mg/kg per day)
- Cyclosporine (1–3 mg/kg per day)
- Methotrexate (0.2–0.4 mg/kg per week)
- Etanercept (0.4 mg/kg per day)

The second-line agents include adalimumab, infliximab, and UVB phototherapy after an adequate cooling-down procedure [8]. Therefore, the recommendations for childhood psoriasis are almost similar to those for adults.

Retinoid use in children should be done with caution, and doses less than 1 mg/kg/day are considered appropriate to avoid the potential for skeletal toxicity. In children, it might be combined with prednisolone to have faster control during the acute phase. Cyclosporin is relatively safe in children as compared to other modalities in the dose of 1–3 mg/kg/day, and they may show improvement after 2–4 weeks. Low-dose methotrexate (0.2–0.4 mg/kg/week) is a useful and effective method, and children as young as 2 years have been treated successfully. In a single case report, etanercept was found to be effective in a case of recalcitrant GPP at the dose of 0.4 mg/kg twice weekly for 2 months [9].

Given the contraindication for pregnancy during acitretin treatment and for 3 years after drug discontinuation, its use in girls must be considered carefully. Additional therapies that may be useful in the treatment of pediatric acute GPP based on case reports include narrowband UVB phototherapy in conjunction with systemic therapy, adalimumab, and infliximab.

Topical corticosteroid therapy may be effective for the treatment of children with annular pustular psoriasis, which exhibits less severe manifestations than acute GPP. In addition, topical compresses, wet wraps, or oatmeal baths may be helpful for soothing the skin lesions. Topical therapy for annular pustular psoriasis is less practical when a large proportion of the body surface is affected. Patients who cannot be managed only with topical therapy can be treated with systemic agents.

MANAGEMENT IN PREGNANCY

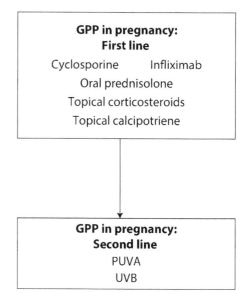

> **GPP in pregnancy:**
> **First line**
> Cyclosporine   Infliximab
> Oral prednisolone
> Topical corticosteroids
> Topical calcipotriene

> **GPP in pregnancy:**
> **Second line**
> PUVA
> UVB

First-line therapy in pregnancy consists of cyclosporine, infliximab, and oral corticosteroids [10]. Despite cyclosporine being a category C drug, no birth defects have been documented, and it can be safely used in pregnancy [11]. Biological agents are category B drugs and are therefore safer to use in pregnancy. Infliximab should be preferentially considered, being a safer and faster-acting alternative. Oral prednisolone in a dose of 30–40 mg per day has shown efficacy, especially when combined with cyclosporine. After control of acute disease, the second-line treatment consists of phototherapy in the form of UVA or narrowband UVB [12].

Biologicals in management of generalized pustular psoriasis

Although cyclosporine, methotrexate, and acitretin are effective medications, each one of them has specific limitations. In pregnancy and hepatic dysfunction, generally acitretin and methotrexate are contraindicated, while in patients with renal dysfunction and hypertension,, cyclosporin is generally contraindicated.

Biologics induce rapid improvement in cases of pustular psoriasis and thus are gaining popularity in the management of GPP, as also there is no absolute contraindication in cases of pregnancy or renal or hepatic impairment.

Among all the biologics, infliximab tops the list as the first choice in treatment of GPP due to an extremely fast onset of action. In some series, the resolution of fever and pustulation occured within 24–72 hours [13]. Concomitant use of methotrexate is advocated to decrease the formation of anti-infliximab antibodies.

Various case reports and series suggest the successful use of etanercept, ustekinumab, adalimumab, and anakinra in psoriasis. The newer biologicals including inhibitors of the Th17 pathway show a promising role in pustular psoriasis and include drugs like secukinumab and ixekizumab.

Secukinumab (150 mg once weekly at baseline; weeks 1, 2, 3, and 4; and then every 4 weeks, with the option to increase the dose to 300 mg in patients who showed minimal or no improvement) has shown good response rates at week 16. Response rates remained high even at 52 weeks [14–17].

Ixekizumab (an anti-IL-17A monoclonal antibody) may be beneficial based on a 52-week open-label study in which four of the five patients with GPP achieved 75% improvement in the Psoriasis Area and Severity Index (PASI) score [18,19].

Biologics being used for GPP are as given in Table 50.5.

Tofacitinib is a newer Janus kinase inhibitor given in the dosage of 5 mg twice a day or 10 mg once a day; it has been shown to be effective in chronic plaque psoriasis and is currently under trial for pustular psoriasis.

A summary of treatment of GPP is provided in Table 50.6.

Table 50.5 Biologics used in generalized pustular psoriasis

1. Infliximab: Dosage 5 mg/kg
2. Etanercept: 50 mg once a week s/c
3. Adalimumab: 80 mg s/c at baseline followed by 40 mg weekly
4. Secukinumab: 150 mg once weekly at baseline; weeks 1, 2, 3, and 4; and then every 4 weeks
5. Ixekizumab: 160 mg at week 0, 80 mg at weeks 2, 4, 6, 8, 10, 12 followed by 80 mg every 4 weeks
6. Apremilast: Standard titration dose (10 mg on day 1 to increase 10 mg daily until reaching 30 mg twice a week on day 6)

Table 50.6 Summary of treatment of generalized pustular psoriasis

Patient category	First line	Second line
Adult	Cyclosporine, acitretin, methotrexate, infliximab	Etanercept, ustekinumab, adalimumab, anakinra
Pregnancy	Cyclosporine, oral prednisolone, infliximab	Etanercept, ustekinumab, adalimumab, phototherapy
Pediatric	Cyclosporine, acitretin, methotrexate, etanercept	Infliximab, ustekinumab, adalimumab, anakinra

KEY POINTS

- Generalized pustular psoriasis can manifest as a dermatological emergency and is associated with life-threatening complications.
- Generalized pustular psoriasis of von Zumbusch is characterized by sudden onset of generalized pustules which can expand and coalesce to form lakes of pus.
- Renal failure, hypoalbuminemia, hypocalcemia, raised liver enzymes, sepsis and ARDS are commonest complications.
- Cyclosporine and infliximab are drugs of choice in severe cute cases while methotrexate and acitretin are good drugs for the less severe subacute cases.

REFERENCES

1. Choon SE et al. Clinical profile, morbidity, and outcome of adult onset generalized pustular psoriasis: Analysis of 35 cases seen in a tertiary hospital in Johor, Malaysia. *Int J Dermatol* 2014;53:676–84.
2. Marrakchi S et al. Interleukin-36-receptor antagonist deficiency and generalised pustular psoriasis. *N Engl J Med* 2011;365(7):620–8.
3. Umezawa Y et al. Therapeutic guidelines for the treatment of generalized pustular psoriasis (GPP) based on a proposed classification of disease severity. *Arch Dermatol Res* 2003;295(Suppl.):S43–54.
4. Mengesha YM, Bennet ML. Pustular skin disorders: Diagnosis and treatment. *Am J Clin Dermatol* 1992;17:257–60.
5. Shupack JL, Webster GF. Pancytopenia following low dose oral methotrexate therapy for psoriasis. *JAMA* 1988;259(24):3594–6.

6. Elewski BE. Infliximab for the treatment of severe pustular psoriasis. *J Am Acad Dermatol* 2002;47:796–7.

7. Rodriguez Garcia F et al. Generalised pustular psoriasis successfully treated with topical tacrolimus. *Br J Dermatol* 2005;152:587–8.

8. Xiao T, Li B, He CD, Chen HD. Juvenile generalised pustular psoriasis. *J Dermatol* 2007;34:573–6.

9. Pereira TM, Viera AP, Fernandes JC, Antunes H, Basto A. Anti-TNF-alpha therapy in childhood pustular psoriasis. *Dermatology* 2006;213:350–2.

10. Robinson A et al. Treatment of pustular psoriasis: From the Medical Board of the National Psoriasis Foundation. *J Am Acad Dermatol* 2012;67(2):279–88.

11. Armenti VT, Ahlswede KM, Ahlswede BA, Jarrel BE, Burke JF. National Transplant Pregnancy Registry— Outcome of 154 pregnancies in cyclosporine treated female kidney transplant recipients. *Transplantation* 1994;57(4):502–6.

12. Vun YY, Jones B, Al-Mudhaffer M, Egan C. Generalised pustular psoriasis of pregnancy treated with narrowband UVB and topical steroids. *J Am Acad Dermatol* 2006;54(Suppl.):528–30.

13. Routhouska SB, Sheth PB, Korman N. Long term management of generalized pustular psoriasis with infliximab: Case series. *J Cutan Med Surg* 2008;12(4):184–8.

14. Levin EC, Gupta R, Brown G, Malakouti M, Koo J. Biologic fatigue in psoriasis. *J Dermatolog Treat* 2014;25(1):78–82.

15. Böhner A et al. Acute generalized pustular psoriasis treated with the IL-17A antibody secukinumab. *JAMA Dermatol* 2016;152:482.

16. Polesie S, Lidholm AG. Secukinumab in the treatment of generalized pustular psoriasis: A case report. *Acta Derm Venereol* 2017;97:124.

17. Cordoro KM et al. Response to interleukin (IL)-17 inhibition in an adolescent with severe manifestations of IL-36 receptor antagonist deficiency (DITRA). *JAMA Dermatol* 2017;153:106.

18. Saeki H et al. Efficacy and safety of open-label ixekizumab treatment in Japanese patients with moderate-to-severe plaque psoriasis, erythrodermic psoriasis and generalized pustular psoriasis. *J Eur Acad Dermatol Venereol* 2015;29:1148.

19. Saeki H et al. Efficacy and safety of ixekizumab treatment for Japanese patients with moderate to severe plaque psoriasis, erythrodermic psoriasis and generalized pustular psoriasis: Results from a 52-week, open-label, phase 3 study (UNCOVER-J). *J Dermatol* 2017;44:355.

51

Psoriatic arthritis

ARUN HEGDE AND RAJESH CHILAKA

INTRODUCTION

Psoriatic arthritis (PsA) is a chronic, systemic inflammatory, heterogenous disease that can characteristically affect various parts of the human body, including the axial skeleton, peripheral joints, skin, nails, enthesis, and tendon sheaths. It can result in joint deformity and severe functional impairment, with poor quality of life and psychosocial disturbances [1]. PsA patients can also have recurrent uveitis and various intestinal complications [2,3]. Premature atherosclerosis as a result of inflammation and associated metabolic syndrome can also cause enhanced cardiovascular mortality [4].

EPIDEMIOLOGY AND DISEASE BURDEN

PsA develops in approximately 30% of patients with psoriasis, with skin changes predating the arthritis by 10 years on average, although in 15% of cases, either both arthritis and psoriasis occur simultaneously or onset of arthritis precedes the skin disease [5,6]. The male-to-female ratio is 1:1. PsA can affect both children and adults. In children, there can be two clinical subtypes: the oligoarticular subtype (predominantly in girls, affecting fewer than four joints and occurring between 1 and 2 years of age) and a polyarticular subtype (M:F = 1:1, affecting more than four joints, age of onset between 6 and 12 years of age).

PATHOGENESIS

It is hypothesized that the most important factors are environmental agents triggering PsA in a genetically susceptible individual leading to pathogenic immunological pathways.

Genetic factors

PsA is a highly heritable polygenic disease. There is a positive family history in first-degree relatives in approximately 40% of patients with psoriasis and PsA [7]. There is also a greater concordance among monozygotic twins as compared to dizygotic twins [8]. Psoriasis and PsA are both associated with class I major histocompatibility complex (MHC) alleles. Unlike human leukocyte antigen (HLA)-Cw*06, which is linked to psoriasis, in PsA, increased frequencies of HLA-B*08, B*27, B*38, and B*39 linkage have been observed. B*38 and B*39 have showed an association with peripheral forms of the disease [9]. The presence of HLA-B27 also correlates with severity of axial disease on magnetic resonance imaging (MRI). HLA antigens may act as antigen presenters. Genome-wide association scans (GWASs) have confirmed associations with genes involved in interleukin (IL)-23 signaling (IL 23A, IL 23R, IL 12B), nuclear factor κB (NF-κB) gene expression (TNIP1 and signaling [TNFAIP3]), and tumor necrosis factor (TNF) expression [10].

Environmental factors

The most commonly reported trigger of PsA is trauma, with studies showing associations with physical as well as psychological trauma (e.g., shifting of house). Studies have also postulated a deep *Koebner phenomenon* at the enthesis, which might trigger the arthritis [11].

Role of gut microbiome

Microbial infections are known triggers of certain forms of spondyloarthritides, and reports of an elevated frequency of subclinical gut inflammation and dysbiosis have been seen in patients with PsA. This has been suggested as a mechanism to generate an autoinflammatory response, comprising IL-23 release, that may precipitate psoriasis and PsA [12,13].

Obesity

Epidemiological studies indicate obesity to be a risk factor for PsA. Adipokines are found to be elevated in the sera of PsA patients, and they fluctuate with disease activity.

Role of cytokines

Recent studies highlight the importance of the IL-23, IL-17, and TNF pathways in the pathogenesis of psoriasis, PsA, and axial spondyloarthropathies [14]. Raised levels of proinflammatory cytokines have also been identified within the joint, including p40 (a common subunit of IL-12 and IL-23), TNF-α, IL-1, IL-6, IL-8, and IL-10 with some relationships noted between cytokine levels and clinical arthritis severity [15].

Role of CD8T cells

It has been shown consistently that T cells are important in psoriasis and PsA. A central role for CD8+ T cells in disease pathogenesis is supported by the association with HLA class I alleles, oligoclonal CD8+ T-cell expansion, and the association of PsA with HIV disease. Type 17 cells, which include CD4+ type 17 helper T (Th17) cells, and type 3 innate lymphocytes (cells that produce IL-17A and IL-22), in addition to CD4+CD8+ lymphocytes, are increased in psoriatic synovial fluid as compared with rheumatoid synovial fluid [16,17].

Synovium

The synovial tissues in patients with PsA are characterized by the presence of more vascularity [18] and more neutrophils, the absence of antibodies to citrullinated peptides, and a lower number of infiltrating T lymphocytes and plasma cells. Th17 cells have been demonstrated in the psoriatic synovium, and mast cells have also been known to express Th17 [19,20].

Role of enthesis

In PsA, the enthesis has been proposed to be the initial site of inflammation. The enthesial interface contains cells expressing the IL-23 receptor. In response to IL-23, the enthesis produce IL-17A, IL-22, and bone morphogenetic factor (Bmp7), resulting in inflammation and bone erosions [21].

Altered bone remodeling in psoriatic arthritis

There is a marked heterogeneity of bone phenotypes in PsA ranging from extensive bone damage in the form of erosions and mutilans variety, to spinal ankyloses and formation of enthesophytes. In psoriatic synovium, there is marked upregulation of the receptor activator of NF-κB (RANK) ligand (RANKL), and low expression of its antagonist, osteoprotegerin, in the adjacent synovial lining. The RANKL cytokine binds to RANK on the surface of osteoclast precursors that are derived from circulating CD14+ monocytes. This ligand-receptor interaction triggers proliferation of the osteoclast precursors and their differentiation into multinucleated osteoclasts, which resorb bone [22]. There is also increased TNF-α, and together with RANK, there is increased osteoclastogenesis and bone erosions.

Enhanced new bone formation that occurs could be due to enhanced bone morphogenetic protein, activation of Wnt signaling pathway and prostaglandin E signaling pathways [23].

CLINICAL FEATURES

Various criteria have been proposed for the diagnosis of PsA, but the criteria proposed in 2006 by CASPAR (Classification Criteria for Psoriatic Arthritis) have been found to have high sensitivity and specificity for classification of cases for clinical research (Table 51.1) [24–26]. However, a diagnosis can still be made if these criteria are not met. Moll and Wright classified PsA into five distinct clinical subtypes [27]:

1. *Arthritis with predominant distal interphalangeal (DIP) joint involvement*: Seen in less than 5% of patients, associations seen with dactylitis and nail dystrophy (Figure 51.1).
2. *Arthritis mutilans*: End-stage, destructive, erosive arthritis leading to flail joints and digital telescoping, also known as "Opera glass finger," seen in less than 5% of patients. Associations with long-standing disease, female sex, and sacroiliac joint inflammation are seen (Figure 51.2).
3. *Symmetric polyarthritis*: Affecting more than five joints symmetrically, resembling rheumatoid arthritis (RA) (Figure 51.3).
4. *Asymmetric oligoarticular arthritis*: Affecting fewer than four joints with a male preponderance (Figure 51.4).
5. *Predominant spondylitis*: Can be symmetric or asymmetric, seen in less than 5% of cases (Figure 51.5).

Enthesitis

Enthesitis can be seen in 20%–40% of patients and can be the presenting feature in 4% [28]. Sites affected are the sites of insertion of plantar fascia and Achilles tendon (Figure 51.6), but pain around the patella, iliac crest, epicondyle, and supraspinatus insertion is also known.

Dactylitis

Also known as "sausage digit," it can occur in both the hands and feet, although the feet are more commonly

Table 51.1 Classification Criteria for Psoriatic Arthritis (CASPAR)

Criterion	Explanation	Points
Evidence of psoriasis		
Current psoriasis	Current psoriatic skin or scalp disease as judged by a dermatologist or rheumatologist	2
Personal history of psoriasis	History of psoriasis according to the patient or a family doctor, dermatologist, or rheumatologist	1
Family history of psoriasis	History of psoriasis in a first- or second-degree relative according to the patient	1
Psoriatic nail dystrophy	Typical psoriatic nail dystrophy (e.g., onycholysis, pitting, or hyperkeratosis) according to observation during current physical examination	1
Negative test for rheumatoid factor	Based on reference range at local laboratory; any testing method except latex, with preference for enzyme-linked immunosorbent assay or nephelometry	1
Dactylitis		
Current dactylitis	Swelling of an entire digit according to observation on current physical examination	1
History of dactylitis	According to a rheumatologist	1
Radiographic evidence of juxta-articular new bone formation	Ill-defined ossification near joint margins (excluding osteophyte formation) on plain radiographs of hand or foot	1

Note: Psoriatic arthritis is considered to be present in patients with inflammatory musculoskeletal disease (disease involving the joint, spine, or enthesis) whose score on the five criteria listed in the table totals at least three points; the "evidence of psoriasis" criterion can account for either one point or two points. The criteria have a specificity of 98.7% and a sensitivity of 91.4%.

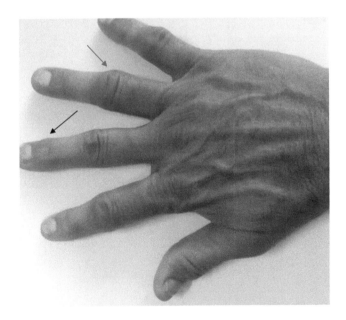

Figure 51.1 Distal interphalangeal joint arthritis in a case of psoriatic arthritis (black arrow) with concomitant proximal interphalangeal joint arthritis (red arrow).

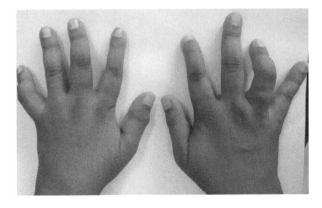

Figure 51.2 Arthritis mutilans presentation in a case of psoriatic arthritis.

Skin changes

There is no correlation between extent of skin disease and total joint scores [30]; however, synchronous flares involving skin and joint are reported in 30%–40% of patients with PsA. Figure 51.8 shows plaque psoriasis in a patient of psoriatic arthritis.

Nail involvement

Involvement of the nail can be seen in 20%–40% of uncomplicated psoriasis, whereas in PsA, it is 60%–80% [31]. Nail changes in PsA include pitting, ridging, onycholysis, and subungual hyperkeratosis (Figures 51.9 through 51.11). Nail

involved (Figure 51.7). It occurs in 30%–40% of patients [29] and can be either acute (associated with swelling and redness) or chronic (without signs of inflammation). Dactylitis is commonly associated with DIP involvement and erosive disease.

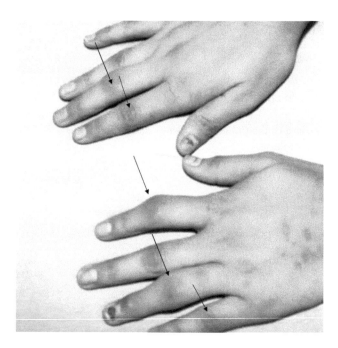

Figure 51.3 Symmetric polyarthritis (arrows) in a case of psoriatic arthritis.

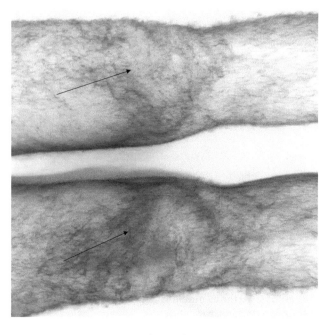

Figure 51.4 Asymmetric oligoarthritis involving both knees (arrows) in a case of psoriatic arthritis.

pits are the most common sign in PsA, affecting almost 68% patients. The potential space formed as a result of onycholysis provides for entry and colonization of organisms and increases infection risk. Nail changes can occur in both fingers and toes.

Extra-articular features

Overlapping clinical features can be seen in spondyloarthritis and PsA, and comprise ocular manifestations of conjunctivitis and iritis, oral ulcers, urethritis, and aortic valve

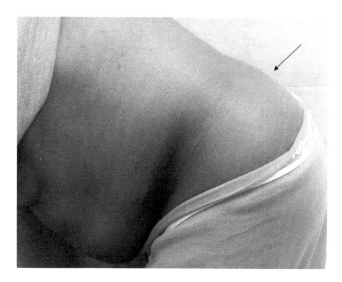

Figure 51.5 Spondylitic subtype in a case of psoriatic arthritis.

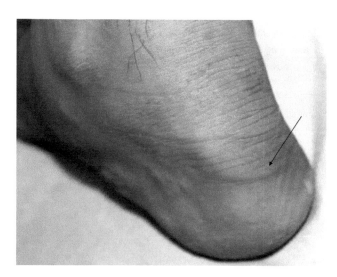

Figure 51.6 Enthesitis (arrow) at insertion of tendo Achillis in a case of psoriatic arthritis.

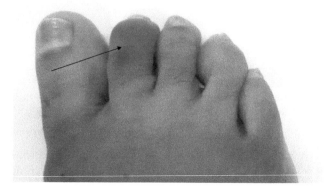

Figure 51.7 Dactylitis (arrow) in second toe in a case of psoriatic arthritis.

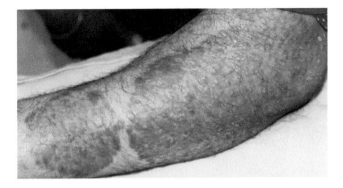

Figure 51.8 Plaque psoriasis in a case of psoriatic arthritis.

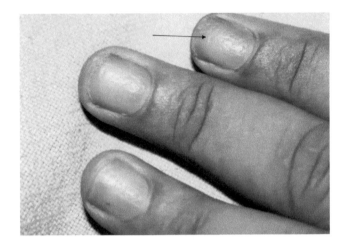

Figure 51.9 Nail pits (arrow) in a case of psoriatic arthritis.

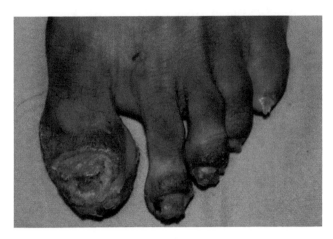

Figure 51.11 Subungual hyperkeratosis in a case of psoriatic arthritis.

during active disease and show good correlation with inflammatory activity in polyarticular disease [33]. Rheumatoid factor positivity can be seen in 5%–10% of patients [33], whereas anticitrullinated protein antibody (ACPA) positivity is seen in 6%–10% of patients [34] and correlates with enthesitis and DIP involvement. Hyperuricemia can be seen in 20% of patients [35]. HLA-B27 positivity can be seen in 25% of patients and correlates with axial disease.

Radiographic changes

Radiographic changes in peripheral joints can be similar to RA and show periarticular soft tissue swelling, erosions, and joint space narrowing (Figure 51.12). DIP joint involvement is characteristic, and the joints tend to be involved asymmetrically in a "ray" pattern. Also, erosions at the wrist are fewer when compared to RA [36]. Arthritis mutilans can cause "pencilling" of heads of metacarpals and metatarsals presenting as a "pencil-in-cup" deformity (Figure 51.13). New bone formation can occur along shafts of metacarpals and metatarsals. When this occurs adjacent to an erosion, it is called *whiskering*.

Changes in the spine are similar to those seen in ankylosing spondylitis, the differentiating feature being paravertebral ossification seen as chunky syndesmophytes (Figure 51.14) [37]. Also, the involvement in the spine tends to be asymmetric with a predilection for the cervical spine and lesser incidence of lumbar spine involvement.

Radiographic changes are late to appear. Hence, early diagnosis can be better picked up on MRI and ultrasonography with power Doppler. MRI can show early changes of asymmetric sacroiliitis in a case of psoriatic spondyloarthritis (Figure 51.15). Power Doppler can depict active enthesitis (Figure 51.16). Enthesitis can also be picked up on bone scan and fluorodeoxyglucose positron emission tomography (FDG PET) scan (Figure 51.17).

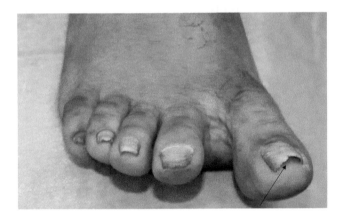

Figure 51.10 Onycholysis (arrow) in a case of psoriatic arthritis.

disease. The prevalence of Crohn disease and microscopic colitis is also increased in these patients [32].

DIAGNOSIS

Laboratory investigations

Acute phase reactants like C-reactive protein (CRP) and erythrocyte sedimentation rate (ESR) can be elevated

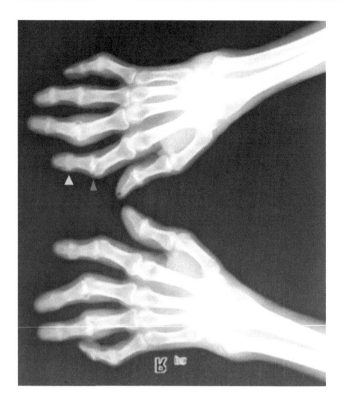

Figure 51.12 X-ray of hands in a patient of psoriatic arthritis showing narrowing of joint space at distal inter-phalangeal joints (green arrowhead) and erosions (red arrowhead).

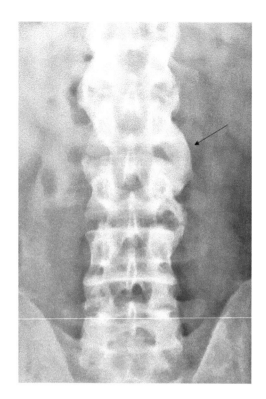

Figure 51.14 Chunky syndesmophytes (arrows) in a case of psoriatic arthritis.

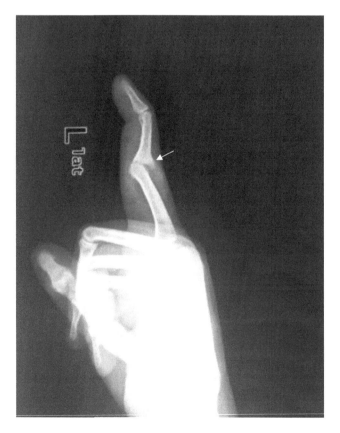

Figure 51.13 "Pencil-in-cup" deformity (white arrow) in a case of psoriatic arthritis.

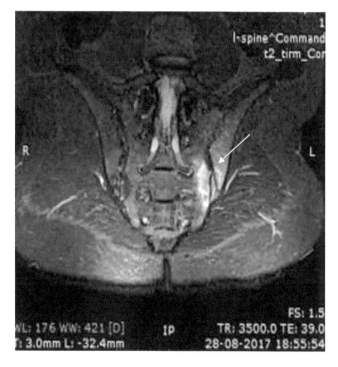

Figure 51.15 Magnetic resonance imaging of the sacroiliac joint (short-tau inversion recovery [STIR] image) showing asymmetric sacroiliitis (arrow) in a case of psoriatic arthritis.

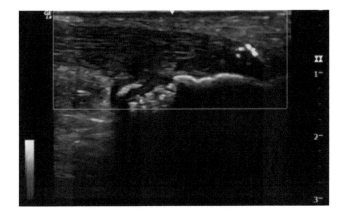

Figure 51.16 The high-frequency (15-MHz) ultrasound image shows enthesitis. The confluent red signals with power Doppler ultrasonography represent hyperemia at the tendon near its insertion into the calcaneus.

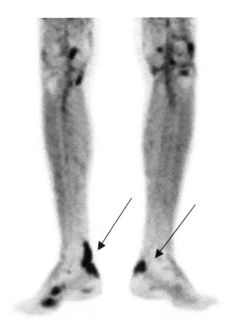

Figure 51.17 Fluorodeoxyglucose positron emission tomography showing enthesitis (arrows) at bilateral tendo Achillis in a case of psoriatic arthritis.

DIFFERENTIAL DIAGNOSIS

PsA needs to be differentiated from RA, gout, osteoarthritis, and ankylosing spondylitis.

RA typically involves the proximal interphalangeal joints while sparing the DIP joint and has a symmetrical pattern at onset. It also affects females predominantly (M:F = 1:3). Gouty arthritis tends to involve similar joints like PsA, the differentiating factor being that erythema in gouty joints extends beyond the joint and tends to involve the periarticular areas. Radiographs are also useful as PsA erosions tend to be marginal, whereas gouty erosions involve a single bone and have sclerotic margins. Osteoarthritis also tends to affect the DIP joints as in PsA; however, the inflammatory features are absent.

Pain in joints is of a mechanical nature, worsening with activity and improving with rest. Psoriatic spondyloarthritis differs from ankylosing spondylitis by way of having asymmetric sacroiliac joint involvement along with chunky paramarginal syndesmophytes and lesser functional restriction.

MANAGEMENT

Since PsA is predated by psoriasis in a majority of cases, the dermatologist carries a unique responsibility to suspect PsA at a very early stage. Assessment of PsA should comprise the domains of skin disease, peripheral arthritis, axial disease, enthesitis, and dactylitis. For treatment aspects, PsA can be classified as mild, moderate, and severe as depicted in Table 51.2. Quality of life assessment is also equally important [38–43].

Various treatment guidelines have been proposed by the Group for Research and Assessment of Psoriasis and Psoriatic Arthritis (GRAPPA) [44], and the European League Against Rheumatism (EULAR) [45]. A treat to target approach has been recommended by GRAPPA and EULAR, since remission is not easy to achieve. The GRAPPA measures of minimal disease activity include achieving five of the following seven targets (Tender joint count <1, Swollen joint count <1, Psoriasis Activity and Severity Index <1, Patient pain visual analogue score <15, Patient global disease activity visual analogue score <20, Health assessment questionnaire ≤0.5, and Tender enthesial point <1).

The various drugs available for the treatment of PsA include nonsteroidal anti-inflammatory drugs (NSAIDs), corticosteroids, conventional synthetic disease-modifying antirheumatic drugs (csDMARDs), targeted synthetic DMARDs (tsDMARDS), TNF agents, and the IL-17 inhibitors. The dosages and side effects of various drugs are as shown in Table 51.3.

Nonsteroidal anti-inflammatory drugs and corticosteroids

NSAIDs are recommended initially for mild joint disease (characterized by noninvolvement of certain joints such as the hip, wrist, ankle, cervical spine joints, and sacroiliac joint) to provide relief from joint pain and stiffness. Studies have been done extensively on only two NSAIDs: nimesulide 200/400 mg and celecoxib [46,47].

Intra-articular corticosteroid injections are recommended only for persistent mono- or oligoarthritis, enthesitis, and occasionally dactylitis. Systemic steroids alone are avoided in PsA, since their sudden withdrawal might precipitate pustular psoriasis. However, good control can be achieved if low-dose steroids (<7.5 g/day) are used in combination with csDMARDs.

Conventional synthetic disease-modifying antirheumatic drugs

csDMARDs are recommended to treat peripheral arthritis but are not effective for axial and enthesial disease.

Table 51.2 Staging of psoriatic arthritis

Parameter	Mild	Moderate	Severe
Peripheral arthritis			
Number of joints	<5 joints	>5 joints (S or T)	>5 joints (S or T)
X-ray findings	No damage	Damage	Severe damage
		NR to mild Rx	NR to mild–moderate Rx
	No LOF	Moderate LOF	Severe LOF
LOF and QoL	QoL minimal impact	Moderate impact on QoL	Severe impact on QoL
Skin disease	BSA <5%, PASI <5, asymptomatic	Nonresponse to topicals, DLQI, PASI <10	BSA >10, DLQI >10, PASI > 10
Spinal disease	Mild pain, no loss of function	Loss of function or BASDAI >4	Failure of response
Enthesitis	One to two sites	>2 sites or loss of function	Loss of function or >2 sites and failure of response
Dactylitis	Pain absent to mild Normal function	Erosive disease or functional loss	Failure of response

Abbreviations: BASDAI, Bath Ankylosing Spondylitis Disease Activity Index; BSA, body surface area; DLQI, Dermatology Life Quality Index; LOF, loss of function; NR, not responding; QoL, quality of life; PASI, Psoriasis Area Severity Index.

Table 51.3 Treatment options available in psoriatic arthritis

Serial Number	Name of drug	Dose for joints	Dose for skin	Side effects
1	**Nonsteroidal anti-inflammatory drugs**			
	1. Naproxen	750–1000 mg/day	Not applicable	Gastrointestinal, renal, and cardiac effects
	2. Diclofenac	100–150 mg/day		
	3. Indomethacin	100–150 mg/day		
2	**Disease-modifying antirheumatic drugs**			
	1. Methotrexate	15–25 mg/wk	15–25 mg/week	Alopecia, nausea, transaminitis
	2. Leflunomide	20 mg/day	Not applicable	Diarrhea, alopecia, hypertension, renal effects
	3. Sulfasalazine	2–3 g/day	Not applicable	Diarrhea, neutropenia
3	**Anti-tumor necrosis factor agents**			
	1. Infliximab (infusion)	5 mg/kg at 0, 2, and 6 weeks and then every 8 weekly	5 mg/kg at 0, 2, and 6 weeks and then every 8 weekly	Infusion reactions, infections
	2. Etanercept (subcutaneous [SC])	50 mg/week	50 mg twice/week	Injection site reactions, infections
	3. Adalimumab (SC)	40 mg/every 2 weeks	80 mg loading dose, 40 mg 1 week later, then 40 mg every 2 weeks	Injection site reactions, infections
	4. Golimumab (SC)	50 mg monthly	Not applicable	Injection site reactions, infections
	5. Certolizumab (SC)	200 mg every 2 weeks or 400 mg every month	Not applicable	Injection site reactions, infections
4	**Anti-interleukin (IL)-17 agents**			
	1. Secukinumab (SC)	150 mg/week from 0–4 weeks then monthly	300 mg/week from 0 to 4 week, then monthly	Candida infections
	2. Ixekizumab (SC)	80 mg every 2 weeks	80 mg every 2 weeks	Candida infections

(Continued)

Table 51.3 (*Continued*) Treatment options available in psoriatic arthritis

S no.	Name of drug	Dose for joints	Dose for skin	Side effects
5	**Anti-IL-12, IL-23 agents**			
	1. Ustekinumab (SC)	45 mg/kg (Body wt < 100 kg) or 90 mg/kg (Body wt > 100 kg) at weeks 0, 4, and 12 and then every 12 weeks	45 mg/kg (Body wt <100 kg) or 90 mg/kg (Body wt > 100 kg) at weeks 0, 4, and 12 and then every 12 weeks	Injection site reactions, infections
6	**Phosphodiesterase-4 inhibitors**			
	1. Apremilast	30 mg twice daily	30 mg twice daily	Weight loss, diarrhea

Methotrexate (MTX) is the first-choice drug, either as monotherapy or in combination, in dosages ranging from 7.5 to 25 mg/week, although the clinical improvements are not significant at doses <15 mg/week [48,49]. Other csDMARDs that can be used are sulfasalazine [50], leflunomide [51], and cyclosporine [52], although there are no head-to-head trials to compare the efficacy among them.

The EULAR recommends MTX as the csDMARD of choice, whereas GRAPPA considers MTX alongside other csDMARDs, with no specific preference.

Tumor necrosis factor inhibitors

TNF inhibitors are effective in both peripheral and axial disease, as well as for resistant enthesitis and dactylitis, and additionally retard radiological progression of disease. They also improve function and quality of life in PsA [53,54]. The various anti-TNF agents approved are infliximab [55], etanercept [56], adalimumab [57], golimumab [58], and certolizumab pegol [59], the pegylated anti-TNF. There is only one randomized control trial that has compared the first three agents and found favorable outcomes to all of these with comparable safety [60]. Biological switching among these agents is another effective strategy that can be employed in case of loss of efficacy to one particular agent [61]. However, PsA is known to relapse on discontinuation of these drugs, and remission can be maintained by maintenance doses with increasing intervals in between doses.

The EULAR recommends anti-TNF agents as first-choice biologic agents after the failure of csDMARDs, whereas GRAPPA includes anti-TNFs with other biologics in the same line as csDMARDs, though they also discuss the potential of using them as first line in case of active severe disease.

Ustekinumab

This is a human monoclonal antibody that binds to the shared p40 subunit of IL-12 and IL-23 and is approved for moderate to severe plaque psoriasis and PsA by the European Medicine Agency and the U.S. Food and Drug Administration (FDA). It has shown efficacy in both anti-TNF naïve [62] and anti-TNF experienced patients [63].

Anti-IL-17 agents

The drugs available are the IL-17 receptor antagonist brodalumab, and the two IL-17A blockers: secukinumab and ixekizumab. Trials of brodalumab have been halted because of safety concerns [64].

Secukinumab is a fully human monoclonal antibody and is effective in the treatment of both psoriasis and PsA. It is also effective in nail psoriasis and has been found to retard radiological progression [65]. Ixekizumab has recently been approved for psoriasis [66].

EULAR recommends the use of anti-IL-17 agents after failure of MTX, but considers anti-TNF as first line, whereas the GRAPPA recommends them alongside the anti-TNF agents.

Apremilast

Apremilast is an oral tsDMARD and works by selective inhibition of phosphodiesterase isoenzyme 4, which is responsible for degradation of cyclic AMP, a key second messenger that controls cytokine production in inflammatory cells. As a result of this, the proinflammatory cytokines TNF, IL17, and IL23 are reduced, and production of anti-inflammatory cytokines such as IL-10 are increased [67]. Skin responses with this drug are similar to that of methotrexate, although joint responses are lower than those seen with other biological agents. Apremilast got approval by the FDA in March 2014 for PsA treatment and in September 2014 for skin psoriasis.

EULAR recommends this drug for patients who do not achieve treatment targets with csDMARDs or where anti-TNFs are not appropriate. GRAPPA recommends apremilast up front for PsA patients with peripheral arthritis unresponsive to csDMARDs.

Abatacept

Abatacept is a fusion protein comprising the extracellular domain of CTLA4 linked to a modified Fc portion of human immunoglobulin, IgG1, and works by the inhibition of T-cell activation. It is moderately effective for PsA [68–70], but not for skin disease, and has received FDA approval for the same in 2017.

Apart from pharmacological treatment, emphasis should also be laid on smoking cessation, weight reduction, physical exercise, and stress management.

CONCLUSIONS

PsA is a medical emergency, and patients with PsA should be diagnosed early and treated promptly and aggressively in order to prevent erosions and joint destruction. The treatment protocol can be individualized once the disease extent and severity have been staged. Therapeutic agents beneficial for the cutaneous manifestations of psoriasis may not necessarily be equally efficacious for PsA, and vice versa. Biologic agents have been impressive in the management of severe PsA. Combined management by the dermatologist and rheumatologist is required for better patient care.

KEY POINTS

- PsA is a musculoskeletal emergency, since delay in initiating treatment can result in disabling deformity and poor quality of life.
- Psoriasis precedes arthritis in the majority of cases, and the responsibility of early diagnosis of such patients rests with the dermatologist.
- Careful selection of drugs is recommended during treatment, since drugs effective for PsA might not be effective against psoriasis, and vice versa.
- A *treat to target* strategy is recommended in the treatment of PsA, with the end point being tight control of the disease.

REFERENCES

1. Gladman DD. Disability and quality of life considerations. Psoriatic arthritis. In: Gordon GB, Ruderman E (Eds), *Psoriasis and Psoriatic Arthritis: An Integrated Approach*. Heidelberg: Springer–Verlag; 2005: 118–23.
2. Scarpa R et al. Microscopic inflammatory changes in colon of patients with both active psoriasis and psoriatic arthritis without bowel symptoms. *J Rheumatol* 2000;27(5):1241–6.
3. Queiro R et al. Clinical features and predictive factors in psoriatic arthritis-related uveitis. *Semin Arthritis Rheum* 2002;31(4):264–70.
4. Gladman DD, Ang M, Su L, Tom BD, Schentag CT, Farewell VT. Cardiovascular morbidity in psoriatic arthritis. *Ann Rheum Dis* 2009;68:1131–5.
5. Gelfand JM et al. The prevalence of psoriasis in African Americans: Results from a population based study. *J Am Acad Dermatol* 2005;52(1):23–6.
6. Veale D, Rogers S, Fitzgerald O. Classification of clinical subsets in psoriatic arthritis. *Br J Rheumatol* 1994;33:133–8.
7. Gladman DD, Anhorn KA, Schachter RK, Mervart H. HLA antigens in psoriatic arthritis. *J Rheumatol* 1986;3:586.
8. Myers A, Kay LJ, Lynch SA, Walker DJ. Recurrence risk for psoriasis and psoriatic arthritis within sibships. *Rheumatology (Oxf)* 2005;44:773.
9. FitzGerald O, Haroon M, Giles JT, Winchester R. Concepts of pathogenesis in psoriatic arthritis: Genotype determines clinical phenotype. *Arthritis Res Ther* 2015;17:115.
10. Stuart PE et al. Genome-wide association analysis of psoriatic arthritis and cutaneous psoriasis reveals differences in their genetic architecture. *Am J Hum Genet* 2015;97(6):816–36.
11. Prinz JC. Psoriasis vulgaris—A sterile antibacterial skin reaction mediated by cross-reactive T cells? An immunological view of the pathophysiology of psoriasis. *Clin Exp Dermatol* 2001;26(4):326–32.
12. Armstrong AW, Harskamp CT, Armstrong EJ. The association between psoriasis and obesity: A systematic review and meta-analysis of observational studies. *Nutrition Diabetes* 2012;2(12):e54.
13. Scher JU et al. Decreased bacterial diversity characterizes the altered gut microbiota in patients with psoriatic arthritis, resembling dysbiosis in inflammatory bowel disease. *Arthritis Rheumatol* 2015;67(1):128–39.
14. Yeremenko N, Paramarta JE, Baeten D. The interleukin-23/interleukin-17 immune axis as a promising new target in the treatment of spondyloarthritis. *Curr Opin Rheumatol* 2014;26:361–70.
15. Szodoray P et al. Circulating cytokines in Norwegian patients with psoriatic arthritis determined by a multiplex cytokine array system. *Rheumatology (Oxf)* 2007;46:417–25.
16. Leijten EF et al. Brief report: Enrichment of activated group 3 innate lymphoid cells in psoriatic arthritis synovial fluid. *Arthritis Rheumatol* 2015;67(10):2673–8.
17. Menon B et al. Interleukin-17+CD8+ T cells are enriched in the joints of patients with psoriatic arthritis and correlate with disease activity and joint damage progression. *Arthritis Rheumatol* 2014;66(5):1272–81.
18. Baeten D et al. Comparative study of the synovial histology in rheumatoid arthritis, spondyloarthropathy, and osteoarthritis: Influence of disease duration and activity. *Ann Rheum Dis* 2000;59(12):945–53.
19. Noordenbos T, Yeremenko N, Gofita I. Interleukin-17–positive mast cells contribute to synovial inflammation in spondylarthritis. *Arthritis Rheum* 2012;64:99–109.
20. Raychaudhuri SP, Raychaudhuri SK, Genovese MC. IL-17 receptor and its functional significance in psoriatic arthritis. *Mol Cell Biochem* 2012;359:419–29.
21. Benjamin M et al. Microdamage and altered vascularity at the enthesis-bone interface provides an anatomic explanation for bone involvement in the HLA-B27-associated spondylarthritides and allied disorders. *Arthritis Rheum* 2007;56(1):224–33.

22. Ritchlin CT, Haas-Smith SA, Li P, Hicks DG, Schwarz EM. Mechanisms of TNF-alpha- and RANKL-mediated osteoclastogenesis and bone resorption in psoriatic arthritis. *J Clin Invest* 2003;111(6):821–31.

23. Beyer C, Schett G. Pharmacotherapy: Concepts of pathogenesis and emerging treatments. Novel targets in bone and cartilage. *Best Pract Res Clin Rheumatol* 2010;24(4):489–96.

24. Wright V. Psoriasis and arthritis. *Ann Rheum Dis* 1956;15:348–56.

25. Blumberg BS, Bunim JJ, Calkins E, Pirani CL, Zvaifler NJ. A nomenclature and classification of arthritis and rheumatism. *Arthritis Rheum* 1964;7:93–7.

26. Taylor W, Gladman D, Helliwell P, Marchesoni A, Mease P, Mielants H. Classification criteria for psoriatic arthritis: Development of new criteria from a large international study. *Arthritis Rheum* 2006;54:2665–73.

27. Moll JM, Wright V. Psoriatic arthritis. *Semin Arthritis Rheum* 1973;3:55–78.

28. Scarpa R. Peripheral enthesopathies in psoriatic arthritis. *J Rheumatol* 1998;25(11);22:88–9.

29. Gladman DD, Shuckett R, Russell ML, PsThorne JC, Schachter RK. Psoriatic arthritis (PsA)—An analysis of 220 patients. *Q J Med* 1987;62(238):127–41.

30. Cohen MR, Reda JD, Clegg DO. Baseline relationship between psoriasis and psoriatic arthritis: Analysis of 221 patients with active psoriatic arthritis. *J Rheumatol* 1999;26(8):1752–6.

31. Jones SM, Armas J, Cohen M, Lovell CR, Evison G, McHugh NJ. Psoriatic arthritis: Outcome of disease subsets and relationship of joint disease to nail and skin disease. *Br J Rheumatol* 1994;33(9):834–9.

32. Gladman DD. Psoriatic arthritis. *Spine* 1990;4:637–56.

33. Torre-Alonso JC, Rodriguez-Perez A, Arribas-Castrillo JM, Ballina-Garcia J, Riestra-Noriega JL, Lopez-Larrea C. Psoriatic arthritis (PA): A clinical, immunological and radiological study of 180 patients. *Br J Rheumatol* 1991;30(4):245–50.

34. Vander Cruyssen B et al. Anti–citrullinated peptide antibodies may occur in patients with psoriatic arthritis. *Ann Rheum Dis* 2005;64:1145–9.

35. Bruce IN, Schentag CT, Gladman DD. Hyperuricemia in psoriatic arthritis: Prevalence and associated features. *J Clin Rheumatol* 2000;6(1):6–9.

36. Van Romunde LKJ et al. Psoriasis and arthritis: III. A cross-sectional comparative study of patients with psoriatic arthritis and seronegative and seropositive polyarthritis: Radiological and HLA aspects. *Rheumatol Int* 1984;4:67–73.

37. Bywaters EGL, Dixon ASTJ. Paravertebral ossification in psoriatic arthritis. *Ann Rheum Dis* 1965;24(4):313–31.

38. Husni ME, Meyer KH, Cohen DS, Mody E, Qureshi AA. The PASE questionnaire: Pilot-testing a psoriatic arthritis screening and evaluation tool. *J Am Acad Dermatol* 2007;57(4):581–7.

39. Gladman DD et al. Development and initial validation of a screening questionnaire for psoriatic arthritis: The Toronto Psoriatic Arthritis Screen (ToPAS). *Ann Rheum Dis* 2009;68:497–501.

40. Gladman DD, Helliwell PS, Khraishi M, Callis Duffin K, Mease PJ. Dermatology screening tools: Project update from GRAPPA 2012 annual meeting. *J Rheumatol* 2013;40(8):1425–7.

41. Ibrahim GH, Buch MH, Lawson C, Waxman R, Helliwell PS. Evaluation of an existing screening tool for psoriatic arthritis in people with psoriasis and the development of a new instrument: The Psoriasis Epidemiology Screening Tool (PEST) questionnaire. *Clin Exp Rheumatol* 2009;27(3):469–74.

42. Khraishi M, Mong J, Mugford G, Landells I. The electronic Psoriasis and Arthritis Screening Questionnaire (ePASQ): A sensitive and specific tool to diagnose psoriatic arthritis patients. *J Cutan Med* 2011;15(3):143–9.

43. Tinazzi I et al. The early psoriatic arthritis screening questionnaire: A simple and fast method for the identification of arthritis in patients with psoriasis. *Rheumatology (Oxf)* 2012;51(11):2058–63.

44. Ritchlin CT et al. Treatment recommendations for psoriatic arthritis. *Ann Rheum Dis* 2009;68(9):1387–94.

45. Gossec L et al. European League Against Rheumatism recommendations for the management of psoriatic arthritis with pharmacological therapies. *Ann Rheum Dis* 2012;71(1):4–12.

46. Sarzi-Puttini P, Santandrea S, Boccassini L, Panni B, Caruso I. The role of NSAIDs in psoriatic arthritis: Evidence from a controlled study with nimesulide. *Clin Exp Rheumatol* 2001;19(Suppl. 22).

47. Kivitz A, Espinoza L, Sherrer Y, Liu-Dumaw M, West CR. A comparison of the efficacy and safety of celecoxib 200 mg and celecoxib 400 mg once daily in treating the signs and symptoms of psoriatic arthritis. *Semin Arthritis Rheum* 2007;37(3):164–73.

48. Ceponis A, Kavanaugh A. Use of methotrexate in patients with psoriatic arthritis. *Clin Exp Rheumatol* 2010;28(5 Suppl. 61):S132–7,

49. Kingsley G et al. A randomized placebo-controlled trial of methotrexate in psoriatic arthritis. *Rheumatology (Oxf)* 2012;51(8):1368–77.

50. Clegg D, Reda D, Abdellatif M. Comparison of sulfasalazine and placebo for the treatment of axial and peripheral articular manifestations of the seronegative spondyloarthropathies: A Department of Veterans Affairs cooperative study. *Arthritis Rheum* 1999;42(11):2325–9.

51. Nash P, Thaci D, Behrens F, Falk F, Kaltwasser J. Leflunomide improves psoriasis in patients with psoriatic arthritis: An in-depth analysis of data from the TOPAS study. *Dermatology* 2006;212(3):238–49.

52. Salvarani C et al. Acomparison of cyclosporine, sulfasalazine, and symptomatic therapy in the treatment of psoriatic arthritis. *J Rheumatol* 2001;28(10):2274–82.

53. D'Angelo S, Palazzi C, Olivieri I. Psoriatic arthritis: Treatment strategies using biologic agents. *Reumatismo* 2012;64(2):113–21.

54. Huynh D, Kavanaugh A. Psoriatic arthritis: Current therapy and future approaches. *Rheumatology (Oxf)* 2015;54:20–8.

55. Kavanaugh A et al. Infliximab maintains a high degree of clinical response in patients with active psoriatic arthritis through 1 year of treatment: Results from the impact 2 trial. *Ann Rheum Dis* 2007;66(4):498–505.

56. Mease P et al. Etanercept treatment of psoriatic arthritis: Safety, efficacy, and effect on disease progression. *Arthritis Rheum* 2004;50(7):2264–72.

57. Mease P et al. Adalimumab for the treatment of patients with moderately to severely active psoriatic arthritis: Results of a double-blind, randomized, placebo-controlled trial. *Arthritis Rheum* 2005;52(10):3279–89.

58. Kavanaugh A et al. Clinical efficacy, radiographic and safety findings through 5 years of subcutaneous golimumab treatment in patients with active psoriatic arthritis: Results from a long-term extension of a randomised, placebo-controlled trial (the Go-Reveal Study). *Ann Rheum Dis* 2014;73(9):1689–94.

59. Mease P et al. Effect of certolizumab pegol on signs and symptoms in patients with psoriatic arthritis: 24-week results of a phase 3 double-blind randomised placebo-controlled study (RAPID-PSA). *Ann Rheum Dis* 2014;73(1):48–55.

60. Atteno M et al. Comparison of effectiveness and safety of infliximab, etanercept, and adalimumab in psoriatic arthritis patients who experienced an inadequate response to previous disease-modifying antirheumatic drugs. *Clin Rheumatol* 2010;29(4):399–403.

61. Fagerli K et al. Switching between TNF inhibitors in psoriatic arthritis: Data from the NOR-DMARD study. *Ann Rheum Dis* 2013;72(11):1840–4.

62. McInnes I et al. Efficacy and safety of ustekinumab in patients with active psoriatic arthritis: 1 year results of the phase 3, multicentre, double-blind, placebo-controlled PSUMMIT 1 trial. *Lancet* 2013;382:780–9.

63. Ritchlin C et al. Efficacy and safety of the anti-Il-12/23 P40 monoclonal antibody, ustekinumab, in patients with active psoriatic arthritis despite conventional non-biological and biological anti-tumour necrosis factor therapy: 6-month and 1-year results of the phase 3, multicentre, double-blind, placebo-controlled, randomized PSUMMIT 2 trial. *Ann Rheum Dis* 2014;73(6):990–9.

64. Mease PJ et al. Brodalumab, an anti-IL17RAmonoclonal antibody, in psoriatic arthritis. *N Engl J Med* 2014;370(24):2295–306.

65. McInnes IB et al. Efficacy and safety of secukinumab, a fully human anti-interleukin-17A monoclonal antibody, in patients with moderate-to severe psoriatic arthritis: A 24-week, randomised, double-blind, placebo-controlled, phase II proof-of-concept trial. *Ann Rheum Dis* 2014;73:349–56.

66. Mease PJ et al. Ixekizumab, an interleukin-17Aspecific monoclonal antibody, for the treatment of biologic-naive patients with active psoriatic arthritis: Results from the 24-week randomised, double-blind, placebo-controlled and active (adalimumab)-controlled period of the phase III trial SPIRIT-P1. *Ann Rheum Dis* 2017;76:79–87.

67. Schafer P. Apremilast mechanism of action and application to psoriasis and psoriatic arthritis. *Biochem Pharmacol* 2012;83(12):1583–90.

68. Altmeyer M, Kerisit K, Boh E. Therapeutic hotline. Abatacept: Our experience of use in two patients with refractory psoriasis and psoriatic arthritis. *Dermatol Ther* 2011;24:287–90.

69. Korman BD, Tyler KL, Korman NJ. Progressive multifocal leukoencephalopathy, efalizumab, and immunosuppression: A cautionary tale for dermatologists. *Arch Dermatol* 2009;145:937–42.

70. Mease PJ, Reich K, Alefacept in Psoriatic Arthritis Study Group. Alefacept with methotrexate for treatment of psoriatic arthritis: Open-label extension of a randomized, double-blind, placebo-controlled study. *J Am Acad Dermatol* 2009;60:402–11.

52

Reactive arthritis

BIJU VASUDEVAN AND ASMITA SINHA

INTRODUCTION

Reactive arthritis is an inflammatory arthritis that arises following a gastrointestinal or urogenital infection, representing the classic interplay of host and environment and with the potential to involve multiple organ systems. The importance lies in the fact that it can be easily overlooked if clinical suspicion is not high at presentation, can develop chronic symptoms and severe debilitating disease, and needs definitive management on an emergency basis to prevent further complications.

The classic syndrome is a triad of symptoms, involving the urethra, conjunctiva, and synovium; however, the majority of patients do not present with this classic triad [1]. It is considered as a form of spondyloarthritis, a group of diseases with inflammatory arthritis, negative rheumatoid factor, and genetic association with HLA-B27 [2].

There are two main types of reactive arthritis, based on antecedent infection, postvenereal and postdysenteric, with no difference in the clinical manifestations, and once the arthritis develops, the microorganism is not found in the joint [3]. The disease is of immunological origin, and bacterial antigens have been detected in synovial or tissue fluid [4].

HISTORY

Hans Reiter first described the triad of arthritis, nongonococcal urethritis, and conjunctivitis in 1916 [5]. Fiessinger and Leroy also described the association in that same year [6]. The disease was thus named Reiter syndrome and Fiessinger-Leroy syndrome [7–11]. However, during recent years the more descriptive term *reactive arthritis*, coined by Ahvonen, Sievers, and Aho in 1969, has become the appropriate term regardless of whether or not the syndrome encompasses the three classic organ systems [12–14].

EPIDEMIOLOGY

The reactive arthritis (ReA) incidence is found to be 5–14/100,000 patients in the age group of 18–60 years, more common in the age bracket of 20–40 years, more common in Caucasians, and found to be equal in males and females in some studies or more prevalent in males in others [3,15,16]. It is less common in young children and the elderly, and when it does occur in these age groups, the antecedent infection is invariably enteric.

The human leukocyte antigen (HLA) B27 positivity in ReA ranges from 30%–70%, which is lowest among the seronegative spondyloarthritis group with the highest positivity (90%) seen in ankylosing spondylitis [17]. Patients of ReA positive for HLA B27 are found to have more extra-articular symptoms, and also the arthritis is more severe and has a higher probability of turning chronic [18].

ETIOPATHOGENESIS

The exact etiopathogenesis of ReA is not clear, but both genetic and environmental factors play a role.

Bacteria that commonly cause ReA are *Salmonella, Shigella, Campylobacter, Yersinia,* and *Chlamydia trachomatis. Chlamydia trachomatis* is the most common etiologic agent associated with genital infection, and most of these patients are asymptomatic. *Ureaplasma urealyticum* is now increasingly being reported to trigger ReA. *Mycoplasma genitalium* has also been rarely associated with the condition. Some bacteria including *Clostridium difficile* and *Escherichia coli* have also been described as the etiological agents, but less commonly [19]. Other microorganisms implicated include *C. pneumoniae*, *U. urealyticum*, and *Helicobacter pylori* (Table 52.1) [3].

It has been postulated that the etiological microorganisms initiate an autoimmune response, via the molecular mimicry shown by HLA B27, which presents the microbial peptides to T cells. Various arthritogenic peptides like chlamydial HSP60, OMP2, DNA primase, *Yersinia* lipopolysaccharide, ribosomal protein L23, etc., have been implicated in the pathogenesis [20–23]. Both toll-like receptors 2 and 4 (TLR2 and TLR4) have been associated with ReA [24]. Some studies also suggest that persistent infection of urogenital organs may be a source of pathogen-associated molecular patterns and damage-associated molecular patterns which in turn stimulate TLRs causing the immune response.

Following the primary infection, the causative bacteria of ReA are incorporated intracellularly into monocytes and trafficked to the synovium [25,26], where the pathogen or the bacterial degradation products persist in the joints. In the chronic state, *Chlamydia* probably evades the immune system by increased expression of HSP60, and downregulation of major OMP1, and surface major histocompatibility complex in infected cells. An imbalance in the cytokine profile may be responsible for persistence of the microbes in the joints and the pathological immune response. It has been postulated that perhaps in ReA, the Th1 and Th2 balance is disturbed. Decreased tumor necrosis factor (TNF) and increased interleukin-10 have been demonstrated in the acute stage of the disease. However, Butrimiene et al. have suggested that TNF-α production is higher in chronic ReA, which suggests that the Th1 response is more dominant in chronic ReA [27].

Table 52.1 Pathogens commonly associated with reactive arthritis

Bacteria associated with enteritis	• *Salmonella enterica*
	  • *S. Typhimurium enteritidis*
	  • *S. Paratyphi*
	• *Shigella* spp.
	  • *S. flexneri*
	  • *S. sonnei*
	  • *S. dysenteriae*
	• *Yersinia* spp.
	  • *Y. enterocolitica*
	  • *Y. pseudotuberculosis*
	• *Campylobacter* spp.
	  • *C. coli*
	  • *C. jejuni*

Bacteria associated with urethritis	*Chlamydia trachomatis* *Mycoplasma genitalium* *Ureaplasma urealyticum*

Source: Carter JD, Hudson AP. *Rheum Dis Clin North Am* 2009;35:21–44.

CLINICAL MANIFESTATIONS

ReA has been reported to present approximately 1–4 weeks after a genitourinary or enteric infection, and the classic triad includes urethritis, conjunctivitis, and arthritis (Table 52.2). It is important to realize that many times the disease may present in the incomplete form, and even asymptomatic initial chlamydial infections can also lead to the appearance of arthritis. The classic triad is found in only one-third of patients [28].

Urethritis and conjunctivitis are usually the first manifestations. Arthritis classically appears 10–14 days later, followed shortly by circinate balanitis. However, circinate balanitis can also be the presenting feature, appearing months before other manifestations in some cases.

Table 52.2 Common clinical manifestations in reactive arthritis

System	Manifestation
Skeletal	Oligoarthritis Polyarthritis Dactylitis Sacroiliitis Enthesitis Planter fasciitis
Genitourinary	Urethritis Prostatitis Cervicitis Vaginitis Cystitis Hydronephrosis
Ocular	Conjunctivitis Anterior uveitis Rare: Keratitis, corneal ulcer, episcleritis, retinal detachment, macular degeneration
Gastrointestinal	Diarrhea
Mucocutaneous	Keratoderma blennorrhagicum Geographic tongue Circinate balanitis Erythema nodosum Nail changes: Onycholysis, onychodystrophy, subungual debris, nail pitting
Cardiac	Electrocardiogram conduction abnormalities Cardiac valve abnormalities Aortic insufficiency Heart failure Pericarditis, myocarditis Heart block
Renal	Proteinurea, microhematuria IgA nephropathy
Central nervous system	Peripheral/cranial nerve palsies Progressive myelopathy

ReA can have a very acute onset and severe manifestations in initial stages. Complications, though rare, need urgent management. Generally it presents acutely with malaise, fatigue, weight loss, and fever, and the different clinical manifestations are described in the following text [29,30].

Arthritis

An asymmetrical oligoarthritis is usually the main presenting symptom; however, arthritis can also be polyarticular or monoarticular. Joint inflammation could be axial, involving lumbar spine or sacroiliac joints, or it could be peripheral with predilection for the weight-bearing joints of the lower limbs (knees, ankles, foot) (Figure 52.1). Alternatively, the upper extremities can be affected less commonly. The arthritis is characteristically nonsuppurative and associated with an inflammatory type of pain that may range from mild arthralgia to severe disabling arthritis, which may resolve spontaneously or persist for months, progressively causing irreversible damage to joints; hence, there is an urgent need for management. The knee joints may show massive effusions up to 100 mL. Rapid development of massive effusions frequently results in popliteal cysts.

A unique manifestation of this disease is enthesitis—the inflammation of the transitional zone where tendons and ligaments insert into the bone. Involvement of the Achilles tendon is most commonly seen, but other enthesitis may also be involved. Plantar fasciitis and posterior tibial tendonitis may also occur.

Sometimes "sausage digits" or dactylitis is also seen, which is a diffuse swelling of the entire finger or toe. However, this feature is common in psoriatic arthritis (PsA) as well. Approximately 50% of patients have acute inflammatory low backache that is worse during the night and

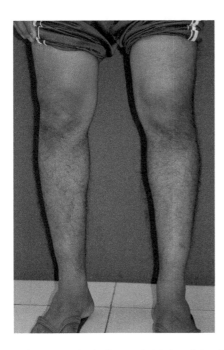

Figure 52.1 Asymmetrical oligoarthritis involving left knee.

radiates to the buttocks [31]. The thoracic and cervical spine are also occasionally involved in chronic ReA.

The PsA pattern is similar to that of ReA, but there are a few differences studied between the two. *First*, PsA has no predilection for lower limbs like ReA. *Second*, ReA has a younger age of onset. *Third*, sacroiliitis is rarer in PsA than ReA. *Finally*, HLA B27 is positive more commonly in ReA than PsA.

Urethritis

Approximately 90% of patients are found to have sterile nongonococcal urethritis that may present with frequency, urgency, meatal erythema or edema, dysuria, and shreds and mucoid material in the first flow of urine. Chronic prostatitis may occur. Women may present with cervicitis, salpingitis, dysuria, vaginitis, bartholinitis, cystitis, and urethritis. However, asymptomatic genital tract infection may also occur in some cases.

Eye lesions

The most common eye manifestation is conjunctivitis that may be unilateral or bilateral and subtarsal. It may be transient and often missed. A more severe presentation is in the form of bilateral uveitis, which occurs with acute-onset pain in the eyes with redness, photophobia, blepharospasm, and miosis. There is generally a period of prodromal eye discomfort for up to 2 days, and it starts as an anterior uveitis. However, repeated episodes can lead to posterior uveitis, complicated cataract, and glaucoma, resulting in severe visual impairment. Hence, it is important to immediately evaluate and treat any suspicious eye complaint. Less commonly, transient keratitis, corneal erosions, episcleritis, retinal detachment, and rarely macular degeneration have been reported [32].

Mucocutaneous manifestations

Approximately 50% of patients present with mucocutaneous lesions, which may appear both before and after the onset of arthritis. The cutaneous lesions resemble that of psoriasis.

Keratoderma blennorrhagicum is a classic cutaneous finding in 5%–30% of patients. The lesions initially start as small vesicles and pustules or erythematous macules that progress to crusted papules and ultimately coalesce to form hyperkeratotic plaques that are found densely scattered on the palms and soles (Figure 52.2) but may also occur on the trunk, scalp, dorsum of fingers and toes, etc. (Figure 52.3).

Circinate balanitis is the most common mucocutaneous finding, observed in 20%–40% of patients and manifesting as painless serpiginous erosions (Figure 52.4) that can coalesce to form a sharply demarcated serpiginous pattern on the glans. If the penis is circumcised, it evolves to form hard crusts and plaques and may involve the penile shaft and scrotum. Females can present with similar lesions in

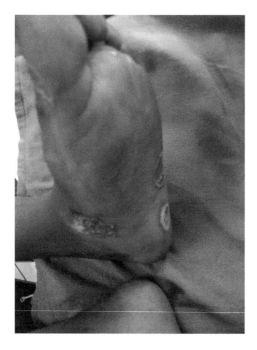

Figure 52.2 Keratoderma blenorrhagicum—soles.

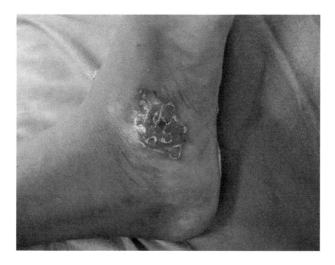

Figure 52.3 Crusted plaque on ankle.

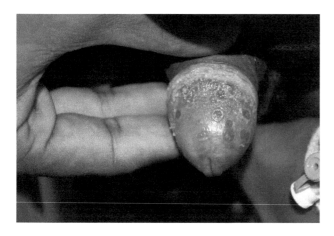

Figure 52.4 Circinate balanitis.

the form of scattered, sharply demarcated, shallow erosions on the vulva, perineum, labia minora, and vestibule [33].

Nails are affected in 20%–30% of patients. There may be subungual thickening and debris, periungual pustules, thickening of nail fold, ridging of nail plate, onychodystrophy, onycholysis, and nail pitting.

Visceral manifestations

There are several case reports about aortic insufficiency developing in patients with ReA, some reporting it as soon as 4 days after diagnosis [34–40]. Cardiac involvement commonly manifests as conduction delays that may progress further, resulting in complete heart block and heart failure. Acute aortitis, myocarditis, and pericarditis may occur rarely. Renal involvement can cause asymptomatic proteinuria, microscopic hematuria, and aseptic pyuria. IgA nephropathy has been found to be associated with ReA in a few cases. There have been rare reports of association of ReA with myelopathy and neurological sequelae [35]. Secondary amyloidosis has also been described as a complication [41].

Reactive arthritis and HIV infection

ReA occurring in AIDS patients is a serious and disabling condition with rapid progression of symptoms and refractoriness to treatment [42,43]. There is need to exercise caution while using immunosuppressants in HIV coinfection, because they have the potential to cause myelosuppression and fatal opportunistic infections. Anti-TNF-α drugs can be useful in patients with HIV and ReA because TNF-α has been implicated in the pathogenesis of ReA, and it also stimulates HIV replication.

INVESTIGATIONS

The diagnosis of ReA is clinical, based on the clinical history and physical examination. No laboratory study or imaging finding is exclusive or diagnostic.

Laboratory and imaging findings: The characteristic findings to look for include the following:

- Serologic or other evidence of antecedent infection
- High acute phase reactants
- Positive HLA-B27
- Inflammatory synovitis
- Imaging abnormalities consistent with enthesitis or arthritis

Plain radiographs of affected joints and entheses are asked for to exclude other causes of joint pain, including other forms of arthritis and stress fractures. Magnetic resonance imaging and scintigraphy can be done as indicated.

In patients with a joint effusion, arthrocentesis and examination of the synovial fluid are carried out, including total and differential white blood cell counts, crystal search, and examination for bacteria by Gram stain and culture to exclude septic arthritis. The synovial fluid can also be sent for nucleic acid amplification technique and polymerase chain reaction (PCR) to look for chlamydia antigens.

In patients with recent diarrhea, stool cultures are obtained to test for *Salmonella*, *Shigella*, *Campylobacter*, and *Yersinia*. Serologic testing for enteric pathogens is generally not indicated because of the limited specificity of such testing [44].

In patients suspected of infection with *Chlamydia trachomatis* and in patients with neither gastrointestinal nor genitourinary symptoms, a urine sample is obtained for testing for *Chlamydia* using nucleic acid amplification techniques.

The prevalence of HLA-B27 in patients with ReA is estimated at approximately 30%–50%.

Rheumatoid factor and anticyclic citrullinated peptide are usually absent in patients with ReA.

Electrocardiography and echocardiography can be done to rule out any cardiac involvement.

Routine laboratory testing: A complete blood count and differential count, acute phase reactants, renal and liver chemistries, and urinalysis to obtain supportive evidence of acute inflammation and to exclude other systemic disorders are usually done.

CLINICAL CRITERIA

The clinical criteria for diagnosis of ReA are provided in Table 52.3 [45,46].

DIFFERENTIAL DIAGNOSIS

The following conditions may be considered in the differential diagnosis:

- Psoriatic arthritis, rheumatoid arthritis, systemic lupus erythematosus, Behçet disease, HIV infection, syphilis

- Enteroviral infection–associated arthritis, inflammatory bowel diseases celiac (sprue) disease, Whipple disease, parasitic infections, intestinal bypass surgery
- Disseminated gonococcal infection or gonococcal arthritis
- Undifferentiated spondyloarthritis, ankylosing spondylitis
- Acute rheumatic fever following streptococcal pharyngitis

TREATMENT

In some patients, especially those with genitourinary infection, treatment of the infection that triggered the arthritis is indicated; arthritis should be treated in patients with symptomatic joint disease. Apart from this, interventions may also be required for the treatment of extraarticular manifestations. The patient is advised restriction of weight-bearing if legs are involved and physiotherapy to prevent muscle wasting.

Treatment of the infection: Antibiotics are not used to treat arthritis specifically but may be indicated for the underlying infection if evidence is detected of ongoing genitourinary infection or carriage of potentially pathogenic organisms. A role for antibiotic therapy for chronic arthritis has not been definitely established.

Enteric infection: In general, antibiotics are not indicated for enteric infections [47–49].

Genitourinary tract infection: Patients with acute *Chlamydia trachomatis* infection of the genitourinary tract and their sexual partners should be given antimicrobial treatment. Antibiotic treatment of the infection may prevent relapses of arthritis in patients with recurrent genitourinary tract symptoms alone [50]. A 3-month course of doxycycline 100 mg is usually advised. Combination antibiotics might be useful in the subset of patients of chronic arthritis with

Table 52.3 Clinical criteria for diagnosing reactive arthritis

Major criteria	Minor criteria
Diagnostic criteria	
Arthritis with two of three of the following: • Asymmetric • Monoarthritis or oligoarthritis • Affecting predominantly lower limbs	Evidence of triggering infection (at least one of the following) • Positive nucleic acid amplification test in the morning urine or urethral/cervical swab for *Chlamydia trachomatis* • Positive stool culture for enteric pathogens
Preceding symptomatic infection with one or two of the following: • Enteritis (diarrhea for at least 1 day, 3 days to 6 weeks before the onset of arthritis) • Urethritis (dysuria or discharge for at least 1 day, 3 days to 6 weeks before the onset of arthritis)	Evidence for persistent synovial infection • Positive immunohistology or polymerase chain reaction for *Chlamydia*

Note: Definite reactive arthritis: Both major criteria and relative minor criterion present. *Probable reactive arthritis*: Both major criteria present but relative minor criterion absent; one major criterion and one or more minor criteria present.

PCR-proven *Chlamydia*-induced arthritis [51]. Rifampicin plus doxycycline is the preferred combination [52–54].

Treatment of arthritis: The treatment of arthritis can be divided into two stages: the treatment of acute ReA and the treatment of refractory (chronic) ReA, defined as disease of greater than 6 months' duration.

The initial treatment goal is to provide symptomatic relief for the arthritis, because the disease is self-limited in quite a number of patients, and joint damage with significant continued symptoms is infrequent.

Acute reactive arthritis

NSAIDs: In patients with acute ReA, treatment is initiated with nonsteroidal anti-inflammatory drugs (NSAIDs), which are the principal form of therapy, followed by intra-articular and/or systemic glucocorticoids in patients with disease resistant to NSAIDs.

Anti-inflammatory doses of NSAIDs (e.g., naproxen 500 mg two to three times a day, diclofenac 50 mg three times a day, or indomethacin 50 mg three to four times a day) provide symptomatic relief for patients of ReA, and form the initial treatment. An adequate trial of a given NSAID is usually at least 2 weeks in duration. A combination of NSAIDs may be needed [55,56].

Intra-articular glucocorticoids: In patients who do not respond adequately to NSAIDs, injection of major affected joints with intra-articular glucocorticoids is recommended. Intra-articular injection with intra-articular triamcinolone acetonide (40 mg for a large joint, such as the knee, and lower doses for smaller joints) is generally effective in reducing joint inflammation and in providing symptomatic relief similar to that seen in other forms of spondyloarthritis.

Systemic glucocorticoids: In patients who do not respond adequately to NSAIDs and intra-articular glucocorticoid injections or in those with a large number of involved joints, low to moderate doses of oral glucocorticoids (e.g., a starting dose of prednisolone 20 mg daily), should be started and reduced gradually to the lowest dose required to control symptoms.

DMARDs: Treatment with a disease-modifying antirheumatic drug (DMARD) is indicated in patients who do not respond well to initial therapies. DMARDs are generally used in patients who have not responded adequately to at least two different NSAIDs over a total of 4 weeks and who require ongoing therapy with more than 7.5 mg prednisolone or equivalent for more than 3–6 months.

Resistant acute arthritis and chronic reactive arthritis

In patients who develop chronic refractory ReA, or who are resistant to initial therapy for acute arthritis with NSAIDs and glucocorticoids, therapy is initiated with a nonbiologic (traditional) DMARD, like sulfasalazine or methotrexate. In patients with disease that is refractory to a nonbiologic DMARD, TNF inhibitors can be tried. The use of these medications for ReA is based on limited data and clinical experience.

Sulfasalazine: Sulfasalazine (SSZ) is used in patients with refractory ReA or with ReA resistant to initial therapy for acute arthritis. Treatment is initiated with 500 mg once daily and the daily dose is increased stepwise (in increments of 500 mg each week) to 1000 mg twice daily. The dose can be increased to 3000 mg/day (taken in two or three divided doses) when required [42].

Methotrexate: Methotrexate (MTX) may be used as an alternative nonbiologic DMARD for patients who are allergic to or intolerant to SSZ or who do not respond to SSZ treatment. The use of MTX is based on clinical experiences with its use for other peripheral spondyloarthritis, including psoriatic arthritis and rheumatoid arthritis. In ReA, MTX is used in the same fashion and doses (15–25 mg given once weekly) as are employed in PsA and in rheumatoid arthritis.

The nonbiologic DMARDs are ideally continued for at least 4 months (SSZ) or 3 months (MTX) at the maximally tolerated therapeutic dose (up to 3 g/day SSZ or up to 25 mg/week MTX) to determine if there is a response to therapy and are then discontinued 3–6 months after the patients have entered into remission.

Anti-TNF agents: For patients who have ReA that is refractory to NSAIDs and glucocorticoids and who do not respond to or have a contraindication to the use of MTX or SSZ, an anti-tumor necrosis factor (TNF) agent (e.g., etanercept 50 mg/week administered by subcutaneous injection or infliximab 3–5 mg/kg administered intravenously on weeks 0, 2, 6 and then every eighth week) can be prescribed. In patients who do not respond initially to one agent after 3 months of therapy, another TNF inhibitor can be tried instead. Effort can be made to discontinue therapy in patients who have been in remission induced by TNF inhibitors for at least 3 months, but retreatment with the medication should be resumed if disease then recurs [57,58].

Treatment of extra-articular manifestations

- *Ocular manifestations*: Patients with abnormal eye findings need to be referred for ophthalmologic evaluation, and a slit-lamp examination may be required to determine if uveitis is present and needs urgent management with steroids to prevent any long-term visual complications.
- *Skin and mucous membrane lesions*: Patients with very mild skin involvement or oral ulcers may not require any intervention. Symptomatic treatment may be sufficient in patients with oral mucosal ulcers, and topical steroids are effective in some patients. More symptomatic involvement with mild to moderate keratoderma blennorrhagica may benefit from the use of topical steroids and salicylates. Patients with more severe keratoderma blennorrhagica and pustular lesions who do not respond to topical medications may require systemic DMARDs, such as MTX [31]. Topical calcipotriol and retinoids may also be helpful.
- *Cardiac*: Definitive management if symptomatic for any cardiac complications, including valve replacement surgeries if required.

PROGNOSIS

ReA has a variable course and may remit spontaneously or progress to chronic illness. According to one study, 75% of patients are in complete remission at the end of the second year after onset [45]. Recurrent exacerbations can cause chronic arthritis and chronic eye symptoms. About 15%–20% of patients may develop chronic disabling symptoms.

CONCLUSION

ReA is an inflammatory arthritis associated with skin and eye lesions. The characteristic involvement is asymmetrical oligoarthritis of lower limb joints, conjunctivitis, uveitis, keratoderma blenorrhagicum, and circinate balanitis. Urethritis or enteritis precedes the arthritis. Treatment involves a course of antibiotics such as doxycycline and immunosuppressants such as MTX. Biologics also have a role to play.

KEY POINTS

- Reactive arthritis is an inflammatory arthritis that arises following a gastrointestinal or urogenital infection, characterized by triad of symptoms, involving the urethra, conjunctiva, and synovium.
- Keratoderma blenorrhagicum, circinate balanitis and crusted heaped up plaques are characteristic mucocutaneous features.
- Asymmetrical lower limb joint arthritis, axial involvement and enthesitis are common.
- HLA B27 and HIV are common associations.
- NSAIDs, Methotrexate and Biologics are treatments of choice.

REFERENCES

1. Parker CT, Thomas D. Reiter's syndrome and reactive arthritis. *J Am Osteopath* 2000;100:101–4.
2. Kim TH, Uhm WS, Inman RD. Pathogenesis of ankylosing spondylitis and reactive arthritis. *Curr Opin Rheumatol* 2005;17:400–5.
3. Carter JD, Hudson AP. Reactive arthritis: Clinical aspects and medical management. *Rheum Dis Clin North Am* 2009;35:21–44.
4. Cox CJ, Kempsell KE, Gaston JS. Investigation of infectious agents associated with arthritis by reverse transcription PCR of bacterial rRNA. *Arthritis Res Ther* 2003;5:R1–8.
5. Reiter H. Uber einebisherunerkannate Spirochaten infektion (Spirochetosis arthritica). *Dtsch Med Wochenschr* 1916;42:1535–6.
6. Fiessinger M, Leroy E. Contribution a l'etuded'uneepidemie de dysenteriedans le somme. *Bull Mem Soc Med Hop Paris* 1916;40:2030–69.
7. Sharp JT. Reiter's syndrome. In: Hollander JH, McCarthy DJ (Eds), *Arthritis and Allied Conditions*. 8th ed. Philadelphia: Lea and Febiger; 1979: 1223–9.
8. Sydenham T. *The Works of Thomas Sydenham, M.D.* Translated by RG Latham. London: Sydenham Society, II; 1848: 257–9.
9. Stoll M. De l'arthritedysenterique. *Arch Med Gen Trop* 1869;14:29–30.
10. Brodie BC. *Pathological and Surgical Observations on Diseases of the Joints.* London: Longman; 1818: 54.
11. Bauer W, Engelmann EP. Syndrome of unknown aetiology characterized by urethritis, conjunctivitis, and arthritis (so-called Reiter's Disease). *Trans Assoc Am Physicians* 1942;57:307–8.
12. Wallace DJ, Weisman M. Should a war criminal be rewarded with eponymous distinction? The double life of Hans Reiter (1881–1969). *J Clin Rheumatol* 2000;6:49–54.
13. Panush RS et al. Retraction of the suggestion to use the term "Reiter's syndrome" sixty-five years later: The legacy of Reiter, a war criminal, should not be eponymic honor but rather condemnation. *Arthritis Rheum* 2007;56:693–4.
14. Leirisalo-Repo M. Reactive arthritis. *Scand J Rheumatol* 2005;34:251–9.
15. Hannu T, Hannu T. Reactive arthritis. *Best Pract Res Clin Rheumat* 2011;25:347–57.
16. Kvien TK et al. Reactive arthritis: Incidence, triggering agents and clinical presentation. *J Rheumatol* 1994;21:115–22.
17. Mcmichael A, Bowness P. HLA-B27: Natural function and pathogenic role in spondyloarthritis. *Arthritis Research* 2002;4:S153–158.
18. Toivanen A. Reactive arthritis. *Best Prac Res Clin Rheumat* 2004;18:689–703.
19. Townes JM et al. Reactive arthritis following culture-confirmed infections with bacterial enteric pathogens in Minnesota and Oregon: A population-based study. *Ann Rheum Dis* 2008;67:1689–96.
20. Alvarez-Navarro et al. Novel HLA B27-restricted epitopes from *Chlamydia trachomatis* generated upon endogenous processing of bacterial proteins suggest a role of molecular mimicry in reactive arthritis. *J Biol Chem* 2013;288(36):25810–25.
21. Deane KH et al. Identification and characterization of a DR4-restricted T cell epitope within *Chlamydia* heat shock protein 60. *Clin Exp Immunol* 1997;109:439–45.
22. Schiellerup P, Krogfelt KA, Locht H. A comparison of self-reported joint symptoms following infection with different enteric pathogens: Effect of HLA-B27. *J Rheumatol* 2008;35:480–7.
23. Reveille J. Genetics of spondyloarthritis—Beyond the MHC. *Nat Rev Rheumatol* 2012;8:296–304.
24. Tsui FW et al. Toll-like receptor 2 variants are associated with acute reactive arthritis. *Arthritis Rheum* 2008;58:3436–8.

25. Gracey E, Inman RD. *Chlamydia*-induced ReA: Immune imbalances and persistent pathogens. *Nat Rev Rheumatol* 2011;8:55–9.

26. Zugel U, Kaufmann SH. Role of heat shock proteins in protection from and pathogenesis of infectious diseases. *Clin Microbiol Rev* 1999;12:19–39.

27. Butrimiene I et al. Different cytokine profiles in patients with chronic and acute reactive arthritis. *Rheumatology (Oxf)* 2004;43:1300–4.

28. Rohekar S, Pope J. Epidemiologic approaches to infection and immunity: The case of reactive arthritis. *Curr Opin Rheumatol* 2009;21:386–90.

29. Shupack JL, Stiller MJ, Haber RS. Psoriasis and Reiter's syndrome. *Clin Dermatol* 1991;9:3–58.

30. Wu IB, Schwartz RA. Reiter's syndrome: The classic triad and more. *J Am Acad Dermatol* 2008;59:113–21.

31. Colmegna I, Cuchacovich R, Espinoza LR. HLA-B27-associated reactive arthritis: Pathogenetic and clinical considerations. *Clin Microbiol Rev* 2004;17:348–69.

32. Kiss S, Letko E, Qamruddin S, Baltatzis S, Foster CS. Long-term progression, prognosis, and treatment of patients with recurrent ocular manifestations of Reiter's syndrome. *Ophthalmology* 2003;110:1764–9.

33. Edwards L, Hansen RC. Reiter's syndrome of the vulva. The psoriasis spectrum. *Arch Dermatol* 1992;128:811–4.

34. Qaiyumi S, Hassan ZU, Toone E. Seronegative spondyloarthropathies in lone aortic insufficiency. *Arch Intern Med* 1985;145:822–4.

35. Good AE. Reiter's disease: A review with special attention to cardiovascular and neurologic sequelae. *Semin Arthritis Rheum* 1974;3:253–86.

36. Paulus HE, Pearson CM, Pitts W, Jr Aortic insufficiency in five patients with Reiter's syndrome. A detailed clinical and pathologic study. *Am J Med* 1972;53(4):464–72.

37. Machado H, Befeler B, Morales AR, Vargas A, Aranda J. Aortic insufficiency in Reiter's syndrome. *South Med J* 1976;69:955–7.

38. Collins P. Aortic incompetence and active myocarditis in Reiter's disease. *Br J Vener Dis* 1972;48:300–3.

39. Cosh JA, Barritt DW, Jayson MI. Cardiac lesions of Reiter's syndrome and ankylosing spondylitis. *Br Heart J* 1973;35:553.

40. Rodnan GP, Benedek TG, Shaver JA, Fennell RH Jr. Reiter's syndrome and aortic insufficiency. *JAMA* 1964;182:889–94.

41. Wakefield D, Charlesworth J, Pussell B, Wenman J. Reiter's syndrome and amyloidosis. *Rheumatology* 1987;26:156–8.

42. Winchester R et al. Implications from the occurrence of Reiter's syndrome and related disorders in association with advanced HIV infection. *Scand J Rheumatol* 1988;74:89–93.

43. Cuellar ML, Espinoza LR. Rheumatic manifestations HIV-AIDS. *Baillieres Best Pract Res Clin Rheumatol* 2000;14:579–93.

44. Sieper J, Rudwaleit M, Braun J, van der Heijde D. Diagnosing reactive arthritis: Role of clinical setting in the value of serologic and microbiologic assays. *Arthritis Rheum* 2002;46:319.

45. Amor B. Reiter's syndrome. Diagnosis and clinical features. *Rheum Dis Clin North Am* 1998;24:677–95.

46. Braun J et al. On the difficulties of establishing a consensus on the definition of and diagnostic investigations of reactive arthritis. Results and discussion of a questionnaire prepared for the 4th International Workshop on Reactive Arthritis, Berlin, Germany, July 3–6, 1999. *J Rheumatol* 2000;27:2185–92.

47. Laasila K, Laasonen L, Leirisalo-Repo M. Antibiotic treatment and long term prognosis of reactive arthritis. *Ann Rheum Dis* 2003;62:655.

48. Lauhio A et al. Double-blind, placebo-controlled study of three-month treatment with lymecycline in reactive arthritis, with special reference to *Chlamydia* arthritis. *Arthritis Rheum* 1991;34:6.

49. Kvien TK et al. Three month treatment of reactive arthritis with azithromycin: A EULAR double blind, placebo controlled study. *Ann Rheum Dis* 2004;63:111.

50. Bardin T et al. Antibiotic treatment of venereal disease and Reiter's syndrome in a Greenland population. *Arthritis Rheum* 1992;35:190.

51. Carter JD et al. Combination antibiotics as a treatment for chronic *Chlamydia*-induced reactive arthritis: A double-blind, placebo-controlled, prospective trial. *Arthritis Rheum* 2010;62:1298.

52. Gerard HC, Schumacher HR, El-Gabalawy H, Goldbach-Mansky R, Hudson AP. *Chlamydia pneumoniae* present in the human synovium are viable and metabolically active. *Microb Pathog* 2000;29:17–24.

53. Engel JN, Pollack J, Perara E, Ganem D. Heat shock response of murine *Chlamydia trachomatis*. *J Bacteriol* 1990;172:6959–72.

54. Carter JD, Valeriano J, Vasey FB. A prospective, randomized 9-month comparison of doxycycline vs. doxycycline and rifampin in undifferentiated spondyloarthritis with special reference to *Chlamydia*-induced arthritis. *J Rheumatol* 2004;31:1973–80.

55. Flores D, Marquez J, Garza M, Espinoza LR. Reactive arthritis: Newer developments. *Rheum Dis Clin North Am* 2003;29:37.

56. Juvakoski T, Lassus A. A double-blind cross-over evaluation of ketoprofen and indomethacin in Reiter's disease. *Scand J Rheumatol* 1982;11:106.

57. Flagg SD et al. Decreased pain and synovial inflammation after etanercept therapy in patients with reactive and undifferentiated arthritis: An open-label trial. *Arthritis Rheum* 2005;53:613.

58. Meyer A et al. Safety and efficacy of anti-tumor necrosis factor α therapy in ten patients with recent-onset refractory reactive arthritis. *Arthritis Rheum* 2011;63:1274.

PART 13

Miscellaneous Dermatological Emergencies

DEBDEEP MITRA

53

Graft versus host disease

SANDEEP ARORA, SANDEEP LAL, AND MANASA SHETTISARA JANNEY

INTRODUCTION

Graft versus host disease (GVHD) is a multisystem disorder that occurs most commonly after allogenic hematopoietic stem cell transplantation (ASCT). It is also observed in transfusion of nonirradiated blood to an immunocompromised host (Wiskott-Aldrich syndrome, ataxia telangiectasia) [1], in donor lymphocyte infusion, solid organ transplant [2], umbilical cord blood transplant, and maternofetal transfusion (Table 53.1). GVHD mirrors allograft rejection caused by the immunocompetent alloreactive donor T lymphocytes that recognize the minor or major histocompatibility antigens on the target tissue of the host, leading to multiorgan involvement. In short, GVHD is a host rejection by the graft. Skin is the earliest and the most common organ to be affected in GVHD. Recognition and treatment of various manifestations of GVHD remain a challenge in transplant medicine, a field that is now being practiced routinely in all major centers across the country.

HISTORY

Transplant medicine has grown leaps and bounds with advances in the harvest of hematopoietic stem cells, various donors, and reduced intensity conditioning regimens (to eliminate tumor cells, and the immunosuppressive component to prevent host immune responses from rejecting the transplanted donor cells) [3,4]. Hematopoietic stem cells are presently being harvested from peripheral blood mobilized stem cells, umbilical cord blood stem cells, in addition to bone marrow hematopoietic stem cells. Stem cell donors can be matched related donors, matched unrelated donors (MUDs), and haploidentical stem cell donors (complete half mismatch (4 of 8 human leukocyte antigen [HLA] loci) from a related

donor) [5]. Donor leukocyte infusions, the administration of additional donor hematopoietic stem cell (HC) to the recipient weeks or even months after hematopoietic stem cell transplantation (HCT), are also frequently utilized to augment the graft versus malignancy effect. These transplants carry a greater risk of GVHD due to mismatch of minor HLA due to MUD.

CLASSIFICATION

Classically, GVHD is divided into acute and chronic, based on the onset of signs from the time of transplant.

Acute GVHD (aGVHD): Defined as disease presenting within 100 days of transplant.

Chronic GVHD (cGVHD): Defined as disease presenting beyond 100 days of transplant.

However, with the newer transplant practices, aGVHD can have a delayed onset or can be persistent or recurrent. Similarly, an overlap of aGVHD and cGVHD is also seen, which is known as overlap syndrome as per the National Institution of Health (NIH) consensus (Table 53.2) [6].

EPIDEMIOLOGY

Various factors that have been implicated in the development of GVHD are HLA mismatch, MUD, gender disparity, multiparous female donor, intensity of conditioning regimen, age factors, use of peripheral blood stem cells as source of stem cells, and the host disease condition [7]. HLA mismatching confers the greatest risk for the development of GVHD.

Approximately 40%–60% of patients of ASCT develop GVHD [8]. Depending on the HLA matching, acute GVHD is seen in around 40%–80% of patients [9]. The incidence of acute GVHD is also further influenced by the various factors

Table 53.1 Etiology of graft versus host disease

1. Bone marrow transplantation
2. Donor lymphocyte infusion
3. Cord blood stem cell transplantation
4. Maternofetal transfusion
5. Blood transfusion associated
6. Peripheral blood stem cell transplantation
7. Solid organ transplantation

Table 53.2 Classification of acute and chronic graft versus host disease

Category	Time of symptoms after ASCT or DLI	Presence of acute GVHD features	Presence of chronic GVHD features
Acute GVHD			
Classic acute GVHD	<100 days	Yes	No
Persistent, recurrent, or late-onset acute GVHD	>100 days	Yes	No
Chronic GVHD			
Classic chronic GVHD	No time limit	No	Yes
Overlap syndrome	No time limit	Yes	Yes

Abbreviations: ASCT, allogenic hematopoietic stem cell transplantation; DLI, donor lymphocyte infusion; GVHD, graft versus host disease.
Source: Filipovich AH et al. Biol Blood Marrow Transplant 2005; 11:945–56.

like donor lymphocyte infusion (DLI), immune status of host, and subsequent allogeneic ASCT. Skin involvement is seen in 80% of cases of aGVHD and is often the presenting sign of GVHD. Gastrointestinal (GI) and hepatic involvement is seen in 50% of aGVHD patients [10].

The incidence of cGVHD is gradually increasing and is one of the important causes of mortality. Previous aGVHD is the most important risk factor for the development of cGVHD. The exact incidence is not known; however, the 5-year cumulative incidence is estimated to range from 9% to 80% [11,12]. Use of peripheral blood stem cell instead of bone marrow has reduced the morbidity of the procedure; however, higher units of blood needed for engraftment have led to greater incidences of cGVHD [13]. Cutaneous involvement is the predominant feature in cGVHD which accounts for 75%, while GI tract, mucosal, hepatic, and ocular involvement are seen in less than 50% of patients [14]. The lichenoid pattern of cutaneous involvement is more common than the sclerotic form.

PATHOGENESIS

Acute GVHD is thought to be mediated by a complex interplay between the host antigens, donor cells, and host immunity [15]. The various phases in the pathogenesis of aGVHD are as follows.

Phase 1: Activation of antigen-presenting cells

Preconditioning chemoradiotherapy induces tissue injury that causes release of endogenous and exogenous inflammatory mediators like interleuking (IL)-1, tumor necrosis factor (TNF), IL-6, interferon (IFN)-γ, IL-2, and lipooligosaccharides (cytokine storm) [16]. These molecules activate host immune response via toll-like receptors and subsequently lead to the interaction between the donor and host antigen-presenting cells (APCs).

Phase 2: Donor T-cell activation

There is donor T-cell activation, differentiation, and migration on the recognition of alloantigens on both host- and donor-type APCs that are present in secondary lymphoid organs. These T cells drive the immune response toward Th1/T-cytotoxic (Tc) and Th17 pathways.

Phase 3: Cellular and inflammatory effector phase

The organs such as the skin, liver, and GI tract are selectively targeted by these cells causing destruction [17].

Chronic GVHD is the most common cause of death in late nonrelapse mortality in hematopoietic stem cell transplant (HSCT) and affects the quality of life adversely. The exact pathophysiology involved in the clinical manifestations of cGVHD is still obscure. However, the concepts of autoimmunity and alloimmunity are widely accepted. The impaired negative selection of the T cells in host's thymus (compromised by conditioning regimens) and escape of these T cells from the peripheral tolerance mechanism are implicated in the proliferation of auto- and alloreactive cells. These T cells are directed against the self-antigens causing autoantibody production, which explains the high incidence of autoantibodies detected in cGVHD [18]. Another model proposes that the donor T cells are chronically activated by the heterogenous host antigens. The success of rituximab (an anti-CD20 antibody) in treatment of GVHD suggests the role of B-cell-mediated autoimmunity in GVHD [19].

CLINICAL FEATURES

Acute graft versus host disease

Acute GVHD usually presents 2–4 weeks after ASCT with a classic triad of morbilliform exanthem, diarrhea, and elevated bilirubin levels. Cutaneous lesions can be preceded by itching or dysesthesias and are often the presenting sign of the disease. Typically, the exanthem starts as folliculocentric blanchable macules over the face, ears, palms, and soles which gradually spread to involve the trunk (Figure 53.1).

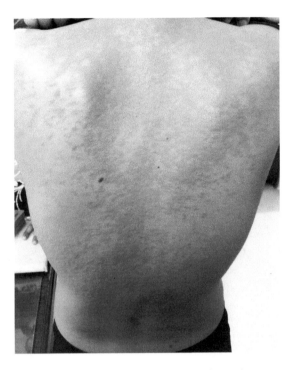

Figure 53.1 Exanthematous graft versus host disease.

The cutaneous manifestation may range from innocuous macules to severe debilitating blistering and erythroderma (Figures 53.2 through 53.4). Rarer manifestations of aGVHD reported are psoriasiform, ichthyosiform, and pityriasis rubra pilaris like eruptions (Figure 53.5) [20–22].

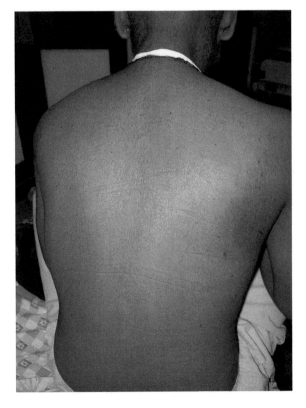

Figure 53.2 Graft versus host disease erythroderma day 33 in a case of acute myeloid leukemia.

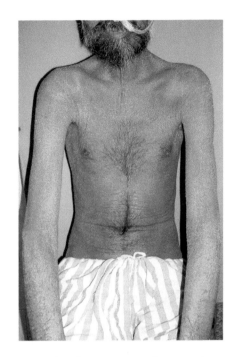

Figure 53.3 Erythroderma post graft versus host disease.

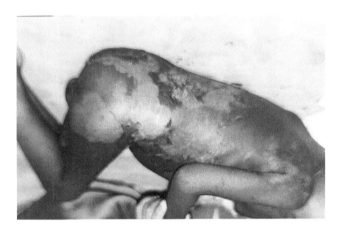

Figure 53.4 Severe graft versus host reaction in a 7-year-old child of acute lymphoblastic leukemia, post bone marrow transplant from a matched sibling donor.

Flexural involvement has been observed not uncommonly by the authors (Figures 53.6 and 53.7). Fine desquamation may resemble pityriasis versicolor like lesions (Figure 53.8). Depending on the organ targeted, the patients may also develop nausea, abdominal pain, diarrhea (GI involvement), thrombocytopenia, transaminitis, cholestasis, and hyperbilirubinemia (hepatic involvement). Glucksberg score is used to stage the severity that is based on the body surface area involvement, level of bilirubin, and GI manifestations (Table 53.3) [23,24].

DIFFERENTIAL DIAGNOSIS

The differential diagnosis involves viral exanthema, drug hypersensitivity reactions, HIV seroconversion, secondary syphilis, and engraftment syndrome.

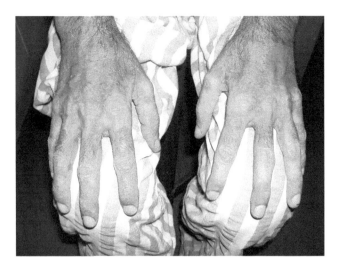

Figure 53.5 Papulosquamous graft versus host disease.

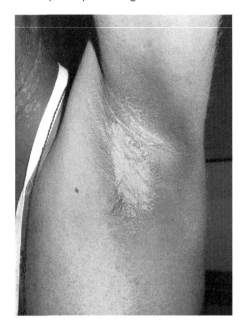

Figure 53.6 Axillary flexural involvement in graft versus host disease.

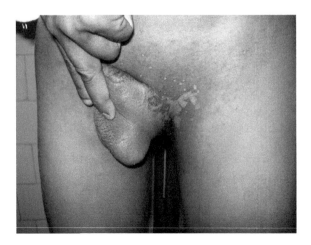

Figure 53.7 Inguinal involvement in graft versus host disease.

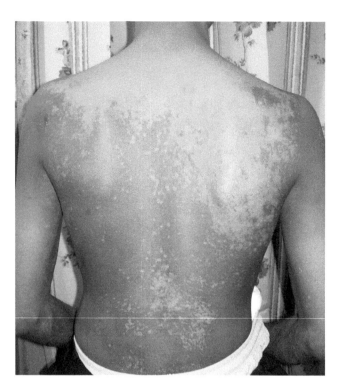

Figure 53.8 Post graft versus host disease desquamation resulting in pityriasis versicolor like appearance at 3 months post bone marrow transplant.

COMPLICATIONS AND COMORBIDITIES

Weight loss due to oral ulceration, dehydration due to diarrhea, and secondary infection due to skin ulceration are the major complications. The severity of disease correlates with prognosis. The mortality rates for grades 0–IV aGVHD are 28%, 27%, 43%, 68%, and 92%, respectively [25].

Chronic graft versus host disease

Chronic GVHD presents usually beyond 100 days of ASCT. Although cGVHD can involve any organ, skin is the most common target. Various cutaneous and extracutaneous manifestations of cGVHD essential for diagnosis are recommended by NIH consensus diagnosis and staging working group (Tables 53.4 and 53.5) [26].

The skin changes can be either sclerotic or nonsclerotic. Lesions resembling lichen planus (cutaneous and oral), morphea, lichen sclerosis, scleroderma, and poikiloderma are considered diagnostic of cGVHD. In cGVHD the lichen planus–like lesions occur on the face, ears, palms, and soles, differentiating it from lichen planus (Figure 53.9). Additional cutaneous manifestations in cGVHD that are not diagnostic by themselves are pigmentary changes, papulosquamous lesions, ichthyosis, xerostomia, oral ulcerations, mucocele, alopecia, and nail dystrophy (Figures 53.10 and 53.11). Extracutaneous manifestations include fasciitis, myositis, keratoconjunctivitis sicca, blepharitis, corneal erosions, bronchiolitis obliterans, esophageal strictures, and exocrine insufficiency.

Table 53.3 Acute graft versus host disease grading criteria

Stage	Skin	Liver (bilirubin)	GI tract (stool output/day)
0	No GVHD rash	<2 mg/dL	Adult: <500 mL/day Child: <10 mL kg/day
1	Maculopapular rash <25% BSA	2–3 mg/dL	Adult: 500–999 mL/day Child: 10–19.9 mL/kg/day or persistent nausea, vomiting, or anorexia, with a positive upper GI biopsy
2	Maculopapular rash 25%–50% BSA	3.1–6 mg/dL	Adult: 1000–1500 mL/day Child: 20–30 mL/kg/day
3	Maculopapular rash >50% BSA	6.1–15 mg/dL	Adult: >1500 mL/day Child: >30 mL/kg/day
4	Generalized erythroderma with bullae formation	>15 mg/dL	Severe abdominal pain with or without ileus

Source: Surjana D et al. *Australas J Dermatol* 2015;56:e21–3; Glucksberg H et al. *Transplantation* 1974;18:295–304.

Abbreviations: BSA, body surface area; GI, gastrointestinal; GVHD, graft versus host disease.
Note: Glucksberg grade:
    I—Stage 1 or 2 skin involvement; no liver or gut involvement.
    II—Stage 1–3 skin involvement; grade 1 liver or gut involvement.
    III—Stage 2 or 3 skin, liver, or gut involvement.
    IV—Stage 1–4 skin involvement; stage 2–4 liver or gut involvement.

Table 53.4 National Institutes of Health recommended classification of clinical manifestations in chronic graft versus host disease (GVHD)

Organ or site	Diagnostic (sufficient to establish the diagnosis of chronic GVHD)	Distinctive (seen in chronic GVHD but insufficient alone to establish a diagnosis)	Other features or unclassified entities	Common (seen with both acute and chronic GVHD)
Skin	Poikiloderma, lichen planus–like features, sclerotic features, morphea-like features, lichen sclerosus–like features	Depigmentation, papulosquamous lesions	Sweat impairment, ichthyosis, keratosis pilaris, hypopigmentation, hyperpigmentation	Erythema, maculopapular rash, pruritus
Nails		Dystrophy; longitudinal ridging, splitting, or brittle features; onycholysis; pterygium unguis; nail loss (usually symmetric, affects most nails)		
Scalp and body hair			Thinning of scalp hair, typically patchy, coarse or dull (not explained by endocrine or other causes), premature gray hair	
Mouth	Lichen planus–like changes	Xerostomia, mucoceles, mucosal atrophy, ulcers, pseudomembranes		Gingivitis, mucositis, erythema, pain

Source: Dignan FL et al. *Br J Haematol* 2012;158:30–45.

COMPLICATIONS AND COMORBIDITIES

Joint mobility is limited by sclerotic disease and fascial contractures, which affects the quality of life of the individual adversely. Oral ulcerations cause dysphagia, while pigmentary involvement causes changes in the appearance. Chronic palmoplantar involvement results in persistent debility (Figure 53.12). GVHD also causes immense psychological distress to the patient who is already affected by malignancy. Among long-term survivors, cGVHD is the major cause of mortality and morbidity.

Table 53.5 Overall chronic graft versus host disease (GVHD) grade according to the National Institutes of Health

Mild chronic GVHD	One or two organs involved, with a score of no more than 1 *plus* lung score 0
Moderate chronic GVHD	Three or more organs involved, with a score of no more than 1 *or* lung score 1
Severe chronic GVHD	At least one organ with a score of 3 *or* lung score of 2 or 3

Source: Dignan FL et al. *Br J Haematol* 2012;158:30–45.

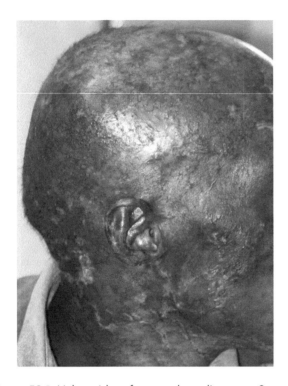

Figure 53.9 Lichenoid graft versus host disease at 8 months posttransplant.

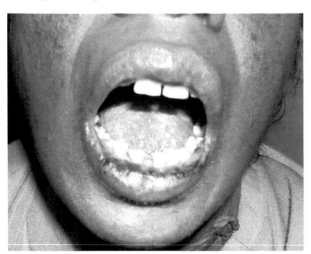

Figure 53.10 Graft versus host disease with lichenoid changes and erosions over lips and oral mucosa.

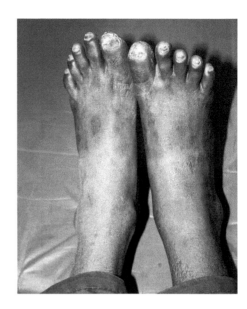

Figure 53.11 Nail dystrophy and residual postinflammatory changes of lichenoid graft versus host disease.

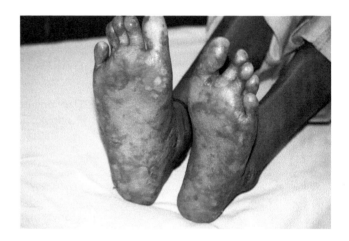

Figure 53.12 Persistent plantar involvement at 6 months.

HISTOPATHOLOGY

In acute stages, the findings are more subtle and the changes may be limited to the hair follicle. In well-developed lesions, aGVHD is characterized by keratinocyte necrosis, basal cell vacuolation, and interface dermatitis. Satellite cell necrosis is the hallmark of aGVHD. In advanced stages there can be complete dermoepidermal separation. The presence of a high number of eosinophils (16 per high-power field) points toward drug reactions [27]. The histopathological grading of aGVHD as proposed by Lerner et al. in 1974 is given in Table 53.6.

Histopathological changes in cGVHD vary depending on the clinical presentation. Lichenoid variant reveals hyperkeratosis, wedge-shaped hypergranulosis, acanthosis, saw-toothed rete ridges, basal cell vacuolation, and band-like infiltrate (Figures 53.13 and 53.14)

Table 53.6 Acute graft versus host disease histopathological grading

Grade	Definition
1	Focal or diffuse vacuolar alteration of basal cells
2	Vacuolar alteration of basal cells; spongiosis and dyskeratosis of epidermal cells
3	Formation of subepidermal cleft in association with dyskeratosis and spongiosis
4	Complete loss of epidermis

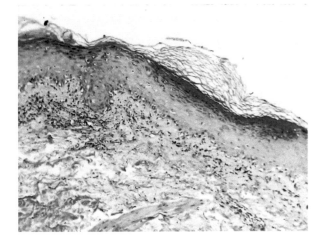

Figure 53.13 Photomicrograph of skin biopsy at day 30 revealing wedge-shaped hypergranulosis, apoptotic epidermal keratinocytes accompanied by lymphocytes with dermal lymphocytic infiltrate H&E 100×. (Photomicrograph from Brigadier [Dr.] Reema Bharadwaj.)

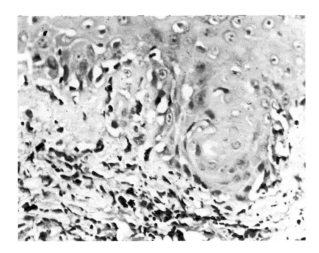

Figure 53.14 Skin biopsy of same patient apoptotic epidermal keratinocytes accompanied by lymphocytes with dermal lymphocytic infiltrate H&E 400×. (Photomicrograph from Brigadier [Dr.] Reema Bharadwaj and Col [Dr.] Aradhana Sood.)

Epidermal atrophy and homogenization of collagen bundles is seen in scleroderma-like, lichen sclerosus et atrophicans (LSEA)-like lesions, and morphea-like cGVHD presentations.

INVESTIGATIONS

The diagnosis of GVHD is clinical but can be challenging in various scenarios like peripheral blood transfusions to an immune competent host or in case of solid organ transplants. Skin biopsy may aid in the diagnosis but can never be conclusive due to the absence of any pathognomic findings. Serum eosinophilia along with elevated levels of serum bilirubin and transaminases may be present. Various serum biomarkers have been tested in the diagnosis of GVHD (Table 53.7).

TREATMENT

Acute graft versus host disease

For limited cutaneous (grade 1) involvement, topical steroids are the preferred line of management. Pruritus can be treated with emollients and antihistamines. In patients with grade II–IV involvement, systemic glucocorticoid therapy is indicated in addition to the posttransplant immunosuppressive regimen. Oral prednisolone 1 mg/kg and IV methyl prednisolone 2 mg/kg are the first-line systemic agents. Second-line therapy with mycophenolate mofetil (MMF), sirolimus, anti-IL-2 receptor antibody (Daclizumab), extracorporeal photophoresis, and etanercept is considered in patients unresponsive to the first-line agents. Third-line therapies include alemtuzumab, pentostatin, methotrexate, and mesenchymal stromal cells (Table 53.8).

Table 53.7 Serum biomarkers for graft versus host disease (GVHD)

Biomarkers	Risk of GVHD	References
Elafin (soluble protein produced by keratinocytes)	Overexpressed in cutaneous GVHD	Paczesny et al. [28]
TNFα, IL-6, and IL-8	Levels increased in acute and chronic GVHD	Dander et al. [29]
Treg, natural killer cells	Levels reduced in chronic GVHD	Pidala et al. [30]
B-cell-activating factor CXCL10 and CXCL11	Predictors for both acute and chronic GVHD	Ahmed et al. [31]
IFNγ, IL-12	Increased levels corelate with chronic GVHD	
ST2, REG3a, TFNR1	Biomarker scoring system to predict 6-month nonrelapse mortality	Levine et al. [32] and Renterie et al. [33]

Table 53.8 Treatment protocols in management of graft versus host disease (GVHD)

Acute GVHD

Grade I	• Topical corticosteroids and calcineurin inhibitors
	• Oral antihistamines
Grade II–IV	First line

- • Optimization of systemic calcineurin inhibitors
  - a. Cyclosporine: 2–3 mg/kg oral, twice daily; dose titrated using serum trough levels of 300 ng/mL initially and a level of 150 ng/mL, 6 weeks posttransplant
  - b. Tacrolimus: 0.02–0.03 mg/kg oral, twice daily; dose titrated using serum trough levels of 8–12 ng/mL initially and a level of 7 ng/mL, 6 weeks posttransplant
- • Methylprednisolone 2 mg/kg/day IV
- • Prednisolone 1 mg/kg/day oral

Second line and third line

- • Extracorporeal photophoresis
- • Phototherapy (UVA1, UVB)
- • Alemtuzumab: 30 mg IV infusion after premedication with antihistamine, antipyretic, and corticosteroid
- • Antilymphocyte globulin: 0.5–1.5 mg/kg/day IV infusion over 4–6 hour period after premedication with antihistamine, antipyretic, and corticosteroid
- • Daclizumab: 1 mg/kg IV infusion on days 1, 4, 8, 15, 22
- • Etanercept: 25 mg twice weekly subcutaneously
- • Methotrexate: 7.5–15 mg/week oral/IV
- • Mycophenolate mofetil: 1–3 g/day, oral, in two divided doses
- • Pentostatin: 1–1.5 mg/m^2/day IV infusion for 3 consecutive days
- • Sirolimus: Loading dose, 6–12 mg, followed by 2–4 mg/day, once daily; dose titrated to attain a level of 4–12 ng/mL

Chronic GVHD

Mild	• Topical corticosteroids and calcineurin inhibitors
	• Oral antihistamines
Sclerodermoid	• Phototherapy (PUVA, NBUVB, UVA1)
	• Physiotherapy
Moderate to severe	First line

- • Prednisolone: 1 mg/kg/day, oral, with tapering
- • Cyclosporine: 5 mg/kg/day, oral

Second line

- • Extracorporeal photophoresis
- • Azathioprine: 1–3 mg/kg/day, oral, total dose not exceeding 200 mg/day
- • Clofazimine: 300 mg, oral, once daily for first 3 months, reduced to 100 mg later on
- • Imatinib mesylate: 100–400 mg/day, oral
- • Ibrutinib: 420 mg/day, oral
- • JAK inhibitors
  - • Ruxolitinib: 5–10 mg twice daily, oral
  - • Tofacitinib: 50 mg/kg twice daily, oral
- • Mycophenolate mofetil: 1–3 g/day, in two divided doses
- • Pentostatin: 4 mg/m^2/day IV infusion, every second week for 3 months
- • Retinoids
  - • Acitretin: 20–30 mg/day
  - • Etretinate: 0.25 mg/kg/day
  - • Isotretinoin: 10 mg/kg/day
- • Rituximab: 375 mg/m^2 IV infusion, weekly for 4 weeks after premedication with antihistamine, antipyretic, and corticosteroid
- • Sirolimus: 2 mg oral, once daily; dose titrated to attain a level of 7–12 ng/mL
- • Thalidomide: 100 mg/day, oral escalated up to 400 mg/day

Chronic graft versus host disease

A multidisciplinary team composed of a dermatologist, hematologist, ophthalmologist, gastroenterologist, and rheumatologist should screen for underlying systemic involvement. Topical steroids and steroid-sparing agents are preferred in mild cGVHD with limited cutaneous involvement along with topical emollients and antihistamines. In case of extensive skin lesions and sclerodermoid changes, phototherapy (PUVA, NBUVB) is the preferred modality. Systemic therapy is warranted in moderate to severe types of cGVHD to address various organ involvements. Tapering doses of oral prednisolone for 8 weeks and cyclosporine 5 mg/kg for 8–12 weeks are the first-line systemic agents. Second-line treatment modalities are considered if there is no clinical improvement with the first-line agents. They include extracorporeal photopheresis, imatinib, sirolimus, pentostatin, and rituximab. The other agents used with varying degrees of success are MMF, pulse high-dose corticosteroid, clofazimine, thalidomide [34], retinoids, azathioprine, and mesenchymal stem cells.

KEY POINTS

- Graft versus host disease is a multisystem disorder that occurs most commonly after allogenic hematopoietic stem cell transplantation.
- Skin is the earliest and the most common organ to be affected in GVHD.
- GVHD is divided into acute and chronic, based on whether the onset of signs from the time of transplant is within 100 days or more.
- Acute GVHD presents 2–4 weeks after ASCT with a classic triad of morbilliform exanthem, diarrhea, and elevated bilirubin levels.
- Lesions resembling lichen planus, morphea, lichen sclerosis, scleroderma, and poikiloderma are considered diagnostic of cGVHD.
- Systemic corticosteroids, cyclosporine and phototherapy are mainline therapies for GVHD.

REFERENCES

1. Desforges JF, Anderson KC, Weinstein HJ. Transfusion-associated graft-versus-host disease. *N Engl J Med* 1990;323:315–21.
2. Zhang Y, Ruiz P. Solid organ transplant-associated acute graft-versus-host disease. *Arch Pathol Lab Med* 2010;134:1220–4.
3. Thomas ED. A history of haemopoietic cell transplantation. *Br J Haematol* 1999;105:330–9.
4. Perry AR, Linch DC. The history of bone-marrow transplantation. *Blood Rev* 1996;10:215–9.
5. Cotliar JA. *Atlas of Graft-versus-Host Disease: Approaches to Diagnosis and Treatment.* Cham, Switzerland: Springer International; 2017.
6. Filipovich AH et al. National Institutes of Health Consensus Development Project on Criteria for Clinical Trials in Chronic Graft-versus-Host Disease: I. Diagnosis and Staging Working Group Report. *Biol Blood Marrow Transplant* 2005;11:945–56.
7. Gale RP et al. Risk factors for acute graft-versus-host disease. *Br J Haematol* 1987;67:397–406.
8. Strong Rodrigues K, Oliveira-Ribeiro C, de Abreu Fiuza Gomes S, Knobler R. Cutaneous graft-versus-host disease: Diagnosis and treatment. *Am J Clin Dermatol* 2017;19(1):33–50.
9. Jagasia M et al. Risk factors for acute GVHD and survival after hematopoietic cell transplantation. *Blood* 2012;119:296–307.
10. Martin PJ et al. A retrospective analysis of therapy for acute graft-versus-host disease: Secondary treatment. *Blood* 1991;77:1821–8.
11. Dignan FL et al. Diagnosis and management of chronic graft-versus-host disease. *Br J Haematol* 2012;158:46–61.
12. Baird K, Pavletic SZ. Chronic graft versus host disease. *Curr Opin Hematol* 2006;13:426–35.
13. Pidala J, Anasetti C, Kharfan-Dabaja M, Cutler C, Sheldon A, Djulbegovic B. Decision analysis of peripheral blood versus bone marrow hematopoietic stem cells for allogeneic hematopoietic cell transplantation. *Boil Blood Marrow Transplant* 2017;15:1415–21.
14. Atkinson K et al. Risk factors for chronic graft-versus-host disease after HLA-identical sibling bone marrow transplantation. *Blood* 1990;75:2459–64.
15. Billingham RE. The biology of graft-versus-host reactions. *Harvey Lect* 1966;62:21–78.
16. Antin JH, Ferrara JL. Cytokine dysregulation and acute graft-versus-host disease. *Blood* 1992;80:2964–8.
17. Choi SW, Levine JE, Ferrara JLM. Pathogenesis and management of graft-versus-host disease. *Immunol Allergy Clin North Am* 2010;30:75–101.
18. Eisenberg RA, Via CS. T cells, murine chronic graft-versus-host disease and autoimmunity. *J Autoimmun* 2012;39:240–7.
19. Cutler C. Rituximab for steroid-refractory chronic graft-versus-host disease. *Blood* 2006;108:756–62.
20. Matsushita T et al. A case of acute cutaneous graft-versus-host disease mimicking psoriasis vulgaris. *Dermatology* 2008;216:64–7.
21. Huang J, Pol-Rodriguez M, Silvers D, Garzon MC. Acquired ichthyosis as a manifestation of acute cutaneous graft-versus-host disease: Acquired ichthyosis in acute cutaneous GVHD. *Pediatr Dermatol* 2007;24:49–52.
22. Surjana D, Robertson I, Kennedy G, James D, Weedon D. Acute cutaneous graft-versus-host disease resembling type II (atypical adult) pityriasis rubra pilaris: GVHD and PRP. *Australas J Dermatol* 2015;56:e21–3.

23. Glucksberg H et al. Clinical manifestations of graft-versus-host disease in human recipients of marrow from HL-A-matched sibling donors. *Transplantation* 1974;18:295–304.

24. Przepiorka D et al. 1994 Consensus Conference on Acute GVHD Grading. *Bone Marrow Transplant* 1995;15:825–8.

25. Dignan FL et al. Diagnosis and management of acute graft-versus-host disease. *Br J Haematol* 2012;158:30–45.

26. Jagasia MH et al. National Institutes of Health Consensus Development Project on Criteria for Clinical Trials in Chronic Graft-versus-Host Disease: I. The 2014 Diagnosis and Staging Working Group report. *Biol Blood Marrow Transplant* 2015;21:389–401.e1.

27. Lerner KG, Kao GF, Storb R, Buckner CD, Clift RA, Thomas ED. Histopathology of graft-vs.-host reaction (GvHR) in human recipients of marrow from HL-A-matched sibling donors. *Transplant Proc* 1974;6:367–71.

28. Paczesny S et al. Elafin is a biomarker of graft-versus-host disease of the skin. *Sci Transl Med* 2010;2:13ra2–13ra2.

29. Dander E, Balduzzi A, Zappa G et al. Interleukin-17–producing T-helper cells as new potential player mediating graft-versus-host disease in patients undergoing allogeneic stem-cell transplantation. *Transplantation* 2009;88:1261–72.

30. Pidala J, Sarwal M, Roedder S, Lee SJ. Biologic markers of chronic GVHD. *Bone Marrow Transplant* 2014;49:324–31.

31. Ahmed SS et al. Identification and validation of biomarkers associated with acute and chronic graft versus host disease. *Bone Marrow Transplant* 2015;50:1563–71.

32. Levine JE et al. A prognostic score for acute graft-versus-host disease based on biomarkers: A multi-centre study. *Lancet Haematol* 2015;2:e21–9.

33. Renteria AS, Levine JE, Ferrara JL. Development of a biomarker scoring system for use in graft-versus-host disease. *Biomark Med* 2016;10:793–5.

34. Nair V, Sharma A, Ghosh I, Arora S, Sahai K, Dutta V. Extensive chronic graft-versus-host disease of skin successfully treated with thalidomide. *J Assoc Physicians India* 2005;53:988–90.

54

Bites and stings

AMBRESH BADAD AND VINAY GERA

INTRODUCTION

Bites and stings are a very common cause of morbidity, and a few cases of mortality are seen throughout the world. The causative agents are also well-known disease vectors worldwide, and personal protection against bites and stings plays a major role in the prevention of disease [1]. A few important bites and stings that can occur as emergencies are as follows:

- Arthropod bites.
- Insect bites: Mosquitoes, flies, fleas, bees, wasps, bugs.
- Arachnid bites and stings: Spiders, scorpions.
- Snakebites.
- Dog bites and stings.
- Sea animal bites and stings: Stingrays, California cones, blue-ringed octopus, sea urchins, box jelly, hydroids, and stinging corals. (These bites and stings are not common in this part of the world and hence are not described here.)

ARTHROPOD BITES

Arthropods produce a wide spectrum of clinical lesions. Classification of arthropods causing bites is as given in Table 54.1.

Mechanisms of skin injury by arthropods

- Mechanical trauma
- Injection of irritant, cytotoxic or pharmacologically active substances
- Injection of potential allergens

- Secondary infection
- Invasion of the host's tissues
- Contact reactions
- Reactions to retained mouthparts

Clinical features of arthropod bites

The type and distribution of skin lesions are different for different arthropods. The most often observed lesion is papular urticaria. Bullous lesions are common on the legs, but may occur in other sites, especially in children. Hemorrhagic or ulcerated lesions have been reported, especially in the presence of lower limb venous hypertension. Cellulitis and lymphangitis may develop. Pseudoangiomatosis-like lesions have been reported [2].

Complications include secondary infection, impetigo, folliculitis, cellulitis, lymphangitis, and anaphylactic shock.

Diagnosis

Diagnosis of arthropod bites is mainly clinical. Patient complains of sudden onset of typical lesions on exposed parts of the body. Patients should be asked about domestic pets or if the patient changed his or her residence recently. Pet animals should be examined for signs of skin disease. Examination of debris from the pet's bedding for cat or dog fleas is important. Flea eggs and feces have a "salt and pepper" appearance. Adult fleas should be examined after treating with 10% potassium hydroxide for 24 hours. Examination of the dust obtained with a vacuum cleaner from bedrooms is helpful.

Table 54.1 Classification of arthropods

Insects	Mosquitoes, flies, beetles, ants, grasshoppers, butterflies
Arachnids	Spiders, scorpions, ticks, mites
Crustaceans	Crabs, shrimps, lobsters, barnacles
Chilopods	Centipedes
Diplopods	Millipedes

CLASS INSECTA

Mosquitoes, gnats, midges, and flies (Diptera)

From the dermatologist's point of view, the Diptera are important as biting insects, cause of myiasis, and their ability to transmit diseases.

FAMILY CULICIDAE (MOSQUITOES)

Mosquitoes are responsible for the transmission of a number of diseases, including malaria, filariasis, West Nile virus, yellow fever, and dengue fever.

The clinical features are variable [3]. The degree of acquired allergic sensitivity to the antigenic substances in the saliva and the nature of the pharmacologically active substances injected are important factors that determine the reaction. The reaction to mosquito bites is determined by previous exposure. Anaphylactic reactions and serum sickness–like reactions to mosquito bites are rare [4,5].

Dengue fever: This is caused by Dengue virus serotypes 1–4, transmitted by *Aedes aegypti, albopictus, polynensiensis*, and *Ascutellaris*. It usually is not as complicated as dengue hemorrhagic fever.

Dengue hemorrhagic fever: This fatal hemorrhagic disease, primarily of children under 15 years of age, is characterized by sudden onset of fever, which usually lasts for 2–7 days. As the fever remits, characteristic manifestations of plasma leakage appear. Common hemorrhagic manifestations include skin hemorrhages such as petechiae, purpuric lesions, and ecchymoses (Figure 54.1). Epistaxis, bleeding gums, gastrointestinal (GI) hemorrhage, and hematuria occur less frequently.

Malaria: This is caused by plasmodium and transmitted by the female anopheles mosquito. Severe malaria complications occur in nonimmune subjects with falciparum malaria and involve the central nervous system (CNS) (cerebral malaria), pulmonary system (respiratory failure), renal system (acute renal failure), and/or hematopoietic system (severe anemia).

Blackwater fever: In this syndrome, the passage of mahogany-colored urine in association with severe intravascular hemolysis can also occur.

Yellow fever: This is caused by the yellow fever virus that is transmitted by the *Aedes aegypti* mosquito. In severe cases it causes high fever, jaundice, epigastric pain with vomiting, prostration, dehydration, deteriorating kidney function, epistaxis, hematemesis, and CNS manifestations such as

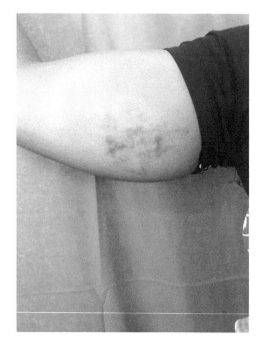

Figure 54.1 Reticulate purpura in dengue hemorrhagic fever.

confusion; coma, seizure, and death may occur within 7–10 days of onset.

MYIASIS

Myiasis is the infestation of body tissues of humans and animals by the larvae (maggots) of Diptera [6–9]. Myiasis can be clinically classified as per the part of the body affected. Cutaneous myiasis includes wound myiasis, furuncular myiasis, and creeping eruption. The flies causing cutaneous myiasis in humans are *Dermatobia hominis, Cuterebra, Cordylobia anthropophaga, Cordylobia (Stasisia) rodhaini, Wohlfahrtia* species, and *Hypodermas* species. The creeping form of myiasis is produced by *Gasterophilus* larvae [10,11].

Cavitary myiasis: This is usually caused by larva deposition in open wounds or external orifices such as nares, ears, and orbit and is characterized by deep tissue larva invasion with secondary infection and extensive tissue necrosis. In nasal myiasis, the patient presents with epistaxis, foul smell, passage of worms, nasal obstruction, discharge, and dysphagia. Ophthalmomyiasis can result in severe eye irritation, redness, foreign-body sensation, pain, lacrimation, swelling of eyelids, and vision loss. Aural myiasis features include otalgia, otorrhea, tinnitus, vertigo, impaired hearing, and perforation of the tympanic membrane.

Intestinal myiasis: This is caused by accidental ingestion of maggot-contaminated food and is characterized by nausea, vomiting, diarrhea, anal pruritus, and rectal bleeding.

Genitourinary myiasis: Dysuria, hematuria, lumbar pain, ureteric obstruction, and pyuria are seen following larval invasion of the urethra or vagina.

Cerebral myiasis: This is characterized by meningitis, encephalitis, intracranial hypertension with hydrocephalus, seizures, motor deficits, and extrapyramidal symptoms.

Treatment: Surgical management is most commonly recommended. The punctum is enlarged by cruciate incisions, and this enables removal of an intact larva [12]. The injection of lignocaine (lidocaine) underneath the nodule may be sufficient to push the larva out [13]. Ivermectin has been used both topically and orally in the management of myiasis [14–17]. Wound myiasis is treated by débridement and irrigation to remove larvae, and by treating secondary infection [18,19].

TUNGIASIS

Tungiasis is caused by the *Tunga penetrans*, a sand flea, also known as a jigger or chigoe, which is common in South America and Africa [20,21].

Clinical features: The most common sites affected are toes, the under surface of nails, and soles, though any part of the body may be affected [22]. The typical lesion is initially a black dot with a surrounding halo of erythema, followed by a pearl-colored papule with a central, dark punctum associated with intense irritation. Itching in turn facilitates bacterial superinfection and frequent abscesses formation.

Fissures, ulcers, lymphangitis, lymphedema, ascending neuritis, tissue necrosis, and septicemia are chronic complications. These result in pain, disability, and mutilation of the feet. These flies may introduce bacteria and viruses into the body resulting in tetanus and gas gangrene.

Treatment: Flea removal is by curettage, cautery, or excision [23].

Bees, wasps, and ants (Hymenoptera)

The bees, wasps, and ants are classified as follows:

- Superfamily Apoidea (bees)
  - Honeybees (Apismellifera)
- Superfamily Vespoidea
  - Family Vespidae (social wasps)
- Superfamily Bethyloidea
- Superfamily Scolioidea
  - Family Formicidae (ants)

Etiopathogenesis: Honeybees have a barbed sting. Allergy to hymenoptera venom is mediated by IgE antibodies [24]. The antigenic substances in the venom of many Hymenoptera are more liable to induce high degrees of hypersensitivity of the immediate type than are the antigens of most other insects. Hymenoptera venom contains vasoactive amines, small polypeptides, and larger protein molecules. Histamine, melittin, phospholipase A2, hyaluronidase acid phosphatase, and mast-cell degranulating peptide form part of this milieu [25,26].

The components of wasp venoms include histamine, serotonin, mast-cell degranulating peptide, wasp kinin, phospholipases, hyaluronidase, and antigen-5. The three major allergens in vespid venoms are phospholipases, hyaluronidase, and antigen-5.

Clinical features: Reactions can be classified as local and systemic [25,26]. The typical local toxic reaction is burning

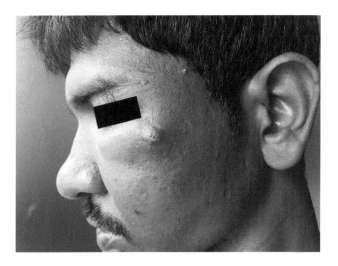

Figure 54.2 Bee sting in periorbital region.

pain, which may be mild to severe, erythema, and edema (Figure 54.2). It subsides in a few hours. In contrast to insect bites, bee and wasp stings are always painful.

The most significant clinical patterns are large local and systemic anaphylactic reactions. The systemic toxic effects include hypotension, severe headache, vomiting, diarrhea, generalized vasodilatation, and shock. Generalized anaphylactic reaction may occur within a few minutes of the sting. Foreign-body granuloma and IgE pseudolymphoma following multiple bee stings have been reported [27].

Treatment: Local reactions may be treated with oral antihistamines [28–30]. The treatment of anaphylaxis includes intramuscular epinephrine (adrenaline) (in adults, a dose of 0.5 mL 1:1,000 solution administered and repeated after 5 minutes in the absence of clinical improvement or if deterioration occurs after the initial treatment), followed by chlorpheniramine (10–20 mg, intramuscular or slow intravenous), and hydrocortisone (100–500 mg, intramuscular or slow intravenous) [30].

Beetles (Coleoptera)

Beetles may harm man by stinging, biting, or transmitting diseases.

Vesicating species [31–34]

a. *Family Meloidae (oil beetles, blister beetles):*
   Lytta vesicatoria: Many species contain the irritant cantharidin which produces an irritant dermatitis and bullae when it comes in contact with the skin.

b. *Family Staphylinidae (rove beetles)* [35–37]: *Paederus* dermatitis is an irritant contact dermatitis characterized by sudden onset of erythemato-bullous lesions on exposed areas of the body. The disease is caused by an insect belonging to the genus *Paederus* (Figure 54.3) [38–40].

Pathogenesis: Many species contain a vesicant called pederin, distinct from cantharidin. Pederin is released

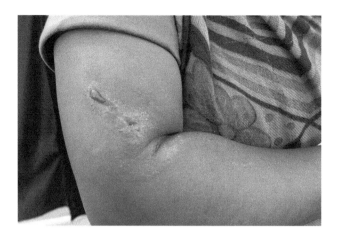

Figure 54.3 Blister due to *Paederus* dermatitis.

when the beetles are crushed, provoking an acute irritant contact dermatitis.

Clinical feature [41–43]: Lesions develop only when the beetle is crushed on the skin. A wheal forms rapidly, followed by a blister after 12–24 hours (Figure 54.4). The blisters are linear forming a "whiplash dermatitis" pattern. Characteristic kissing lesions, where a blister comes into contact with another area, may be present (Figure 54.5).

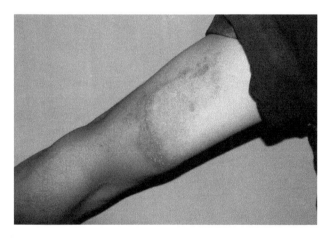

Figure 54.4 Characteristic blistering beetle dermatitis.

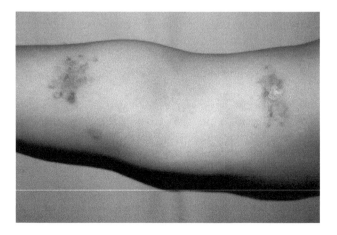

Figure 54.5 Kissing lesions of blistering beetle dermatitis.

Ocular involvement usually presents with unilateral periorbital dermatitis or keratoconjunctivitis and is called *Nairobi eye*. Severe cases are characterized by more extensive skin involvement and systemic features such as fever, arthralgia, neuralgia, rhinitis, and tympanitis.

An atypical variant of *Paederus* dermatitis is characterized by diffuse erythematous and desquamative lesions predominantly occurring in the upper body.

Treatment: It initially involves removing the irritant by washing the area with soap and water. The blistered site should be treated with cool wet soaks, followed by a strong topical steroid. Oral ciprofloxacin in addition to a topical steroid for treating concurrent bacterial infection and oral corticosteroids in case of severe involvement also are of benefit [44,45].

ARACHNIDS

Brown recluse spider bite: *Loxosceles spiders*

INTRODUCTION

Brown recluse spiders (*Loxosceles reclusa*) are principally nocturnal but can be observed in daylight. They are found most often at night in corners, under furniture, under piles of clothing on the floor, in attics and basements, under or in boxes, and in pantries or cellars [46]. Brown recluse spiders are most common in the South Central United States, from Tennessee and Missouri to Oklahoma and Texas. Bites from *L. reclusa* (the brown recluse spider), *L. laeta*, *L. rufescens*, *L. deserta*, and *L. arizonica* can cause skin necrosis (Figure 54.6). Systemic reactions in the form of shock, hemolysis, renal insufficiency, and disseminated intravascular coagulation have been reported.

DIAGNOSIS

Confirmation of diagnosis can either be by enzyme immunoassay to detect *Loxosceles* venom in a biopsied skin or plucked hairs (obtained within 4 days of bite) or by a passive hemagglutination inhibition test (within 3 days of the bite).

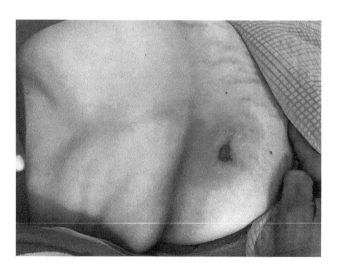

Figure 54.6 Brown recluse spider bite.

PATHOGENESIS

Sphingomyelinase D is the major toxin in brown recluse venom, and it interacts with serum amyloid protein. Neutrophils activation due to interaction between the venom and endothelial cells can be seen.

CLINICAL FEATURES

Local pain is commonly delayed until several hours after the bite, which mostly occurs on an extremity. The majority of bites do not cause serious reactions. Cutaneous lesions typically begin with erythema and central vesiculation or duskiness, later develop blanched halo, and can evolve into hemorrhagic bullae and necrosis. Necrotic eschars and ulceration can also be seen. Upper airway obstruction caused by envenomation of the neck by brown recluse spiders has been reported. Systemic reactions include disseminated intravascular coagulation (DIC) and Coombs positive hemolytic anemia [47,48].

HISTOPATHOLOGY

Early biopsy features a neutrophilic infiltrate. Later changes show "mummified" coagulative necrosis of the epidermis, adnexal epithelium, and superficial dermis. A neutrophilic band between viable skin and eschar can be seen. Small vessel vasculitis and thrombosis are seen near the neutrophilic band [49,50].

Preventive measures: Pest control with use of 2% DDT and 2% chlordane mix, lindane, diazinon, and DDVP sprays are effective for the control of the brown recluse spider [46].

Treatment: Rest, ice application, and elevation help in most bites. Intradermal injection of polyclonal anti-*Loxosceles* Fab antibody fragments and antivenin may reduce the size of the necrotic area [51]. Hyperbaric oxygen therapy may decrease the size of ulceration. Dapsone, colchicine, triamcinolone, prednisone, and intralesional triamcinolone can be tried [52]. Surgical intervention helps in symptomatic relief when medical therapy fails [53].

Scorpion sting

INTRODUCTION

Scorpions belong to class Arachnida, order Scorpiones. Scorpions are typically found in woodpiles, in shoes, and in damp areas. They sting when threatened or disturbed and accidentally trapped by a hand or foot.

CLINICAL FEATURES

Local symptoms in the form of pain, tingling sensation, paresthesia, and systemic symptoms are out of proportion to cutaneous signs like erythema and edema (Figure 54.7).

TREATMENT

Antivenin is available in endemic areas and, along with supportive care, has been shown to reduce morbidity and mortality from severe scorpion envenomation [54,55]. However, application of ice is sufficient for most minor scorpion envenomations [56].

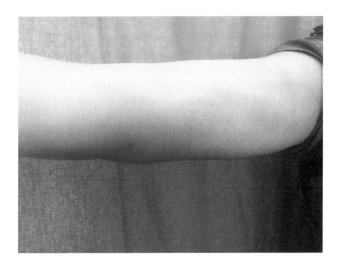

Figure 54.7 Scorpion sting.

SNAKEBITES

Introduction

Snakebites occur mainly in individuals who engage in outdoor activities. Occupational bite injuries may also affect those who raise snakes and are common in those who extract venom. Approximately 3,000 known species of snakes are found worldwide, of which only 15% are known to be venomous.

Epidemiology

The incidence of snakebites is highest in South Asia, Southeast Asia, and sub-Saharan Africa. Approximately 5.4 million snakebites, 2.5 million envenomations, and 125,000 deaths occur annually. According to the World Health Organization, the incidence of snakebites in India is 83,000 per annum with around 11,000 deaths, which is the maximum fatality rate in the world [57].

Clinical features

The most common initial symptoms include panic, fear, and emotional instability, which may lead to nausea, vomiting, diarrhea, vertigo, fainting, tachycardia, and cold, clammy skin. Marked edema within an hour of a snakebite is typical. Hemorrhage, necrosis, and paired bite marks are commonly seen [58].

SNAKE VENOMS

- Cobra and krait venoms: Neurotoxic and cardiotoxic
- Viper venom: Vasculotoxic
- Sea snakes and elapid venom: Neurotoxic

Hemostatic abnormalities: Persistent bleeding from fang puncture wounds or injection sites, spontaneous systemic hemorrhage, hemoptysis, epistaxis, and subconjunctival retroperitoneal and intracranial hemorrhage are reported.

Neurotoxicity: Paralysis is first detectable as ptosis and external ophthalmoplegia appearing as early as 15 minutes. Airway obstruction or paralysis of intercostals muscles and diaphragm causes respiratory failure. Neurotoxic effects are completely reversible, and it is important to note that neurotoxins do not cross the blood-brain barrier and do not alter consciousness.

Myotoxicity: Sea snake venom contains myotoxins that cause myalgias, myopathy, and rhabdomyolysis.

Cardiotoxicity: Viper and elapid venom cause direct myocardial damage presenting as arrhythmias, bradycardia, tachycardia, or hypotension.

Nephrotoxicity: Renal failure is secondary to ischemia in viper bites.

Diagnosis

History of snakebite and presence of bite marks help in the diagnosis. Identification of the biting snake and time of bite helps in determining the progression of signs and symptoms. A 20-minute whole blood clotting test (20 WBCT) is a reliable bedside test of coagulation.

Treatment

The patient of a snakebite should be kept under observation for a minimum period of 24 hours. Antivenin therapy is very important in the management. Adverse reactions to antivenin are seen in the form of serum sickness or anaphylaxis. Hypersensitivity to antivenin is common in those who have been previously treated. The evaluation of antivenin reactions is complicated, because serum sickness and snakebites share some signs and symptoms. Thrombocytopenia induced by rattlesnake venom (Crotalidae) is only partially reversed by antivenin polyvalent administration. DIC caused by crotalid snakebites can occur even after antivenin treatment. DIC is also seen in envenomation by some exotic vipers. In India, where the cost of antivenin therapy is a critical factor, low-dose regimens have been shown to be an effective alternative. Tourniquets have been associated with tissue ischemia if improperly applied. Tourniquet application appears to be of little benefit according to some studies [59].

DOG AND CAT BITES

Introduction

Dog bites account for 85% of all bites due to mammals. Cat bites are commonly provoked, whereas the majority of dog bites are unprovoked [60].

An estimated 5 million dog bites occur per year in the United States, of which 800,000 require medical attention [61]. Dog bites are particularly common in children in the age group of 5–9 years, and the dog is usually a family pet or a neighbor's dog [62]. Rabies still occurs almost everywhere in the world. Rabies associated with dog bites remains a problem in low-income countries.

Clinical features

Common pathogens associated with bite wounds include streptococci, staphylococci, *Pasteurella* spp., *Capnocytophaga canimorsus*, and anaerobes. Breast implant infection and lung abscesses due to *Pasteurella multocida* have both been linked to cats, and staphylococcal endocarditis has been reported after a cat bite. Brain abscess formation has been observed following a dog bite. In immunocompromised patients, there is a significant risk of *Pasteurella* or *Capnocytophaga* sepsis. *Capnocytophaga canimorsus* sepsis has a high mortality rate and has been associated with purpura fulminans. Human bites have a higher likelihood of infections with *Staphylococcus aureus* and *Eikenella corrodens*.

The most common pathogens associated with bite wound infections are listed in Table 54.2.

Treatment

Animal bite wounds are considered grossly contaminated; therefore, proper wound treatment is essential to prevent secondary infection. The affected skin surface should be cleansed, and the wound should be copiously irrigated with water, normal saline, or dilute Povidine iodine solution. A 20 mL or larger syringe should be used to generate high pressure required for adequate cleaning. Cautious débridement of devitalized tissue further decreases potential for infection.

Table 54.2 Pathogens causing secondary infections in human and animal bites

Bite	Pathogens
Human bites	*Staphylococcus aureus*
	Streptococcus pyogenes
	Eikenella corrodens
	Various anaerobes
Cat bite	*Pasteurella multocida* (75%)
	Moraxella spp.
	Neisseria weaver
	Bergeyella zoohelcum
	Various anaerobes
Dog bite	*Pasteurella* spp. (canis > multocida) (50%)
	S. aureus (20%)
	S. pyogenes
	N. weaver
	Capnocytophaga canimorsus
	B. zoohelcum
	Various anaerobes
Horse and sheep bites	*Actinobacillus* spp.
	Pasteurella spp.
	Various anaerobes
Marine animal bites	*Vibrio* spp.
	Aeromonas hydrophila
	Pseudomonas spp.
	Plesiomonas shigelloides

Oral antibiotics in the form of β-lactam antibiotic and a β-lactamase inhibitor (e.g., amoxicillin/clavulanic acid) provide good coverage for most organisms associated with dog and cat bites [63–66]. Other drugs such as second-generation cephalosporins, penicillin plus a first-generation cephalosporin, and clindamycin plus a fluoroquinolone are also efficacious.

Hospitalization of patients due to *Pasteurella*-infected animal bite wounds is strongly associated with initial use of suboptimal antibiotic therapy.

The antirabies vaccine is very important in the prevention of rabies. Postexposure prophylaxis is indicated in all persons exposed to a rabid animal. Prophylaxis consists of immunoglobulins at presentation and rabies vaccination on days 0, 3, 7, and 14. Immunoglobulin is infiltrated around the bite wound, and any additional volume is administered at a site distant to the vaccination site, usually in the opposite arm as compared to the rabies vaccine. If the patient already received preexposure prophylaxis before the animal bite, no immunoglobulin is needed, and the rabies vaccine is administered only on days 0 and 3.

Preexposure prophylaxis should be considered in persons with higher risk of exposure; it consists of three vaccines given on days 0, 7, 21, and 28.

Tetanus vaccination is recommended after an animal bite if it has been more than 5 years since the patient has been immunized.

KEY POINTS

- Bites and stings are common causes of morbidity and sometimes mortality globally.
- Arthropod bites, snakebites, dog bites and sea animal bites and stings are commonest among them.
- Arthropod bites can lead to complications like secondary infection, cellulitis, lymphangitis and anaphylactic shock.
- Poisonous snake bites can cause hemostatic abnormalities, cardiotoxicity, myotoxicity, neurotoxicity, nephrotoxicity is and death.
- Dog and cat bites can lead to rabies.

REFERENCES

1. Elston DM. Life-threatening stings, bites, infestations, and parasitic diseases. *Clin Dermatol* 2005;23:164–70.
2. Restano L et al. Eruptive pseudoangiomatosis caused by an insect bite. *J Am Acad Dermatol* 2005;52:174–5.
3. Allen JR. Mosquitoes and other biting flies. In: Parish CL, Nutting WB, Schwartzman RM (Eds), *Cutaneous Infestations of Man and Animal*. New York: Praeger, 1983:344–55.
4. Galindo PA et al. Mosquito bite hypersensitivity. *Allergol Immunopathol (Madr)* 1998;26:251–4.
5. Gaig P et al. Serum sickness-like syndrome due to mosquito bite. *J Invest Allergol Clin Immunol* 1999;9:190–2.
6. Zumpt F. *Myiasis in Man and Animals in the Old World*. London: Butterworth, 1965.
7. Hall MJR, Smith KGV. Diptera causing myiasis in man. In: Lane RP, Crosskey RW (Eds), *Medical Insects and Arachnids*. London: Chapman and Hall, 1993:429.
8. Kettle DS. *Medical and Veterinary Entomology*. 2nd ed. Wallingford: CAB International, 1995:268–91.
9. Burns DA. Myiasis. In: Faber WR, Hay RJ, Naafs B (Eds), *Imported Skin Diseases*. Maarssen: Elsevier; 2006:251–8.
10. Lane RP et al. Human cutaneous myiasis—A review and report of three cases due to *Dermatobia hominis*. *Clin Exp Dermatol* 1987;12:40–5.
11. Spigel GT. Opportunistic cutaneous myiasis. *Arch Dermatol* 1988;124:1014–5.
12. Richards KA, Brieva J. Myiasis in a pregnant woman and an effective, sterile method of surgical extraction. *Dermatol Surg* 2000;26:955–7.
13. Nunzi E, Rongioletti F, Rebora A. Removal of *Dermatobia hominis* larvae. *Arch Dermatol* 1986;122:140.
14. Jelinek T et al. Cutaneous myiasis: Review of 13 cases in travellers returning from tropical countries. *Int J Dermatol* 1995;34:624–6.
15. Denion E et al. External ophthalmomyiasis caused by *Dermatobia hominis*. A retrospective study of nine cases and a review of the literature. *Acta Ophthalmol Scand* 2004;82:576–84.
16. Osorio J et al. Role of ivermectin in the treatment of severe orbital myiasis due to *Cochliomyia hominivorax*. *Clin Infect Dis* 2006;43:e57–9.
17. Clyti E et al. Myiasis owing to *Dermatobia hominis* in a HIV-infected subject: Treatment by topical ivermectin. *Int J Dermatol* 2007;46:52–4.
18. Alexander JO. Flea bites and other diseases caused by fleas. In: *Arthropods and Human Skin*. Berlin: Springer-Verlag; 1984: 159–71.
19. Dickey RF. Papular urticaria—Hordes of fleas in the living room. *Cutis* 1967;3:345–8.
20. Douglas-Jones AG, Llewelyn MB, Mills CM. Cutaneous infection with *Tunga penetrans*. *Br J Dermatol* 1995;133:125–7.
21. Feldmeier H, Heukelbach J. Tungiasis. In: Faber WR, Hay RJ, Naafs B (Eds), *Imported Skin Disease*. Maarssen: Elsevier; 2006:233–41.
22. Alexander JO. Tungiasis. In: *Arthropods and Human Skin*. Berlin: Springer-Verlag; 1984:171–6.
23. Heukelbach J. Revision on tungiasis: Treatment options and prevention. *Expert Rev Anti Infect Ther* 2006;4:151–7.
24. Green AW, Reisman RE, Arbesman CE. Clinical and immunological studies of patients with large local reactions following insect stings. *J Allergy Clin Immunol* 1980;66:186–9.
25. Hoffman DR et al. Allergens in Hymenoptera venom. XXI. Cross-reactivity and multiple reactivity between fire ant venom and bee and wasp venoms. *J Allergy Clin Immunol* 1988;82:828–34.

26. Nugent JS et al. Cross-reactivity between allergens in the common striped scorpion and the imported fire ant. *J Allergy Clin Immunol* 2004;114:383–6.

27. Hermes B, Haas N, Grabbe J, Czarnetzki BM. Foreign-body granuloma and IgE pseudolymphoma after multiple bee stings. *Br J Dermatol* 1994;130:780–4.

28. Ewan PW. Venom allergy. *BMJ* 1998;316:1365–8.

29. Reisman RE. Venom hypersensitivity. *J Allergy Clin Immunol* 1994;94:651–8.

30. Project Team of the Resuscitation Council (UK). Emergency medical treatment of anaphylactic reactions. *J Accid Emerg Med* 1999;16:243–7.

31. Theodorides J. The parasitological, medical and veterinary importance of Coleoptera. *Acta Trop* 1950;7:48–60.

32. Alexander JO. *Arthropods and Human Skin*. Berlin: Springer-Verlag; 1984:75–85.

33. Nicholls DSH, Christmas TI, Greig DE. Oedemerid blister beetle dermatosis: A review. *J Am Acad Dermatol* 1990;22:815–9.

34. Southcott RV. Injuries from Coleoptera. *Med J Aust* 1989;151:654–9.

35. Kerdel-Vegas F, Goihman-Yahr M. Paederus dermatitis. *Arch Dermatol* 1966;94:175–85.

36. George AO. Paederus dermatitis—A mimic. *Contact Dermatitis* 1993;29:212–3.

37. Brazzelli V et al. Staphylinid blister beetle dermatitis. *Contact Dermatitis* 2002;46:183–4.

38. Jere J. Mammino-Paederus dermatitis: An outbreak in a medical mission boat on the Amazon River. *J Clin Aesthet Dermatol* 2011;4(11):44–6.

39. Frank JH, Kanamitsu K. *Paederus sensulato* (Coleoptera: Staphylinidae): Natural history and medical importance. *J Med Entomol* 1987;24:155–91.

40. Zargari O, Kimyai-Asadi A, Fathalikhani F, Panahi M. Paederus dermatitis in Northern Iran: A report of 156 cases. *Int J Dermatol* 2003;42:608–12.

41. Weedon D. *Skin Pathology*. 2nd ed. Edinburgh: Churchill Livingstone; 2005:738–49.

42. Calnan CD. Persistent insect bites. *Trans St John's Hosp Dermatol Soc* 1969;55:198–201.

43. Ploysangam T, Breneman DL, Mutasim DF. Cutaneous pseudolymphomas. *J Am Acad Dermatol* 1998;38:877–95.

44. Rahman S. Paederus dermatitis in Sierra Leone. *Dermatol Online J* 2006;12:9.

45. Karthikeyan K, Kumar A. Paederus dermatitis. *Indian J Dermatol Venereol Leprol* 2017;83:424–31.

46. Sandidge JS, Hopwood JL. Brown recluse spiders: A review of biology, life history and pest management.

47. McDade J, Aygun B, Ware RE. Brown recluse spider (*Loxosceles reclusa*) envenomation leading to acute hemolytic anemia in six adolescents. *J Pediatr* 2010;156:155–7.

48. Parekh KP, Seger D. Systemic loxoscelism. *Clin Toxicol (Phila)*. 2009;47:430–1.

49. Elston DM et al. Histological findings after brown recluse spider envenomation. *Am J Dermatopathol* 2000;22:242–6.

50. Eckermann JM et al. Arterial thrombosis and gangrene secondary to arachnidism. *Vascular* 2009;17:239–42.

51. Pauli I et al. Analysis of therapeutic benefits of antivenin at different time intervals after experimental envenomation in rabbits by venom of the brown spider (*Loxosceles intermedia*). *Toxicon* 2009;53:660–71.

52. Elston DM et al. Comparison of colchicine, dapsone, triamcinolone, and diphenhydramine therapy for the treatment of brown recluse spider envenomation. A double blind, controlled study in a rabbit model. *Arch Dermatol* 2005;141:595–7.

53. Delasotta LA, Orozco F, Ong A, Sheikh E. Surgical treatment of a brown recluse spider bite: A case study and literature review.

54. Sofer S, Bawaskar HS, Gueron M. Antivenom for children with neurotoxicity from scorpion stings. *N Engl J Med* 2009;361:631–2.

55. Deshpande SB, Pandey R, Tiwari AK. Pathophysiological approach to the management of scorpion envenomation. *Indian J Physiol Pharmacol* 2008;52:311–14.

56. Holve S. Venomous spiders, snakes, and scorpions in the United States. *Pediatr Ann* 2009;38:210–7.

57. Kasturiratne A et al. The global burden of snake bite: A literature analysis and modelling based on regional estimates of envenoming and deaths. *PLOS Med* 2008;5(11):e218.

58. Warell DA. WHO/SEARO Guidelines for the clinical management of snakebite in the Southeast Asian Region. *Southeast Asian J Trop Med Pub Health* 1999;30:1–85.

59. Indian National Snakebite Protocols 2007. Indian National Snakebite Protocol Consultation Meeting, August 2, 2007, Delhi.

60. Kaye AE, Belz JM, Kirschner RE. Pediatric dog bite injuries: A 5-year review of the experience at the Children's Hospital of Philadelphia. *Plast Reconstr Surg* 2009;124:551–8.

61. Centers for Disease Control and Prevention (CDC). Nonfatal dog bite–related injuries treated in hospital emergency departments—United States, 2001. *MMWR Mob Mortal Wkly Rep* 2003;52(26);605–10.

62. Gilchrist J, Sacks JJ, White D, Kresnow MJ, Dog bites: Still a problem? *Inj Prev* 2008;14(5):296–301.

63. Brook I. Management of human and animal bite wound infection: An overview. *Curr Infect Dis Rep* 2009;11:389–95.

64. Patronek GJ, Slavinski SA. Animal bites. *J Am Vet Med Assoc* 2009;234:336–45.

65. Dendle C, Looke D. Review article: Animal bites: An update for management with a focus on infections. *Emerg Med Australas* 2008;20:458–67.

66. Oehler RL et al. Bite-related and septic syndromes caused by cats and dogs. *Lancet Infect Dis* 2009;9:439–47.

55

Angioedema and anaphylaxis: Angioedema

VIJAY ZAWAR AND MANOJ PAWAR

INTRODUCTION

Angioedema is an abrupt, localized and often asymmetric nonpitting swelling of skin, mucous membranes, or both, including respiratory and gastrointestinal (GI) tracts. It is caused by temporarily increased endothelial permeability with localized plasma extravasation in the deep dermis and subcutis/submucosa. Loose facial tissue, especially periorbital, lip, and genital skin, is often involved, but hands, feet, airways, and abdomen may also be involved. Angioedema without urticaria is quite rare and should alert the physician to think of other types of angioedema, such as idiopathic angioedema, hereditary or acquired angioedema, or angioedema associated with angiotensin-converting enzyme (ACE) inhibitors.

PREDISPOSING/TRIGGERING FACTORS

1. Foods, especially peanuts, tree nuts, shellfish, milk, eggs
2. Drugs, especially penicillin and sulfa drugs and their derivatives, ACE inhibitors (ACEIs) or angiotensin receptor blockers (ARBs), nonsteroidal anti-inflammatory drugs (NSAIDs), aspirin, muscle relaxants, calcium channel blockers, β-blockers, estrogens, fibrinolytic agents, numerous chemotherapy agents
3. Anaphylactoid reactions, radiocontrast agents
4. Venoms (insects such as bees, yellow jackets, hornets, wasps, and fire ants)
5. Latex (contained in medical devices, air balloons, condoms, among others)
6. Physical: Cholinergic, vibratory angioedema, and exercise-induced anaphylaxis
7. Associated with chronic urticaria, either autoimmune or idiopathic
8. Urticaria associated with connective tissue diseases, vasculitis, and idiopathic urticarial vasculitis
9. C1 INH deficiency (hereditary, acquired)
10. Mild trauma to the face (especially dental trauma), stress/anxiety, *Helicobacter pylori* infection, Parvovirus infection, menstruation

CLASSIFICATION

Hereditary angioedema

Hereditary angioedema (HAE) is a rare autosomal dominant genetic disorder resulting from an inherited deficiency or dysfunction of the C1 inhibitor (a plasma protease inhibitor that regulates several proinflammatory pathways) (Figure 55.1).

Two main types of HAE have been defined: type I and type II. Type I HAE is characterized by low C1 inhibitor levels and function (85% of cases). Type II is associated with normal or even elevated C1 inhibitor levels but low function (15% of cases). Rarely, a form of HAE with normal C1 INH concentration is seen, which is occasionally referred to as HAE type III and also known as estrogen-dependent hereditary angioedema.

Acquired angioedema

Acquired angioedema (AAE) is another rare C1 inhibitor deficiency syndrome that is most commonly associated with B-cell lymphoproliferative diseases (type 1 AAE). It may also be related to the presence of an autoantibody

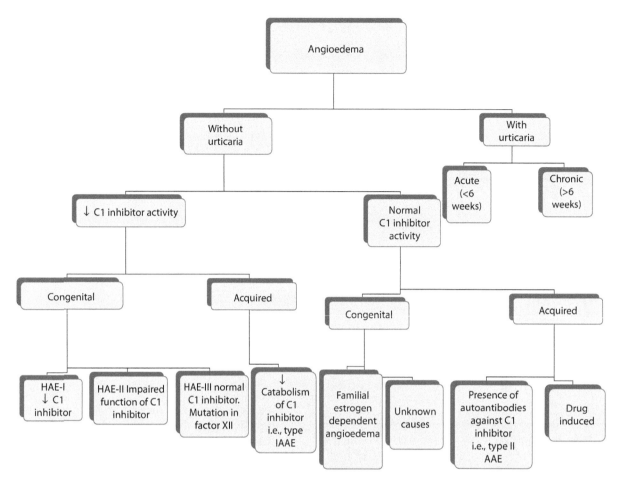

Figure 55.1 Classification of angioedema.

directed against the C1 inhibitor molecule (type II AAE). Unlike HAE, C1q levels are low in AAE.

Idiopathic angioedema

This is the most common diagnosis among patients of angioedema. The definition is a minimum of three angioedema episodes within a period of 6–12 months without a cause being identified despite thorough medical examination and regular reevaluations.

Rare forms of angioedema

Acquired C1 INH deficiency occurs secondary to malignant or autoimmune disease. The clinical profile resembles that of HAE, and it is characterized by increased catabolism of C1 INH.

Isolated angioedema also occurs in approximately 0.1%–6% of individuals using ACE inhibitors.

Angioedema associated with eosinophilia is of two types: episodic and nonepisodic. Episodic angioedema with eosinophilia (Gleich syndrome) is recognized by recurrent episodes of angioedema with weight gain (18% of total body weight), raised IgM, fever, peripheral eosinophilia (>1500/

mm³) and, in some cases, urticaria. Nonepisodic angioedema with eosinophilia has edema of bilateral upper or lower extremities with eosinophilia.

Systemic capillary leak syndrome (Clarkson disease) involves sudden inexplicable attacks of massive angioedema. It has a poor prognosis. Hemoconcentration, hypoalbuminemia and monoclonal gammopathy, and sometimes myelomatosis are common findings on laboratory investigations. The different types of angioedema with decreasing frequency are as given in Table 55.1.

Table 55.1 Types of angioedema in decreasing frequency

Serial number	Type of angioedema
1	Associated with anaphylaxis
2	Associated with urticaria
3	Idiopathic
4	Drug induced, mainly angiotensin-converting enzyme inhibitor

5	Rare forms
	    Clarkson syndrome
	    Gleich syndrome

6	Hereditary angioedema

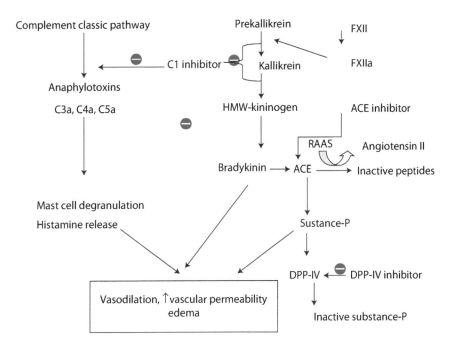

Figure 55.2 Pathogenesis of angioedema.

PATHOGENESIS

The pathophysiology of angioedema consists of rapid onset of local increase in permeability of the submucosal or subcutaneous capillaries and postcapillary venules, causing local plasma extravasation and consequent ephemeral swelling (Figure 55.2). A variety of vasoactive molecular mediators cause plasma extravasation. Among them, of prime importance is the preformed mast cell–derived mediators, namely, histamine, and proteases such as tryptase. The pathophysiology of angioedema is broadly divided according to the type of mediator involved in the process.

Mast cell–mediated angioedema

Mast cell–mediated angioedema usually begins within minutes of exposure to the allergen, builds over a few hours, and resolves in 24–48 hours. In the sensitization phase, the allergen is taken up by antigen-presenting cells, which activate T-helper cells. These then release IL-4, which stimulate the synthesis of IgE antibodies. The second contact with the allergen results within minutes in the IgE-mediated degranulation of mast cells and basophils. This cascade results in release of vasoactive and proinflammatory mediators, such as histamine.

Nonhistamine/bradykinin-mediated angioedema

It has a somewhat more prolonged time course, usually developing over 24–36 hours and resolving within 2–4 days. The vasoactive peptide hormone bradykinin is formed by the kallikrein-kinin system, with C1 INH acting as an inhibitor. In patients with ACE inhibitor–induced angioedema, a degradation enzyme of bradykinin is inhibited, which triggers edema development. Estrogen can induce coagulation factor XII and kallikrein, as well as reduce C1 INH, which raises the bradykinin level causing edema.

NSAIDs-induced angioedema is thought to be caused by cyclo-oxygenase (COX) pathway inhibition with overproduction of cysteinyl leukotrienes.

CLINICAL FEATURES

Mast cell–induced angioedema presents with urticaria (Figure 55.3), flushing, generalized pruritus, bronchospasm, throat tightness, and/or hypotension. Bradykinin-induced angioedema is not associated with urticaria, bronchospasm, or other symptoms of allergic reactions.

The clinical features of angioedema vary according to its location:

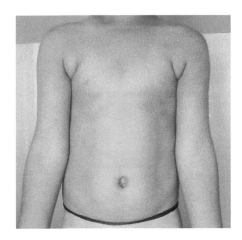

Figure 55.3 Erythematous urticarial weals in a child.

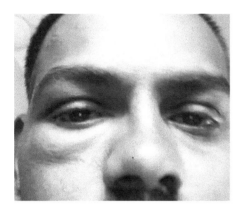

Figure 55.4 Angioedema of the right eyelid.

- *Subcutaneous angioedema*: It is nonpitting and nonpruritic, mainly affecting the face, hands, feet, and genitalia, but can involve any part of the body (Figure 55.4).
- *Intestinal angioedema*: Angioedema affecting the bowel wall presents as colicky abdominal pain, sometimes accompanied by vomiting and/or diarrhea. Intestinal angioedema is seen in patients on ACE inhibitors and in those with hereditary or acquired C1 inhibitor deficiency.
- *Laryngeal angioedema*: Angioedema of the larynx, upper airway, or tongue (of any mechanism) can progress to airway obstruction and asphyxiation. Dyspnea, dysphagia, and dysphonia are the suggestive features of laryngeal angioedema.

In patients presenting with angioedema affecting the airway, airway protection must be given priority over a comprehensive diagnostic evaluation.

Features of hereditary and acquired angioedema are summarized in Table 55.2.

DIAGNOSIS

Clinical history

To secure a correct diagnosis, the most important assessment factor is a precise and comprehensive anamnesis, especially with reference to location, severity, duration, and trigger factors. The patient should be questioned about any unusual exposures (e.g., insect stings), activities (e.g., exercise), foods, or other ingestions in the 24 hours before the onset of symptoms. Patients should be asked about activities, exposures, or travel preceding the episodes of angioedema/anaphylaxis, to see if any pattern is apparent. A review of the patient's medications is important. Patients should be asked about family members with similar episodes of cutaneous or laryngeal angioedema or with recurrent abdominal pain, to identify families with HAE. Patients with recurrent orofacial angioedema after dental work or episodes of unexplained abdominal pain may have hereditary or acquired C1 inhibitor deficiency.

Physical examination

As mentioned previously, the presence of signs and symptoms such as urticaria, flushing, generalized pruritus, bronchospasm, throat tightness, hypotension, and features of an allergic reaction (i.e., of mast cell activation) is helpful in narrowing down the list of possible causes.

INVESTIGATIONS

These are influenced by the presence of other signs and symptoms and by the suspected cause. The following investigations should be considered in all patients with new-onset angioedema:

- Complete blood count with differential.
- Basic chemistry panel with liver function tests.
- C4 and C3 levels. Depressed C4 levels should prompt further evaluation for complement-mediated angioedema, and low C3 and C4 levels suggest an immune complex–mediated process, such as systemic lupus erythematosus.
- Complement studies that should be ordered for patients with suspected HAE and AAE include C4 (the natural substrate for C1) level, C1q level, C1 inhibitor antigenic level, and C1 inhibitor functional level. These studies should be performed when the patient is off treatment, since the use of drugs for AAE or HAE can alter laboratory results.
- If complement studies are normal, ACE-inhibitor-induced angioedema should be considered.
- Patients with AAE should also be evaluated for an underlying B-cell lymphoproliferative disorder at the time of diagnosis.

Table 55.2 Features of hereditary and acquired angioedema

			Complement levels			
Angioedema type	Age of onset	Family history	C1q	C4	C1 inhibitor	C1 inhibitor function
HAE Type I	Early	Present	N	↓	↓	↓
HAE Type II	Early	Present	N	↓	N/↑	↓
HAE Type III	Late	Absent	N	N	N	N
AAE	Late	Absent	↓	↓	N/↑	↓

Abbreviation: AAE, acquired angioedema; HAE, hereditary angioedema.

- If there is reason to suspect trigger agents such as food or medication, a provocation test should be performed while providing anaphylaxis preparedness. It is, however, important to distinguish between allergic reactions and nonhistaminergic angioedema caused by, e.g., ACE inhibitors, DPP-IV inhibitors, or estrogen, as these are class related and consequently should not be provocation tested.

If diagnostic clarification is still not achieved, the condition will have to be ascribed to the group of idiopathic angioedema.

TREATMENT

Mast cell–mediated angioedema responds to epinephrine (if severe), glucocorticoids, and antihistamines. In contrast, bradykinin-mediated angioedema responds to C1-inhibitor concentrate, fresh frozen plasma, and other agents that interfere with the production or action of bradykinin.

First aid

At the first signs of any clinical manifestations of anaphylaxis, the patient should self-administer epinephrine, if available (adult dose, 0.3 mL of 1:1,000 intramuscular; pediatric dose, 0.01 mL/kg of 1:1,000 intramuscular). Susceptible patients may even use aerosolized epinephrine from a metered-dose inhaler (10–20 doses) to counteract the effects of laryngeal edema, bronchoconstriction, and other manifestations of anaphylaxis.

1. Angioedema in or near the airway and angioedema in anaphylaxis (in-hospital management)
   - The patient with angioedema near or involving the tongue, uvula, soft palate, or larynx must be immediately assessed for airway patency, breathing, and circulation. Establish IV access.
   - The airway should be managed by the expert intensivist, as intubation in the presence of laryngeal angioedema can be difficult due to distortion of the normal anatomy. Due to the risk of aspiration, an oral airway should never be used to maintain clear airways in awake patients. The favored options will often be awake nasal intubation guided by a flexible nasendoscope.
   - Aqueous epinephrine (1:1,000), in a dose of 0.3–0.5 mL for adults and 0.01 mL/kg (not exceeding 0.3 mL) for children, should be given. Epinephrine is the most important drug for the treatment for anaphylaxis owing to its vasoconstriction and bronchodilation effects; rapid administration of epinephrine can lead to a good prognosis and alleviate symptoms and stabilize mast cells to prevent progression.
   - In case of profound hypotension, skin perfusion is hampered. In such cases, 2–5 mL of epinephrine (1:10,000) should be given slow IV or an IV infusion

can be set up by mixing 1 mg of epinephrine in 250 mL saline and be given at the rate of 0.25–1 mL/min. If IV access cannot be established, epinephrine can be given through endotracheal tube, intralingually, or intramuscularly.
   - IV methylprednisolone (125–250 mg) or IV hydrocortisone can be used. Reviews have reported a nonspecific membrane stabilizing effect within 10–30 minutes after the administration of high doses of glucocorticoids (500–1000 mg in adults).
   - In case of hypotension, IV crystalloids should be given. Vasopressors such as dopamine and norepinephrine may be needed for persistent hypotension. Antihistaminics should be used in addition to epinephrine and not as its substitute. Diphenhydramine in a dosage of 50 mg IV can be given.
   - Nebulized β2 agonist, salbutamol (2.5 mg diluted to 3 mL saline), can be used to relieve bronchospasm.
   - Patients on ß-blockers may respond poorly to epinephrine; glucagon is given to such patients to counteract the ß-blockade. Dose: 1–5 mg IV over 5 minutes followed by 5–15 mcg/min infusion.
   - The approved daily dose of the antihistamine can be recommended as a single/individual dose. In individual cases, oral antihistamines can be increased up to four times the daily single dose.
2. Acute allergic angioedema (less severe than anaphylaxis)
   - Antihistamines and glucocorticoids are the main therapies for isolated angioedema that appears to be allergic (i.e., mast-cell mediated). H1 and H2 antihistamines at standard doses are useful along with prednisone (20–40 mg daily) in adults or prednisolone (0.5–1 mg/kg/day) in children, tapered over 5–7 days.
   - Antihistamines and glucocorticoids will likely be ineffective if the angioedema is bradykinin mediated.
3. Severe acute attacks of HAE and AAE
   - The treatment of laryngeal attacks, which are the leading cause of mortality in patients with HAE, must always begin with immediate measures to keep the airway patent, regardless of the therapies available.
   - Those with respiratory distress or stridor may require intubation, because even the first-line therapies take approximately 30 minutes or more to show effect.
   - First-line therapies for the treatment of HAE include C1 inhibitor replacement therapy, ecallantide, and icatibant.
   - C1 inhibitor replacement therapy is the most well-studied first-line therapy. The current recommended dose is 20 U/kg body weight IV at a rate of 4 mL/minute; patients with AAE may require higher doses. Some patients with AAE may become refractory to this treatment over time; in these patients ecallantide and icatibant should be used.

- Ecallantide is an inhibitor of plasma kallikrein (the enzyme that releases bradykinin, the primary mediator of angioedema). It has been approved by the U.S. Food and Drug Administration (FDA) for the treatment of acute angioedema attacks in patients with HAE. The recommended dose is 30 mg (3 mL) subcutaneously in three 10 mg (1 mL) injections. If the attack persists, an additional dose of 30 mg (3 mL) may be administered within a 24-hour period.
- Icatibant is a bradykinin receptor blocker that has been approved in the European Union for the treatment of acute attacks of HAE. The usual recommended dose for adults is 30 mg (3 mL) injected subcutaneously in the abdominal area. If the attack persists, additional injections of 30 mg (3 mL) may be administered at intervals of ≥6 hours. No more than three injections in 24 hours are to be administered.
- Attenuated androgens, such as danazol and stanozolol (maximum long-term recommended doses are 200 mg daily for danazol and 2 mg daily for stanozolol), increase C4 and C1 inhibitor levels and are effective for both the short- and long-term prophylaxis of HAE and AAE. Although generally well tolerated by most patients, adverse effects with long-term androgen administration are a matter of concern. Therefore, the lowest effective dose should be utilized and the patient's complete blood count, liver enzymes, and lipid profile should be monitored regularly (every 6 months) while on therapy.
- The antifibrinolytic agent, tranexamic acid (used at a daily dose of 4 g [1 g four times daily] for adults or 2 g [500 mg four times daily] for children), has also been shown to be more effective for the prophylactic treatment of AAE than HAE. Tranexamic acid is well-tolerated and is generally preferred for long-term prophylaxis in pregnant women, children, and patients who do not tolerate androgens.
4. ACE inhibitor–induced and ARB-induced angioedema
   - Acute airway evaluation and management are the first important steps in the approach to a patient with ACEI angioedema in the emergency department setting. Nasotracheal intubation usually is preferred to secure the airway, since nonpitting edema can make oral intubation difficult or even impossible.
   - The next step is discontinuation of the drug. Angioedema due to ACEIs usually is self-limiting and resolves in 12–48 hours after discontinuation.
   - Fresh frozen plasma (2 U at 1–12 hours before the event), ecallantide, and icatibant are potential treatments in investigational studies for ACEI-induced angioedema.
5. Recurrent, idiopathic angioedema
   - Patients with idiopathic recurrent angioedema without urticaria can be treated with nonsedating antihistamines initially (i.e., either cetirizine 10 mg twice daily or desloratadine 5 mg twice daily) for at least 1 month.

FOLLOW-UP

Patients whose angioedema has a systemic cause should be followed up vigilantly. Educating the patient forms a significant part of the treatment.

ANAPHYLAXIS

Introduction

Anaphylaxis is the maximal variant of an acute allergic reaction involving several organ systems. It is a severe, life-threatening allergic reaction in presensitized individuals that is rapid in onset; characterized by life-threatening airway, breathing, and/or circulatory problems; and usually associated with skin and mucosal changes.

Triggering factors

In young children, the most common triggers of food-related anaphylaxis are milk protein, hen's egg protein, and wheat, while among adolescents, peanuts and tree nuts are the most common triggers. In adults, the most common food allergens are wheat, celery, and seafood.

Latex proteins in medical devices, toys, and condoms can induce severe clinical pictures of anaphylaxis in susceptible people. Atopy is a risk factor for latex sensitization. Latex allergy is more frequent among health-care professionals who usually work using gloves, such as surgeons, nurses, and technicians, and patients who have undergone multiple surgeries.

Exercise-induced anaphylaxis can occur isolated or associated with previous ingestion of certain foods or medications.

In some crises, it is not possible to identify the causative agent, thus characterizing idiopathic anaphylaxis.

Pathogenesis

The mechanisms for mast cell activation and mediator release are dependent on the binding of IgE to FcεRI (Figure 55.5). Upon antigen binding to IgE, these receptors aggregate and

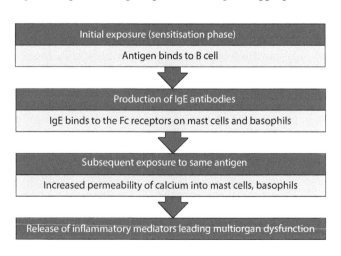

Initial exposure (sensitisation phase)

Antigen binds to B cell

Production of IgE antibodies

IgE binds to the Fc receptors on mast cells and basophils

Subsequent exposure to same antigen

Increased permeability of calcium into mast cells, basophils

Release of inflammatory mediators leading multiorgan dysfunction

Figure 55.5 Pathogenesis of anaphylaxis.

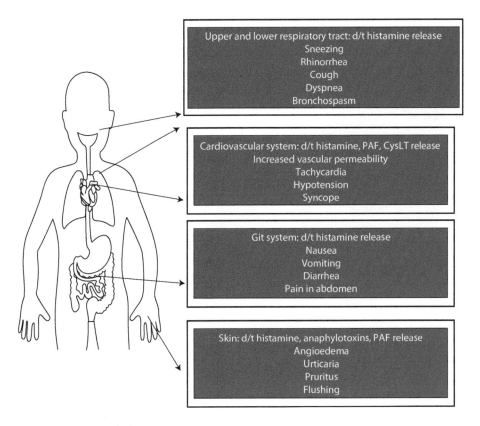

Figure 55.6 Symptomatology of anaphylaxis.

initiate the signaling cascade, resulting in rapid degranulation of mast cells, the generation of arachidonic acid metabolites (lipid mediators), and later production of cytokines and chemokines such as histamine, tryptase, carboxypeptidase A3, chimase, and proteoglycans. Histamine is the critical mediator of symptoms arising in the immediate phase of anaphylaxis. Tryptase produced can activate the kallikrein-kinin system, resulting in production of bradykinin and causing angioedema.

Clinical features

One of the following symptoms occurs rapidly (within a few hours) after exposure to a suspected allergen: (1) involvement of skin-mucosal tissues, (2) respiratory symptoms, (3) reduced blood pressure or associated symptoms, and (4) persistent GI symptoms (crampy abdominal pain, vomiting, and diarrhea) (Figure 55.6). According to the severity of anaphylaxis, i.e., mild, moderate, or severe, the symptoms vary (Table 55.3). Mild anaphylaxis is limited to skin or mucosal symptoms, involving urticaria, erythema, and edema near the eyes or angioedema and combined mild symptoms of other organs. In moderate anaphylaxis, there is involvement of respiratory, cardiovascular, and GI systems causing dyspnea, wheezing, vertigo, nausea, vomiting, and abdominal pain. Severe anaphylaxis is defined as reactions involving cyanosis (Figure 55.7), hypotension, and neurological symptoms with oxygen saturation <92% or systolic blood pressure <90 mm Hg.

Diagnosis

Anaphylaxis diagnosis is usually based on clinical findings. Generally, the history is characteristic. Sudden onset of signs and symptoms, such as urticaria, angioedema, diffuse erythema, pruritus, difficulty breathing, nausea, vomiting, abdominal colic, hypotension, bronchospasm, dizziness, or syncope raise the suspicion of anaphylactic reaction. Levels of tryptase remain elevated for a prolonged time (4–6 hours) and can be used for confirming the diagnosis of anaphylaxis. The identification of allergen-specific IgE antibodies can be made by skin prick

Table 55.3 Grading of anaphylaxis severity

Grade I	Symptoms limited to skin	Erythema, itching, angioedema, wheals, and plaques
Grade II	Mild systemic signs and symptoms	Above plus cough, dyspnea, stridor, rhinorrhea, nausea, vomiting, tachycardia, hypotension
Grade III	Moderate systemic signs and symptoms	Above plus cyanosis, bronchospasm, shock
Grade IV	Severe systemic signs and symptoms	Above plus cardiorespiratory arrest

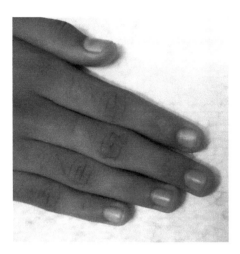

Figure 55.7 Cyanosis as evident by bluish discoloration of the nails.

testing (puncture) to evaluate allergies to food, venom of insects, and certain medications.

Treatment

Immediately after quick examination, the patient should be positioned horizontally, and further physical exercise and getting up from the sitting position should be avoided. In cases of cardiac arrest, cardiopulmonary resuscitation with cardiac massage and aided ventilation in a ratio of 30:2 must be started. Airway should be secured to achieve adequate oxygenation. IV (intramuscular if IV route is not accessible) adrenaline is the drug of choice in anaphylaxis. Then 1 mL adrenaline (1 mg/mL) is diluted in a ratio of 1:10 to a volume of 10 mL (0.1 mg/mL), and it is given as a 1 mg bolus in 2–5 minute intervals until circulation is established.

IV fluid with an electrolyte solution (5–10 mL/ kg within 5 minutes) via large-bore IV cannula (>8 gauge) is essential to restore the blood pressure and intravascular fluid. Short-acting $\beta2$ sympathomimetics, e.g., salbutamol, terbutaline at a dose of two to four puffs, are useful in the treatment of bronchial obstruction.

The only H1 antihistamines given via IV application in the acute treatment of anaphylaxis are the first-generation substances dimetindene (0.1 mg/kg) and clemastine (0.05 mg/kg). Second-generation antihistamines can be used in severe and treatment-resistant anaphylaxis orally.

Glucocorticoids are only useful in the treatment of protracted or biphasic anaphylactic reactions.

CONCLUSION

All patients who have experienced anaphylaxis should be equipped with an anaphylaxis emergency action plan, one or more epinephrine autoinjectors, a plan for arranging further evaluation, and printed information about anaphylaxis and its treatment.

KEY POINTS

- Angioedema is an abrupt and short-lived nonpitting swelling of lax skin, mucous membranes, or both, including the upper respiratory and intestinal epithelial linings.
- Angioedema is subcategorized into mast cell–mediated and bradykinin-mediated edema. Mast cell–mediated angioedema, in contrast to bradykinin-mediated angioedema, often goes hand in hand with urticaria and pruritus.
- HAE and AAE are rare disorders that result from a deficiency or dysfunction of the C1 inhibitor and are characterized by angioedema in the absence of urticaria. They are associated with life-threatening upper airway swelling.
- Angioedema may be life threatening when it causes airway obstruction or when it represents a component of anaphylaxis. Immediate assessment of the airway patency is critical in any patient with angioedema near or affecting the larynx, mouth, soft palate, or tongue.
- ACE inhibitors should be discontinued in any individual who presents with angioedema as they are associated with life-threatening upper airway angioedema.

BIBLIOGRAPHY

1. An overview of angioedema: Clinical features, diagnosis, and management. Clifton O Bingham. http://www.uptodate.com (Accessed October 24, 2017).
2. Kanani A, Schellenberg R, Warrington R. Urticaria and angioedema. *Allergy Asthma Clin Immunol* 2011;7(Suppl. 1):S9.
3. Radonjic-Hoesli S, Hofmeier KS, Micaletto S, Schmid-Grendelmeier P, Bircher A, Simon D. Urticaria and angioedema: An update on classification and pathogenesis. *Clin Rev Allergy Immunol* 2018;54:88–101.
4. Hahn J, Hoffmann TK, Bock B, Nordmann-Kleiner M, Trainotti S, Greve J. Angioedema: An interdisciplinary emergency. *Dtsch Arztebl Int* 2017;114:489–96.
5. Rye Rasmussen EH, Bindslev-Jensen C, Bygum A. Angioedema: Assessment and treatment. *Tidsskr Nor Laegeforen* 2012;132(21):2391–5.
6. Ring J et al. Guideline for acute therapy and management of anaphylaxis – S2 Guideline of DGAKI, AeDA, GPA, DAAU, BVKJ, ÖGAI, SGAI, DGAI, DGP, DGPM, AGATE and DAAB. *Allergo J Int* 2014;23:96–112.
7. Kaplan AP, Greaves MW. Angioedema. *J Am Acad Dermatol* 2005;53(3):373–88; quiz 389–92. Review.
8. Bernstein JA, Moellman J. Emerging concepts in the diagnosis and treatment of patients with undifferentiated angioedema. *Int J Emerg Med* 2012;5(1):39–40.

56

Dermatological emergencies in pregnancy

RITI BHATIA, NEIRITA HAZARIKA, AND RUBY BHATIA

INTRODUCTION

Pregnancy is a state of complex immunological, endocrinological, metabolic, and vascular changes. These changes can manifest on the skin in the form of various disorders. Apart from dermatoses specific to pregnancy, a number of other disorders can present during pregnancy. Dermatological emergencies in pregnancy are often a challenge in terms of both making a diagnosis and choosing the treatment modality. Consideration of the well-being of both mother and fetus is of prime importance. The focus of this chapter is common dermatological emergencies encountered in pregnancy.

DISORDERS SPECIFIC TO PREGNANCY

The specific dermatoses of pregnancy are a heterogenous group of inflammatory skin diseases characterized by severe itching with skin lesions of varying morphology, occurring exclusively during pregnancy and the postpartum period. The revised classification by Rudolph et al. includes pemphigoid gestationis, polymorphic eruption of pregnancy, atopic eruption of pregnancy, and intrahepatic cholestasis of pregnancy [1]. Although considered benign, severe manifestations of any of these may be seen.

Polymorphic eruption of pregnancy/ pruritic urticarial papules and plaques of pregnancy, toxemic rash of pregnancy/ Bourne toxic erythema of pregnancy

Polymorphic eruption of pregnancy is a benign, self-limited pruritic inflammatory disorder that usually affects primigravidae in the last weeks of pregnancy or immediately postpartum.

Clinically there are intensely pruritic, nonfollicular, erythematous urticarial papules, plaques, and sometimes, vesicles on the striae (Figures 56.1 and 56.2). There may be spreading of papules to buttocks, proximal thighs, and rarely legs (Figure 56.3). Often the eruption remains localized to these sites but can quickly generalize in severe cases. Approximately 50% of cases develop polymorphous lesions, including papulovesicles, annular or polycyclic urticarial lesions, targetoid lesions, and rarely, small bullae. Histopathology shows a spongiotic tissue reaction pattern, and immunofluorescence is negative. Maternal and fetal prognoses are excellent. In very severe generalized cases, a short course of systemic steroids in tapering doses is effective.

Atopic eruption of pregnancy

Atopic eruption of pregnancy is the most common cause of pruritus in pregnancy. Severe cases require a short course of systemic corticosteroids. Phototherapy with narrowband UVB is safe, particularly for severe recalcitrant cases [2]. Maternal prognosis is good even in severe cases, as skin lesions respond quickly to therapy. Apart from increased risk of developing atopic skin changes in later life, fetal prognosis is unaffected.

Pemphigoid gestationis

Pemphigoid gestationis is a rare autoimmune blistering disorder that presents mainly in the second or third trimester of pregnancy. The reported incidence is 1 in 20,000–50,000 pregnancies [1]. It was found to be associated with human leukocyte antigen (HLA)-haplotypes DR3 in 61% and DR4 in 43% of 23 cases in a study [3]. Pathogenesis involves production of IgG antibodies directed against the extracellular noncollagenous 16A (NC16A) domain of the transmembrane hemidesmosomal glycoprotein, BP180, a transcellular

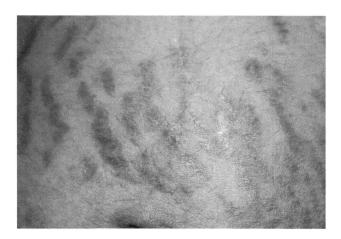

Figure 56.1 Pruritic urticarial papules and plaques of pregnancy on striae.

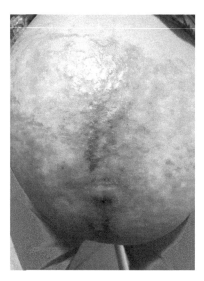

Figure 56.2 Extensive PUPPP on striae.

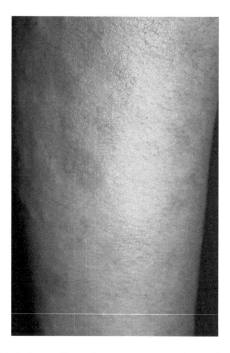

Figure 56.3 Spreading of pruritic urticarial papules and plaques of pregnancy onto lower limbs.

Treatment depends on the disease severity. In mild pre-blistering pemphigoid, topical corticosteroids with or without oral antihistamines are sufficient. All other cases require systemic corticosteroids. Prednisolone given in a dose of 0.5–1 mg/kg/day is usually effective. IVIg has been used to treat severe pemphigoid gestationis not responding to 1 mg/kg/day of prednisolone given for 2 weeks. A rapid response has been seen within 48 hours of first infusion [6]. A total dose of 2 g/kg given over 3 days is adequate. Plasmapheresis is another safe and effective therapeutic option for severe cases. Immunosuppressive agents such as azathioprine, cyclosporine, and rituximab have been successfully used in isolated cases. These are best avoided due to the risk of fetal immunosuppression [4,7,8].

Intrahepatic cholestasis of pregnancy

Intrahepatic cholestasis of pregnancy is a reversible form of hormonally triggered cholestasis that typically develops in genetically predisposed individuals in late pregnancy. The prevalence ranges from 0.7% in the United Kingdom, 1.2% in Asians of Indian origin in the United Kingdom, 2% in China, to 4% in Chile [9–11]. A defect in excretion of bile salts results in elevated bile acids in the serum. This leads to severe pruritus in the mother and may have deleterious effects on the fetus due to acute placental anoxia and cardiac depression. Etiology is multifactorial, involving genetics, hormones, environmental, dietary, and underlying liver, biliary, or pancreatic conditions. Approximately half of affected individuals have a positive family history. Mutations of genes encoding for transport proteins for bile excretion, i.e., *ABCB4* gene (multidrug resistance gene 3), *ATP8B1*, and *ABC11* have been implicated.

glycoprotein in the basement membrane zone of the skin and the amniotic sac. This may be induced by abnormal expression of paternal MHC class II antigens in the placenta. The immune complexes formed lead to complement activation, influx of eosinophils, and blister formation.

Pemphigoid gestationis usually starts during the second or third trimester of pregnancy. Clinically, it manifests with periumbilical itchy urticarial papules and erythematous plaques which spread to the rest of abdomen, back, and limbs. Development of tense blisters occurs in the next 1–2 weeks over preexisting erythematous plaques. Skin biopsy from bulla shows subepidermal blister with eosinophils. Direct immunofluorescence shows linear C3 and IgG deposition along the dermoepidermal junction. The disease usually remits within 6 months after delivery with frequent recurrences in subsequent pregnancies. Recurrence occurs in 90% of cases in subsequent pregnancies [4]. There is a slight risk of premature and small-for-date babies [5]. Passive transfer of maternal IgG antibodies can lead to mild, self-resolving skin lesions in about 10% of newborns [6].

Typically the patient presents with sudden onset of severe pruritus in the final trimester that may start on the palms and soles and becomes generalized in some cases. The pruritus is worse at night and often precedes laboratory abnormalities. It is not associated with primary skin lesions. Secondary skin lesions in the form of excoriations and prurigo-like nodules develop later. Hyperbilirubinemia (up to 5 mg/dL) occurs in approximately 10% of patients after 2–4 weeks, complicating more severe episodes.

There is a risk of developing cholelithiasis, steatorrhea, and rarely bleeding complications, due to malabsorption of fat-soluble vitamins. Serum bile acids are elevated 3 to 100 times the normal level (>11.0 nmol/L). ALT and γ-glutamyltransferase are raised in 20%–60% and 30% of cases, respectively, with a 2- to 10-fold elevation in levels. Histopathology is nonspecific, and immunofluorescence is negative.

Maternal prognosis is good. However, fetal complications such as prematurity, bradycardia, meconium staining of amniotic fluid, intrapartal fetal distress, and stillbirths are seen, which correlate with higher bile acid levels, particularly exceeding 40 μmol/L. There is a risk of fetal demise after 37 weeks of gestation; hence, induction of labor is recommended at or just prior to 37 weeks [12]. Cases with jaundice and vitamin K deficiency have an increased risk of intra- and postpartum hemorrhage.

An interdisciplinary management of intrahepatic cholestasis of pregnancy by dermatologists, hepatologists, gynecologists, and pediatricians is advised. Ursodeoxycholic acid (UDCA) is the only treatment that has been shown to reduce maternal pruritus and improve fetal prognosis. It is administered in a dose of 15 mg/kg/day, up to 1 g/day either as single dose or divided into two to three doses until delivery. UDCA is a category B drug [13]. Other drugs including antihistamines, S-adenosyl-L-methionine (SAM), dexamethasone, and cholestyramine have been tried without any effect on fetal prognosis. Close obstetric surveillance with weekly fetal cardiotocographic (CTG) monitoring is recommended from 34 weeks of gestation. Approximately 70% of patients have a recurrence during future pregnancies or while taking oral contraceptives.

OTHER DISEASES PRESENTING AS DERMATOLOGICAL EMERGENCIES

Impetigo herpetiformis

Impetigo herpetiformis or generalized pustular psoriasis of pregnancy is a rare, life-threatening pustular dermatosis related to pregnancy. Factors such as high progesterone during the last trimester of pregnancy, low calcium, and reduced epidermal skin–derived antileukoproteinase/elafin activity are implicated in formation of epidermal pustules.

The onset occurs in the second half of pregnancy, typically during the third trimester. Clinically, it manifests as widespread, tiny, superficial pustules on erythematous background on trunk and extremities with sparing of hands and feet. These pustules are arranged in rings or groups at margins of lesions, described as an herpetiform pattern. The pustules break down in the center, followed by crusting and impetiginization. Constitutional symptoms such as pain, fever, chills, vomiting, delirium, tetany (due to hypocalcemia), and lymphadenopathy are often present. In addition, severe dehydration, prostration, and convulsions can occur.

Skin biopsy shows subcorneal spongiform pustules filled with neutrophils, and perivascular infiltrates with lymphocytes and neutrophils. Parakeratosis and psoriasiform hyperplasia are seen in old cases. Other features include leukocytosis with neutrophilia; elevated erythrocyte sedimentation rate; low maternal serum calcium, phosphate, and vitamin D; hypoalbuminemia; and iron deficiency anemia. Early diagnosis and treatment are essential to prevent complications. Fetal adverse effects include stillbirth, neonatal death, and congenital abnormalities. Continuous monitoring for fetal anoxia is essential. When present, fetal anoxia is an indication for induction of labor, even if the fetus is premature [14].

Systemic corticosteroids are the first line of treatment. Oral prednisolone is usually started at a dose of 20–30 mg per day, and the dose can be increased to 40–60 mg per day. Narrowband ultraviolet B (NBUVB) and cyclosporine are useful in patients who have no or limited benefit from high doses of corticosteroids [15,16]. After delivery, other agents such as retinoids, psoralen plus ultraviolet A phototherapy, and methotrexate may be used, either as single agents or in combination with oral corticosteroids.

Systemic lupus erythematosus in pregnancy

Systemic lupus erythematosus (SLE) is associated with a high risk of intrauterine growth retardation, preterm labor, fetal loss (25% cases), and perinatal mortality. The increased risk of fetal death is attributed to immune complex deposition on the trophoblast basement membrane or the transplacental passage of antiphospholipid antibodies. The presence of anticardiolipin antibody or the lupus anticoagulant antibodies is associated with recurrent fetal loss, fetal growth restriction, congenital heart block, and neonatal cutaneous lupus [17]. There is an increased risk of flareup of SLE, especially in the second trimester of pregnancy. Active lupus during pregnancy leads to increased premature birth and a decrease in live births [18]. Pregnancies in lupus patients must be closely watched for pregnancy-induced hypertension (preeclampsia) and proteinurea.

Neonatal lupus occurs due to passive transfer of autoantibodies from the mother to the fetus. The major features are cardiac and cutaneous. Of these, congenital complete heart block is the most serious complication. It is reported in 2% of children born to primigravida women with anti-Ro/SSA antibodies [19,20]. Approximately 20% of affected neonates have an associated cardiomyopathy at the initial diagnosis or develop it later [21].

Hydroxychloroquine should be continued in pregnancy. A flare-up of disease is managed with a short course of prednisolone, in a dose of 0.5–1 mg/kg/day. Cyclosporine has been used safely in SLE in pregnancy [22]. Although there are reports of safe use of azathioprine, it is best avoided due to risk of fetal prematurity and congenital anomalies. Agents not recommended are mycophenolate mofetil, leflunomide, cyclophosphamide, and methotrexate.

Antiphospholipid antibody syndrome

Antiphospholipid antibody (APLA) syndrome is an autoimmune condition characterized by antibodies that recognize and attack phospholipid-binding proteins. Clinical manifestations include vascular thrombosis and pregnancy complications including recurrent abortions.

Diagnosis of APLA syndrome is based on clinical criteria of thromboembolism or pregnancy morbidity and laboratory findings of raised titers of antiphospholipid antibodies that are present on two or more occasions at least 12 weeks apart. Severe thrombocytopenia is seen in 5%–10% of cases.

Combinations of treatments are typically used, including anticoagulation with heparin. Immunomodulatory therapies including plasmapheresis, IV human IgG, corticosteroids, and rituximab have been used. Pregnant women with APLA syndrome and thrombocytopenia often require treatment to ensure adequate hemostasis at the time of delivery. In these cases, IV immunoglobulins and early delivery, if possible, are preferred [23].

Pemphigus vulgaris in pregnancy

Predominance of Th2 cytokines in pregnancy may promote autoantibody production against desmosomal glycoproteins Dsg1 and Dsg3, manifesting as first time onset or exacerbation of preexisting pemphigus. Severe pemphigus in pregnancy may be associated with adverse fetal outcomes, including immaturity and death and neonatal pemphigus. A flare-up of disease is usually seen in the first and second trimesters and immediate postpartum period due to low chorionic corticosteroid level as compared with the third trimester. Abortion was seen in 9.6% (five cases) in a study from Iran [24].

Systemic steroids are considered the first line of treatment, as in other autoimmune diseases. A safe and effective modality is IVIg. It has been used with good outcomes in severe and widespread disease without any adverse neonatal outcomes [25].

Psoriatic erythroderma in pregnancy

The majority of patients (40%–60%) with preexisting psoriasis improve in pregnancy, and few patients (10%–20%) deteriorate [26]. More than half of patients have a flare-up of disease in the immediate postpartum period [27]. Psoriasis does not affect fertility or rate of miscarriage, birth defect, or premature birth. Severe disease is best managed by NBUVB therapy. The drug of choice for erythroderma is cyclosporine [27].

Cutaneous adverse drug reactions

TOXIC EPIDERMAL NECROLYSIS

The occurrence of toxic epidermal necrolysis (TEN) during pregnancy can affect the fetus adversely. Isolated reports of TEN in pregnancy affecting the fetus simultaneously leading to premature death reflect the significant impact of this disease in pregnancy [28].

In a series of 22 HIV-infected pregnant females with Stevens-Johnson syndrome (SJS)/TEN, nevirapine was the most frequently implicated drug. Adverse fetal outcomes reported were fetal distress, miscarriage, intrauterine fetal death, and low birth weight [29].

Critical care management including immediate discontinuation of suspected drug, care of fluid and electrolytes, prevention of infection, daily wound care, mucosal care, systemic antibiotics in case of secondary infection, nutritional support, and frequent obstetric ultrasound evaluations are the mainstay of management. The role of steroids is established to be more when given in the first 3 days of disease onset. Tapering should be done rapidly, stopping within the next 1 week to 10 days. Systemic steroids are not favored in the first trimester but may be useful in the third trimester as they help to increase the lung maturity of the fetus, especially in preterm labor. IV immunoglobulin and cyclosporine can also be used [30].

Drug reaction with eosinophilia and systemic symptoms syndrome

Drug reaction with eosinophilia and systemic symptoms (DRESS) syndrome in pregnancy is complicated by unpredictable systemic toxicity in the mother and adverse fetal outcomes. Management includes systemic steroids in a dose of 1 mg/kg/day with slow tapering. Oral betamethasone in a single dose followed by cesarean section was successfully used in an HIV-infected pregnant female with DRESS secondary to nevirapine at 32 weeks' gestation [31]. The patient was given prednisolone 60 mg daily in the postpartum period [31]. Continuous monitoring for systemic involvement in mother and fetal well-being is a must.

Type 2 leprosy reactions in pregnancy

Leprosy in pregnancy shows a biphasic course of disease, with deterioration and downgrading of disease during pregnancy, increased risk of type 2 reaction especially in the third trimester, and prolonged type 1 reaction following delivery. There is an increased risk of relapse, reactions, and nerve damage, both in patients on treatment and those released from treatment [32]. Up to 20% of children born to mothers with leprosy may develop leprosy by puberty. Awareness regarding these adverse effects is essential for early diagnosis. The standard multidrug therapy for leprosy is safe and should be continued unchanged in pregnancy and lactation. Short courses of systemic steroids are effective in managing severe reactions. Thalidomide should not be used because of its teratogenicity [33,34].

Ehler–Danlos syndrome

Ehler–Danlos syndrome (EDS) can affect the pregnancy outcome adversely. The rate of preterm premature rupture of membranes (PPROM) and preterm birth is reported to be 25%–75%. Cervical insufficiency and fetal growth restriction are commonly reported. A multidisciplinary approach involving specialists from rheumatology, ophthalmology, neurosurgery, obstetrics, and cardiology should be employed in managing such cases. Implications for obstetric management are in accordance with the type of EDS in an individual case. The hypermobility type of EDS is associated with relatively benign musculoskeletal problems, including joint dislocation and pain. There are no contraindications to pregnancy in this type of EDS. Vascular and classical types of EDS are reported to have serious complications. Vaginal delivery is associated with an increased risk of extensive perineal trauma. Cesarian section is associated with a risk of developing incisional hernia and poor skin healing. Meticulous hemostasis and retention sutures should be ensured to avoid obstetric hemorrhage, especially in cases with uterine atony and lacerations. The neonate may be affected by floppy baby syndrome and congenital hip dislocation. Management includes use of ß-blockers to control blood pressure, avoidance of strenuous activity, vitamin C supplementation to strengthen collagen cross-linking, and early hospital admission [35].

Pseudoxanthoma elasticum

Pseudoxanthoma elasticum (PXE) is an autosomal recessive disorder characterized by calcified fragmented elastic fibers in skin, retina, and arteries. In a study involving 306 respondents with PXE who had ever been pregnant, there were 795 pregnancies. Of these, 83% ended in live births and 1% in stillbirth. There was a very low incidence of low birth weight for gestation (1%), hypertension (10%), gastric bleeding and retinal complications (<1%), and worsening of skin manifestations (12%). Hence, it was concluded that most pregnancies in PXE are uncomplicated [36].

Nevertheless, it is essential for the treating physician to be aware of potential complications. A multidisciplinary approach should be taken, with regular monitoring of cardiac and renal function, blood pressure, changes in the retina, and any evidence of signs or symptoms that could be the consequence of gastrointestinal bleeding. PXE is not an absolute indication for elective cesarean section. This should be restricted to patients with visual deficits proven by a choroidal neovascularization examination of the eye [37].

Trichothiodystrophy

Patients affected by trichothiodystrophy (TTD) have sulfur-deficient brittle hair and developmental abnormalities due to DNA repair and transcription gene defects. Pregnancies with affected fetuses are reported to have complications in the form of preeclampsia, decreased fetal movement, and HELLP (hemolysis, elevated liver enzymes, and low platelets) syndrome. In a study involving 27 TTD patients and their 23 mothers, 81% of the pregnancies had complications. These included preterm delivery (56%), preeclampsia (30%), placental abnormalities (19%), HELLP syndrome (11%), and fetal distress (4%). Other reported abnormalities include oligohydramnios, stillbirth, and placental asphyxiation. Prenatal diagnosis using fetal hair biopsy and DNA repair measurements is possible [38].

Erythromelalgia

Erythromelalgia is characterized by high platelet counts (>4 lacs/uL) leading to erythema, warmth, congestion, and pain involving palms and soles. This may progress to ischemic acrocyanosis and, sometimes, gangrene. Skin biopsy shows arterioles with fibromuscular proliferation and occasional thrombotic occlusion. Pregnancy is a secondary cause of erythromelalgia [39]. Oral aspirin is usually helpful. A complete blood cell count, platelet count, urinalysis, and immunologic survey are recommended.

Rosacea fulminans

Rosacea fulminans is a rare disease of unknown cause that occurs exclusively in women. Hormonal factors in pregnancy may be responsible for its trigger. Involvement is in the form of inflammatory nodules and pustules with perilesional erythema on cheeks. Conventional treatment with systemic corticosteroids is usually successful. Topical 0.75% metronidazole cream should not be used in the first trimester but may be employed thereafter [40].

Melanoma

Pregnancy is a state of immunosuppression. This is associated with reduced tumor surveillance that should worsen the prognosis of melanoma. Contrary to this belief, most small, controlled studies and large, population-based cohort studies have reported no significant influence of pregnancy on survival in women diagnosed with malignant melanoma compared with women not pregnant at the time of diagnosis [41]. Early detection is critical, and prompt biopsy of suspicious lesions is important and should not be deferred until after pregnancy. Biopsies and wide local excisions can be performed safely during pregnancy. Placental and fetal metastasis is exceptionally rare. Sentinel lymph node (SLN) biopsy is recommended using radiocolloid due to the risk of rare but potentially catastrophic anaphylaxis with isosulfan blue dye. However, in women in middle to late pregnancy who have undergone narrow excision of their primary melanoma with clear histologic margins, definitive wide local excision and SLN biopsy may be delayed until after delivery, with close clinical follow-up during pregnancy [42].

Pyogenic granuloma/pregnancy tumor/lobular capillary hemangioma

The pregnancy tumor most frequently develops on the areas of frequent trauma including gingiva, tongue, lips, and buccal mucosa. It is characterized by an exophytic pedunculated fleshy growth with a tendency to bleed on manipulation. It rarely reaches more than 2 cm in size (Figure 56.4). It usually develops in the second or third trimester, and rapid growth accompanies the steady increase of circulating estrogens and progesterones. Partial or complete regression is common after delivery.

Various modalities of treatment have been documented for treatment of this lesion. These include surgical excision (Figure 56.5), laser excision using diode or neodymium:yttrium-aluminum-garnet (Nd:YAG) lasers, and cryotherapy.

Infections during pregnancy

VARICELLA/CHICKEN POX

Varicella, caused by varicella zoster virus (VZV; human herpesvirus 3), in pregnancy may cause maternal mortality or serious morbidity. Awareness of potential complications including hepatitis, pneumonia, and encephalitis is essential. It may also cause fetal varicella syndrome, congenital varicella syndrome, and neonatal varicella. The UK Advisory Group on Chickenpox recommends oral acyclovir for pregnant women with chicken pox if they present within 24 hours of the onset of the rash and if they are more than 20 weeks of gestation [43]. Use of acyclovir before 20 weeks should also be considered. However, in cases of severe maternal infection, IV acyclovir should be administered.

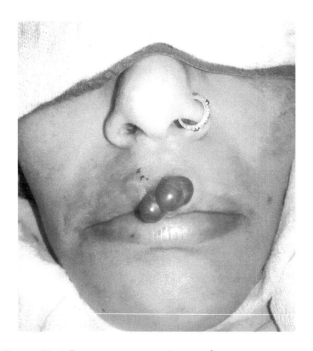

Figure 56.4 Pregnancy pyogenic granuloma.

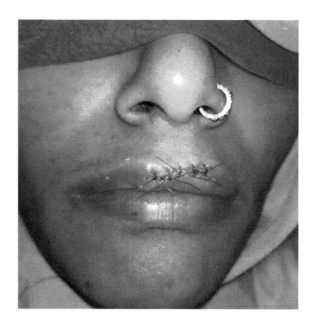

Figure 56.5 Removal of pyogenic granuloma by excision.

VZIG is recommended for postexposure prophylaxis and is not appropriate treatment for patients with clinical chickenpox [44].

CYTOMEGALOVIRUS

Primary cytomegalovirus (CMV) infection should be suspected in a pregnant woman with influenza-like symptoms not attributable to another specific infection; who shows signs of hepatitis with negative serology for hepatitis A, B, and C; and when imaging findings are suggestive of fetal cytomegalovirus infection. Fetal CMV is associated with significant morbidity in the form of microcephaly, hepatosplenomegaly, and retinitis. Diagnosis of primary maternal CMV infection in pregnancy is based on *de novo* appearance of virus-specific IgG in the serum of a previously seronegative woman, or on detection of specific IgM antibody. In case of primary maternal infection, parents should be informed about a 30%–40% risk for intrauterine transmission, and a risk of 20%–25% for development of postnatal sequelae. Prenatal diagnosis of fetal CMV infection can be confirmed by amniocentesis, which should be done at least 7 weeks after presumed time of maternal infection and after 21 weeks of gestation. In cases of fetal CMV infection, serial ultrasound examinations should be performed every 2–4 weeks to detect sonographic abnormalities to determine prognosis of the fetus [45]. Once the diagnosis of congenital CMV infection is confirmed, one option is pregnancy termination. A second proposed option has been treatment of the mother with antiviral agents such as ganciclovir, foscarnet, and cidofovir. However, they are not of proven value in preventing or treating congenital CMV infection.

RUBELLA

Rubella virus is an enveloped RNA virus classified as a Rubivirus in the Togaviridae family. Patients present with maculopapular exanthema with fever. Arthralgia occurs in up to 70% of cases. Rare complications include thrombocytopenia, encephalitis, stillbirths, miscarriages, and severe birth defects known as congenital rubella syndrome. The most common congenital defects are cataracts, heart defects, and hearing impairment. Patients with rubella should be isolated for 7 days after they develop rash. Detection of specific IgM antibodies can provide presumptive evidence for infection. The optimum period for collection of serum is 5 days after the onset of symptoms when greater than 90% of cases will be IgM positive [46].

Sexually transmitted diseases

HERPES SIMPLEX VIRUS

Herpes simplex virus (HSV) infection has been rising in prevalence in the developed world. The manifestations of neonatal or congenital HSV infection include involvement of eye, mouth, central nervous system, and disseminated disease. The latter is the most serious form of infection, with an approximate 90% mortality rate if untreated.

Women with recurrent HSV should be offered a cesarean section if there are prodromal symptoms or in the presence of lesions suggestive of HSV. Women with known recurrent genital HSV infection as well as primary genital herpes in the third trimester should be offered acyclovir or valacyclovir suppression at 36 weeks' gestation to decrease the risk of viral shedding at the time of delivery and therefore decrease the need for cesarean section [47].

CHLAMYDIA

Chlamydia infection in pregnancy is associated with maternal morbidity in the form of puerperal infection and PROM. Fetal complications include preterm birth, low birth weight, ophthalmia neonatorum, and chlamydial pneumonitis. Testing for chlamydia should be done in all women with lower genital tract symptoms. Endocervical swabs should be tested with nucleic acid amplification tests (NAATs) for chlamydia detection. Azithromycin 1 g oral stat is recommended as first-line treatment for chlamydia in pregnancy [48].

GONORRHEA

Gonococcal cervicitis is associated with increased risk of PROM, preterm birth, low birth weight, ophthalmia neonatorum, and disseminated gonococcal infection. Gonorrhea testing should be performed on women with lower genital tract symptoms, intrapartum or postpartum fever, and mothers of infants with ophthalmia neonatorum. Endocervical swabs are tested with NAATs and culture for *Neisseria gonorrhoeae*. Due to emerging reports of resistance to cefixime, ceftriaxone 250 mg intramuscularly is the recommended treatment for gonococcal infection at any genital or extragenital site. Concomitant treatment with azithromycin 1 g orally is imperative to cover for asymptomatic chlamydia infection [48].

SYPHILIS

The transmission risk of early syphilis in pregnancy is up to 100%. About half of these pregnancies will result in preterm birth or perinatal death. In women with late infection, 10% of infants are affected. Congenital syphilis can result in stillbirth, neonatal death, and long-term disability with affection of multiple organs. Penicillin is the treatment of choice, and the treatment regimen is the same as for nonpregnant cases. In cases with penicillin allergy, the Centers for Disease Control and Prevention recommend penicillin desensitization, as alternative treatments have high failure rates. The Jarisch-Herxheimer reaction can complicate up to 45% of cases treated in pregnancy. Maternal fever may result in uterine contractions, preterm labor, and fetal heart rate decelerations. Fetal monitoring should be considered in women receiving treatment after 26 weeks of gestation. Management of the Jarisch-Herxheimer reaction is supportive. Monthly VDRL testing is done to monitor treatment response. In case delivery occurs less than 30 days after completion of treatment, the neonate should be administered empirical treatment [48].

Table 56.1 U.S. Food and Drug Administration (FDA) pregnancy category classification for common dermatological therapies

Drug name	FDA pregnancy category
Topical steroids	C
Oral corticosteroids	C
Topical calcineurin inhibitors	C
Dapsone	C
Isotretinoin	X
Acitretin	X
Cyclosporine	C
Cyclophosphamide	D
Azathioprine	D
Mycophenolate mofetil	D
Methotrexate	X
Rituximab	C
IVIg	C
Psoralens	C
NBUVB phototherapy	–
Chlorpheniramine	B
Cyproheptadine	B
Dexchlorpheniramine	B
Hydroxyzine	C
Promethazine	C
Tripelennamine	B
Cetrizine	B
Fexofenadine	C
Loratidine	B
Levocetrizine	B
Desloratadine	C

CONCLUSION

To conclude, a dermatologist often encounters a pregnant female with cutaneous disorders. When these conditions present as emergencies, the management can be challenging. Apart from distinguishing disorders with overlapping features, taking therapeutic decisions promptly after holistic consideration of maternal and fetal well-being is of utmost importance. Data regarding safety and efficacy of most commonly used medications in these disorders are limited to isolated case reports or animal studies. In most of these scenarios, management is done with a multidisciplinary approach, keeping the obstetrician, dermatologist, physician/rheumatologist, and pediatrician in the loop. FDA pregnancy categories for common dermatological drugs are as provided in Table 56.1.

KEY POINTS

- The specific dermatoses of pregnancy includes pemphigoid gestationis, polymorphic eruption of pregnancy, atopic eruption of pregnancy, and intrahepatic cholestasis of pregnancy.
- Other emergencies which can occur commonly in pregnancy include APLA, SLE complications, type 2 lepra reactions and impetigo herpetiformis.
- Other diseases which can present as emergencies in pregnancy include Pemphigus, severe cutaneous drug reactions and erythroderma.
- Infections like herpes simplex, varicella, rubella and STD's need to be given special importance in pregnancy and treated accordingly.

REFERENCES

1. Ambros-Rudolph CM, Müllegger RR, Vaughan-Jones SA, Kerl H, Black MM. The specific dermatoses of pregnancy revisited and reclassified: Results of a retrospective two-center study on 505 pregnant patients. *J Am Acad Dermatol* 2006;54:395–404.
2. Weatherhead S, Robson SC, Reynolds NJ. Eczema in pregnancy. *BMJ* 2007;335:152–4.
3. Shornick JK, Stastny P, Gilliam JN. High frequency of histocompatibility antigens HLA-DR3 and DR4 in herpes gestations. *J Clin Invest* 1981;68:553–5.
4. Jenkins RE, Hern S, Black MM. Clinical features and management of 87 patients with pemphigoid gestationis. *Clin Exp Dermatol* 1999;24:255–9.
5. Intong LRA, Murrell DF. Pemphigoid gestationis: Pathogenesis and clinical features. *Dermatol Clin* 2011;29:447–52.
6. Gan DCC, Welsh B, Webster M. Successful treatment of a severe persistent case of pemphigoid gestationis with antepartum and postpartum intravenous immunoglobulin followed by azathioprine. *Australas J Dermatol* 2012;53:66–9.
7. Hern S, Harman K, Bhogal BS, Black MM. A severe persistent case of pemphigoid gestationis treated with intravenous immunoglobulins and cyclosporin. *Clin Exp Dermatol* 1998;23:185–8.
8. Cianchini G, Masini C, Lupi F, Corona R, De Pità O, Puddu P. Severe persistent pemphigoid gestationis: Long-term remission with rituximab. *Br J Dermatol* 2007;157:388–9.
9. Humberto R. Sex hormones and bile acids in intrahepatic cholestasis of pregnancy. *Hepatology* 2008;47:376–9.
10. Abedin P, Weaver JB, Egginton E. Intrahepatic cholestasis of pregnancy: Prevalence and ethnic distribution. *Ethn Health* 1999;4:35–7.
11. Luo X-L, Zhang W-Y. Obstetrical disease spectrum in China: An epidemiological study of 111,767 cases in 2011. *Chin Med J (Engl)* 2015;128:1137–46.
12. Ovadia C, Williamson C. Intrahepatic cholestasis of pregnancy: Recent advances. *Clin Dermatol* 2016;34:327–34.
13. Bacq Y et al. Efficacy of ursodeoxycholic acid in treating intrahepatic cholestasis of pregnancy: A meta-analysis. *Gastroenterology* 2012;143:1492–501.
14. Wolf R, Tartler U, Stege H, Megahed M, Ruzicka T. Impetigo herpetiformis with hyperparathyroidism. *J Eur Acad Dermatol Venereol* 2005;19:743–6.
15. Bozdag K, Ozturk S, Ermete M. A case of recurrent impetigo herpetiformis treated with systemic corticosteroids and narrowband UVB. *Cutan Ocul Toxicol* 2012;31:67–9.
16. Patsatsi A et al. Cyclosporine in the management of impetigo herpetiformis: A case report and review of the literature. *Case Rep Dermatol* 2013;5:99–104.
17. Rahman A, Isenberg DA. Systemic lupus erythematosus. *N Engl J Med* 2008;358:929–39.
18. Clowse MEB, Magder LS, Witter F, Petri M. The impact of increased lupus activity on obstetric outcomes. *Arthritis Rheum* 2005;52:514–21.
19. Ambrosi A, Wahren-Herlenius M. Congenital heart block: Evidence for a pathogenic role of maternal autoantibodies. *Arthritis Res Ther* 2012; 14:208.
20. Buyon JP et al. Autoimmune-associated congenital heart block: Demographics, mortality, morbidity and recurrence rates obtained from a national neonatal lupus registry. *J Am Coll Cardiol* 1998; 31:1658.
21. Stainforth J, Goodfield M, Taylor P. Pregnancy-induced chilblain lupus erythematosus. *Clin Exp Dermatol* 1993;18:449–51.

22. Østensen M et al. Update on safety during pregnancy of biological agents and some immunosuppressive anti-rheumatic drugs. *Rheumatol Oxf Engl* 2008;47(Suppl. 3):iii28–31.

23. Myers B, Pavord S. Diagnosis and management of antiphospholipid syndrome in pregnancy. *Obstet Gynaecol (RCOG)* 2011;13:15–21.

24. Daneshpazhooh M et al. Pemphigus and pregnancy: A 23-year experience. *Indian J Dermatol Venereol Leprol* 2011;77:534.

25. Ahmed AR, Gürcan HM. Use of intravenous immunoglobulin therapy during pregnancy in patients with pemphigus vulgaris. *J Eur Acad Dermatol Venereol* 2011;25(9):1073–9.

26. Tauscher AE, Fleischer AB, Phelps KC, Feldman SR. Psoriasis and pregnancy. *J Cutan Med Surg* 2002;6:561–70.

27. Weatherhead S, Robson SC, Reynolds NJ. Management of psoriasis in pregnancy. *BMJ* 2007;334:1218–20.

28. Rodriguez G, Trent JT, Mirzabeigi M, Zaulyanov L, Bruce J, Vincek V. Toxic epidermal necrolysis in a mother and fetus. *J Am Acad Dermatol* 2006;55:S96–8.

29. Knight L, Todd G, Muloiwa R, Matjila M, Lehloenya RJ. Stevens-Johnson syndrome and toxic epidermal necrolysis: Maternal and foetal outcomes in twenty-two consecutive pregnant HIV infected women. *PLOS ONE* 2015;10:e0135501.

30. Gupta LK et al. Guidelines for the management of Stevens-Johnson syndrome/toxic epidermal necrolysis: An Indian perspective. *Indian J Dermatol Venereol Leprol* 2016;82:603.

31. Knudtson E, Para M, Boswell H, Fan-Havard P. Drug rash with eosinophilia and systemic symptoms syndrome and renal toxicity with a nevirapine-containing regimen in a pregnant patient with human immunodeficiency virus. *Obstet Gynecol* 2003;101:1094–7.

32. Ozturk Z, Tatliparmak A. Leprosy treatment during pregnancy and breastfeeding: A case report and brief review of literature. *Dermatol Ther* 2017;3.

33. Rochael MC et al. Sweet's syndrome: Study of 73 cases, emphasizing histopathological findings. *An Bras Dermatol* 2011;86:702–7.

34. Sankar M, Kaliaperumal K. Pregnancy-associated Sweet's syndrome: A rare clinical entity. *J Obstet Gynaecol India* 2016; 66: 587–9.

35. Lind J, Wallenburg HC. Pregnancy and the Ehlers-Danlos syndrome: A retrospective study in a Dutch population. *Acta Obstet Gynecol Scand* 2002;81:293–300.

36. Bercovitch L, Leroux T, Terry S, Weinstock MA. Pregnancy and obstetrical outcomes in pseudoxanthoma elasticum. *Br J Dermatol* 2004;151:1011–8.

37. Camacho M et al. Approach to the management of pregnancy in patients with pseudoxanthoma elasticum: A review. *J Obstet Gynecol* 2016;36:1–6.

38. Tamura D, Merideth M, DiGiovanna JJ. High risk pregnancy and neonatal complications in the DNA repair and transcription disorder trichothiodystrophy: Report of 27 affected pregnancies. *Prenat Diagn* 2011;31:1046–53.

39. Hart JJ. Painful, swollen, and erythematous hands and feet. *Arthritis Rheum* 1996; 39:1761–2.

40. Ferahbas A, Utas S, Mistik S, Uksal U, Peker D. Rosacea fulminans in pregnancy: Case report and review of the literature. *Am J Clin Dermatol* 2006;7:141–4.

41. Driscoll MS et al. Pregnancy and melanoma. *J Am Acad Dermatol* 2016; 75:669–78.

42. Schwartz JL, Mozurkewich EL, Johnson TM. Current management of patients with melanoma who are pregnant, want to get pregnant, or do not want to get pregnant. *Cancer* 2003;97:2130–3.

43. Nathwani D, Maclean A, Conway S, Carrington D. Varicella infections in pregnancy and the newborn. A review prepared for the UK Advisory Group on Chickenpox on behalf of the British Society for the Study of Infection. *J Infect* 1998;36:59–71.

44. Chickenpox in pregnancy. RCOG Greentop guidelines, https://www.rcog.org.uk/globalassets/documents/guidelines/gtg13.pdf (Accessed August 1, 2018).

45. Yinon Y, Farine D, Yudin MH. Cytomegalovirus infection in pregnancy. *J Obstet Gynaecol Can* 2010;32:348–54.

46. Centers for Disease Control and Prevention Guidelines 2015. https://www.cdc.gov/rubella/hcp.html (Accessed August 1, 2018).

47. Money D, Steben M. Guidelines for the management of herpes simplex virus in pregnancy. *J Obstet Gynaecol Can* 2008;30:514–9.

48. Allstaff S, Wilson J. The management of sexually transmitted infections in pregnancy. *Obstet Gynaecol (RCOG)* 2012;14:25–32.

Emergencies in Leprosy

ANUPAM DAS

Lepromatous leprosy

ANUPAM DAS

INTRODUCTION

Lepromatous leprosy is a multibacillary form of the disease characterized by poor cell-mediated immunity toward the disease and the presence of numerous bacilli in the body. It is rightly designated as the highly infectious spectrum of the disease. The high bacillary load, vulnerability of close contacts to contract the disease, and multisystem involvement of this spectrum all make it a dermatological emergency that requires early diagnosis and prompt intervention.

IMMUNOLOGY

Lepromatous leprosy is characterized by T-cell unresponsiveness to lepra bacilli [1,2]. There is reduced production of interleukin (IL)-12, leading to a reduced Th1 response. This eventually leads to reduced stimulation of macrophages and impaired cell-mediated immunity. A dominant Th2 response produces IL-4, IL-5, and IL-10, which suppresses the activation of macrophages [3,4].

CLINICAL FEATURES

In this pole of leprosy, the host immunity toward lepra bacilli is very poor, and the disease is manifested throughout the body [5]. The earliest findings include nasal stuffiness and epistaxis. Cutaneous findings include bilateral symmetrically arranged macules, papules, nodules (Figure 57.1), and diffuse or ulcerative lesions. Sensory loss is usually absent, except for glove and stocking anesthesia. Nerves are symmetrically thickened, tender, and fibrotic. Diffuse infiltration of the skin of the forehead, chin, nose, and ears leads to development of "leonine facies" [6].

Besides saddle nose, Hertoghe sign (loss of eyebrows), loss of eyelashes, perforation of nasal septum, lagophthalmos, and trophic ulcers on the legs, thighs, and upper limbs are also found. Oral manifestations occur in 20%–60% of cases, characterized by formation of multiple nodules (lepromas) progressing to necrosis and ulceration [7]. Isolated presentation with a leg ulcer is also possible [8].

Systemic involvement is very common. Hoarseness of voice (leprous huskiness) and stridor are due to involvement of the larynx. Lepromatous lesions can develop in the oral cavity, gums, tongue, and palate, leading to erosion and perforation. Ocular involvement can lead to iris pearls (microgranuloma deposits), reduced visual acuity, pain, and photophobia. Ciliary body involvement can lead to iridocyclitis and gradual loss of vision. Involvement of Vth and VIIth cranial nerves leads to loss of corneal and conjunctival sensations, lagophthalmos, exposure keratitis, corneal ulceration, and blindness. Musculoskeletal involvement is characterized by bone cysts, aseptic necrosis, dactylitis, periostitis, Charcot joints, etc. Generalized lymphadenopathy, hepatosplenomegaly, mesangioproliferative glomerulonephritis, and renal amyloidosis are among the other complications. Atrophy of testes, impotence, and gynecomastia are some of the other troublesome features of lepromatous leprosy. Secondary atrophy of seminiferous tubules has also been reported. Hormonal imbalance in association with reduced plasma testosterone levels, and elevated urinary gondatrophins has also been reported [9].

Bony involvement is characterized by punched out radiolucent lesions of nasal bones and small bones of hands and feet. Histology shows trabecular erosions by acid-fast bacilli (AFB)–laden macrophage granulomas. The eventual result of these changes is osteomyelitis, periostitis, and concentric resorption of bones (Figures 57.2 and 57.3).

Renal involvement is not due to deposits of granulomas. This is attributed to extensive load of bacilli and deposition of immune complexes. Renal failure is thought to be one of the major causes of death in patients of leprosy.

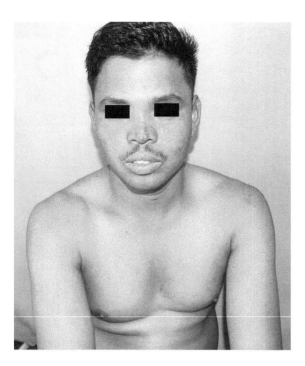

Figure 57.1 Nodules on the nose; early lepromatous leprosy.

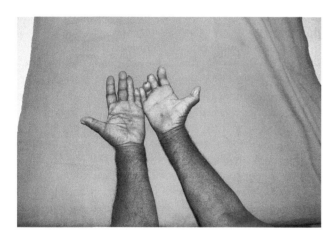

Figure 57.2 Resorption of hand bones.

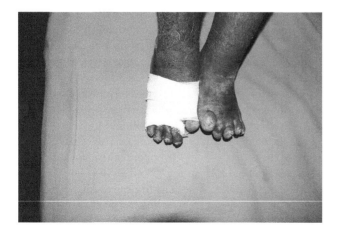

Figure 57.3 Resorption of feet.

Mesangioproliferative glomerulonephritis, glomerulonephritis, and membranous glomerulonephritis are the common conditions encountered, apart from amyloid deposits.

Hepatic manifestations are due to involvement of Kupffer cells. Small lepromatous deposits containing macrophages have also been observed in close vicinity of the portal tract.

DIAGNOSIS

Slit skin smear

This usually shows plenty of AFB, and the diagnosis is obvious in a background of the classical clinical features.

Histopathology

It is characterized by an extensive cellular infiltrate, separated from the overlying atrophic epidermis by a clear-cut Grenz zone. There is destruction of cutaneous appendages. In severe cases, there is an abundant presence of dermal histiocytes laden with AFB (Virchow cells/lepra cells/foam cells). Plasma cells may also be found. Epithelioid cells are usually absent [10].

Variants

- *Leonine leprosy*: Lepromatous leprosy due to diffuse nodular infiltration; this is also called *nodular lepromatous leprosy.*
- *Lucio leprosy or lepra bonita or beautiful leprosy or pretty leprosy*: This is usually seen in Mexico and Central America. It is characterized by diffuse infiltration of skin by lepra bacilli and loss of body hairs, eyebrows, and eyelashes, partly from widespread loss of sensation and sweating. The lesions never transform into nodules. The patient looks younger for his or her age. Rarely, the patient may develop a reaction (Lucio phenomenon) [11].
- *Histoid leprosy*: In this variant, there is an absence of diffuse infiltration of the skin. Instead, we find dome-shaped discrete reddish to skin-colored firm papulonodules (Figure 57.4). Biopsy typically shows a well-circumscribed lesion surrounded by a pseudo-capsule, epidermal atrophy, Grenz zone, and classical spindle-shaped histiocytes and foam cells [12].
- *Lazarine leprosy*: This is seen in undernourished patients, clinically presenting with diffuse ulcerations of the skin [13,14].

TREATMENT

- Rifampicin 600 mg once monthly supervised
- Dapsone 100 mg once daily
- Clofazimine 50 mg once daily or 100 mg alternate day

Management of nerve function deficits is done by continuing multidrug therapy, standard course of oral corticosteroids, and surgical decompression of nerve trunks (if required) [15,16].

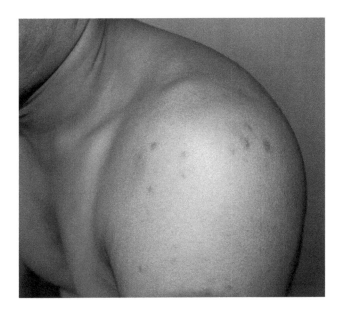

Figure 57.4 Papules of histioid leprosy.

Management of eye problems is crucial to prevent the development of disabilities. Patients with corneal anesthesia should be strictly asked to protect their eyes from foreign bodies using spectacles or eyeshades. Application of artificial eye drops is also advised. Iridocyclitis is managed using mydriatics, topical corticosteroid drops, and occasionally systemic steroids. Surgeries include lateral tarsorrhaphy or temporalis transfer, for correction of lagophthalmos.

Gynecomastia is managed by simple mastectomy by an intra-areolar incision (Webster operation) [17].

KEY POINTS

- The high bacillary load, vulnerability of close contacts to contract the disease, and multisystem involvement makes lepromatous leprosy an emergency condition that requires early diagnosis and prompt intervention.
- Nasal stuffiness, epistaxis, bilateral symmetrically arranged macules, papules, nodules, diffuse or ulcerative lesions, glove and stocking anesthesia, "leonine facies", saddle nose, madarosis, perforation of nasal septum, lagophthalmos, and trophic ulcers may manifest.
- Hoarseness of voice, stridor, palate perforation, iridocyclitis, lagophthalmos, exposure keratitis, corneal ulceration, blindness, periostitis, mesangioproliferative glomerulonephritis, atrophy of testes, impotence, and gynecomastia may occur.

CONCLUSION

Lepromatous leprosy is characterized by multisystem involvement. Early diagnosis is the key to better management.

REFERENCES

1. Nath IMC. Immunological aspects. In: Kar HK and Kumar B (Eds), *Textbook of Leprosy*. Mubai: Jaypee Brothers Medical Publishers; 2010: 60–73.
2. Haregewoin A, Godal T, Mustafa AS, Belehu A, Yemaneberhan T. T-cell conditioned media reverse T-cell unresponsiveness in lepromatous leprosy. *Nature* 1983;303:342–4.
3. Nath I, Saini C, Valluri VL. Immunology of leprosy and diagnostic challenges. *Clin Dermatol* 2015;33:90–8.
4. Salgame PR, Birdi TJ, Mahadevan PR, Antia NH. Role of macrophages in defective cell mediated immunity in lepromatous leprosy. I. Factor(s) from macrophages affecting protein synthesis and lymphocyte transformation. *Int J Lepr Other Mycobact Dis* 1980;48:172–7.
5. Fischer M. Leprosy: An overview of clinical features, diagnosis, and treatment. *J Dtsch Dermatol Ges* 2017;15:801–27.
6. Murthy PK. Clinical manifestations, diagnosis and classification of leprosy. *J Indian Med Assoc* 2004;102:678–9.
7. Chimenos KE, Pascual CM, Pinol DC, Vinals IH, Rodríguez de Rivera Campillo ME, López López J. Lepromatous leprosy: A review and case report. *Med Oral Patol Oral Cir Bucal* 2006;11:E474–9.
8. de O Fernandes TRM, dos Santos TSS, de M Lopes RR. Leg ulcer in lepromatous leprosy— Case report. *Anais Brasileiros de Dermatologia* 2016;91:673–5.
9. Walker SL, Lockwood DNJ. The clinical and immunological features of leprosy. *Br Med Bull* 2006;77:103–21.
10. Massone C, Belachew WA, Schettini A. Histopathology of the lepromatous skin biopsy. *Clin Dermatol* 2015;33:38–45.
11. Ramal C et al. Diffuse multibacillary leprosy of Lucio and Latapí with Lucio's phenomenon, Peru. *Emerg Infect Dis* 2017;23:1929–30.
12. Karthikeyan K. Histoid leprosy. *Am J Trop Med Hyg* 2015;92:1085–6.
13. Thappa DM. What is lazarine leprosy? Is it a separate entity? *Indian J Lepr* 2005;77:179–81.
14. Nanda S, Bansal S, Grover C, Garg V, Reddy BS. Lazarine leprosy—Revisited? *Indian J Lepr* 2004;76:351–4.
15. Reibel F, Cambau E, Aubry A. Update on the epidemiology, diagnosis, and treatment of leprosy. *Médecine et Maladies Infectieuses* 2015;45:383–93.
16. Britton WJ, Lockwood DN. Leprosy. *Lancet* 2004;363:1209–19.
17. Moschella SL. An update on the diagnosis and treatment of leprosy. *J Am Acad Dermatol* 2004;51:417–26.

58

Lepra reactions

TANMAY PADHI AND MITANJALI SETHY

INTRODUCTION

Leprosy is a chronic infectious disease caused by *Mycobacterium leprae*, an acid-fast bacillus (AFB), and is characterized by cutaneous and neural manifestations. The progress of the disease is often considered to be slow and indolent. However, skin or nerve lesions may suddenly flare up in a state of immunological reaction (lepra reaction), and the resultant systemic inflammatory complications such as severe neuritis, high fever, episcleritis, epididymo-orchitis, and sudden onset of neurological impairment such as foot drop and wrist drop usually need emergency medical and occasionally surgical measures.

In lepra reaction, the infected nerves and surrounding tissues are damaged as the host mounts an immune response to bacterial antigens. Leprosy reactions play a significant role in the morbidity associated with the disease. Reactions are responsible for most of the permanent nerve damage, deformity, disability, and death in leprosy.

Two major types of reactions are recognized in leprosy. Type 1 lepra reaction is a delayed-type hypersensitivity reaction (type IV hypersensitivity reaction); type 2 lepra reaction, erythema nodosum leprosum (ENL), is thought to be an immune complex disorder. The reactions can occur during the natural course of untreated disease, during therapy, or after completion of multidrug therapy (MDT).

If the reactions are not managed promptly and appropriately, the patient experiences permanent nerve damage, which may result in severe permanent disability, for example, claw hands, claw toes, and/or foot drop. Deformities further lead to physical disabilities, and the associated social stigma often impairs the patient's ability to earn a living throughout his or her life. Even with adequate treatment, 40% of patients with T1LR may present with permanent nerve damage [1].

TYPE 1 LEPRA REACTION

Epidemiology

The prevalence rate of type 1 lepra reaction (T1LR) varies from 8.9% to 35.7% in various prospective and retrospective studies [2,3]. Type 1 reactions are known to occur in approximately 30% of patients in the borderline spectrum of leprosy [3]. Approximately 95% of T1LR cases are diagnosed simultaneously with leprosy or during the first 2 years of MDT [4,5].

Nerve function impairment (NFI) is the most dreaded complication of T1LR. Clinically detectable NFI occurs in approximately 10% of paucibacillary and 40% of multibacillary leprosy patients in patients with T1LR [6].

Etiopathogenesis

T1LR, also described as a "reversal" reaction, is a type IV hypersensitivity reaction that mainly occurs in borderline leprosy (BT, BB, BL) patients and those with cellular immune responses to *M. leprae* antigenic determinants, and it rarely occurs in polar lepromatous leprosy (LL) [7].

The natural tendency for borderline leprosy patients (not on any antileprosy treatment) is to downgrade slowly toward lepromatous pole. Therefore, T1LR associated with rapid increase in specific CMI, particularly seen in those receiving MDT, is known as upgrading or reversal reaction, and when there is evidence of T1LR with associated reduction in CMI, it is known as downgrading reaction [8–10].

Clinical features

Type 1 lepra reactions typically occur within the first 6 months after the start of MDT, although they can occur at any stage of the disease process even after completion of

MDT [11,12]. Risk factors for development of type 1LR are given in Box 58.1.

There may be redness, pain, swelling, and burning in pre-existing lesions. Lesions desquamate as they subside. Edema or erythema may develop over existing lesions (Figures 58.1 and 58.2) [13]. There may be an appearance of new lesions in previously uninvolved skin (Figures 58.3 and 58.4).

There may be rapid swelling of one or more nerves with serious motor disturbances such as palsy and deformities. Most at risk are the ulnar, lateral popliteal, and facial nerves. The involvement of the ulnar nerve in type ILR may lead to claw hand deformity (Figure 58.5), involvement of lateral popliteal nerve may lead to foot drop, and facial nerve involvement may cause facial palsy. Rarely, severe inflammation may result in a nerve abscess manifested as a fluctuant swelling, attached to the affected nerve (Figure 58.6) [8].

Edema of hands and feet with or without tenderness of the palms and soles is usually associated with T1LR [8].

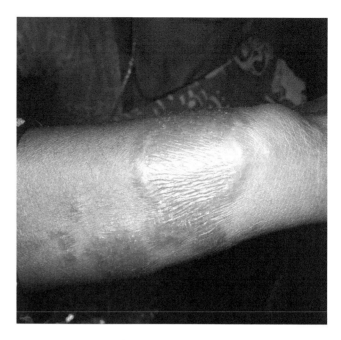

Figure 58.2 Type 1 lepra reaction over the elbow joint.

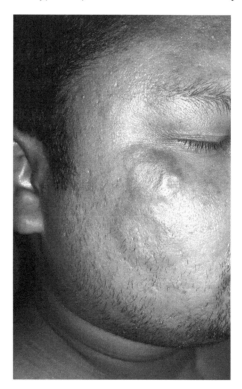

Figure 58.3 Type 1 lepra reaction over the face with appearance of new lesions.

MILD-TYPE 1LR

There is marked erythema, edema, pain, and tenderness in a few of the skin lesions.

SEVERE-TYPE 1LR

There is marked erythema, edema, pain, and tenderness in most of the skin lesions along with the appearance of new lesions over previously normal skin, nerve pain and

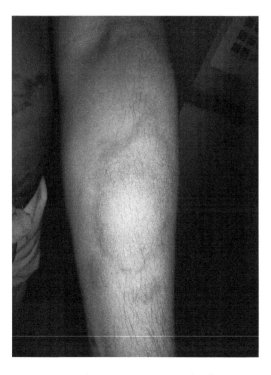

Figure 58.1 Type 1 lepra reaction over the forearm.

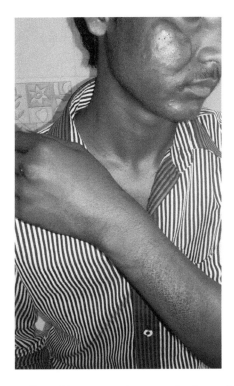

Figure 58.4 Type 1 lepra reaction over the face with a patch on left forearm

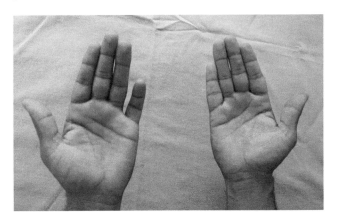

Figure 58.5 Ulnar claw.

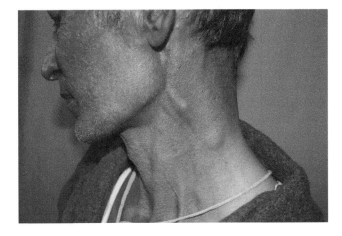

Figure 58.6 Nerve abscess—greater auricular nerve.

BOX 58.2: Complications of type 1 lepra reaction

- Facial palsy including lagophthalmos
- Iritis, scleritis, blindness
- Wrist drop
- Claw hand
- Foot drop

Source: van Brakel WH et al. *Lepr Rev* 2005;76:14–34; BrittonWJ,LockwoodDN.*Lancet*2004;363:1209–19.

tenderness, systemic symptoms like fever, arthralgia, edema of hands and feet, and ulcerative skin lesions. Complications of type 1LR are as given in Box 58.2.

Diagnosis

HISTOPATHOLOGY

The presence of granuloma edema (extracellular edema in and around the granuloma), dermal edema, plasma cells, and giant cells in the biopsy specimen suggests that a T1LR is taking place. In severe reaction, there can be breakdown and dispersal of the granuloma [13–15].

Treatment

The treatment of T1LRs is aimed at controlling the acute inflammation, relieving pain, and reversing nerve damage.

1. *Treatment of mild-type 1LR*
   a. Mild reaction may be treated with anti-inflammatory and nonsteroidal anti-inflammatory drugs (NSAIDS) for a few weeks.
   b. MDT should be initiated in those presenting with a T1LR or continued in those who develop a reaction while on MDT.
2. *Treatment of severe-type 1LR*
   a. *Bed rest*: Admission and bed rest for 2 weeks or more is usually advised. Rest to the affected nerve using a static splint may be tried. The splint is applied involving the joint in the vicinity of the affected nerve.
   b. *NSAIDs*: NSAIDs relieve symptoms by their analgesic and antipyretic effects.
   c. *Corticosteroids*: Individuals with severe inflamed skin lesions, neuritis, or nerve function impairment are treated with oral corticosteroids. Steroids cause inhibition of both the early and late phenomenon of inflammation. The early changes include edema, capillary dilation, influx of leukocytes, and phagocytic activity [16]. The later events of inflammation, which occur after several hours, like capillary and fibroblast proliferation, are also inhibited. They also help by their immunosuppressive action.

   Prednisolone is the most preferred drug. It should be started at a dose of 1 mg/kg of body weight and continued until the skin lesions improve, and nerve tenderness and pain subside. After the reaction/inflammation is controlled, prednisolone is tapered by 5 mg every 1–2 weeks. A maintenance dose of around 15–20 mg should be given for several weeks/months. After this, the dose should be cut by 5 mg every 2–3 months. Total duration of corticosteroids as advised by the World Health Organization (WHO) Global Strategy is 3–6 months [17].

Despite prolonged oral prednisolone, only 60% show improvement in nerve function. It has been seen that it is the duration rather than dose of treatment with prednisolone which is more important in controlling T1LR [18]. The treatment of patients with steroids is not beneficial if their NFI has been present for longer than 6 months [19].

d. *Other drugs*
   i. *Azathioprine*: In a trial, azathioprine in combination with a short course of prednisolone was as effective as a 12-week course of prednisolone in the management of T1LR [20].
   ii. *Cyclosporin A*: Cyclosporin A has been used in some studies with some success in T1LRs. It is administered with a starting dose of 5 mg/kg/day followed by gradual tapering of dose [21,22].
   iii. *Methotrexate*: Methotrexate has some efficacy in controlling reaction because of its anti-inflammatory properties.

e. *Surgical management*: The presence of abscess along the course of a nerve needs surgical intervention. In some cases, despite treatment with steroids for 2–4 weeks, pain along the affected nerve persists, and there is no improvement in motor function. To relieve nerve pain and restore nerve function, nerve pressure is relieved by surgery called *nerve decompression*. In nerve decompression, the affected nerve trunk is exposed at the point of maximum thickness. A longitudinal incision is given up to the epineurium layer.

TYPE 2 LEPRA REACTION

Epidemiology

ENL is the most common manifestation of type 2 LR (T2LR). The prevalence of ENL in BL and LL cases has wide geographic variation, varying from 19% to 26% in Asia to 37% in Brazil [2].

ENL reactions have been reported to occur in more than 50% of LL cases and in about 25% of borderline lepromatous (BL) cases in the pre-MDT era [23,12].

Etiopathogenesis

The type 2 lepra reaction is mediated by immune complexes and is therefore an example of type III hypersensitivity reaction. There is an increase in number of lymphocytes, mainly CD4 + Th2 cells, leading to an increase in the

---

BOX 58.3: Risk factors for type 2 lepra reaction

1. Lepromatous leprosy
2. Pregnancy and lactation
3. High bacteriological index (>4)
4. Bacterial or viral infection or parasitic infestation such as malaria, filariasis, and streptococcal infection
5. Emotional and psychological stress
6. History of surgery in recent past
7. Immunization

---

pro-inflammatory cytokines such as tumor necrosis factor alpha (TNF-α) and interferon gamma (IFN-γ) which induce cytotoxic activity and bacillary destruction, followed by the intensification of cytokine secretion like IL-4, IL5, IL-10, and IL-13, which activates the immune response.

There is a high concentration of IL-1 and TNF-α in T2LR. During episodes of reaction, the presence of cytokines like IL-4, IL-5, TNF-α and IFN-γ is responsible for the associated rise in temperature [24,25].

Risk factors: The risk factors for type 2LR are provided in Box 58.3.

Clinical features

In T2LR, the preexisting lesions of leprosy usually remain unaffected. ENL is the most common manifestation of T2LR. ENL can appear during different stages in the natural history of patients with the BL or LL form of disease, although these reactions often emerge when patients are taking MDT. Some patients continue to experience episodes of ENL reactions for many years even after stoppage of MDT. Most of the T2LRs occur during the first year of institution of MDT [26].

Symptoms of ENL are diverse. ENL presents with red, firm, painful, and tender cutaneous or subcutaneous lesions. Lesions appear in crops, preferentially on cooler parts of the skin (on the face and outer surfaces of limbs) and less frequently on the trunk. Warmer body sites such as the scalp, axillae, groin, and perineum are usually spared. Lesions are palpable rather than visible. Mostly lesions are distributed bilaterally and symmetrically (Figure 58.7). Lesions appear usually in the evening when the level of endogenously produced cortisol is very low.

These nodule crops are evanescent, melting away in 7–10 days. Sometimes pustular (Figure 58.8), vesicular, bullous, or necrotic lesions (Figures 58.9 and 58.10) may develop.

There may be associated fever, malaise, headache, joint pain, and other systemic inflammation affecting the nerves, eyes, testes, and lymph nodes [26]. There may be swelling of the hands and feet.

Ocular involvement can manifest as red, watery, and painful eyes. The pupil becomes constricted and nonreactive. The patient complains of photophobia. Involvement of

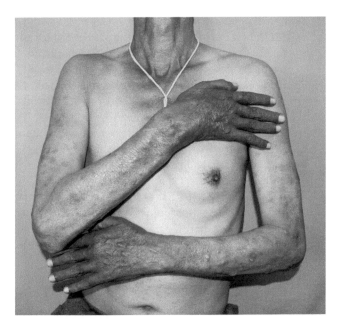

Figure 58.7 Symmetrical nodules on forearm in erythema nodosum leprosum.

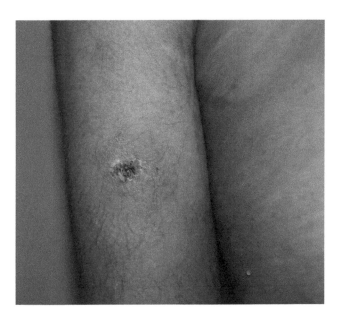

Figure 58.9 Necrotic erythema nodosum leprosum.

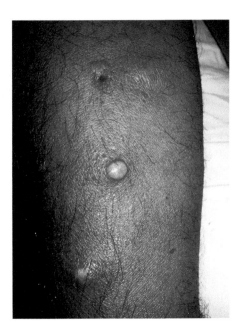

Figure 58.8 Pustular erythema nodosum leprosum.

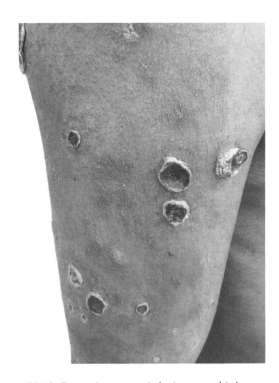

Figure 58.10 Extensive necrotic lesions on thighs.

the eyes in T2LR can be an emergency as there can be iridocyclitis, glaucoma, or even blindness. All such cases need immediate referral to an ophthalmologist.

In ENL, due to inflammatory edema, the peripheral nerves may be swollen, painful, or tender. However, in type 2 lepra reaction, the motor conduction abnormalities are not prominent and occur late [27].

Bone changes include periosteitis of the tibia, which clinically manifests as severe bone pain and swelling in the anterior aspect of the tibia. There may be osteoporosis due to excretion of calcium in urine during the reaction phase.

Other associated features in T2LRs are acute myositis and arthritis involving the knee, and metacarpophalangeal, interphalangeal, wrist, and ankle joints. There may be rhinitis, epistaxis, and laryngitis.

Other organs like liver, kidney, suprarenal glands, and testis may be involved resulting in features like hepatitis, glomerulonephritis, and epididymo-orchitis. In severe T2LR, the larynx may be affected, which may lead to death due to glottis edema. The systemic involvement in type 2LR is depicted in Box 58.4.

BOX 58.4: Multisystem involvement in type 2 lepra reaction

Skin: Classical erythema nodosum leprosum (painful tender nodules appearing in crops); bullous, pustular, ulcerative, or necrotic lesions
Nerve: Peripheral neuritis (swollen and tender nerves)
Bone: Periosteitis, osteoporosis
Eyes: Iritis, scleritis
Liver: Hepatitis
Genitourinary: Glomerulonephritis, renal amyloidosis, epididymoorchitis
Nose and respiratory system: Rhinitis, epistaxis, laryngitis

Diagnosis

HISTOPATHOLOGY

Histopathology of classical type 2 leprosy reaction (ENL) is characterized by dead (fragmented) bacilli, a large influx of neutrophils in the dermis, which is permeated by groups of vacuolated histiocytes containing bacilli. Neutrophils are distributed predominantly in the reticular portion of the dermis, in the dermohypodermic junction, and in the subcutaneous tissue. Vasculitis may be seen [28].

Differential diagnosis

ENL should be differentiated from lesions of erythema nodosum and other forms of panniculitis. ENL lesions differ from erythema nodosum by their evanescent nature and the large number of lesions involving sites other than the lower legs. ENL may also mimic Sweet syndrome and septicemia.

Bullous ENL can be considered in the differential diagnosis of immunobullous disorders. Ulcerated lesions should be differentiated from pyoderma gangrenosum. Chronic ENL may also mimic connective tissue disorders or lymphoreticular malignancies.

Investigations

- *Complete blood count*: Leukocytosis varies from 20,000 to 50,000. Erythrocyte sedimentation rate is elevated, and anemia may be seen.
- *Routine and microscopic examination of urine*: There may be the presence of red blood cells, pus cell, cast, or albumin.
- *Liver function test*: Raised serum bilirubin and transaminases.

Treatment

Type 2 reactions tend to be more dangerous than type 1 reactions, because of their systemic nature and the chances of recurrent episodes.

1. *Treatment of mild-type T2LR*
   a. *MDT*: MDT is to be started if the patient has come for the first time and MDT was not taken previously. Patients on MDT must continue their treatment. However, those who have completed their course of MDT do not need antileprosy treatment while on treatment for reaction.
   b. *Analgesics and anti-inflammatory agents*: Patients should be treated symptomatically with NSAIDs such as aspirin and paracetamol.
2. *Treatment of moderate T2LR*: Medication with anti-inflammatory properties has been used successfully.
   a. *Antimalarials*: Chloroquine is given in a dose of 250 mg thrice daily for a week, then tapered to 250 mg twice daily for the next week, and 250 mg daily for maintenance.
   b. *Colchicine*: Colchicine is given at a dose of 0.5 mg three times a day. It inhibits neutrophil chemotaxis, thereby preventing vascular injury [9].
3. *Treatment of severe T2LR*: The main aims in the management of ENL are the control of inflammation, pain relief, and prevention of further episodes.
   a. *Corticosteroids*: Prednisolone is commonly used for the management of moderate to severe ENL. It relieves pain and inflammation in the nerve and the skin. The usual adult dose of steroids is 0.5–1 mg/kg body weight. Duration of treatment is 12–24 weeks depending on the severity of reaction and response to the therapy. If inflammation of skin and nerve subsides and there is no new nerve involvement, the dose of prednisolone is gradually reduced by 10 mg fortnightly until the dose of 20 mg/day. Thereafter, prednisolone is tapered by 5 mg/day, fortnightly until withdrawal.
   b. *Thalidomide*: Thalidomide is very effective in the treatment of moderate to severe ENL. It has a rapid onset of action, and improvement is seen in 48–72 hours [30–35]. Treatment with thalidomide has also been shown to reduce the prednisolone requirement of patients with chronic ENL [36].

      Thalidomide is a potent inhibitor of *in vitro* TNF production, enabling the control of the diseases caused by this cytokine [24].

      Teratogenicity is the most important side effect. The use of thalidomide in women of childbearing age is restricted [25,31,37]. A negative pregnancy test should be obtained before starting thalidomide therapy. During use of thalidomide in women of the reproductive age group, it is absolutely mandatory to ensure contraception by two reliable methods for a period of 4 weeks before starting the drug, during the administration of the drug, and 4 weeks after administration of the drug.

      Another major side effect of thalidomide is peripheral neuropathy, mainly sensory [38,39]. A nerve conduction study of peripheral neuropathy induced by thalidomide reveals reduction of sensory nerve action potential amplitude and relative conservation of nerve conduction velocities.

Dosage: In severe ENL, thalidomide should be started at a dose of 400 mg at night. This dose controls reaction within 48 hours in most of the cases. Then the dose should be reduced to 300 mg as soon as possible. This dose can then be reduced by 100 mg per month, but a maintenance dose may be required in those with chronic disease. Every 6 months, attempts should be made to discontinue the drug after gradual tapering of the dose. Controlling ENL by replacing the steroid with thalidomide is more difficult than using thalidomide from the beginning [40].

c. *Clofazimine*: Clofazimine is an anti-inflammatory agent. It can be used for the treatment of mild to moderate ENL at a dose of up to 300 mg daily orally for a period of 1 month followed by 200 mg daily for 3–6 months and 100 mg daily as maintenance [41]. This higher dose should not be continued for more than 12 months.

d. *Other drugs*
   i. *NSAIDs*: NSAIDs have also been tried in reactions of leprosy. They relieve symptoms by their analgesic and antipyretic effects.
   ii. *Pentoxifylline*: Pentoxifylline interferes in the TNF-α and IL-1 levels, which act against leprosy reactions, and should therefore be considered an alternative drug in the management of ENL [42].
   iii. *Cyclosporine*: The use of immune-suppressive drugs such as cyclosporine has been shown to be helpful for patients who develop intolerance to steroids or who experience severe side effects from steroids [11].
   iv. *Methotrexate*: Methotrexate has shown some efficacy in management of ENL [11].
   v. *Mycophenolate mofetil*: Mycophenolate mofetil is a reversible inhibitor of inosine monophosphate dehydrogenase. It causes immune suppression by affecting both B- and T-lymphocyte activity.
   vi. *Etanercept*: Etanercept, a TNF-α antagonist, has shown good results on the treatment of the type II reaction of leprosy [43].
   vii. *Infliximab*: Infliximab used in patients with ENL that was nonresponsive to prednisone, pentoxifylline, and thalidomide in a dose of 5 mg/kg has shown significant reduction in symptoms. After two administrations of infliximab during weeks 2 and 6, and with a follow-up of 1 year, no further episodes of ENL were described [44,45].
   viii. *Azathioprine*: Some success has been reported for the use of the drug azathioprine in patients with frequent ENL recurrences [46].
   ix. *Plasmapheresis*: Plasmapheresis has been employed in the treatment of type 2 lepra reactions and involves replacement of plasma of the patient with sterile albumin solution. Its possible mechanism includes dilution of

BOX 58.5: Treatment approach to type 2 lepra reaction (T2LR)

	Mild T2LR	Moderate T2LR	Severe T2LR
Erythema nodosum leprosum (ENL) lesions	Few ENL lesions	Few ENL lesions	Pustular/necrotic ENL lesions
Fever	Absent	Mild (<100°F)	High-grade fever
Organ involvement	NIL	Some organs involved except nerve, eye, and testis	Neuritis Arthritis Orchitis Iridocyclitis Albuminuria
Treatment	1. Reassurance 2. Initiation/continuation of multidrug therapy 3. Nonsteroidal anti-inflammatory drugs (NSAIDs)	1. NSAIDs 2. Antimalarials (chloroquine) 3. Antimonials (sodium stibogluconate) 4. Colchicine	1. Corticosteroids 2. Thalidomide 3. Chloroquine 4. Clofazimine 5. Pentoxifylline 6. Cyclosporine 7. Methotrexate 8. Etanercept 9. Infliximab 10. Plasmapheresis

immune complex and/or free antigens and antibodies [29].

An approach to treatment of type 2LR is provided in Box 58.5. [47,48]

Lucio phenomenon

This is an uncommon third type of lepra reaction seen in Lucio leprosy. Here the patient presents with recurrent multiple ischemic and necrotic ulcers on the extremities. Pathogenesis is immune complex deposition triggered by a huge endothelial cell infiltration by the bacilli, leading to vasculitis and thrombosis. Secondary infection can lead to sepsis. Treatment is with oral corticosteroids along with MDT.

CONCLUSION

Leprosy reactions are medical emergency conditions, and their management continues to be a major challenge. If not managed immediately, leprosy reactions may lead to serious consequences like permanent disability, blindness, multiorgan involvement, and death. So, early detection and management of lepra reactions are very important in preventing nerve function impairment, disability, deformity, and death. Patients should be educated to recognize symptoms of reaction, seek medical advice immediately, and undergo regular follow-up examinations.

KEY POINTS

- Type 1 lepra reaction is a delayed-type hypersensitivity reaction while type 2 lepra reaction is an immune complex disorder.
- Nerve function impairment is the most dreaded complication of T1LR.
- Facial palys, lagophthalmos, iritis, scleritis, blindness, wrist drop, claw hand and foot drop may occur in type 1 Lepra reaction
- ENL presents with crops of red, firm, painful, and tender cutaneous or subcutaneous lesions.
- Peripheral neuritis, periosteitis, iritis, scleritis,
- hepatitis, glomerulonephritis, renal amyloidosis, epididymoorchitis, rhinitis, epistaxis and laryngitis may occur as part of type 2 lepra reaction.
- Steroids are the drugs of choice for lepra reactions while Thalidomide is very useful in type 2 reaction.

REFERENCES

1. Verhagen CE, Wierenga EA, Buffing AA, Chand MA, Faber WR, Das PK. Reversal reaction in borderline leprosy is associated with a polarized shift to type 1-like *Mycobacterium leprae* T cell reactivity in lesional skin: A follow-up study. *J Immunol* 1997;159:4474–83.

2. Kahawita IP, Walker SL, Lockwood DNJ. Leprosy type 1 reactions and erythema nodosum leprosum. *An Bras Dermatol* 2008;83:75–82.

3. Walker SL, Lockwood DNJ. Leprosy type 1 (reversal) reactions and their management. *Lepr Rev* 2008;79:372–86.

4. Pandhi D, Chhabra N. New insights in the pathogenesis of type 1 and type 2 lepra reaction. *Indian J Dermatol Venereol Leprol* 2013;79:739.

5. Scollard DM et al. Risk factors for leprosy reactions in three endemic countries. *Am J Trop Med Hyg* 2015;92:108–14.

6. Richardus JH, Finlay KM, Croft RP, Smith WC. Nerve function impairment in leprosy at diagnosis and at completion of MDT: A retrospective cohort study of 786 patients in Bangladesh. *Lepr Rev* 1996;67:297–305.

7. Scollard DM, Smith T, Bhoopat L, Theetranont C, Rangdaeng S, Morens DM. Epidemiologic characteristics of leprosy reactions. *Int J Lepr Other Mycobact Dis* 1994;62:559–67.

8. Jopling WH, Mcdougall AC (Eds). *Handbook of Leprosy*. 5th ed. CBS; 2013:82–91.

9. Kar HK, Kumar B (Eds), *IAL Textbook of Leprosy*. New Delhi: Jaypee Brothers Medical Publishers; 2010:269–89.

10. Skoff AM, Lisak RP, Bealmear B, Benjamins JA. TNF-alpha and TGF-beta act synergistically to kill Schwann cells. *J Neurosci Res* 1998 15;53:747–56.

11. Franco-Paredes C, Jacob JT, Stryjewska B, Yoder L. Two patients with leprosy and the sudden appearance of inflammation in the skin and new sensory loss. *PLOS Negl Trop Dis* 2009;3:e425.

12. Kumar B, Dogra S, Kaur I. Epidemiological characteristics of leprosy reactions: 15 years experience from North India. *Int J Lepr Other Mycobact Dis* 2004;72:125–33.

13. van Brakel WH et al. The INFIR Cohort Study: Investigating prediction, detection and pathogenesis of neuropathy and reactions in leprosy. Methods and baseline results of a cohort of multibacillary leprosy patients in north India. *Lepr Rev* 2005;76:14–34.

14. Britton WJ, Lockwood DN. Leprosy. *Lancet* 2004;363:1209–19.

15. Adhe V, Dongre A, Khopkar U. A retrospective analysis of histopathology of 64 cases of lepra reactions. *Indian J Dermatol* 2012;57:114–7.

16. Haynes RCLJ Jr. Pharmacological basis of therapeutics. In: Gilman AG, Goodman LS (Eds), *Pharmacological Basis of Therapeutics*. 5th ed. London: Macmillan; 1975:1487–8.

17. World Health Organization. Global Strategy for Further Reducing the Leprosy Burden and Sustaining Leprosy Control Activities. 2006.

18. Rao PSSS, Sugamaran DST, Richard J, Smith WCS. Multi-centre, double blind, randomized trial of three

steroid regimens in the treatment of type-1 reactions in leprosy. *Lepr Rev* 2006;77:25–33.

19. Richardus JH et al. Treatment with corticosteroids of long-standing nerve function impairment in leprosy: A randomized controlled trial (TRIPOD 3). *Lepr Rev* 2003;74:311–8.

20. Marlowe SN, Hawksworth RA, Butlin CR, Nicholls PG, Lockwood DN. Clinical outcomes in a random-ized controlled study comparing azathioprine and prednisolone versus prednisolone alone in the treat-ment of severe leprosy type 1 reactions in Nepal. *Trans R Soc Trop Med Hyg* 2004;98:602–9.

21. Marlowe SNS et al. Response to ciclosporin treat-ment in Ethiopian and Nepali patients with severe leprosy type 1 reactions. *Trans R Soc Trop Med Hyg* 2007;101:1004–12.

22. Sena CBCD, Salgado CG, Tavares CMP, Da Cruz CAV, Xavier MB, Do Nascimento JLM. Cyclosporine A treat-ment of leprosy patients with chronic neuritis is asso-ciated with pain control and reduction in antibodies against nerve growth factor. *Lepr Rev* 2006;77:121–9.

23. Van Brakel WH, Khawas IB, Lucas SB. Reactions in leprosy: An epidemiological study of 386 patients in west Nepal. *Lepr Rev* 1994;65:190–203.

24. Santos JRS et al. Etanercept in erythema nodosum leprosum. *An Bras Dermatol. Sociedade Brasileira de Dermatologia* 2017;92:575–7.

25. Sampaio EP, Malta AM, Sarno EN, Kaplan G. Effect of rhuIFN-gamma treatment in multibacillary leprosy patients. *Int J Lepr Other Mycobact Dis* 1996;64:268–73.

26. Pocaterra L et al. Clinical course of erythema nodo-sum leprosum: An 11-year cohort study in Hyderabad, India. *Am J Trop Med Hyg* 2006;74:868–79.

27. Singh S, Gupta S, Mukhija R, Thacker A. Electrophysiological study of nerves in type-II reac-tion in leprosy. *Indian J Dermatol* 2017;62:644–8.

28. Sarita S et al. A study on histological features of lepra reactions in patients attending the Dermatology Department of the Government Medical College, Calicut, Kerala, India. *Lepr Rev* 2013;84:51–64.

29. Girdhar BK. Immuno pharmacology of drugs used in leprosy reactions. *Indian J Dermatol Venereol Leprol* 1990;56:354–63.

30. Diggle GE. Thalidomide: 40 years on. *Int J Clin Pract* 2001;55:627–31.

31. Barnes PF, Chatterjee D, Brennan PJ, Rea TH, Modlin RL. Tumor necrosis factor production in patients with leprosy. *Infect Immun* 1992;60:1441–6.

32. Foss NT, de Oliveira EB, Silva CL. Correlation between TNF production, increase of plasma C-reactive protein level and suppression of T lymphocyte response to concanavalin A during erythema nodosum leprosum. *Int J Lepr Other Mycobact Dis* 1993;61:218–26.

33. Sales AM, de Matos HJ, Nery JAC, Duppre NC, Sampaio EP, Sarno EN. Double-blind trial of the efficacy of pentoxifylline vs thalidomide for the treatment of type II reaction in leprosy. *Brazilian J Med Biol Res Rev Bras Pesqui Medicas E Biol* 2007; 40:243–8.

34. Iyer CG et al. WHO co-ordinated short-term double-blind trial with thalidomide in the treatment of acute lepra reactions in male lepromatous patients. *Bull World Health Organ* 1971;45:719–32.

35. Putinatti MSMA, Lastória JC, Padovani CR. Prevention of repeated episodes of type 2 reaction of leprosy with the use of thalidomide 100 mg/day. *An Bras Dermatol* 2014;89:266–73.

36. Vázquez-Botet M, Sánchez JL. Erythema nodosum leprosum. *Int J Dermatol* 1987;26:436–7.

37. Lary JM, Daniel KL, Erickson JD, Roberts HE, Moore CA. The return of thalidomide: Can birth defects be prevented? *Drug Saf* 1999;21:161–9.

38. Fullerton PM, O'Sullivan DJ. Thalidomide neuropa-thy: A clinical electrophysiological, and histologi-cal follow-up study. *J Neurol Neurosurg Psychiatry* 1968;31:543–51.

39. Clemmensen OJ, Olsen PZ, Andersen KE. Thalidomide neurotoxicity. *Arch Dermatol* 1984;120:338–41.

40. Walker SL, Waters MFR, Lockwood DNJ. The role of thalidomide in the management of erythema nodosum leprosum. *Lepr Rev* 2007;78:197–215.

41. Mason GH, Ellis-Pegler RB, Arthur JF. Clofazimine and eosinophilic enteritis. *Lepr Rev* 1977;48:175–80.

42. Talhari S, Orsi AT, Talhari AC, Souza FH, Ferreira LC. Pentoxifylline may be useful in the treatment of type 2 leprosy reaction. *Lepr Rev* 1995;66:261–3.

43. Ramien ML, Wong A, Keystone JS. Severe refractory erythema nodosum leprosum successfully treated with the tumor necrosis factor inhibitor etanercept. *Clin Infect Dis* 2011;52:e133–5.

44. Faber WR, Jensema AJ, Goldschmidt WFM. Treatment of recurrent erythema nodosum leprosum with infliximab. *N Engl J Med* 2006;355:739–739.

45. Mahajan PM, Jadhav VH, Patki AH, Jogaikar DG, Mehta JM. Oral zinc therapy in recurrent erythema nodosum leprosum: A clinical study. *Indian J Lepr* 1994;66:51–7.

46. Vikram Jitendra SS, Bachaspatimayum R, Devi AS, Rita S. Azathioprine in chronic recalcitrant erythema nodosum leprosum: A case report. *J Clin Diagnostic Res* 2017;11:FD01–2.

47. Verhaegen H, De Cree J, De Cock W, Verbruggen F. Restoration by levamisole of low E-rosette form-ing cells in patients suffering from various diseases. *Clin Exp Immunol* 1977;27:313–8.

48. Girdhar A, Chakma JK, Girdhar BK. Pulsed cortico-steroid therapy in patients with chronic recurrent ENL: A pilot study. *Indian J Lepr* 2002;74:233–6.

59

Leprosy: Therapy-related emergencies

G. K. SINGH AND ANUJ BHATNAGAR

INTRODUCTION

The World Health Organization (WHO) has recommended the use of multidrug therapy (MDT) constituting dapsone (DDS), rifampicin, and clofazimine since 1981 [1]. Initially, MDT for multibacillary patients (MB-MDT) was recommended for a 24-month period. Subsequently, the WHO Expert Committee on Leprosy (1998) recommended shortening MB-MDT to 12 months. The introduction of MDT by the WHO was aimed to control primary and secondary resistance to drug monotherapy, to prevent further resistance of *Mycobacterium leprae* to other antibiotics, and also to prevent relapses [2].

It is not uncommon to find adverse effects of MDT during routine therapy. Different studies indicate that almost 30%–40% patients of leprosy will have adverse effects [3–5]. There are instances when the treating physician or dermatologist encounters life-threatening adverse effects, for example, dapsone hypersensitivity syndrome, methemoglobinemia, hemolytic anemia, agranulocytosis, thrombocytopenia, hepatitis, fatal enteropathy, etc. [10,11]. Alternative drugs such as minocycline, ofloxacin, and clarithromycin are infrequently used or their serious side effects are very rare; so these conditions are not covered in this chapter. Three common drugs used as MDT with their brief pharmacological properties and adverse effects are presented in Table 59.1.

Drug hypersensitivity syndrome due to dapsone

(*Synonyms*: Sulfone syndrome, dapsone hypersensitivity syndrome, fifth-week dapsone dermatitis)

Drug hypersensivity syndrome (DHS) is an idiosyncratic multiorgan disease characterized by some or all of the following features: exfoliative dermatitis and/or other skin rashes, generalized lymphadenopathy, fever, hepatitis, and hepatosplenomegaly [12]. The term *drug reaction* *with eosinophilia and systemic symptoms* (DRESS) is interchangeably used in the literature.

The exact incidence of DHS is not known, but it is reported to occur in less than 1% of patients treated with dapsone, and gradually this condition is showing a rising trend [13–18].

DDS gets metabolized by either N-acetylation or N-hydroxylation. The N-acetylation pathway has no role in any of the adverse effects. Hydroxylamine, which is a toxic intermediate metabolite formed by the N-hydroxylation pathway, is responsible for hemolytic anemia, methemoglobinemia, and DHS [7,19]. An association between HLA-B*13:01 and DHS, which has overlapping clinical features with DRESS, has been found in a genome-wide Chinese study [20].

The onset of DHS usually occurs within 2–6 weeks of start of therapy, so it is also known as *fifth-week dapsone dermatitis*. Erythroderma (Figure 59.1), morbilliform eruption, erythema multiforme, toxic epidermal necrolysis (TEN), and Stevens-Johnson syndrome–like eruptions may be the cutaneous presentation [21,22]. It is not difficult to diagnose DHS in the setting of leprosy. However, lepra reaction, other causes such as TEN, Stevens-Johnson syndrome, and viral exanthem need to be excluded [22,23].

On investigation, these patients of DHS may have the following features: (1) leukocytosis with eosinophil counts >700/microL; (2) atypical lymphocytosis with large activated lymphocytes, lymphoblasts, or mononucleosis-like cells; (3) increased serum alanine aminotransferase; (4) reactivation of human herpesvirus-6 (HHV-6) and other viruses; and (5) other features depending on the organ involved, for example, hepatitis, interstitial nephritis, etc. [24,25]. It may ultimately lead to multiorgan failure.

The first and most important aspect in the management of DHS is discontinuation of dapsone. Supportive treatment should include fluid and electrolyte balance, regulation of body temperature, nutritional support, and antibiotics when necessary. The addition of drugs should be avoided. Skin care with emollients and avoidance of irritants are

Table 59.1 Summary of adverse effects of multidrug therapy in leprosy

Multidrug therapy drug	Common or less serious adverse effects	Serious adverse effects
Dapsone	Gastrointestinal irritation, headache, nervousness, insomnia, blurred vision, paresthesia, reversible neuropathy, skin rashes, psychoses, and hepatitis	Drug hypersensitivity syndrome, hemolytic anemia, agranulocytosis, methemoglobinemia
Clofazimine	Reversible skin discoloration, discoloration of the hair, cornea, conjunctiva, tears, sweat, sputum, feces and urine, dose-related gastrointestinal symptoms include pain, nausea, vomiting, and diarrhea	Enteropathy (clofazimine-induced histiocytosis)
Rifampicin	Gastrointestinal intolerance, skin rashes, fever, influenza-like syndrome	Thrombocytopenia, hemolytic anemia, hepatitis, acute renal failure

equally important. There are no well-controlled trials to evaluate the effectiveness of any drug to treat such a serious condition. However, traditionally, systemic glucocorticoid in a dose of 1–2 mg/kg/day is recommended. Considering the long retention period (35 days) of dapsone in the human body, which may be due to hepatic storage and enterohepatic circulation, the corticosteroids should be administered for 2–3 months and tapered gradually [22–25].

Dapsone-induced methemoglobinemia

Methemoglobin is an abnormal form of hemoglobin resulting from the oxidation of iron in the normal heme molecule from the ferrous form ($Fe2+$) to the ferric ($Fe3+$) form. The presence of ferric heme molecules causes a structural change in the hemoglobin, resulting in reduced oxygen-carrying capacity and impaired oxygen delivery at the tissue [26,27]. Naturally, red blood cells maintain a steady-state level of methemoglobin

of less than 1% via two main enzymatic pathways. Patients with G6PD deficiency are at increased risk of oxidative stress because of depletion of reduced glutathione. Exogenous oxidizing agents can challenge the cytochrome b5 reductase system, leading to increased production of methemoglobin [26].

Clinical symptoms of methemoglobinemia depend on the serum concentration of methemoglobin. Peripheral and central cyanosis are usually seen at a serum methemoglobin level of 15% (Figure 59.2). Methemoglobin levels of 30%–45% result in tachycardia, weakness, headache, fatigue, and dizziness, while levels above 60% result in dyspnea, seizures, cardiac arrhythmia, and coma. Mortality happens at methemoglobin levels greater than 70% [28].

Diagnosis of methemoglobinemia is normally based on characteristic clinical symptoms and raised serum methemoglobin level. Serum methemoglobin levels are not routinely available in a resource-poor setup. Therefore, the typical oxygen "saturation gap" observed between arterial blood gas analysis and pulse oximetry readings is very helpful for making the diagnosis of methemoglobinemia. Once other forms of

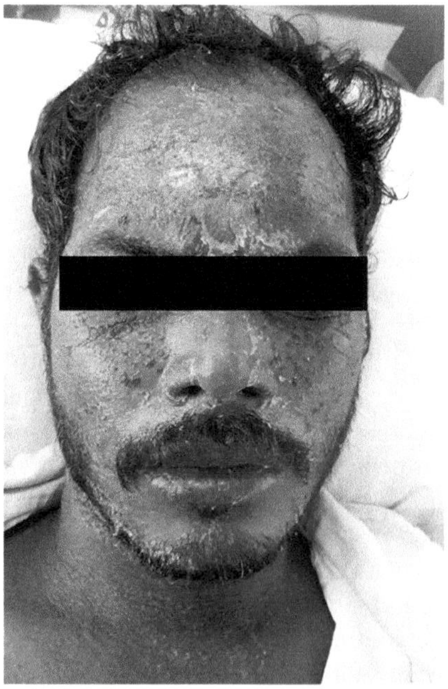

Figure 59.1 Drug hypersensitivity syndrome to dapsone in a patient of Hansen disease (borderline tuberculoid). Severe erythema and scaling involving the face can be noted.

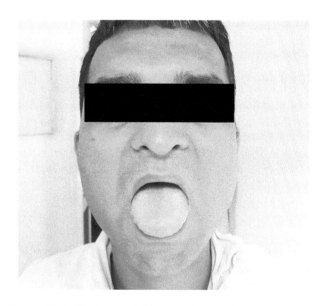

Figure 59.2 Methemoglobinemia due to dapsone seen as cyanosis of the tongue in a patient of Hansen disease (borderline tuberculoid). (Image courtesy of Joyjit Das, Dermatologist, 158 Base Hospital.)

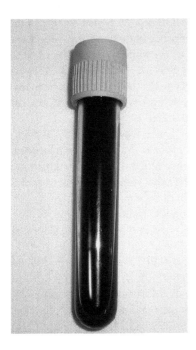

Figure 59.3 Chocolate-brown color of venous blood in a patient of methemoglobinemia. (Image courtesy of Joyjit Das, Dermatologist, 158 Base Hospital.)

hemoglobin such as methemoglobin rise, the oxygen saturation on pulse oximetry falls and plateaus at 85%. This situation, where oxygen saturation levels measured with pulse oximetry are substantially lower than arterial blood gas oxygen saturation levels, should alarm the treating physician. Also, in cases of methemoglobinemia, arterial blood samples will have a typical chocolate-brown color (Figure 59.3) [28,29]. Since its advent, the carbon monoxide (CO) oximeter has become the gold standard in diagnosing methemoglobinemia [29].

Initial management of patients with methemoglobinemia is supportive care with discontinuation of the offending agent. In asymptomatic patients, usually those with methemoglobin levels <20%, no therapy other than discontinuation of the DDS is required. For patients with signs of hypoxia or methemoglobin levels exceeding 30%, administration of IV methylene blue at 1–2 mg/kg is required. Methylene blue should not be administered to patients with known G6PD deficiency, since the reduction of methemoglobin by methylene blue is dependent on NADPH generated by G6PD [26,28]. The appropriate treatment for such patients is ascorbic acid. Severely affected patients may benefit from adjunctive treatment with blood transfusion, exchange transfusion, and/or hyperbaric oxygen [30,31]. Cimetidine, an inhibitor of cytochrome P450, can be used as a prophylactic drug when a higher dosage of dapsone is required [32].

Dapsone-induced hemolytic anemia and agranulocytosis

Leprosy patients who are deficient in glucose-6–phosphate dehydrogenase (G6PD) are at risk of severe and potentially fatal hemolysis due to dapsone. Hemolytic anemia is one of the causes, which often leads to stoppage of dapsone during treatment [7,33,34]. Agranulocytosis is a rare but very serious complication of DDS. It has been reported to occur in 0.2%–0.4% of patients treated with dapsone. Agranulocytosis is an acute condition characterized by a sudden drop in white cell production leaving the body susceptible to bacterial infection and septicemia. Though reversible, it can be fatal if timely management is not started. The mechanism is the same as for methemoglobinemia and hemolytic anemia, that is, formation of hydroxylamine, the toxic metabolite of dapsone that ultimately leads to depression of bone marrow. Agranulocytosis due to dapsone is not dose related, and when severe, can also involve platelets causing thrombocytopenia [35,36]. It is neutropenia, which is noticed earliest, usually at 3 weeks. Fever, pallor, and pharyngitis in a patient of leprosy on the first few months of dapsone should be taken as warning symptoms. Agranulocytosis should be excluded at the earliest in such cases [35,37]. Prompt treatment with antibiotics and G-CSF is essential for the survival of the patient.

To monitor any adverse effects of MDT, total leukocyte count with differential counts and hemoglobin levels along with liver and renal function tests with enzymes should be done weekly for the first month of therapy, twice monthly for the next 2 months, and periodically thereafter [35–37].

Clofazimine-induced enteropathy

Clofazimine is a lipophilic iminophenazine dye, having both antimicrobial and anti-inflammatory activities. Being lipophilic, it concentrates well in the lipid-rich tissues, particularly the reticuloendothelial system and intestine, breast, and liver. The skin, gastrointestinal tract, and eyes are the most common sites affected by clofazimine. It has a long half-life of approximately 70 days. Clofazimine in the usual recommended dosage (50 mg OD or 100 mg alternate day) as a component of MDT is well tolerated. However, the higher dosage commonly used in lepra reactions can cause enteritis [6,8,9]. In a review of 14 cases of clofazimine enteropathy, 10 patients (71.4%) had to undergo exploratory laparotomy [38].

Patients present with epigastric distress, occasional vomiting unrelated to meals, intermittent abdominal pain, malabsorption, and abdominal rebound tenderness. Barium swallow shows coarsening of the mucosal pattern and segmentation of barium in the ileum and distal jejunum. Biopsy of the jejunum demonstrates red crystals in the lamina propria accompanied by a moderate number of plasma cells [38–40]. Clofazimine has been reported to induce three types of enteropathy:

1. Eosinophilic/allergic pattern
2. Crohn disease–like pattern with granulomas
3. Clofazimine-induced crystal-storing histiocytosis [41]

Cessation of clofazimine induces clinical improvement in most cases; however, abdominal symptoms may persist for several months to years [42].

Emergencies due to rifampicin

A single dose of rifampicin every month is very rarely reported to cause any side effects in cases of leprosy. Hepatotoxicity is the most common serious adverse effect. However, the treating physician should be watchful for serious side effects such as hemolysis, renal failure, and thrombocytopenia. Multiple ecchymoses, bleeding from gums, and very low platelet count (<20,000/cmm) can be the presentations of thrombocytopenia. Rifampicin should be discontinued and replaced with alternative MDT such as ofloxacin and minocycline. It generally recovers in 2–3 weeks. For major or life-threatening bleeding, platelet transfusions should be administered without delay [43,44].

CONCLUSION

The introduction of MDT in the treatment of leprosy has been one the greatest boons to mankind. Millions of leprosy patients have been cured of the disease. MDT and even alternative drugs are usually very safe, even in the long term. However, drugs used in leprosy may rarely cause life-threatening emergencies. Understanding the pharmacology of the drugs, monitoring their use, watching for subtle alarming signs and symptoms, and having a high index of suspicion can save many valuable lives.

KEY POINTS

- Treatment of leprosy is usually very safe. However, rarely the treatments can cause serious, life-threatening adverse effects due to MDT.
- Dapsone is the most common drug to cause serious adverse effects such as dapsone hypersensitivity syndrome, methemoglobinemia, hemolytic anemia, and agranulocytosis. Clofazimine can cause enteropathy, and rifampicin can lead to hepatotoxicity and thrombocytopenia.
- Awareness of clinical features of such serious conditions, routine baseline investigations, follow-up investigations, G6PD testing before starting dapsone, and prompt management can save patients of leprosy from having life-threatening emergencies.

REFERENCES

1. World Health Organization. Global leprosy update 2015. *Wkly Epidemiol Rec* 2016;91:405–20.
2. Morel CM. *Foreword. Multi Drug Therapy against Leprosy. Development and Implementation over the Past 25 Years.* Geneva: World Health Organization; 2004:vii.
3. Goulart IMB et al. Adverse effects of multidrug therapy in leprosy patients: A five-year survey at a Health Centre of the Federal University of Uberlândia. *Rev Soc Bras Med Trop* 2002;35:453–60.
4. Deps PD et al. Adverse effects from multi-drug therapy in leprosy: A Brazilian study. *Lepr Rev* 2007;78.3:216–22.
5. Singh H, Nel B, Dey V, Tiwari P, Dulhani N. Adverse effects of multi-drug therapy in leprosy, a two years' experience (2006–2008) in tertiary health care centre in the tribal region of Chhattisgarh State (Bastar, Jagdalpur). *Lepr Rev* 2011;82:17.
6. Jacobson RR. Treatment of leprosy. In: Hastings RC (Ed), *Leprosy.* 2nd ed. London: Churchill Livingstone; 1994:317–49.
7. Sago J, Hall RP. Dapsone. *Dermatol Ther* 2002;15:340–51.
8. Arbiser JL, Moschella SL. Clofazimine: A review of its medical uses and mechanisms of action. *J Am Acad Dermatol* 1995;32:241–7.
9. Morrison NE, Morley GM. The mode of action of clofazimine: DNA binding studies. *Int J Lepr* 1976;44:133–5.
10. Hardman JG, Limbird LE, Gilman AG (Eds). *"Rifampin." The Pharmacological Basis of Therapeutics.* 10th ed. New York: McGraw-Hill; 2001;1277–79.
11. Girling DJ. Adverse effects of antituberculosis drugs. *Drugs* 1982;23.1–2:56–74.
12. Uetrecht JP. Idiosyncratic drug reactions: Possible role of reactive metabolites generated by leukocytes. *Pharm Res* 1989;6:265–73.
13. Lowe J, Smith M. The chemotherapy of leprosy in Nigeria. *Int J Lepr* 1949;17:181–95.
14. Alldy EJ, Barnes J. Toxic effects of diaminodiphenyl sulphone in the treatment of leprosy. *Lancet* 1951;2:205–6.
15. Millikan LE, Harrell ER. Drug reactions to the sulfones. *Arch Dermatol* 1970;102:220–4.
16. Mohamed KN. Hypersensitivity reaction to dapsone: Report from Malaysia. *Lepr Rev* 1984;55:385–9.
17. Rao PN, Lakshmi TS. Increase in the incidence of dapsone hypersensitivity syndrome—An appraisal. *Lepr Rev* 2001;72:57–62.
18. Kumar RH, Kumar MV, Thappa DM. Dapsone syndrome—A five-year retrospective analysis. *Indian J Lepr* 1998;70:271–6.
19. Kosseifi SG et al. The dapsone hypersensitivity syndrome revisited: A potentially fatal multisystem disorder with prominent hepatopulmonary manifestations. *J Occup Med Toxicol* 2006;1:9.
20. Zhang FR et al. HLA-B*13:01 and the dapsone hypersensitivity syndrome. *N Engl J Med* 2013;369:1620.
21. Gokhale NR, Sule RR, Gharpure MB. Dapsone syndrome. *Indian J Dermatol Venereol Leprol* 1992;58:376–8.

22. Thappa DM, Sethuraman G. Dapsone (sulfone) syndrome (CME). *Indian J Dermatol Venereol Leprol* 2000;66:117–20.

23. Prussik R, Shear NH. Dapsone hypersensitivity syndrome. *J Am Acad Dermatol* 1996;35:346–9.

24. Cacoub P et al. The DRESS syndrome: A literature review. *Am J Med* 2011;124:588.

25. Kardaun SH et al. Drug reaction with eosinophilia and systemic symptoms (DRESS): An original multisystem adverse drug reaction. Results from the prospective RegiSCAR study. *Br J Dermatol* 2013;169:1071.

26. Zosel A, Rychter K, Leikin JB. Dapsone-induced methemoglobinemia: Case report and literature review. *Am J Ther* 2007;14:585–7.

27. Ash-Bernal R, Wise R, Wright SM. Acquired methemoglobinemia: A retrospective series of 138 cases at 2 teaching hospitals. *Medicine (Baltim)* 2004;83:265–73.

28. Ashurst JV, Wasson MN, Hauger W, Fritz WT. Pathophysiologic mechanisms, diagnosis, and management of dapsone-induced methemoglobinemia. *J Am Osteopath Assoc* 2010;110:16–20.

29. Das J, Katyal A, Naunwaar D. Dapsone-induced methemoglobinemia in a patient of leprosy. *Indian J Dermatol* 2015;60:108.

30. Nitzan M, Romem A, Koppel R. Pulse oximetry: Fundamentals and technology update. *Med Devices (Auckl)* 2014;7:231–9.

31. Park SY, Lee KW, Kang TS. High-dose vitamin C management in dapsone-induced methemoglobinemia. *Am J Emerg Med* 2014;32:684.

32. Scheinfeld N. Cimetidine: A review of the recent developments and reports in cutaneous medicine. *Dermatol Online J* 2003;9:4.

33. Deps P, Guerra P, Nasser S, Simon M. Hemolytic anemia in patients receiving daily dapsone for the treatment of leprosy. *Lepr Rev* 2012;83:305.

34. Grossman S, Budinscki R, Jollow D. Dapsone-induced hemolytic anemia: role of glucose-6-phosphatodehydrogenase in the hemolytic response of rat erythrocytes to N-hydroxydapsone. *J Pharmacol Exp Ther* 1995;272:870–77.

35. Woodbury GR, Fried W, Ertle JO, Malkinson FD. Dapsone associated agranulocytosis and severe anemia in a patient with leukocytoclastic vasculitis. *J Am Acad Dermatol* 1993;28:781–3.

36. Jacobus DP. Dapsone. In: Millikan LE (Ed), *Drug Therapy in Dermatology*. New York: Marcel Dekker; 2000:445–75.

37. Bhat RM, Radhakrishnan K. A case report of total dapsone induced agranulocytosis in an Indian mid-borderline leprosy patient. *Lepr Rev* 2003;74:167–70.

38. Pais AV, Pereira S, Garg I, Stephen J, Antony M, Inchara YK. Intra-abdominal, crystal storing histiocytosis due to clofazimine in a patient with lepromatous leprosy and concurrent carcinoma of the colon. *Lepr Rev* 2004;75:171–6.

39. Sukapanichnant S et al. Clofazimine-induced crystal-storing histiocytosis producing chronic abdominal pain in a leprosy patient. *Am J Surg Pathol* 2000;21:129–35.

40. Singh H, Azad K, Kaur K. Clofazimine-induced enteropathy in a patient of leprosy. *Indian J Pharmacol* 2013;45:197–8.

41. Szeto W, Garcia-Buitrago MT, Abbo L, Rosenblatt JD, Moshiree B, Morris MI. Clofazimine enteropathy: A rare and under recognized complication of mycobacterial therapy. *Open Forum Infect Dis* 2016;3(3):w004.

42. Chong PY, Ti TK. Severe abdominal pain in low dose clofazimine. *Pathology* 1993;25:24–6.

43. Aster RH, Curtis BR, McFarland JG, Bougie DW. Drug-induced immune thrombocytopenia: Pathogenesis, diagnosis, and management. *J Thromb Haemost* 2009;7:911.

44. Das S, Roy A, Maiti A. Rifampicin induced thrombocytopenia. *Indian J Dermatol* 2006;51:222.

PART 15

Emergencies in STD

SRIDHAR JANDYALA

60

Sexually transmitted disease related emergencies

K. LEKSMI PRIYA AND AFREEN AYUB

INTRODUCTION

Sexually transmitted diseases (STDs) are commonly encountered in the dermatology practice. Many of these diseases when untreated can develop systemic complications, which may present to an emergency department. The complication itself may be the initial presentation of the condition; hence, it is pertinent to have adequate knowledge of these so as to arrive at a correct diagnosis.

The emergency medical conditions related to STDs are as follows:

1. Neurosyphilis
2. Cardiovascular syphilis
3. Jarisch-Herxheimer reactions
4. Gonococcal meningitis
5. Gonococcal endocarditis
6. Perihepatitis (Fitz-Hugh-Curtis syndrome)
7. Herpes genitalis–associated meningitis

1. *Neurosyphilis*
   a. *Acute syphilitic meningitis*: Seen in 6% of all cases of neurosyphilis.
      i. Etiopathogenesis. This infection is caused by the spirochete *Treponema pallidum* acquired through sexual contact. The central nervous system (CNS) is invaded by the spirochete during early syphilis (Figure 60.1). In case of untreated syphilitic infection, it persists as asymptomatic syphilitic meningitis or progresses to acute syphilitic meningitis and subsequently leads to meningovascular syphilis.

         The inflammatory infiltrate consisting of lymphocytes and plasma cells is located in the perivascular spaces of the meninges as well as the ependyma. Acute syphilitic hydrocephalus develops as a result of obstruction of cerebrospinal fluid (CSF) flow by the infiltrate. Cranial nerve abnormalities are due to compression by basilar exudate or due to increased intracranial pressure.
      ii. Clinical features. Symptoms are generally seen 3–7 months after primary infection.
         - Cranial nerve palsies (seen in 40%) involve multiple cranial nerves, usually the third, sixth, seventh, and eighth.
         - Reversible sensorineural deafness to higher frequencies is seen in 20%.
         - Signs of increased intracranial pressure include headache, nausea, vomiting, and photophobia.
         - Acute syphilitic hydrocephalus may occur, leading to papilledema.
      iii. Investigations
         - CSF analysis includes reactive venereal disease research laboratory (VDRL) test, elevated pressure, raised cell count with mononuclear pleocytosis, raised protein concentration (up to 200 mg/dL) with elevated globulin level, and minimal reduction in glucose.
         - Serological tests for syphilis are positive.
   b. Meningovascular syphilis
      i. Etiopathogenesis. This usually occurs 5–12 years after initial syphilitic infection. Any part of the CNS may be involved, but the territory of the middle cerebral artery is most commonly involved. The underlying pathology is syphilitic endarteritis of medium and large arteries (Heubner arteritis) or small arteries and arterioles (Nissl arteritis) leading to thrombosis, vascular occlusion, and cerebral infarction.

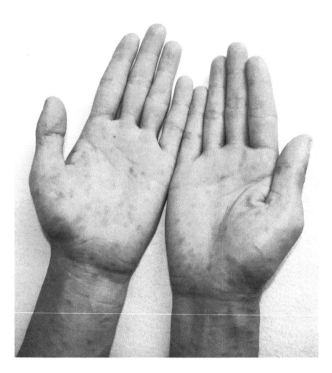

Figure 60.1 Palmar syphilides in secondary (early) syphilis.

Infiltration by lymphocytes and plasma cells of the vasa vasorum, the adventitia, and the media of large and medium-sized arteries lead to destruction of the smooth muscle and elastic tissue of the media. Concentric proliferation of subintimal fibroblasts causes narrowing of the lumen.

ii. Clinical features. Onset may be sudden or may be preceded by prodromal symptoms such as headache, dizziness, insomnia, memory loss, or mood disturbances.

The common presentations are as follows:
– Hemiparesis or hemiplegia
– Aphasia
– Seizures

Other presentations include the following:
– Psychiatric manifestations such as personality and behavioral changes and slowing of mentation and speech
– Cerebellar ataxia, homonymous hemianopia

iii. Investigations
– *Serum rapid plasma reagin (RPR)*: Positive
– *CSF-VDRL test*: Positive in most.
  -Lymphocytic pleocytosis may be seen
– *Angiographic changes*
  – *Anterior and middle cerebral arteries*: Diffuse irregularity and "beading"
  – *Pericallosal artery*: Segmental dilatation
  – *Changes in the supraclinoid portion of the internal carotid artery*
  – Absence of stenotic changes at the carotid bifurcation

– *Computed tomography (CT)*: Low-density areas with variable degrees of contrast enhancement
– *Magnetic resonance imaging*: Focal regions of high signal intensity on T2-weighted sequences, suggestive of foci of ischemia

c. Meningovascular syphilis of the spinal cord
i. Etiopathogenesis. This condition is rare, seen in only 3% of cases of neurosyphilis. The basic underlying process is chronic spinal meningitis causing parenchymatous degeneration of the cord.

ii. Clinical features
– *Syphilitic meningomyelitis*: Usually occurs after a latent period of 20–25 years
  – Weakness or paresthesias of the legs
  – Paraparesis or paraplegia (spastic, deep tendon reflexes are hyperactive)
  – Urinary and fecal incontinence
  – Sensory abnormalities such as loss of position and vibratory sense in the lower extremities
– *Spinal vascular syphilis*: Presents with transection of the spinal cord causing sudden onset of
  – Flaccid paraplegia
  – Sensory level on the trunk
  – Urinary retention

iii. Investigations
– *Blood serologic tests for syphilis*: Positive
– *CSF examination*: Positive VDRL and raised cell count

iv. Treatment of neurosyphilis (with or without HIV infection)
– IV aqueous crystalline penicillin-G 18–24 million units (3–4 MU 4 hourly) daily for 10–14 days

or

– Intramuscular procaine penicillin-G 2.4 million units plus probenecid 500 mg per orally four times daily for 10–14 days

– In patients with penicillin allergy
– Ceftriaxone 1 g IV OD for 10–14 days

Follow-up
– Clinical (including CSF) examination should be done 3 months and then at 6-month intervals, until the CSF findings return to normal.
– Failure of CSF cell count or VDRL to return to normal 1 year after completion of therapy is considered as treatment failure and has to be retreated.

2. **Cardiovascular syphilis**. It occurs after a latent period of 15–30 years. Men are three times prone than women, and age of onset is generally 40–55 years. It is seen in 10% or less of patients with tertiary disease.

a. Etiopathogenesis. *Treponema pallidum* spreads to the heart through the lymphatics during early syphilis, lodges in the aortic wall, and remains dormant for years. They cause endarteritis of proximal aorta by specifically affecting the vasa vasorum of the aorta. Endarteritis also involves the proximal portions of the coronary arteries near the ostia.

The aortic media develops patchy necrosis with subsequent focal scarring. Aortic dilation and aneurysm formation occur due to destruction of the important elastic tissue of the media. The adventitia undergoes fibrous thickening. There are atherosclerotic changes involving the intimal surface of the affected aorta resulting in extensive plaque formation.

b. Clinical features. The main presentations are
   - Aortic aneurysm (Figure 60.2)
   - Aortic insufficiency
   - Coronary artery stenosis
   - Myocarditis

Aortic aneurysm. This is the most common manifestation. It mainly involves the thoracic aorta (60% involve the ascending portion and 25% involve the transverse arch). Aneurysms are characteristically fusiform or saccular in type and do not dissect. They remain asymptomatic for many years. Symptoms usually occur when an aneurysm encroaches on surrounding structures or ruptures. The common symptoms are persistent chest pain, hoarseness from recurrent laryngeal nerve pressure, cough, hemoptysis, dyspnea, and dysphagia. A chest wall mass can occur due to erosion of the aneurysm through the chest wall.

Coronary artery disease. Only the ostia or the most proximal few millimeters of the coronary arteries are affected by obliterative endarteritis. It

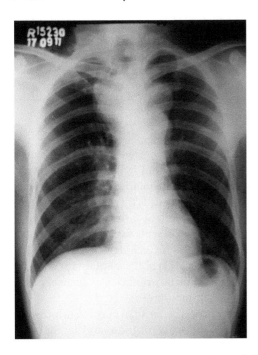

Figure 60.2 Aortic aneurysm in cardiovascular syphilis.

may present as ischemic heart disease, angina pectoris, or sudden death.

Aortic regurgitation. The characteristic feature is pure aortic regurgitation without stenosis. This is due to aortic root dilation with stretching of the aortic valve leading to widening of the aortic valve commissures, thickening of the aortic valve leaflets, and aortic valve incompetence. The signs are mainly diastolic blowing along the lower left sternal border and increased aortic second sound having a tambour-like quality (due to aortic root dilation).

c. Investigations
   - *Chest radiograph*: Mediastinal mass with typical eggshell calcification outlining the aneurysm
   - *Electrocardiogram (ECG)*
   - *Two-dimensional echo*: Hypertrophied and dilated left ventricle
   - *Coronary angiography*: Isolated right or left main coronary ostial narrowing without atherosclerosis in the rest of the coronary tree
   - *Aortic root angiography*: For achieving definition of aneurysm
   - *Serology*: VDRL reactive only in three-fourths of cases

d. Treatment of cardiovascular syphilis (with or without HIV infection)
   - Three doses each of 2.4 million units benzathine penicillin deep intramuscularly at weekly intervals
   - Definitive management
     Aortic aneurysm: Surgical resection
     Aortic regurgitation: Valve replacement

3. *Jarisch-Herxheimer reactions*
   a. Etiopathogenesis
      - Usually seen after treatment for primary or secondary syphilis
      - Due to sudden release of treponemal constituents and increase in circulating levels of tumor necrosis factor (TNF)-α and interleukins
   b. Clinical features
      - Onset is within 4–6 hours after treatment with penicillin and subsides within 24 hours
      - Reaction characterized by chills, fever, malaise, flushing, arthralgias, headache, and transiently increased prominence of primary and secondary lesions
   c. Management
      - Fluids, aspirin or ibuprofen, short-term steroid therapy

4. *Gonococcal meningitis*
   a. Etiopathogenesis
      - *Neisseria meningitides* can cause colonization of mucosal sites: Oropharyngeal, genital, anorectal, urethral, cervical

b. Clinical features
  – Present with features of acute bacterial meningitis
c. Investigations
  – Stained smears (Gram stain, methylene blue stain) of genital discharge (Figure 60.3) and CSF for demonstration of gonococci
  – Culture of organism on selective media
  – Nucleic acid amplification tests (NAATs)
  – Polymerase chain reaction (PCR)
  – *Serologic tests*: Complement fixation, immunofluorescence
d. Treatment
  – Injectable ceftriaxone 1–2 g IV 12 hourly for 10–14 days

5. *Gonococcal endocarditis*
  ○ Seen in 1%–3% of patients with disseminated gonococcal infection
  ○ Rapidly progressive valvular damage involving aortic valve leading to aortic valve incompetence and acute heart failure within 6 weeks
  ○ Management consists of injectable ceftriaxone 1–2 g IV 12 hourly for 4 weeks

6. *Perihepatitis (Fitz-Hugh-Curtis syndrome)*
  a. Etiopathogenesis
    – *Neisseria gonorrhoea* (10%)
    – *Chlamydia trachomatis*, more common (50%)
  b. Clinical features. Usually seen in young, sexually active women. Presents with right-upper-quadrant pain, fever, nausea, or vomiting. There is evidence of salpingitis associated with extensive tubal scarring, adhesions, and inflammation.

7. Herpes genitalis–associated meningitis
  a. Etiopathogenesis. Herpes genitalis is caused by HSV1 and HSV2 and is sexually transmitted. The virus is inoculated onto the mucosal surfaces. There is focal necrosis and ballooning degeneration of cells, formation of mononucleated giant cells, and eosinophilic intranuclear inclusions.

b. Clinical features. *Aseptic meningitis*: Occurs 3–12 days after onset of genital lesions that are transient vesicles and painful erosions. Presents with fever, headache, neck rigidity, vomiting, and photophobia.
  – *Autonomic nervous system dysfunction*: Can present with hyperesthesia or anesthesia of the perineal and sacral regions, urinary retention, and constipation. On examination, there is large bladder, decreased sacral sensation, and poor rectal and perineal sphincter tone, impotence, and absent bulbocavernous reflexes.
  – *Transverse myelitis*: Characterized by decreased deep-tendon reflexes and muscle strength in the lower extremities along with autonomic nervous system signs and symptoms.
c. Investigations
  – *CSF*: Usually clear. White blood cell counts range from 10 to over 1000 cells per cubic millimetre. Pleocytosis is predominantly lymphocytic, glucose is usually more than 50% of the blood glucose, and CSF protein is slightly elevated.
  – *PCR assay*: Helps in HSV DNA detection.
  – *Serology*: Enzyme-linked immunosorbent assay, complement fixation.
  – *Electromyography*: Shows slowed nerve conduction velocities and fibrillation potentials.
  – *Urinary cystometric examination*: Reveals a large atonic bladder.
d. Treatment. IV Acyclovir 5–10 mg/kg 8 hourly for 7 days followed by oral acyclovir until 10 days.

CONCLUSION

STDs can have a plethora of extragenital clinical manifestations, many of which may present as emergency. The possibility of a STD leading to these manifestations in a susceptible individual must be borne in mind when such a condition is encountered.

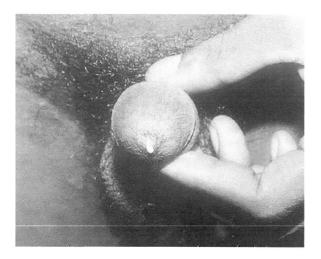

Figure 60.3 Urethral discharge in gonococcal infection.

KEY POINTS

- STD related emergencies include neurosyphilis, cardiovascular syphilis, jarisch-herxheimer reactions, gonococcal meningitis, gonococcal endocarditis, perihepatitis (fitz-hugh-curtis syndrome) and Herpes genitalis–associated meningitis.
- CNS syphilis presents as either meningovascular or acute syphilitic meningitis.
- Cardiovascular syphilis manifests as aortic aneurysm, aortic insufficiency, coronary artery stenosis or myocarditis.
- Prevention is better than cure in such cases with counselling, early diagnosis and appropriate treatment of early stages of disease.

61

HIV-related dermatological emergencies

S. YOGESH MARFATIA AND J. RUCHI SHAH

INTRODUCTION

Human immunodeficiency virus (HIV) is associated with several life-threatening emergencies that need quick intervention. Due to underlying immunosuppression and low CD4 counts, HIV-infected cases are more prone to develop complications due to opportunistic infections (OIs). With the free availability of combined antiretroviral therapy (cART) under the National AIDS Control Organization (NACO), the number of people living with HIV (PLHIV) is on the rise, and mortality due to AIDS has decreased. The life expectancy of PLHIV has increased significantly postintroduction of antiretroviral therapy (ART). Since 2005, AIDS-related death has declined by nearly 54%. It is estimated that the scale-up of free cART since 2004 has saved cumulatively around 4.5 lakhs lives in India until 2014 [1].

Increased life expectancy leads to a greater number of people presenting with various noninfectious complications and other emergencies. With the introduction of cART, the pattern of critical illnesses in HIV-infected cases has observed a subtle shift. The most common cause of intensive care unit (ICU) admission in HIV-infected cases remains acute respiratory failure due to pneumonia. However, post-ART, the most common causative agent is bacterial rather than pneumocystis [2].

With increasing use of cART, the incidence of its adverse drug reactions, such as severe cutaneous adverse drug reactions (Stevens-Johnson syndrome/toxic epidermal necrolysis [SJS/TEN]) and lactic acidosis, is also on the rise. cART-related immune reconstitution inflammatory syndrome (IRIS) can give rise to medical emergencies.

Though HIV-related dermatological emergencies may be smaller in number, many medical emergencies have dermatological manifestations as presenting symptoms, making the role of dermatologists crucial.

CAUSE OF EMERGENCIES IN HIV INFECTED

1. Acute skin failure due to dermatological conditions
2. OIs
3. Complications of antiretroviral therapy (cART), including adverse drug reactions and drug interactions
4. IRIS
5. Malignancies associated with AIDS
6. Epidemiologic emergencies (Table 61.1)

ACUTE SKIN FAILURE

Acute skin failure in HIV can occur due to various dermatological conditions (Table 61.2) [3]. Seborrheic dermatitis is a marker of early HIV infection with CD4 counts more than 500/cu mm. Up to 85% PLHIV experience seborrheic dermatitis at some point of time during their life span. In addition to the seborrheic areas such as the scalp, eyebrows, eyelashes, and beard, rash also appears over chest, back, axilla, and groin in HIV-infected cases. Kaposi varicelliform eruption can develop in such PLHIV with extensive seborrheic dermatitis (Figure 61.1) and atopic dermatitis. Psoriasis in HIV-infected cases can be more florid, severe, and atypical. Both seborrheic dermatitis as well as psoriasis can lead to erythroderma and acute skin failure commonly in HIV (Figures 61.2 and 61.3).

Table 61.1 Classification of HIV-related emergencies

1. Acute skin failure due to dermatological conditions	Erythroderma due to • Psoriasis (Figures 61.2 and 61.3) • Seborrheic dermatitis • Pityriasis rubra pilaris
2. Emergencies due to opportunistic infections	Ocular emergencies: • Cytomegalovirus retinitis[a] • Varicella zoster[a] Central nervous system emergencies: • Cerebral toxoplasmosis • Cryptococcal meningitis[a] Pulmonary emergencies: • Tuberculosis[a] • Bacterial pneumonia • *Pneumocystis carinii* pneumonia Gastrointestinal emergencies[a] Penicilliosis[a]
3. Emergencies due to cART	• Abacavir hypersensitivity reaction • Maculopapular rash/Stevens-Johnson syndrome by nonnucleoside reverse transcriptase inhibitor (nevirapine/efavirenz) • Lactic acidosis • Cardiac emergencies due to antiretroviral therapy • Drug interactions
4. Emergencies related to immune reconstitution syndrome	• Worsening of pulmonary tuberculosis • Development of cerebral masses (tuberculoma) • Acute respiratory distress syndrome • Tubercular and cryptococcal meningitis • Kaposi sarcoma • *Pneumocystis carinii* pneumonia
5. Emergencies related to malignancies associated with HIV/AIDS	• Kaposi sarcoma • Human papillomavirus oropharyngeal carcinoma
6. Epidemiologic emergencies	• Needlestick injury • Unprotected sexual exposure to people living with HIV/AIDS

[a] These infections may have dermatological manifestations that serve as a marker of impending life-threatening emergency.

Table 61.2 Causes of acute skin failure in HIV/AIDS cases

1. Extensive seborrheic dermatitis
2. Psoriasis, pityriasis rubra pilaris
3. Stevens-Johnson syndrome/toxic epidermal necrolysis
4. Exfoliative drug rash

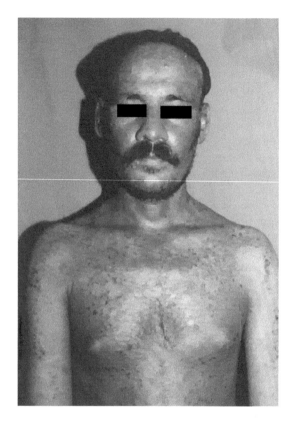

Figure 61.1 Kaposi varicelliform eruption in a case of extensive seborrheic dermatitis.

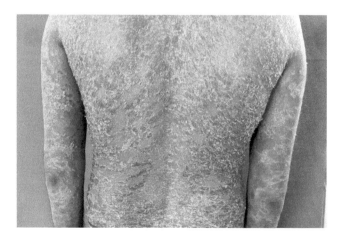

Figure 61.2 Psoriatic erythroderma manifesting as extensive scaling and erythema of the trunk and upper limbs.

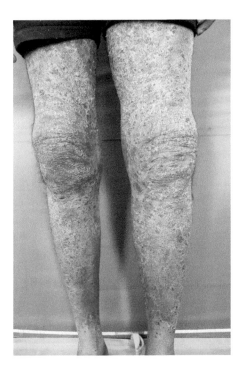

Figure 61.3 Psoriatic erythroderma with extensive scaling and erythema visible on lower limbs.

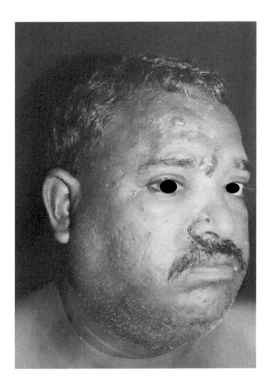

Figure 61.4 Herpes zoster ophthalmicus.

DERMATOLOGICAL MANIFESTATIONS OF OPPORTUNISTIC INFECTIONS AS A MARKER OF MEDICAL EMERGENCIES

Initial manifestations of HIV-related emergencies can be dermatologic. It is essential that dermatologists are well versed with them so that early referral to the relevant physician can save the life of the patient.

Ocular emergencies

CYTOMEGALOVIRUS RETINITIS

This is the most important cause of vision loss in those infected with HIV. Patients present with complaints of blind spots, flashing lights, floaters, and blurred vision. Early and quick intervention with administration of high doses of ganciclovir, foscarnet, or cidofovir is essential to prevent the progression of disease and development of permanent blindness.

Cutaneous involvement by opportunistic cytomegalovirus (CMV) infection may present with a variety of clinical features ranging from localized ulcers, maculopapular rash with terminal petechiae, pruritic rash, hyperpigmented indurated lesions, and perianal ulcers [4].

Cutaneous lesions due to CMV can thus serve as an early marker prior to development of severe systemic complications in immunocompromised patients and provide an opportunity for early diagnosis and better prognosis.

VARICELLA ZOSTER EYE INFECTION

The incidence of herpes zoster ophthalmicus (Figure 61.4) is higher in those with HIV infection than in those who are not infected. Retinal involvement can occur in the form of acute retinal necrosis and progressive outer retinal necrosis syndrome, which can progress to retinal detachment resulting in poor vision. Varicella zoster infection of the eye can later progress to involve the optic nerve and lead to development of herpes encephalopathy presenting as viral meningitis.

Disseminated, hemorrhagic, and multiple dermatomal involvement in herpes zoster was commonly noticed among HIV-positive cases when compared to HIV-negative cases (Figure 61.5) [5]. The development of herpes zoster in otherwise young, asymptomatic individuals at high risk for HIV represents an early clinical sign that should alert the physician to consider the possibility of the impending development of an immune deficiency [6].

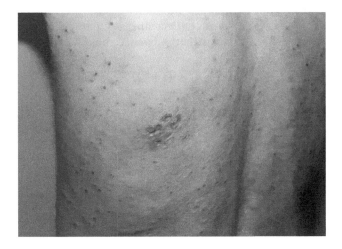

Figure 61.5 Disseminated herpes infection.

Central nervous system emergencies

CRYPTOCOCCAL MENINGITIS

Chronic meningitis caused by *Cryptococcus neoformans* is one of the most frequent fungal infections seen in PLHIV. It can present as a life-threatening complication in the form of raised intracranial pressure due to acute cryptococcal meningitis.

Disseminated cryptococcus infection may present as herpes-like vesiculation, umbilicated lesions, and cellulitis, which evolve into areas of blistering and ulceration in immunocompromised patients. India ink preparations of aspirates from areas of cellulitis or Tzanck preparations from blisters may show characteristic organisms and makes possible an immediate diagnosis of cutaneous cryptococcosis [7].

Gastrointestinal emergencies with mucocutaneous manifestations

Oral and esophageal candidiasis manifesting as dysphagia, odynophagia, or chest pain is commonly seen in HIV-infected cases. Esophagitis in AIDS cases can be caused by *Candida*, HSV, CMV, Kaposi sarcoma, mycobacterium avium complex, or can occur due to reflux esophagitis [8]. Antiretroviral agents have a high incidence of gastrointestinal side effects, too.

Infections

PENICILLIOSIS

Penicilliosis due to *Penicillium marneffei* is a common OI seen in HIV-infected cases [9]. It can present with multiple erythematous, discrete papules, and nodules with umblication over the face, trunk, and proximal parts of the extremities [10]. Oral *P. marneffei* lesions usually occur in patients with disseminated infections, presenting as erosions or shallow ulcers covered with whitish-yellow, necrotic slough that may be found on the palate, gingival, labial mucosa, tongue, and oropharynx [11]. Acute disseminated penicilliosis is associated with high mortality unless prompt diagnosis is made and effective antifungal treatment is initiated.

Disseminated infection with the fungal pathogen *Penicillium marneffei* is, after extrapulmonary tuberculosis and cryptococcal meningitis, the third most common OI in HIV.

EMERGENCIES DUE TO OPPORTUNISTIC INFECTIONS NOT HAVING DERMATOLOGIC MANIFESTATIONS

The following emergency conditions do not have dermatological manifestations, but dermatologists should be aware of their presentation so that prompt physician referral can be made.

Central nervous system emergencies

CEREBRAL TOXOPLASMOSIS

Toxoplasma gondii is the most common infective cause of space-occupying lesions in the brain of those who are HIV infected. Patients complain of headache, altered mental status, confusion, seizures, and occasionally even stroke. The presence of IgG antibodies against toxoplasma, low T-cell count, and hypointense mass on magnetic resonance imaging of the brain and computed tomography scan are diagnostic of cerebral toxoplasmosis. Skin manifestations are not reported.

Pulmonary emergencies

TUBERCULOSIS

HIV infection modifies the clinical presentation of tuberculosis (TB) and is associated with more frequent extrapulmonary dissemination [12]. TB meningitis is a frequent complication of patients with HIV infection in areas of endemic TB [13–16]. Pulmonary basal involvement, TB pneumonia, hilar or mediastinal lymphadenopathies, and miliary TB are seen more frequently in severely immunocompromised HIV-infected patients. These manifestations occur due to reactivation of latent infection, and some of them require emergency management. Cutaneous TB is common in HIV-infected cases. Its presentation is diverse, ranging from scrofuloderma, scattered violaceous papules, nodules, tuberculides, palmoplantar keratoderma, to TB cutis miliaris acuta generalisata. Cultures from such atypical lesions are often negative, since they are typically paucibacillary.

BACTERIAL PNEUMONIA

The degree of immunosuppression estimated by CD4 counts directly correlate with the incidence of bacterial pneumonia in HIV-infected cases. Cases present with fever with chills, shortness of breath, cough with expectoration, and an abnormal chest x-ray.

PNEUMOCYSTIS CARINII PNEUMONIA

This is perhaps one of the most characteristic and most common causes of emergency in AIDS cases. Extreme fatigue, fever, and increasing shortness of breath are the most common presenting features. Chest x-ray and sputum examination remain the main modality for diagnosis and help in guiding treatment for *Pneumocystis carinii* pneumonia (PCP).

DERMATOLOGICAL EMERGENCIES DUE TO COMBINED ANTIRETROVIRAL THERAPY

HIV-infected cases are more prone to develop adverse drug reactions due to altered drug metabolism, immune dysregulation, polypharmacy, genetic predisposition, and oxidative stress [17]. Various drugs are administered for prophylaxis or treatment of coexisting OIs, increasing the potential for drug toxicities and interactions [18] (Table 61.3). The pathophysiology of drug hypersensitivity is based on a variety of factors—immunological, host, and viral. It is postulated to be immune mediated, leading to involvement and recruitment of T cells in the skin, which can be demonstrated on immunohistochemical analysis.

Table 61.3 Antiretroviral drugs causing emergencies

Antiretroviral therapy	Emergencies
Nucleoside reverse transcriptase inhibitor:	
• Abacavir	Abacavir hypersensitivity syndrome
• Zidovudine	Bone marrow suppression
• Lamivudine	Anaphylaxis (rarely)
• Stavudine	Lactic acidosis
• Didanosine	Stevens-Johnson syndrome/ toxic epidermal necrolysis (SJS/TEN)
Nonnucleoside reverse transcriptase inhibitor:	SJS/TEN Drug hypersensitivity syndrome
• Efavirenz	
• Nevirapine	
Protease inhibitor	Acute generalized exanthematous pustulosis
Integrase inhibitor (Raltegravir)	Hypersensitivity reaction

Severe cutaneous adverse drug reactions

HIV significantly increases the risk of SJS/TEN and thereby mortality. TEN has the highest mortality (30%–35%); SJS has less extensive skin detachment and a lower mortality (5%–15%). Hypersensitivity syndrome, sometimes called drug reaction with eosinophilia and systemic symptoms (DRESS), has a mortality rate evaluated at about 10%.

Stevens-Johnson syndrome/toxic epidermal necrolysis

SJS and TEN are severe cutaneous reactions that can be caused by ART. Nevirapine is the most common cause among them. HIV also increases the chances of occurrence of TEN due to the requirement of multiple drugs for various manifestations. They manifest as widespread targetoid skin lesions and mucosal involvement (eyes, mouth, upper gastrointestinal tract, upper airway), usually preceded by a prodrome of fever, nausea, vomiting, malaise, myalgia, and arthralgia. Multiple organs including the kidneys, lungs, and heart can be involved, leading to increased mortality [19].

Early diagnosis and prompt withdrawal of the culprit drug are essential for a favorable outcome [20,21]. Topical recombinant bovine basic fibroblast growth factor allowed faster granulation tissue formation and epidermal regeneration than placebo [22]. The prevention of ocular sequelae requires daily examination by an ophthalmologist. Eye drops, physiologic saline, or antibiotics, if needed, are instilled every 2 hours, and developing synechiae are disrupted by a blunt instrument [23].

A short course of high-dose corticosteroids in the absence of any potential source of infection is proven to be beneficial in SJS/TEN. Cyclosporine is found to be safe and effective in cases of SJS and TEN at a dose of 3–5 mg/kg/day orally or intravenously for 7 days. It is associated with a rapid epithelialization rate and a lower mortality rate in patients with severe TEN [24].

DRUG HYPERSENSITIVITY REACTION

Hypersensitivity syndrome usually refers to a specific, severe, idiosyncratic reaction, defined by a widespread and long-lasting papulopustular or erythematous skin eruption often progressing to exfoliative dermatitis with fever, lymphadenopathy, facial edema (hallmark), and visceral involvement in the form of hepatitis, pneumonitis, myocarditis, pericarditis, and nephritis.

Hypersensitivity reaction occurs after initiation of abacavir in approximately 3.7% patients on cART [25]. Abacavir hypersensitivity is strongly associated with major histocompatibility complex allele and human leukocyte antigen (HLA) B*5701 [26]. Screening for allele is thus recommended prior to initiation of the drug. Prompt stoppage of the drug, IV hydration, and administration of a short course of systemic steroids in the dose of 0.5–1 mg/kg/day rapidly improves the symptoms as well as the laboratory parameters.

NONNUCLEOSIDE REVERSE TRANSCRIPTASE INHIBITOR INDUCED CUTANEOUS ADVERSE DRUG REACTION

Drugs implicated in erythema multiforme/SJS/TEN in HIV/AIDS cases include abacavir, nevirapine, and efavirenz. Other drugs used in the treatment and prophylaxis of OIs, including cotrimoxazole, isoniazid, phenytoin, carbamazepine, clarithromycin, fluconazole, griseofulvin, vancomycin, etc., can also lead to severe cutaneous adverse drug reactions.

Maculopapular rashes are characterized by widespread, pruritic, confluent pink-to-red macules and papules usually on the trunk and proximal extremities (Figure 61.6). Rash appears within 2–10 weeks of first exposure to the culprit drug and may take up to 2 weeks to resolve after its

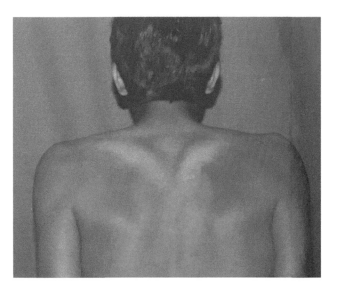

Figure 61.6 Nevirapine-induced maculopapular rash.

discontinuation. The maculopapular reaction may progress to exfoliative dermatitis. Reexposure to the offender, however, may trigger the reaction in as early as 1–2 days. Grades III and IV rash involving more than 50% of the body surface area with ulceration and mucosal involvement and SJS/TEN require emergency management.

Other antiretroviral therapy–related emergencies

The dermatologist may be the first contact physician facing a patient having life-threatening drug toxicities. The diagnosis and referral are in the domain of the dermatologist.

LACTIC ACIDOSIS

Lactic acidosis is an uncommon, yet serious complication of ART. The reported incidence rates vary from 1.3 to 10 per 1000 person-years on ART. Asymptomatic hyperlactatemia is seen in 9%–16% PLHA on ART.

Only 1% of cases have severe hyperlactatemia, that is, serum lactate >5 mmol/L. Drugs such as stavudine (d4 T) and didanosine (ddI) induce more mitochondrial DNA inhibition than others [27,28].

CARDIAC EMERGENCIES DUE TO ANTIRETROVIRAL TREATMENT

Antiretroviral drugs cause dyslipidemia and metabolic derangements leading to increased risk of coronary artery disease (CAD) in HIV-infected patients [29]. Among ART, protease inhibitors (Pis) are associated with hyperlipidemia with elevated total and LDL cholesterol levels and insulin resistance [30]. Other components of metabolic syndrome, including hypertension and obesity, are also found to be associated with ART. These factors increase the risk for CAD in AIDS cases.

The HIV Outpatient Study (HOPS), a large prospective study, found an increased risk of myocardial infarction (MI) in the HIV-infected postintroduction of protease inhibitors [31]. The Data Collection on Adverse Events of Anti-HIV drugs Study Group also showed that the incidence of MI increased with increased exposure to cART [32]. Another study showed an increased risk of MI after exposure to nucleoside reverse transcriptases abacavir and didanosine [33].

Although long-term survival rates are good in HIV-infected patients with acute coronary syndrome (ACS), an increased rate of revascularization and recurrent ischemic events is noted [34,35]. The prevalence of pericardial effusions and dilated cardiomyopathy has decreased significantly in the post-ART era [36].

Emergencies due to drug interactions

A patient infected with HIV-1 who was treated with ritonavir and saquinavir then experienced a prolonged effect from a small dose of methylenedioxymethamphetamine (MDMA or Ecstasy) and a nearly fatal reaction from a small dose of γ-hydroxybutyrate (GHB). ART can lead to midazolam overdose due to increased availability and can lead the patient to develop coma. These are a few of the many instances reported.

EMERGENCIES DUE TO IMMUNE RECONSTITUTION INFLAMMATORY SYNDROME

Initiation of ART in PLHA results in paradoxical worsening of an existing infection or disease process or appearance of a new infection/disease process as a result of substantial reconstitution of the host's immune responses. This phenomenon is referred to as IRIS. It appears to be the result of unbalanced reconstitution of effector and regulatory T cells, leading to an exuberant inflammatory response in patients receiving ART.

IRIS may manifest as various infective and noninfective conditions. Various infective conditions include relapse of CMV retinitis, acute hepatitis associated with HCV infection, relapse of pulmonary tuberculosis, *Mycobacterium avium* disease, mucocutaneous herpes, inflamed cutaneous warts or molluscum contagiosum, and reactions in Hansen disease [37]. Other noninfective IRIS events include sarcoidosis, foreign-body granulomas, dyshidrosis, and lichen planus.

Patients with CNS involvement with raised intracranial pressures in cryptococcal and tubercular meningitis have poor prognosis and require aggressive management, including administration of corticosteroids. Acute respiratory failure can recur after initiation of antiretroviral therapy in patients being treated for severe PCP. A short course of steroid therapy may suppress this reaction [38]. Patients who developed life-threatening pulmonary IRIS due to PCP after initiation of ART have been reported.

In a study conducted among 196 patients with 260 OIs, 21 (11%; 95% confidence interval, 7%–16%) developed paradoxical IRIS in the first year of ART [39]. The three most common OIs among study patients were *Pneumocystis* pneumonia, candidal esophagitis, and Kaposi sarcoma (KS). Morbidity and mortality were highest in those with visceral KS-IRIS compared with other types of IRIS.

Management of immune reconstitution inflammatory syndrome

The key to management is accurate diagnosis and ruling out of alternative diagnoses such as drug toxicity and new infection. If IRIS has been provoked by an opportunistic infection, this should be optimally treated. Nonsteroidal anti-inflammatory agents and corticosteroids have been used widely in patients with IRIS to control the inflammatory response, particularly in those with severe manifestations. ART should be continued unless IRIS becomes life threatening.

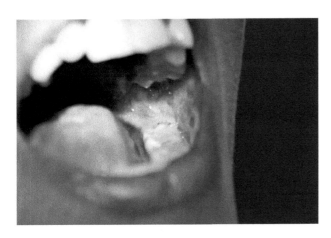

Figure 61.7 Kaposi sarcoma.

MALIGNANCY-ASSOCIATED EMERGENCIES IN HIV INFECTED

In immunocompromised patients, Kaposi sarcoma is commonly seen over oromucosal surfaces (Figure 61.7) and may occasionally present with upper airway obstruction that needs urgent emergency manipulation and radiotherapy [40].

Oropharyngeal carcinoma due to HPV is more common and aggressive in AIDS cases [41]. This can also lead to pressure symptoms and medical emergency.

EPIDEMIOLOGIC EMERGENCIES: ROLE OF DERMATOLOGISTS

Epidemiologic emergencies where dermatologists may be involved are as follows:

- Needlestick injury
- Unprotected sexual exposure with PLHA
- Psychological trauma due to disclosure of positive status, particularly in young adolescents

KEY POINTS

- The introduction of cART in management of AIDS has resulted in significant changes in the profile of complications and emergencies seen in HIV-infected cases.
- Dermatologic emergencies in HIV-infected cases can be due to acute skin failure due to dermatological conditions, opportunistic infections, severe drug reactions due to cART, IRIS, and AIDS-related mucocutaneous malignancies.
- Exfoliative dermatitis due to psoriasis, PRP, seborrheic dermatitis, and drugs can give rise to acute skin failure.
- The dermatologist is the first-contact physician for many PLHA presenting with life-threatening

systemic opportunistic infections. Early diagnosis and prompt referral can save the lives of such cases.
- cART-induced severe cutaneous adverse drug reactions such as SJS/TEN, DRESS, and exfoliative dermatitis require a multidisciplinary approach.
- HIV-related malignancies such as mucosal Kaposi sarcoma and HPV-related oropharyngeal carcinoma can cause upper airway obstruction and thus can be life threatening.
- Dermatologists have a crucial role in identifying and managing dermatologic and nondermatologic emergencies related to HIV/AIDS and cART.

REFERENCES

1. Annual report 2016–17. Department of AIDS Control. National AIDS Control Organization. Ministry of Health and Family Welfare. Government of India. Available from: http://naco.gov.in/sites/default/files/NACO%20ANNUAL%20REPORT%202016-17.pdf.
2. Kathleen et al. Critical Illness in HIV infected patients in the era of combination antiretroviral therapy. *Proc Am Thorac Soc* 2011;8:301–7.
3. Inamdar AC, Patil A. Acute skin failure: Concept, causes, consequences and care. *Indian J Dermatol Venereol Leprol* 2005;71:379–85.
4. Feldman PS et al. Cutaneous lesions heralding disseminated cytomegalovirus infection. *J Am Acad Dermatol* 1982;7:545–8.
5. Vora RV et al. Study of clinical profile of herpes zoster in human immunodeficiency virus positive and negative patients at a rural-based tertiary care center, Gujarat. *Indian J Sex Transm Dis* 2017;38:65–8.
6. Glesby MJ, Moore RD, Chaisson RE. Clinical spectrum of herpes zoster in adults infected with human immunodeficiency virus. *Clin Infect Dis* 1995;21:370–5.
7. Schupbach CW, Wheeler CE, Briggaman RA, Warner NA, Kanof EP et al. Cutaneous manifestations of disseminated cryptococcosis. *Arch Dermatol* 1976;112:1734–40.
8. Marco CA, Rothman RE. HIV infection and complications in emergency medicine. *Emerg Med Clin N Am* 2008;26:367–87.
9. Dahiya P, Kamal R, Puri A, Saini G, Arora A. Penicillinosis in a HIV-positive individual. *Indian J Sex Transm Dis* 2012;33:38–40.
10. Maniar JK, Chitale AR, Miskeen A, Shah K, Maniar A. *Penicillium marneffei* infection: An AIDS defining illness. *Indian J Dermatol Venereol Leprol* 2005;71:202–4.
11. Nittayananta W. *Penicilliosis marneffei*: Another AIDS defining illness in southeast Asia. *Oral Dis* 1999;5:286–93.

12. Aaron L et al. Tuberculosis in HIV-infected patients: A comprehensive review. *Clin Microbiol Infect* 2015;10:388–98.

13. Berenguer J et al. Tuberculous meningitis in patients infected with human immunodeficiency virus. *N Engl J Med* 1992;326:668–72.

14. Sharma R et al. Tubercular meningitis with hydrocephalus with HIV co-infection: Role of cerebrospinal fluid diversion procedures. *J Neurosurg* 2015;122:1087–95.

15. Perlman DC et al. Variation of chest radiographic patterns in pulmonary tuberculosis by degree of human immunodeficiency virus-related immunosuppression. The Terry Beirn Community Programs for Clinical Research on AIDS (CPCRA). The AIDS Clinical Trials Group (ACTG). *Clin Infect Dis* 1997;25:242–6.

16. Smith RL, Yew K, Berkowitz KA, Aranda CP. Factors affecting the yield of acid-fast sputum smears in patients with HIV and tuberculosis. *Chest* 1994;106:684–6.

17. Marfatia YS, Shah RJ. Cutaeous ADRs in HIV infected and AIDS cases. In: *IADVL's Textbook on Cutaneous Adverse Drug Reactions*, 2nd edition. Balani Publishers, 2017: 1213–1220.

18. Chaponda M, Pirmohamed M. Hypersensitivity reactions to HIV therapy. *Br J Clin Pharmacol* 2005;71:659–67.

19. Ghislain P-D, Roujeau J-C. Treatment of severe drug reactions: Stevens-Johnson syndrome, toxic epidermal necrolysis and hypersensitivity syndrome. *Dermatol Online J* 2002;8(1):5.

20. Peng YZ, Yuan ZQ, Xiao, GX. Effects of early enteral feeding on the prevention of enterogenic infection in severely burned patients. *Burns* 2001;27:145–9.

21. Revuz J et al. Toxic epidermal necrolysis. Clinical findings and prognosis factors in 87 patients. *Arch Dermatol* 1987;123:1160–5.

22. Fu X et al. Randomised placebo-controlled trial of use of topical recombinant bovine basic fibroblast growth factor for second-degree burns. *Lancet* 1998;352:1661–4.

23. Romero-Rangel T, Stavrou P, Cotter J, Rosenthal P, Baltatzis S, Foster CS. Gas permeable scleral contact lens therapy in ocular surface disease. *Am J Ophthalmol* 2000;130:25–32.

24. Jose et al. Treatment of toxic epidermal necrolysis with cyclosporine A. *J Trauma Acute Care Surg* 2000;48:473–8.

25. Ross GH. Abacavir hypersensitivity reaction. *Clin Infect Dis* 2002;34:1137–42.

26. Yunihastuti E, Widhani A, Harjono Karjadi T. Drug hypersensitivity in human immunodeficiency virus-infected patient: Challenging diagnosis and management. *Asia Pacific Allergy* 2014;4:54–67.

27. Arenas-Pinto A, Grant AD, Edwards S, Weller IVD. Lactic acidosis in HIV infected patients: A systematic review of published cases. *Sex Transm Infect* 2003;79:340–4.

28. Marfatia YS, Talwar M, Agrawal M, Sharma A, Mehta K. Mitochondrial toxicities of nucleoside analogue reverse transcriptase inhibitors in AIDS cases. *Indian J Sex Transm Dis* 2014;35:96–9.

29. Mishra R. Cardiac emergencies in patients with HIV. *Emerg Med Clin N Am* 2010;28:273–82.

30. Mulligan K et al. Hyperlipidemia and insulin resistance are induced by protease inhibitors independent of changes in body composition in patients with HIV infection. *J Acquir Immune Defic Syndr* 2000;23:35–43.

31. Holmberg SD et al. Protease inhibitors and cardiovascular outcomes in patients with HIV-1. *Lancet* 2002;360:1747–8.

32. Friis-Moller N et al. Class of antiretroviral drugs and the risk of myocardial infarction. *N Engl J Med* 2007;356:1723–35.

33. Sabin CA et al. Use of nucleoside reverse transcriptase inhibitors and risk of myocardial infarction in HIV-infected patients enrolled in the D:A:D study: A multi-cohort collaboration. *Lancet* 2008;371: 1417–26.

34. Ambrose JA et al. Frequency of and outcome of acute coronary syndromes in patients with human immunodeficiency virus infection. *Am J Cardiol* 2003;92:301–3.

35. Boccara F, Cohen A. Coronary artery disease and stroke in HIV-infected patients: Prevention and pharmacological therapy. *Adv Cardiol* 2003;40:163–84.

36. Pugliese A et al. Impact of highly active antiretroviral therapy in HIV-positive patients with cardiac involvement. *J Infect* 2000;40:282–4.

37. French MA et al. Immune restoration disease after the treatment of immunodeficient HIV infected patients with highly active antiretroviral therapy. *HIV Med* 2000;1:107–15.

38. Marie W et al. Acute respiratory failure following HAART introduction in patients treated for *Pneumocystis carinii* pneumonia. *Am J Respir Crit Care Med* 2001;164(5):847–51.

39. Sharm SK, Soneja M. Human immunodeficiency virus and immune reconstitution inflammatory syndrome. *Indian J Med Res* 2011;134:866–77.

40. Roy TM[1], Dow FT, Puthuff DL. Upper airway obstruction from AIDS-related Kaposi's sarcoma. *J Emerg Med* 1991;9:23–5.

41. Bharti AH, Marfatia YS. An update on oral human papillomavirus infection. *Indian J Sex Transm Dis* 2013;34:77–82.

PART 16

Procedure-related Emergencies

C. MADURA

62

Emergencies in dermatosurgery

B. R. HARISH PRASAD, C. MADURA AND M. R. KUSUMA

INTRODUCTION

Emergencies can occur any time in dermatosurgery, irrespective of the patients' laboratory profiles. The operating surgeon should be well versed in identifying these complications and their timely management. In the era of modern dermatosurgery, the operating rooms should be well equipped with emergency medications and equipment, and the staff should be well trained in emergency medicine. Dermatosurgical emergencies can be of two types: (1) emergencies encountered during dermatosurgical procedures (Table 62.1) and (2) dermatosurgical conditions that require emergency interventions (Table 62.2).

PREPAREDNESS FOR EMERGENCY IN DERMATOSURGERY SETUP

Preoperative patient evaluation

A complete and thorough examination and evaluation of the patient by the dermatosurgeon are of prime importance like for any other surgery, irrespective of whether the procedure is as simple as a skin biopsy or a major case such as flap surgeries or hair restoration surgeries. The patient should be evaluated for psychological (appearance, mood, orientation, thought process, insights, and thoughts), physical (demography data, allergies, medication and supplements, tobacco, alcohol, and family history), and medical profiles (complete systems evaluation). The best indicator of surgical complications is a history of previous surgical complications. A complete hemogram with organ profiles are a must, which completes the comprehensive preoperative evaluation.

Patient education during preoperative evaluation is very important. Well-educated patients who know precisely what to expect before, during, and after their surgery tend to be less apprehensive and better able to participate in their own care.

Operating room

The operating room is a dynamic and complicated area, where the safety of the patients undergoing surgery takes utmost priority. Emergency equipment must be checked regularly to determine whether they are in perfect condition. An emergency trolley with resuscitation medications, syringes, needles, and IV infusions with different IV sets must be available at all times. A monitor with a defibrillator must be available in the recovery room for tackling emergencies. An anesthetic machine/ventilator and monitors must be permanent occupants of the recovery room. Make sure sufficient oxygen supply, masks, airways, and intratracheal tubes as well as a laryngoscope are available. Check that the suction apparatus is connected and in working condition. The crash cart inventory should be periodically reviewed and renewed as necessary.

Emergency care

Contact details of the emergency medical system, anesthetist, physician, vascular and plastic surgeons, nearby hospitals, intensive care unit (ICU), and ambulance should all be maintained, and every team member should be aware of the same.

The team

The ultimate goal of the team should be to stabilize the patient. Each staff member should have a prearranged, clearly defined role for an effective office emergency plan. Cardiopulmonary resuscitation (CPR) is initiated if indicated, while an assigned staff member activates the emergency medical service (EMS)

Table 62.1 Emergencies presenting in a dermatosurgical operating room

1. Anaphylaxis
2. Vasovagal syncope
3. Lidocaine "allergy" and toxicity
4. Hypertensive crisis
5. Hypotension
6. Cardiac arrhythmias
7. Status epilepticus
8. Motor nerve injury
9. Retrobulbar hematoma
10. Hemorrhage

Table 62.2 Dermatosurgical conditions that require emergency interventions

1. Hemorrhage
2. Abscess
3. Bleeding of varicose vein
4. Blister drainage
5. Burns and scalds
6. Paraphimosis
7. Fournier gangrene
8. Impacted finger ring
9. Frenulum tear
10. Traumatic nail avulsion
11. Pyogenic granuloma
12. Thrombophlebitis
13. Cryoblister

system. Another staff member can serve as the designated recorder of events and duration, serial vital sign measurements, and administered medications. Further roles can include obtaining IV access, greeting and escorting the arriving EMS team to the patient, and communicating with family.

Role of dermatosurgeon

Every dermatosurgeon must and should undergo 2–4 weeks of rotational postings in the anesthesia and plastic surgery departments to get well versed with the skills of managing emergency situations. They should also get certificate training in CPR, basic life support (BLS), and advanced cardiac life support (ACLS) from the American Heart Association. These should be mandatory, as it is here that health-care professionals learn to recognize several life-threatening emergencies, provide CPR to victims of all ages, use an automated external defibrillator (AED), and relieve choking in a safe, timely, and effective manner.

IMPORTANT EMERGENCIES FACED IN A DERMATOSURGERY UNIT

Anaphylaxis

Anaphylaxis is defined as a serious, life-threatening, generalized or systemic hypersensitivity reaction that is rapid in

onset and might cause death. The World Allergy Organization (WAO) Guidelines emphasize risk factors related to age (infancy, adolescence, advanced age); physiologic state (pregnancy); concomitant diseases including asthma, cardiovascular diseases (CVDs), and mastocytosis; and concurrent medications such as ß-blockers and angiotensin-converting enzyme (ACE) inhibitors. Cofactors such as exercise, emotional stress, acute infection, fever, concomitant ingestion of ethanol or a nonsteroidal anti-inflammatory drug (NSAID), disruption of routine, and perimenstrual status can act as significant cofactors [1–5].

The manifestation may vary from pruritus, urticaria in milder cases, to inspiratory stridor, laryngeal edema, bronchospasm, hypotension, and cardiac arrhythmias in more severe cases. Classic anaphylaxis manifests with a massive cardiovascular collapse within minutes of exposure to the offending antigen. The outcome in such events depends mainly on the preparedness of the team to treat anaphylaxis and other measures, such as rapid assessment of the patient, removing the trigger if possible, and calling for help. It is recommended to position the patient in supine (or semireclining) position if the patient is dyspneic or vomiting, with elevation of the lower extremities [6].

Epinephrine injection, calling for help, and positioning the patient appropriately are important initial steps in management [2,3]. Recommendations for prompt initial treatment of anaphylaxis includes epinephrine (adrenaline) injected intramuscularly in the mid-outer thigh, and repeating the epinephrine dose after 5–15 minutes if the response to the first injection is not optimal [2,4].

Supplemental oxygen, IV fluid resuscitation with a crystalloid such as 0.9% (isotonic) saline, and cardiopulmonary resuscitation should be started without delay [7–9]. If patients with anaphylaxis are refractory to epinephrine, supplemental oxygen, IV fluids, and second-line medications, they should be transferred to the care of a specialist team for ventilatory and inotropic support and continuous electronic monitoring. Interventions for cardiopulmonary arrest, airway management, and IV administration of vasopressors including epinephrine, dopamine, and vasopressin should be undertaken when required [3].

Syncope

Syncope is a transient loss of consciousness due to transient global cerebral hypoperfusion characterized by rapid onset, short duration, and spontaneous complete recovery.

VASOVAGAL SYNCOPE

Vasovagal syncope is one of the very commonly seen emergency situations in the dermatosurgery setup. The clinical features of vasovagal episode may include a characteristic prodrome composed of anxiety, diaphoresis, nausea, tachypnea, tachycardia, or confusion. The skin tends to become pale and cool. Subsequent vagal-induced bradycardia in the setting of decreased systemic vascular resistance can initiate circulatory collapse. Blood pressure may initially decrease but is restored with recumbency. There are often no associated cardiac or neurological abnormalities. Conversely, anaphylaxis features warm, erythematous, dry, pruritic skin with tachycardia and recumbent hypertension [10].

Risk factors for vasovagal syncope are emotional stress, fear of pain, fear of injection room, fear of blood; and sometimes even the smells, sights, and sounds of the operating room trigger this response in a few.

Immediate identification of the condition and shifting the patient to more comfortable surroundings is the first step. Monitoring vitals and clinical examination help to differentiate it from more serious causes. Foot end elevation, loosening the clothes, and providing appropriate ventilation make the patient more comfortable. Placing cool water-soaked gauze and providing cool air are often helpful.

Vasovagal syncope can be minimized by following these simple steps:

1. Provide prior explanation of the procedure to reduce anxiety.
2. Always do procedures or injections with patient in supine position.
3. Make the patient with prior syncopal attack history comfortable with his or her surroundings.
4. Place a gauze or towel over the eyes to avoid the sight of blood, syringes, biopsy specimens, or surgical trolleys.
5. Use talkesthesia or a distracting conversation to help distract the patient's mind and hence lessen the chances of syncopal attacks.
6. After any procedure, advise the patient to slowly turn to one side and then slowly sit up while the operating surgeon or the assistant has a watchful eye on the patient.
7. Should a vasovagal reaction develop, promptly restore the patient to recumbency, preferably in the Trendelenburg position [11].
8. For certain susceptible patients, distract the patient or prevent the patient from viewing the procedure by blocking the field of view.
9. In those with vasovagal hypotension, consider using benzodiazepines for prophylaxis, although selective serotonin reuptake inhibitors and ß-blockers may also be effective. Vasovagal events may occur more frequently when the patient misses a meal before the procedure.

Managing the patient with vasovagal syncope includes the following measures:

1. Place the patient in supine and preferably in a head down (Trendelenburg) position.
2. Monitor vital parameters such as heart rate, blood pressure, and pulse oximetry.
3. Reassure the patient; that may be all that is necessary in addition to the recumbent posture.
4. Start IV access.
5. Administer injection atropine 1 mg if heart rate is less than 40 per minute and IV fluids if blood pressure

continues to be low. If alone, one should call for help and step up the monitoring [13].

6. In addition, application of a cool water washcloth placed on the forehead with a low-power fan directed toward the face may be helpful. Some have proposed that crossing the legs combined with tensing the muscles at the onset of prodromal symptoms can abort vasovagal syncopes.

Lidocaine "allergy" and toxicity

Allergy due to lignocaine is a rare entity that has to be clearly differentiated from vasovagal reaction due to injections and lignocaine toxicity [12]. The breakdown products of the amide local anesthetics do not include a basic amine in the para position as seen with p-aminobenzoic acid; therefore, this may account for the rarity of sensitization reactions. Consequently, cross-hypersensitivity among amide anesthetics or between amide and ester anesthetics is not seen. Lignocaine toxicity occurs due to high dosages, an excessively rapid systemic uptake [13,14], impaired hepatic metabolism [15], from drug interactions [16], or when lignocaine is inadvertently infiltrated directly into the intravascular compartment.

The main cause of allergy is additives in local anesthetic preparations: the parabens, which are used as preservatives for the anesthetic solution, and sodium bisulfite, an antioxidant for the vasoconstrictor.

Toxic reactions to lidocaine resulting from overdosage or vasovagal reactions should be distinguished to avoid confusion with allergy. Symptoms of lidocaine toxicity begin at serum lidocaine concentrations of about 1–5 mcg/mL with subjective sensory alterations, starting with complaints of dizziness and lightheadedness, followed by tinnitus, circumoral paresthesia, blurred vision, and a metallic taste. With higher serum concentrations (5–8 mcg/mL), nystagmus, slurred speech, localized muscle twitching, and fine tremors may occur. At 8–12 mcg/mL, focal seizure activity begins and may progress to tonic-clonic seizures, and at even higher concentrations, to respiratory depression, cardiac arrest, and coma [17].

Among common nonlidocaine local anesthetics, bupivacaine exhibits the smallest therapeutic range, and acutely elevated plasma levels may result in cardiac manifestations that can include ventricular tachyarrhythmias and asystole, even before central nervous system symptoms [18]. This usually occurs from direct intravascular injection of the anesthetic. True allergic reactions do occur, with anaphylaxis being the greatest concern: its onset is rapid and may be fatal.

The prick test is valuable in diagnosis because it is accurately reproduced, and even though a full-strength anesthetic is used, it is estimated that only 3×10^6 mL is injected [19]. There are no known fatalities using the prick test.

The scratch test may be performed, but it is 100 times less sensitive than the intradermal test and not as accurately reproduced as the prick test [20].

Allergy testing gives an indication of the patient's hypersensitivity. Although a negative skin reaction is thought to be conclusive, it is suggested that the best way to determine if a patient can tolerate a given local anesthetic is to actually administer it in a clinical trial, because skin tests do not always elicit a reaction. One must always be prepared for adverse reactions.

The management goals are to correct arterial hypoxemia, inhibit further release of endogenous chemical mediators, and maintain the vital signs.

The patient should be placed in supine position with the legs elevated to help maintain the blood pressure. Administration of oxygen and epinephrine (0.3–0.5 mg IV) is imperative. Subcutaneous or intramuscular epinephrine (0.3 mg) may be administered as an alternative. Diphenhydramine (0.5 mg/kg body wt IV) is administered to reduce the effects of circulating histamine by competing for unoccupied H1-receptors. An anti-inflammatory steroid is often given, as it may stabilize lysosomal membranes, decrease capillary permeability, and suppress T cells that may be involved in delayed hypersensitivity reactions. If bronchospasm is still a problem, aminophylline can be administered intravenously [21–23].

Bupivacaine-induced asystole and ventricular tachyarrhythmias may be treated with prolonged CPR (often 1 hour), with Bretylium being preferable over lidocaine to correct bupivacaine-induced ventricular tachyarrhythmias [24].

Hypertensive crisis

In chronic hypertensive patients undergoing surgery, stress, greater intraoperative bleeding [25], decreased duration of activity of local anesthesia [25], and greater risk of intraoperative serious adverse events [26] can occur, leading to a hypertensive crisis.

Dermatosurgeons thus should be aware that elevations of systolic blood pressure (SBP above 180 mm Hg) and diastolic blood pressure (DBP above 120 mm Hg) constitute a hypertensive crisis [25,27].

Hypertensive emergency can lead to hypertensive encephalopathy, cerebral infarction, intracranial hemorrhage, acute left ventricular failure, acute pulmonary edema, aortic dissection, or renal failure [27].

Zampaglione et al. [28] reported that the most frequent presenting signs in patients with hypertensive emergencies were chest pain (27%), dyspnea (22%), neurologic deficits (21%), faintness (10.0%), paraesthesias (8.0%), vomiting (3.0%), and headache (3.0%) [29].

At times, procedure-related anxiety may lead to elevation of blood pressure above normal limits [30,31].

In asymptomatic patients, relaxation exercises or the use of an anxiolytic, where appropriate, may help relieve anxiety and lower blood pressure. In spite of basic measures, if the pressure is high and patients are symptomatic, the emergency medical system should be activated immediately [31].

Hypotension

Hypotension could be because of vasovagal syncope or orthostatic hypotension, both of which are transient, and there is complete recovery of the patient. Risk of potential trauma associated with loss of postural integrity or if the patient does not completely recover from consciousness are two situations that require active medical intervention [32].

Orthostatic hypotension may be encountered in the dermatological surgery setting during the prone position. Patients who rapidly sit up after completion of a procedure can become predisposed to a hypotensive event. Strictly speaking, orthostatic hypotension is defined as a reduction in blood pressure by 20/10 within 3 minutes of standing [33].

The symptoms associated with orthostatic hypotension are similar to those of vasovagal syncope, the major difference being that the occurrence of the former is preceded by standing.

Adequate hydration can be both treatment and prevention in both vasovagal and orthostatic hypotension, because dehydration exacerbates both etiologies [34]. Despite efforts at rehydration, medications may still be needed to decrease the likelihood of a prolonged hypotensive event, especially in patients with a known history.

Cardiac arrhythmias

Cardiac arrhythmias can be life-threatening emergencies with impending cardiac arrest. Even though rarely encountered in dermatosurgery practice, the dermatologist should be aware of cardiac arrhythmias.

Dermatosurgeons should be aware of risk factors for arrhythmias related to dermatological procedures (chemical cautery and chemical peels with phenol). Conscious victims, especially those with a heart rate 150 beats per minute or symptoms of hypotension, altered mental status, ischemic chest discomfort, or symptoms of acute heart failure should be transferred to the nearest EMS system because of the difficulty in distinguishing tachyarrhythmia (e.g., sinus tachycardia and atrial fibrillation) without an electrocardiogram [35].

While it may be prudent to preemptively identify a high heart rate from easily reversible causes (e.g., anxiety), this is not always a simple determination, and clinical judgment should err on the side of patient safety.

Circulation, airway, and breathing is assessed by testing for a response to voice, observing respiratory movements, noting skin color, and simultaneously palpating major arteries for a pulse [31]. The absence of a carotid or femoral pulse, particularly if it is confirmed by the absence of an audible heartbeat, is a primary diagnostic criterion [31]. The absence of respiratory efforts or the presence of agonal breathing, in conjunction with an absent pulse, is diagnostic of cardiac arrest [31]. Once a life-threatening incident has been suspected or confirmed, it is essential to contact EMS.

Survival from ventricular fibrillation or cardiac arrest may require both basic life support and ACLS, with integrated post-cardiac-arrest care [35].

Motor nerve injury

The nerves at greatest risk for transection, trauma, ligation, or electrical injury during cutaneous surgery are the temporal branch of the facial nerve, the marginal mandibular branch of the facial nerve, and the spinal accessory nerve at Erb point [36]. Transection of the buccal and zygomatic branches rarely leads to a clinically noticeable deficit because of the robust cross innervation and arborization of the distal portions of these nerves [37–39]. Cases of nerve transection during cutaneous surgery have been reported in association with resection of large cutaneous tumors in this "danger zone"

Management of nerve transection is often conservative, including exercises, physiotherapy, or other noninvasive methods to keep patients actively engaged in the recovery process. In cases without eventual return of function, nerve reconstruction by a microvascular surgeon may be required. This includes either reapproximation of the severed nerve or placement of a nerve graft [40].

Retrobulbar hematoma

Retrobulbar hematoma or hemorrhage (RBH) is an ocular emergency that can result in permanent vision loss [41]. With prompt treatment, vision impairment is often reversible [42]. The incidence of orbital hemorrhage associated with cosmetic eyelid surgery is 0.055% (1 in 2000 patients). Permanent vision loss occurs in 0.0045% (1 in 10,000 patients) [41]. Blindness after blepharoplasty is a documented complication and can occur because of RBH [43].

Status epilepticus

Continuous or rapid sequential seizure activity for 30 minutes or more is a medical emergency with a high mortality rate in both children and adults. Prompt and effective treatment is the key. Status epilepticus (SE) is associated with a 6%–18% mortality and higher morbidity [44,45].

Though a rarely encountered emergency, a dermatosurgeon should be careful while operating on certain dermatological disorders with potential risk factor for seizures, such as neurofibromatosis, Sturge-Weber syndrome, tuberous sclerosis, and lupus erythematosus. If a patient is on antiepileptic treatment, he or she should be advised to continue the treatment until the day of surgery.

Fulminant tonic-clonic movements with frothing and dysautonomic features with loss of consciousness are important indicators of the diagnosis of SE.

As with any critically ill patient, the first step in the management of a patient with SE would be to ensure an adequate airway and to provide respiratory support [46,47]. The patient should be positioned such that self-injury is prevented during seizure activity. As the patient is not breathing during a generalized tonic-clonic seizure, the patient is not at high risk for aspiration until the event ends. Immediately following the seizure, patients usually take a deep breath. Therefore, the patient should be rolled over onto his or her side immediately after the motor activity ceases. Likewise, to prevent injury to the patient, suction of the oropharynx can wait until the end of the seizure. A few key management steps are as follows:

- The ongoing procedure should be stopped and secured to prevent any local area complications.
- The patient's surrounding area should be cleared of any sharps and medical devices.
- Stabilize the patient with airway breathing circulation assessment and neurological examination.
- Assess oxygenation, give oxygen via nasal canula or mask or nasopharyngeal airway.
- Time the seizure activity from its onset, and monitor vitals.
- To avoid injuries to oral structures, one should resist the urge to forcibly introduce a tongue depressor or other hard object between locked teeth. Gentle suction can be applied to remove saliva and blood, if any.
- Two large-gauge IV catheters should be inserted to facilitate fluid resuscitation, blood sample collection for glucose, serum electrolytes, and pharmacotherapy.
- Benzodiazepines such as midazolam or lorazepam 1–2 mg or diazepam 5–10 mg intravenously will stop the seizures.
- Call for the physician and evaluate for seizures etiology and further management options.

DERMATOSURGICAL CONDITIONS THAT REQUIRE EMERGENCY INTERVENTIONS

Dermatosurgical emergences are not only those faced during procedural interventions but also those that present as emergencies to the dermatosurgery department for active intervention.

Hemorrhage

Bleeding is always a concern for dermatosurgeons as it can change the outcome of various procedures. Postoperative bleeding can lead to the development of a hematoma, which subsequently can lead to surgical complications such as wound infection, dehiscence, and necrosis. Such adverse events may ultimately result in a poor outcome with suboptimal scar formation. There are multiple factors that can affect bleeding during or after a surgical procedure. These include age of the patient, medications, medical comorbidities, and poor knowledge of anatomy of vessels. The source of bleeding can be capillary, venous, or arterial (Table 62.3).

Preoperative evaluation of patients will help in recognizing patients at risk of bleeding. Common drugs that increase the risk of bleeding are aspirin, NSAIDs, warfarin [48], or other newer antiplatelet agents and anticoagulants [49]. Several herbal or over-the-counter (OTC) medications including garlic, ginseng, ginger, feverfew, vitamin E, *Ginkgo biloba*, and many others can have intended or unintended effects on the coagulation pathway. Hence, investigate the patients for risk of bleeding, which include bleeding and clotting time, prothrombin time, and activated partial thromboplastin time.

Table 62.3 Types of hemorrhage

Primary hemorrhage	It is the bleeding during intra-operative period
Reactionary hemorrhage	It is the bleeding which occurs within 24 hours post-operatively
Secondary hemorrhage	It usually occurs after 1 week of surgery which may be due to infection. This type of bleeding is rare in dermatosurgery

Hypertension carries a risk of intraoperative bleeding [50]. Surgical procedures should be done under the supervision of a physician once blood pressure is more than 180 mm Hg systolic or 100 mm Hg diastolic. For patients with blood pressure exceeding 200 mm Hg systolic or 110 mm Hg diastolic, it may be prudent to defer the surgical procedure until after his or her primary medical physician properly evaluates the patient.

The majority of operative cutaneous lesions are located on the head or neck. It is important to know the "danger zones" for arterial bleeding in procedural dermatology, all located on the head and neck [51]: (1) the frontal branch of the temporal artery located at the temple, (2) the facial artery at its crossing over the mandibular rim, and (3) the angular artery adjacent to the nose. Knowing this anatomy makes the surgeon confident in putting an incision of the proper depth and undermine in the correct plane to minimize bleeding complications.

MANAGEMENT OF HEMORRHAGE

Intraoperative management

One of the first steps taken to help minimize intraoperative bleeding is the addition of epinephrine to the local anesthetic. The concentration of epinephrine added to the local anesthetic is usually either 1:100,000 or 1:200,000. The three major benefits are prolonged activity of the anesthetic agent, decreased volume of anesthetic required, and better control of bleeding [52].

Frank bleeding can be arterial/venous or arteriolar/venular [53]. The superficial/dermal oozing is managed with 10 minutes of manual pressure. Electrosurgery and hemostatic agents such as aluminum chloride, 20% ferric sulfate (Monsel solution), and 10%–50% silver nitrate can also be used. If the oozing is deeper and more muscular, the same techniques of pressure and/or electrosurgery may be used to control the hemorrhage. Arterial/venous hemorrhage is best managed using electrosurgery (electrodessication and electrocoagulation) or heat cautery. Regardless, any electrosurgery should be precise to minimize excessive and unnecessary charring of surrounding tissue. Larger arterial or venous bleeding requires ligation of the vessels using absorbable sutures. The simplest and most commonly used stitch is the figure-of-eight stitch [54].

Occasionally, the surgeon will encounter a surgical wound where oozing and bleeding continues despite multiple attempts at homeostasis. In such a case, it may be more practical to leave the wound partially open or consider placing a Penrose drain to allow for drainage. If a drain is used in the wound, it is important to remove it in a timely fashion (usually after 24 hours) to prevent infection.

Postoperative management

Once the cutaneous surgery is completed, the postoperative phase of patient care and instructions begins. There are two key components to the postoperative period:

1. *Bandaging the wound/surgical repair site:* A typical pressure dressing involves the placement of a nonadherent film followed by one or more layers of cotton gauze, and finally, securing the dressing with adhesive tape. A pressure dressing is probably not effective beyond 24 hours, and therefore, the patient has to come for follow-up after 1 day.
2. *Educating the patient and family:* Providing education to the patient and the family about proper care of the site with verbal and written instructions on wound care is important. Avoiding any strenuous exercise, bending, lifting heavy objects, or physical activity that could potentially lead to direct trauma to the surgical site is important for healing and prevention of hemorrhagic complications. In addition, sites that are in constant motion due to daily activities, such as the lips or the perioral area, require specific instructions such as minimizing talking/laughing, eating soft or well-cooked foods, avoiding sucking action via a straw, and taking care when inserting or removing dentures and also while brushing the teeth.

Abscess (infection)

Abscesses require emergency drainage to not only alleviate pain but also to prevent the spread of infection. The most fearful abscesses faced in the dermatosurgery department are palmar abscess, periungual abscess, and abscess in danger zones of the face. Cellulitis may precede or occur in conjunction with an abscess if not treated early. It is caused mainly by *Staphylococcus* and *Streptococcus*. Enteric organisms commonly cause perianal abscesses. Treatment is primarily through incision and drainage (Figure 62.1). Smaller abscesses (<5 mm) may resolve spontaneously with the application of warm compresses and topical antibiotic therapy.

Blister

Blister is a small pocket of fluid, either serum or plasma, within the upper layers of the skin, caused by friction, burning, freezing, chemical exposure, or infection. It will be asymptomatic most of the time, but if it is painful and if risk of infection is noticed, then it has to be drained.

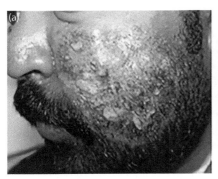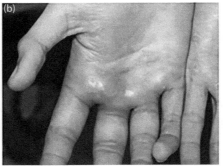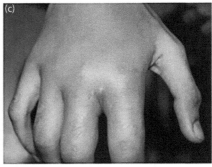

Figure 62.1 (a) Carbuncle over left cheek. (b and c) Hand abscess. (Courtesy of Cutis Academy.)

Under aseptic precautions, using a sterile needle, the blister should be punctured to drain the fluid, and the overlying skin is to be left in place so that it acts as a biological dressing. The area is to be inspected for infection in the follow-up period.

Bleeding from varicose vein

Bleeding is one of the rare complications of varicose veins that present to a dermatosurgery department. It occurs due to rupture of the varicose veins (Figure 62.2). It can be due to minor trauma to the skin or can occur spontaneously. If a varicose vein bleeds, the bleeding can be stopped by making the patient lie flat on a hard surface, raise the leg high, and apply pressure with a clean cloth or dressing onto the bleeding area for at least 10 minutes. Sclerotherapy has proven to be one of the best treatments to prevent repeat bleeding episodes. Wearing stockings of class II will act as a preventive measure and help to avoid such complications.

Burns and scalds

Chemical burns involving smaller body surface area and epidermis and superficial dermis will be handled by dermatosurgeons and for larger area involvement must be referred to a higher center for management. Burns cases are treated in the following manner:

- Cool the burnt area with cool or lukewarm running water for 20 minutes—do not use ice, iced water, or any creams or greasy substances such as butter.
- Remove any clothing or jewelry that is near the burnt area of skin, including babies' diapers, but do not move anything that is stuck to the skin.
- Make sure the person keeps himself or herself warm, but take care not to rub anything hot against the burnt area.
- Use painkillers such as paracetamol or NSAIDs to treat any pain. Systemic antibiotics can prevent secondary infection.
- If the face or eyes are burnt, have the patient sit up as much as possible, rather than lie down. This helps to reduce swelling. Those with chemical burns, electrical burns, large or deep burns, and burns on the face, hands, arms, feet, legs, or genitals that cause blisters should be admitted to the hospital and treated under strict asepsis with monitoring.
- Prefer regular closed dressings for deeper wounds and open dressings for superficial wounds with topical antibiotic creams.

Cryoblister

A cryoblister is a temporary and expected side effect with cryotherapy. It usually occurs due to the tissue damage caused by the cryogen, i.e., liquid nitrogen (Figure 62.3).

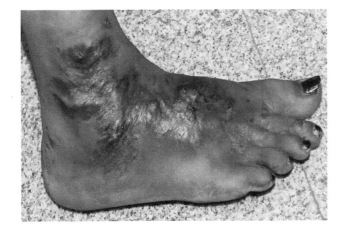

Figure 62.2 Bleeding from varicose veins. (Courtesy of Cutis Academy.)

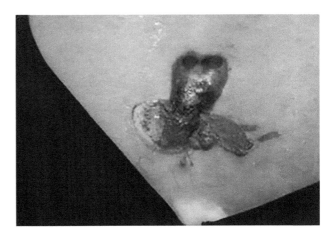

Figure 62.3 Cryoblister following surface cryotherapy. (Courtesy of Cutis Academy.)

It usually manifests 24–48 hours following cryotherapy. Patients are usually counseled about it, and treatment includes topical antibiotics with blister drainage.

Traumatic nail avulsion

Most of the fingernail injuries are caused by crush trauma. It is common in children and young adults. Effective emergency treatment of traumatic nail injuries is important to prevent secondary deformities. If subungual hematoma is present involving more than 50% of the nail, then it has to be evacuated. It is done by making two small holes in the nail plate. If the avulsed nail plate is intact, then it can be placed over the nail bed as a biological dressing. If it is too damaged, then nail substitutes can be used. If there are wounds or laceration present on the nail bed/matrix, then it can be closed using absorbable sutures. In case of avulsion of the nail bed or matrix and if the avulsed tissue is available, then it can be repositioned and sutured. If the avulsed tissue is not available, then conservative or reconstructive surgeries should be done. If there is associated distal phalanx fracture, nail bed repair is done, and a simple splint can be given in case of a nondisplaced fracture. In case of a displaced fracture, K-wire is inserted and fixed *in situ*.

CONCLUSION

A well-equipped emergency operating room, a good knowledge of dermatosurgery, and training in emergency BLS and ACLS courses make a dermatosurgeon more confident in identifying and managing these emergencies.

KEY POINTS

- Dermatosurgical emergencies can be of two types: emergencies encountered during dermatosurgical procedures and dermatosurgical conditions that require emergency interventions.
- A complete and thorough examination and evaluation of the patient by the dermatosurgeon are of prime importance like for any other surgery, irrespective of whether the procedure is as simple as a skin biopsy or a major case such as flap surgeries or hair restoration surgeries.
- Anaphylaxis, Vasovagal syncope and Lidocaine "allergy" and toxicity are the commonest emergencies we face in a dermatosurgery set up.
- Hemorrhage, bleeding of varicose vein, paraphimosis, Fournier gangrene, traumatic nail avulsion, thrombophlebitis and cryoblister may also occur.

REFERENCES

1. Worm M et al. Symptom profile and risk factors of anaphylaxis in Central Europe. *Allergy* 2012;7:691–8.
2. Tejedor-Alonso MA et al. Incidence of anaphylaxis in the city of Alcorcon (Spain): A population-based study. *Clin Exp Allergy* 2012;7:578–89.
3. Wood RA et al. Anaphylaxis in America: The prevalence and characteristics of anaphylaxis in the United States. *J Allergy Clin Immunol* 2014;7:461–7.
4. Simons FER et al. For the World Allergy Organization. World Allergy Organization guidelines for the assessment and management of anaphylaxis. *J Allergy Clin Immunol* 2011;7:587–93.
5. Lieberman P et al. The diagnosis and management of anaphylaxis practice parameter: 2010 update. *J Allergy Clin Immunol* 2010;7:477–80.
6. Muraro A et al. On behalf of EAACI Food Allergy and Anaphylaxis Guidelines Group. Anaphylaxis: Guidelines from the European Academy of Allergy and Clinical Immunology. *Allergy* 2014;69:1025–45.
7. Choo KJL, Simons FER, Sheikh A. Glucocorticoids for the treatment of anaphylaxis. *Cochrane Database Syst Rev* 2012;7:CD007596.
8. Sheikh A, Ten-Broek V, Brown SGA, Simons FER. H₁ antihistamines for the treatment of anaphylaxis: Cochrane systematic review. *Allergy* 2007;7:830–7.
9. Ellis BC, Brown SGA. Parenteral antihistamines cause hypotension in anaphylaxis. *Emerg Med Australas* 2013;7:92–3.
10. Nurmatov U, Rhatigan E, Simons FER, Sheikh A. H₂-antihistamines for the treatment of anaphylaxis with and without shock: A systematic review. *Ann Allergy Asthma Immunol* 2014;7:126–31.
11. Soto-Aguilar MC, deShazo RD, Waring NP. Anaphylaxis: Why it happens and what to do about it. *Postgrad Med* 1987;82:154–70.
12. Gordon BR. Prevention and management of office allergy emergencies. *Otolaryngol Clin North Am* 1992;25:119–134.
13. Martin JB, Ruskin J. Faintness, syncope, and seizures. In: Wilson JD et al. (Eds), *Harrison's Principles of Internal Medicine*. 12th ed. New York: McGraw-Hill; 1991:134–140.
14. Covino BG. Systemic toxicity of local anesthetic agents. *Anesth Analg* 1978;57:387–8.
15. Albright GA. Cardiac arrest following regional anesthesia with etidocaine or bupivacaine. *Anesthesiology* 1979;51:285–7.
16. Thomson PD et al. Lidocaine pharmacokinetics in advanced heart failure, liver disease, and renal failure in humans. *Ann Intern Med* 1973;78:499–508.
17. Feely J, Wilkinson GR, McAllister CB, Wood AJ. Increased toxicity and reduced clearance of lidocaine by cimetidine. *Ann Intern Med* 1982;96:592–4.
18. Sobanko JF, Miller CJ, Alster TS. Topical anesthetics for dermatologic procedures: A review. *Dermatol Surg* 2012;38:709–21.
19. Lubarsky DA, Moy R. Complications of anesthesia (local, topical, general). In: Nouri K (Ed), *Complications in Dermatologic Surgery*. Philadelphia: Elsevier; 2008.

20. Martin EW. *Techniques of Medication*. Philadelphia: JB Lippincott, 1969; 116–9.

21. Poplawski F, Zweig BE. Evaluation and management of allergy to local anesthesia. *Compend Cont Ed Dent* 1980;1:319–22.

22. Bennett CR. *Monheim's Local Anesthesia and Pain Control in Dental Practice*. 7th ed. St. Louis, MO: CV Mosby; 1984, 225.

23. Raj PP, Winnie AP. Immediate reactions to local anesthetics. In: Orkin F, Cooperman LH (Eds), *Complications in Anesthesiology*. Philadelphia: JB Lippincott; 1983: 51–74.

24. Roesch RP. The immune system. In: Stoelting RK and Dierdorf SF (Eds), *Anesthesia and Co-Existing Disease*. New York: Churchill Livingstone, 1983; 645–61.

25. Kasten GW, Martin ST. Successful cardiovascular resuscitation after massive intravenous bupivacaine overdosage in anesthetized dogs. *Anesth Analg* 1985;64:491–7.

26. Fader DJ, Johnson TM. Medical issues and emergencies in the dermatology office. *J Am Acad Dermatol* 1997;36:1–16.

27. Howell SJ, Sear YM, Yeates D, Goldacre M, Sear JW, Foex P. Hypertension, admission blood pressure and perioperative cardiovascular risk. *Anaesthesia* 1996;51:1000–4.

28. Mancia G et al. 2013 ESH/ESC guidelines for the management of arterial hypertension: The Task Force for the management of arterial hypertension of the European Society of Hypertension (ESH) and of the European Society of Cardiology (ESC). *J Hypertens* 2013;31:1281–357.

29. Rodriguez MA, Kumar SK, De Caro M. Hypertensive crisis. *Cardiol Rev* 2010;18:102–7.

30. Chobanian AV et al. The seventh report of the Joint National Committee on Prevention, Detection, Evaluation, and Treatment of High Blood Pressure: The JNC 7 report. *JAMA* 2003;289:2560–72.

31. Calhoun DA, Oparil S. Treatment of hypertensive crisis. *N Engl J Med* 1990;323:1177–83.

32. Varon J, Fromm RE Jr. Hypertensive crises. The need for urgent management. *Postgrad Med* 1996;99:189–91.

33. Woo E, Ball R, Braun M. Fatal syncope-related fall after immunization. *Arch Pediatr Adolesc Med* 2005;159:1083.

34. Hancox JG, Venkat AP, Coldiron B, Feldman SR, Williford PM. The safety of office-based surgery: Review of recent literature from several disciplines. *Arch Dermatol* 2004;140:1379–82.

35. Raj SR, Coffin ST. Medical therapy and physical maneuvers in the treatment of the vasovagal syncope and orthostatic hypotension. *Prog Cardiovasc Dis* 2013;55:425–33.

36. Calhoun DA, Oparil S. Treatment of hypertensive crisis. *N Engl J Med* 1990;323:1177–83.

37. Moffat DA, Ramsden RT. The deformity produced by a palsy of the marginal mandibular branch of the facial nerve. *J Laryngol Otol* 1977;91:401–6.

38. Ishikawa Y. An anatomical study on the distribution of the temporal branch of the facial nerve. *J Craniomaxillofac Surg* 1990;18:287–92.

39. Wiater JM, Bigliani LU. Spinal accessory nerve injury. *Clin Orthop Relat Res* 1999;(368):5–16.

40. Grabski WJ, Salasche SJ. Management of temporal nerve injuries. *J Dermatol Surg Oncol* 1985;11:145–51.

41. Hausamen JE, Schmelzeisen R. Current principles in microsurgical nerve repair. *Br J Oral Maxillofac Surg* 1996;34:143–57.

42. Hass AN, Penne RB, Stefanyszyn MA, Flanagan JC. Incidence of post blepharoplasty orbital hemorrhage and associated visual loss. *Ophthal Plast Reconstr Surg* 2004;20:426–32.

43. Klapper SR, Patrinely JR. Management of cosmetic eyelid surgery complications. *Semin Plast Surg* 2007;21:80–93.

44. Anderson RL. Bilateral visual loss after blepharoplasty. *Arch Ophthalmol* 1981;99:2205.

45. Selbst SM. Office management of status epilepticus. *Pediatr Emerg Care* 1991;7:106–9.

46. Brodie M. Status epilepticus in adults. *Lancet* 1990;336:551–2.

47. Bleck TP. Management approaches to prolonged seizures and status epilepticus. *Epilepsia* 1999;40:S59–63.

48. Delgado-Escueta AV et al. Management of status epilepticus. *N Engl J Med* 1982;306:1337–40.

49. Alcalay J. Cutaneous surgery in patients receiving warfarin therapy. *Dermatol Surg* 2001;27(8):756–8.

50. Kargi E, Babuccu O, Hosnuter M, Babuccu B, Altinyazar C. Complications of minor cutaneous surgery in patients under anticoagulant treatment. *Aesthetic PlastSurg* 2002;26(6):483–5.

51. Larson MJ, Taylor RS. Monitoring vital signs during outpatient Mohs and post-Mohs reconstructive surgery performed under local anesthesia. *Dermatol Surg* 2004;30(5):777–83.

52. Robinson JK. Anatomy for procedural dermatology. In: Robinson JK, Hanke CW, Siegel DM, Fratila A (Eds) *Surgery of the Skin*. New York: Mosby Elsevier; 2010: 3–27.

53. Hruza GJ. Anesthesia. In: Bolognia JL, Jorrizo JL, Rapini RP (Eds), *Dermatology*. 2nd ed. New York: Mosby Elsevier; 2008: 2173–81.

54. Goldman G. Wound closure materials and instruments. In: Bolognia JL, Jorizzo JL, Rapini RP (Eds), *Dermatology*. 2nd ed. New York: Mosby Elsevier; 2008: 2183–93.

63

Emergencies associated with cosmetological procedures

RASYA DIXIT

INTRODUCTION

A cosmetic procedure is often a clinic-based procedure. Presented as quick "lunchtime" procedures, patients walk in and walk out of the dermatologist's office, hoping to be rejuvenated and renewed. To note, most of them do not have any medical issues but seek help for enhancing their beauty or appearance. Therefore, common side effects that may be very acceptable in other dermatosurgical techniques may be unacceptable to the cosmetic patient. Therefore, it is important to establish three primary criteria: a sound knowledge of the procedure, placing standard operating protocols for all cosmetic procedures, and identifying and treating emerging complications at the earliest. This chapter presents the common emergencies and the approaches to prevention and management of the same.

CONCEPT: FROM START TO FINISH

The golden step in the management of complications and emergencies is prevention of the complication itself. This can be achieved in the following steps:

1. *Patient counseling, informed consent forms, and photography*: The patient has to have a clear understanding of the procedure, be aware of the possible complications, and be aware of the normal recovery time postprocedure. Also the patient should be allowed to share his or her treatment goals, and the patient's social engagements and events must be taken into account. This step of going over the treatment objectives and social program needs to be done at each visit as the patient may have forgotten the explanation given the previous time. An informed consent form stating the common and rare side effects has to be signed by the patient in a language understood by the patient. Photography can be used as a tool to document the pretreatment baseline.

2. *Intraprocedure observations and documentation*: A well-prepared dermatologist is as aware of the steps of the procedure as well as the possible complications that may arise and the ways to deal with them. A standard operating protocol has to be defined for each procedure and should list all of the steps of the procedure. It should also encompass the steps needed in case of a complication. The setup for the procedure therefore should not only include the instruments and devices needed for the procedure, but also emergency equipment needed to manage a complication. The procedure needs to be documented in detail. In case of a complication or emergency, the treatment offered also needs to be documented in detail.

3. *Postprocedure counseling and proactive follow-up*: After the procedure, a brief recap of what to expect is explained to the patient, and the postprocedure care is given. A printed sheet of the postprocedure care can be given to the patient. If a complication arises, the dermatologist should offer reassurance and discuss the potential cause of the same, as well as the management plan.

Now we can consider a few common cosmetic treatments in the dermatological outpatient department, and the dermatological emergencies that may arise.

CHEMICAL PEEL

1. *Complications associated with chemical peels*:
Complications (Table 63.1) are usually minor and can be easily treated. Most of the complications occur due to improper patient selection or due to inadequate priming. Sometimes the priming agents are not withdrawn adequately before the peel, causing the skin to be dry and the peeling agent to penetrate deeper than indicated. Perioral and periorbital areas often have lines or creases where the peel agent can accumulate and avoid being neutralized adequately and cause a chemical burn (Figure 63.1) or a scab that is discovered the next day [1]. Usually these are superficial scabs and they resolve without incident. However, if there is a social event on the next few days, it needs to be treated as an emergency.
   Clinical tips:
   - Always do the peel in a well-lit room.
   - Examine the patient's skin after it has been cleansed, avoid peel if the skin is dry.
   - Check when the priming agent has been stopped.
   - Protect the sensitive areas, such as the angle of the lips, the nasal folds, and the under-eye area, with petroleum jelly to prevent pooling of the chemical peel agent [1].
   - Start the peel on the areas where the skin is generally more resistant to treatment before applying peel on the more sensitive areas; for example, the forehead is followed by the cheek, chin and then the eyelids.
   - Explain to the patient what to expect during the peel. Some amount of irritation and stinginess is expected in a peel. However, to assess the sensation, ask the patient to grade the sensation of stinging on a scale of 1–10, with 1 being very tolerable to 10 being the skin feels like it is on fire. This helps us to understand when to terminate the peel, especially in darker skin patients where the appearance of erythema might not be recognized easily.
   - Neutralize the peel when the patient reports sensation more than 6 on the 10-point scale. Wash with cold normal saline until the patient reports that the skin feels normal, and examine for erythema or blistering.
   - If you note blistering or significant erythema after the treatment, direct the patient to frequently apply bland emollient and a medium-potency topical steroid for the next 2–3 days.
   - Examine the skin daily until the scabs fall off.

2. *Chemical burn of the eye*: The most serious complication of any chemical peel is a chemical burn of the eye from an accidental splash [2].
   - Make sure that when you are doing the chemical peel, you cover the eyes with protective gauze. Tell the patient to keep his or her eyes closed throughout the procedure.
   - Always arrange the procedure tray to avoid accidental spillage.
   - Make sure that you or your assistant does not pass the container containing the chemical peel over the patient's face or body.
   - An eyewash station should be maintained whenever a chemical peel is done. It should contain a bottle of normal saline that can be flushed immediately into the eyes to neutralize the effect of the peel.
   - Immediate evaluation by an ophthalmologist is warranted should an accidental spillage occur.

3. *Hypersensitivity or allergic reactions to the agent used*: Hypersensitivity, both immediate and delayed, is more common than allergic reactions to chemical peels [3]. It may present as a minor reaction or as severe as an anaphylactic reaction. Laryngeal edema has been reported as a hypersensitivity reaction to phenol peel and presents as stridor, hoarseness, and or tachypnea and can occur as late as 24 hours. These have to be treated with oral steroids under hospitalization.

4. *Systemic toxicity to salicylic acid*: A rare complication, systemic toxicity to salicylic acid [4] occurs when salicylic acid peels are done on a large body surface area. Symptoms are seen when the levels in the blood are ≥ 35 mg/dL. The common presentation includes nausea, vomiting, dizziness, psychosis, stupor, tinnitus, and finally, coma and death. Patients who have preexisting uremia can develop hypoglycemia if they have systemic absorption of salicylates.

5. *Rare complications*: Rare complications such as toxic shock syndrome have been rarely reported with chemical peels. They may involve the hematological, hepatorenal, and central nervous systems. There should be

Table 63.1 Complications of chemical peel

Complications due to wrong patient selection
Complications due to wrong peel selection
Accidental spillage
Allergy and hypersensitivity to peel agents
Toxicity

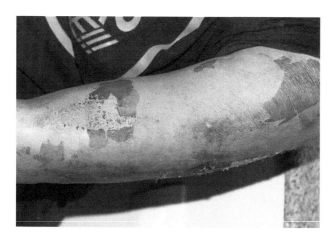

Figure 63.1 Postchemical peel burn. (Courtesy of Cutis Academy.)

no delay in recognition of the condition and in starting treatment. Hydration by administering IV fluids should be done, and if required, antibiotics targeting *Staphylococcus aureus* should be used [5,6].

MICRODERMABRASION

During and after the procedure, a persistent urticarial rash can be seen in some patients almost like a physical dermographism. This usually resolves by itself. Improper usage or nonusage of eye protection can lead to ocular complications such as irritation, chemosis, photophobia, and punctate keratitis if the aluminum crystals enter the eye. The crystals should not be rubbed out, but instead flushed out with copious amounts of normal saline. An immediate referral to an ophthalmologist is indicated to diagnose and treat the above complications [7,8].

MICRONEEDLING RADIOFREQUENCY

Electromagnetic interference (EMI) of implantable electronic devices is a rare complication with office-based electrosurgery procedures, especially after the introduction of newer implantable electronic devices [9].

- *Cochlear implants*: There may be irreparable damage to the cochlear device needing a reimplantation of a new device. It can also cause necrotization of the cells of the basilar membrane. This is an irreversible complication, and future implants will also not work.
- *Implanted cardiac device*: Caution should be exercised in patients who are pacemaker dependent [10–13]. One report described EMI from a monopolar device causing battery depletion and eventual "voltage control oscillator lock-out," with subsequent pacemaker failure in a 15-year-old patient after cardiac surgery.

PLATELET-RICH PLASMA

This is generally considered a safe procedure because autologous blood is used. However, there is a case report of unilateral visual loss in a patient who underwent PRP in the glabellar region for rhytides [14].

DERMAL FILLERS

1. Inappropriate placement of filler, such as superficial placement, is one of the most frequent reasons for patient dissatisfaction. The action of some fillers, including hyaluronic acid (HA), are reversible with hyaluronidase, and these complications can be easily corrected.
2. Hypersensitivity to current U.S. Food and Drug Administration approved products is rare and can most often be managed with anti-inflammatory agents.
3. Infection is also uncommon and is managed with antibiotics.

4. Vascular and ischemic complications occur due to intra-arterial injections. Although they can occur at any site where vessels are present, intra-arterial injections are most common in the glabellar and nasal region, though filler injection in the nasolabial area, forehead, and chin causing these complications has been described [15,16]. The incidence of vascular occlusion is 3 in 1000 injections. An intra-arterial injection can lead to either soft tissue ischemia or visual compromise.
   - Thorough knowledge of the anatomy and the vasculature of the face are imperative to the injecting doctor.
   - Do the treatment in a well-lit room, and inject small amounts at a time.
   - Before injecting a bolus, always withdraw and wait for a few seconds with negative pressure to look for any blood in the hub of the syringe. This may not be a foolproof method as the viscosity of the filler may prevent blood from entering the syringe even if the needle is intravascular. If blood enters the hub of the needle, then withdraw the needle, discard the needle and blood, and start again with a fresh needle.
   - Inject one small bolus at a time.
   - Do not inject if you feel resistance to the injection.
   - If the patient reports severe pain, stop the injection.

Stop injecting if you observe blanching, as soft tissue ischemia presents as pain, mottling, and blanching at the site of injection immediately postinjection. Features that may appear later are formation of vesicles and bulla, bluish discoloration, and necrosis [16]. If you notice blanching, gauze soaked in warm saline should then be applied to facilitate vasodilation [17,18]. If the filler used is a HA-based one, hyaluronidase should be injected, and the whole area should be flooded with the product and massaged. The risk of allergic reaction to hyaluronidase (which may be of ovine or bovine or human recombinant sources) must be taken into consideration [19,20,21]. Special caution must be taken with those patients who have allergy to bee stings, as the hyaluronidase shares 30% sequence identity with bee venom. The availability of hyaluronidase in the clinic should be confirmed before starting treatment. Typically, a range of 8–16 units of hyaluronidase 0.5 mL of HA will dissolve the cosmetically imperfect swelling. For emergency situations when occlusion or ischemia is suspected, use more. As per the literature, it is an exceedingly rare situation where native HA had to be dissolved with hyaluronidase. Immediate application of nitroglycerin paste to facilitate vascular dilatation and blood flow to the area should be done. Additionally, anticoagulants such as aspirin and nonsteroidal anti-inflammatory agents, as well as vitamins that inhibit platelet aggregation, should be encouraged in any protocol to treat cutaneous tissue ischemia [22–25].

Given that hyperbaric oxygen has proven successful in healing nasal tip grafting in cases of cancer or trauma reconstruction, administration of oxygen via nasal cannula is suggested, or in the form of hyperbaric oxygen for ischemia secondary to cosmetic filler injection. For cases with severe, unremitting swelling, oral antihistamines may also be employed. Finally, treatment with low molecular weight heparin (5000 IE daily) has been reported to treat impending necrosis after HA injection in the treatment of frown lines of the glabella due to occlusion or compression of the supratrochlear vessels [26,27,28].

BOTULINUM TOXIN INJECTIONS

Serious side effects are rare when botulinum toxin (BT) injections are used for a cosmetic purpose. The side effects caused by distant spread or systemic absorption are usually dose related and occur when more than 600 U of BT is used or when the frequency of injections is high. Allergic and anaphylactic reactions can occur either due to the BT or to one of the other constituents, such as albumin or lactose [29,30].

Patients in whom there has been a systemic spread of toxin present with botulism-like symptoms, including redness of the eye, accommodation difficulty, xerostomia, gastrointestinal disturbances, dysphagia, hoarseness, and breathing difficulties and the possibility of death [30]. This complication has not been seen when botulinum toxin is used for cosmetic purposes, except when used for hyperhidrosis.

CONCLUSION

Emergencies in cosmetic practice are rare. But one must be equipped with the knowledge to identify symptoms and signs that might indicate an emergent condition.

KEY POINTS

- Common side effects that may be very acceptable in other dermatosurgical techniques may not be acceptable in cosmetic procedures and are therefore considered as emergencies.
- During chemical peeling, wrong patient selection, wrong peel selection, accidental spillage, allergy and hypersensitivity to peel agents and irritant potential may all cause unforgiving adverse effects.
- Incorrect placement, hypersensitivity reactions, intra-arterial injections and secondary infections can complicate the administration of fillers.
- Botulinum toxin can rarely cause botulism too.

REFERENCES

1. Khunger N, IADVL Task Force. Standard guidelines of care for chemical peels. *Indian J Dermatol Venereol Leprol* 2008(Suppl);74:S5–12.
2. Resnick SS, Resnick BI. Complications of chemical peeling. *Dermatol Clin* 1995;13:309–12.
3. Duffy DM. Avoiding complications. In: Rubin MG (Ed), *Chemical Peels. Procedures in Cosmetic Dermatology*. New York: Elsevier; 2006:137–69.
4. Landau M. Cardiac complications in deep chemical peels. *Dermatol Surg* 2007;33:190–3.
5. LoVerme WE, Drapkin MS, Courtiss EH, Wilson RM. Toxic shock syndrome after chemical face peel. *Plast Reconstr Surg* 1987;80:115–8.
6. Levy LL, Emer JJ. Complications of minimally invasive cosmetic procedures: Prevention and management. *J Cutan Aesthet Surg* 2012;5:121–32.
7. Farris PK, Rietschel RL. An unusual acute urticarial response following microdermabrasion. *Dermatol Surg* 2002;28:606–8; discussion 608.
8. Spencer JM. Microdermabrasion. *Am J Clin Dermatol* 2005;6:89–92.
9. Voutsalath MA, Bichakjian CK, Pelosi F, Blum D, Johnson TM, Farrehi PM. Electrosurgery and implantable electronic devices: Review and implications for office-based procedures. *Dermatol Surg* 2011;37:889–99.
10. Smalley PJ. Laser safety: Risks, hazards, and control measures. *Laser Ther* 2011;20:95–106.
11. Zhang AY, Obagi S. Diagnosis and management of skin resurfacing—Related complications. *Oral Maxillofacial Surg Clin N Am* 2009;21:1–12.
12. Alam M, Warycha M. Complications of lasers and light treatments. *Dermatol Ther* 2011;24:571–80.
13. Batra RS, Jacob CI, Hobbs L, Arndt KA, Dover JS. A prospective survey of patient experiences after laser skin resurfacing: Results from 2 ½ years of follow-up. *Arch Dermatol* 2003;139:1295–9.
14. Kalyam K, Kavoussi SC, Ehrlich M, Teng CC, Chadha N, Khodadadeh S, Liu J. Irreversible blindness following periocular autologous platelet-rich plasma skin rejuvenation treatment. *Ophthal Plast Reconstr Surg* 2017;33(3S Suppl 1):S12–16.
15. Cohen JL. Understanding, avoiding, and managing dermal filler complications. *Dermatol Surg* 2008;34(Suppl 1):S9209.
16. Grunebaum LD et al. The risk of alar necrosis associated with dermal filler injection. *Dermatol Surg* 2009;35:1635–40.
17. Winslow C. The management of dermal filler complications. *Facial Plast Surg* 2009;25:124–8.
18. Bolognia J, Jorizzo J, Rapini R (Eds). *Dermatology*. 2nd ed. St. Louis, MO: Mosby;2007.
19. Bailey SH, Cohen JL, Kenkel JM. Etiology, prevention and treatment of dermal filler complications. *Aesthetic Surg J* 2011;31:110–21.
20. Cohen JL. Understanding, avoiding and managing dermal filler complications. *Dermatol Surg* 2008;34:s92–9.
21. Cohen JL, Brown MR. Anatomic considerations for soft tissue augmentation of the face. *J Drugs Dermatol* 2009;8:13–6.
22. Glaich D, Cohen J, Goldberg L. Injection necrosis of the glabella: Protocol for prevention and treatment after use of dermal fillers. *Dermatol Surg* 2006;32:276–81.

23. Grunebaum LD, Elsaie ML, Kaufman JY. Six-month, double-blind, randomized, split-face study to compare the efficacy and safety of calcium hydroxylapatite (CaHA) mixed with lidocaine and CaHA alone for correction of nasolabial fold wrinkles. *Dermatol Surg* 2008;36:760–5.

24. Sclafani A, Fagien S. Treatment of injectable soft tissue filler complications. *Dermatol Surg* 2009;35:1672–80.

25. Nichter LS, Morwood DT, Williams GS, Spence RJ. Expanding the limits of composite grafting: A case report of successful nose replantation assisted by hyperbaric oxygen. *Plast Reconstr Surg* 1991;87:337–40.

26. Rapley JH, Lawrence WT, Witt PD. Composite grafting and hyperbaric oxygen therapy in pediatric nasal tip reconstruction after avulsive dog bite injury. *Am Plast Surg* 2001;46:434–8.

27. Sanchz S et al. Arterial embolization caused by injection of hyaluronic acid (Restylane). *Br J Dermatol* 2002;146:928–9.

28. Van Loghem JA, Fouché JJ, Thuis J. Sensitivity of aspiration as a safety test before injection of soft tissue fillers. *J Cosmet Dermatol* 2017;7.

29. Niamtu J. Complications in fillers and Botox. *Oral Maxillofacial Surg Clin N Am* 2009;21:13–21.

30. Omprakash HM, Rajendran SC. Botulinum toxin deaths: What is the fact? *J Cutan Aesthet Surg* 2008;1:95–7.

64

Emergencies due to laser and light-based devices

M. KUMARESAN

INTRODUCTION

Different types of lasers are often used in dermatology clinic–based practice. The applications of lasers and light devices have grown exponentially. With increasing applications, the incidence of clinical emergencies arises consequently, and knowledge about these emergency situations becomes essential. It is therefore imperative to establish standards for the practice of laser safety. The purpose is to establish the safety guidelines for the dermatologist and the team. It is recommended that laser safety practices be meticulously followed by all surgical personnel who are involved in the use of lasers in order to protect themselves and their patients. The emergency situations in lasers and light-based applications are categorized into medical and nonmedical emergencies. Medical emergencies are usually eye injuries. The nonmedical emergencies include fire accidents, device explosion, and laser plume effects.

EYE INJURIES

Eye injuries are a potential hazard in laser and light-based devices, and the eye is the most sensitive organ to laser irradiation. Almost all of the structures of the eye are susceptible to laser-induced injuries [1]. Various host and light characteristics determine the nature of the injury to the eye (Tables 64.1 through 64.3) [1–3].

Clinical features of eye injury

The common signs and symptoms are pain and soreness of the eye, sudden loss of vision, pigmentary cells in the chambers of the eye, synechiae, distorted pupils, reduced visual acuity, and photophobia, either immediately or a few days

later [2,4–8]. Retinal injuries are manifested as sudden loss of vision followed by gradual recovery over a few days and weeks, usually with associated complications [2,4–8]. Corneal and retinal burns, uveitis, and cataract can also occur.

Long-wavelength lasers: The target chromophore for long-wavelength lasers such as CO_2 and erbium:yttrium-aluminum-garnet (Er:YAG) is water. When the laser beam comes in contact with the eye, it is absorbed by the tear layer covering and cornea, which gets evaporated, and further exposure leads to corneal burns. Even though such burns are treatable and do not lead to permanent loss of vision, they are painful and can cause temporary visual loss [10].

Midrange lasers: Exposure to a laser beam from midrange wavelength lasers can damage both the cornea and the lens.

Short wavelengths: Exposure to a beam of short wavelength is the most dangerous, as it can reach all the anterior structures of the eye. The target chromophore for these rays in the eye is the hemoglobin present in the retina, and this can lead to irreversible visual loss [4,12].

Risk factors

The injuries are seen among the operators and the subjects undergoing laser treatment. The most common risk factor is lack of proper protective eyewear. The other reasons could be slippage of the eye shield and incidental exposure to laser light due to reflection from bone or any reflecting surface [4].

Incidence

Laser epilation around the eyebrow has led to the most complications. Several cases of posterior synechiae, conjunctival hyperemia, photophobia, reduced visual acuity, pigmentary cells in the chambers of the eye, anterior uveitis, iris atrophy,

Table 64.1 Various factors of the light that determine damage to the eye

Light characteristics	Extent of eye damage
Wavelength	Determines depth of penetration
Exposure duration	The longer the duration of light exposure, the greater is the damage to the eye
Pulse duration	Shorter pulses produce more damage due to high energy
Fluence	Higher fluence causes greater injury

Source: Pierce JS et al. J Occup Environ Med 2011;53:1302–9.

Table 64.2 Various host factors that influence damage to the eye structures

Host factors	Extent of eye damage
Pupil size	Dilated pupil allows more light to penetrate, causing greater damage
Retinal pigmentation	Heavily pigmented retina gets damaged more due to greater absorption of light

Source: Barkana Y, Belkin M. Serv Opthamolol 2000;44:459–78.

Table 64.3 Wavelength of the light and eye damage

Wavelength	Eye damage
UV-C 290–300 nm	Photokeratitis
UV-B 290–320 nm	Photokeratitis
UV-A 320–400 nm	Photochemical cataract
Visible/near infrared 400–1400 nm	Photochemical and thermal retinal injury
Infrared 760–100,000 nm	Aqueous flare, corneal burn, cataract

Source: Kochevar IE et al. In: Goldsmith L et al. (Eds), Fitzpatrick's Dermatology in General Medicine. 8th ed. New York: McGraw-Hill; 2011.

and cataract have been reported as sequelae to the laser epilation around the eyebrows [4,10]. There are reports of macular hole and vitreous floaters among the laser operators who had slippage of the protective eyewear [7,8]. Exposure to the Q-switched 1064 nm neodymium-doped yttrium-aluminium-garnet (Nd:YAG) laser is particularly dangerous and may initially go undetected because of the invisibility of the main laser beam, the lack of a visible secondary aiming beam, and the absence of sensory nerves on the retina [12].

Prevention

The laser physician and other operators should exercise caution in ensuring proper eye protection for themselves and their staff when working with lasers. A warning sign should

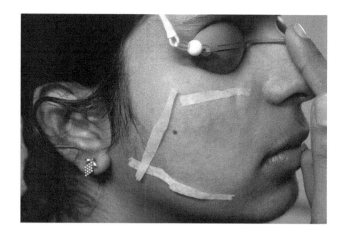

Figure 64.1 External eye shield.

be displayed on the external door of any room in which lasers are used.

Protective eyewear is chosen based on the wavelength of light emitted by the laser. Each pair of laser safety goggles is designated with a central wavelength of rejection, or a rejection band composed of a range of wavelengths, and the optical density afforded by the lens. The higher the optical density, the greater is the protection. Adequate eyewear has an optic density of ≥4 for the wavelength of the laser [12].

Eye shields protect the chromophores within the eye from the laser. Eye shields can be internal (i.e., placed between the globe and eyelid) or external [13]. External shields are used routinely (Figure 64.1). Internal eye shields are generally considered more protective and are used when procedures are performed very close to the eye (Figure 64.2). Internal

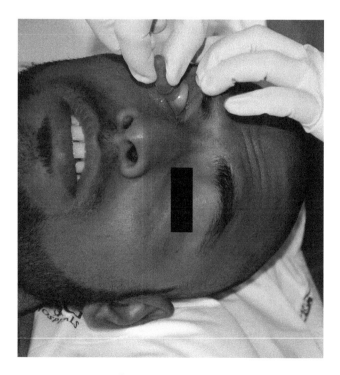

Figure 64.2 Internal eye shield for ocular safety.

eye shields do not cover the patient's entire eye and may shift with movement; the operator must ensure that ocular pigmented structures, including the iris, are fully protected at all times. Caution should be exercised with the use of internal eye shields, because minor injuries, most commonly corneal abrasions, can occur [13].

Although eye protection is essential, laser eye injury can occur even if protection is used. Goggles and shields can shift during use, and laser light can penetrate through to exposed, unprotected surfaces. It has also been postulated that light can reflect off of the cheekbone or orbital rim and enter the eye indirectly [12].

Treatment

When eye injuries are suspected, they should be promptly treated by stopping the laser treatment immediately and referring the subject to an ophthalmologist for complete evaluation. Corticosteroids, antioxidants, and vasodilators are used based on the extent of the injury. Hemorrhages resolve spontaneously within a relatively short time, from 2 weeks to a few months [12].

FIRE ACCIDENTS

A fire accident during laser surgery is a rare but potentially life-threatening complication. A flash fire caused by a pulsed-dye laser that resulted in a partial-thickness burn and second- and third-degree burns after the inadvertent firing of a carbon dioxide laser that ignited a smoldering spot on a surgical towel has been reported in the literature [14,15].

Risk factors

The three elements required to initiate fire are a source of ignition, fuel, and an oxidizer. Laser devices are the source of ignition with a CO_2 laser carrying the highest risk. Numerous materials ubiquitous in the health-care setting can serve as fuels. Gauze, drapes, towels, underpads, skin degreasers, and cotton have all been experimentally shown to be potential fuel sources [12]. Supplemental oxygen is a common oxidizer in surgical fires, but ambient oxygen can also be sufficient as an oxidizer [1].

Alcohol-based skin preparations have been reported to act as fuel to initiate a fire accident [16,17]. Aluminum chloride, chlorhexidine, and isopropyl alcohol may also fuel fires, where these materials have not fully dried [16,17].

Prevention

Less flammable equipment and materials (e.g., phenol polymer drape, water-based prepping gents, and red rubber endotracheal tubes [when using a carbon dioxide laser]) may be substituted for more flammable equipment and materials (e.g., a cotton/polyester drape, alcohol-based prepping agents, and polyvinylchloride endotracheal tubes) [1]. Staff should also ensure that water and fire

extinguishers are readily available [11]. The use of moistened towels or sponges to drape the perimeter of laser treatment areas, and avoiding or protecting hairlines that might have hair spray or flammable prep solutions dried in the hairline is recommended.

A warning sign board indicating that laser surgery is in progress and caution is advised should be displayed prominently in the door of the laser room (Figure 64.3). The instructions regarding fire safety to all health-care personnel and checklists, time-outs, or procedures to identify and remove potential fuel sources should all be available at hand and rehearsed. Fire extinguishers should be mounted on the wall just outside the laser room for easy access, and all the laser operators should have a working knowledge of how to use the fire extinguisher (Figure 64.4) [12]. Solutions that contain iodophors (Hibiclens, Betadine, etc.) must be thoroughly dry before firing the laser, as heat can cause a chemical burn to the skin if it interacts with a wet solution [9].

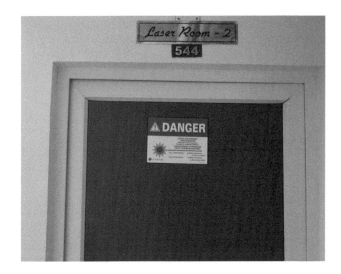

Figure 64.3 Laser in use warning sign.

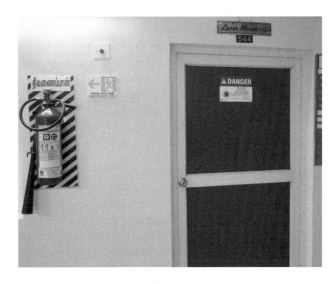

Figure 64.4 Fire extinguisher outside the laser room.

Flammable gases, such as oxygen or nitrous oxide, will be used only if necessary during laser cases, at concentrations less than 40%, and the laser operator will examine the gas delivery system setup to minimize any fire risks. Minimum concentrations of oxygen below the 40% required to adequately oxygenate the patient will be used.

PREVENTIVE MEASURES

- Care should be taken to not have any reflective surfaces in the laser room, such as a mirror or metal, including metallic instruments.
- All areas other than those being treated should be draped with a nonflammable material like wet gauze to prevent any burns.
- Special attention is given to the perianal area as methane gas explosions can occur. Use a wet gauze in the rectum prior to the procedure.
- It should be made certain that the target area is dry before starting the procedure. Decontaminating solutions such as alcohol or betadine are flammable, and so one should wait for these to dry before starting the procedure.
- If the forehead is being targeted, the patient's hair should be covered with a nonflammable material to make sure no hair cosmetics such as hair sprays or gels come in the way of the laser beam.

Treatment

A proper fire management plan should be developed in conjunction with a safety officer and should be rehearsed by all operative personnel on regular intervals to be familiar with the protocol. A laser surgical fire can spread rapidly; prompt action should be taken to extinguish the fire [12]. Large fires may require a more comprehensive response, such as stopping the flow of oxidizers, removing the burning materials, extinguishing them, and attending to the care of the patient [14]. If the fire cannot be extinguished by materials available nearby, other means may include fire extinguishers, fire blankets, sprinkler systems, or evacuation and handover to firefighters [14]. Local wound care is based on the degree of the burn, the percentage of body surface area involved, and specific patient and wound characteristics.

MISCELLANEOUS COMPLICATIONS

Mild, short-term complications of laser treatment include erythema, edema, urticaria, crusting or erosion, ecchymoses, blistering, and infection, such as reactivation of herpes simplex virus (HSV). An active search for these preexisting conditions (HSV) and watchfulness during treatment preempt these minor complications. If the treatment is being administered by an assistant, the dermatologist should supervise the treatment and observe the skin changes during the session. The assistants also must be trained on observing these changes and bring them to the attention of the doctor.

KEY POINTS

- Eye injury is a potential hazard while using laser devices.
- Eye injuries might lead to permanent vision loss.
- Protective eyewear is selected based on the wavelength of the laser.
- Fire accidents are rare but a potential threat in the laser room.
- Fire safety must be practiced by all staff handling the lasers.

REFERENCES

1. Pierce JS, Lacey SE, Lippert JF, Lopez R, Franke JE, Colvard MD. An assessment of the occupational hazards related to medical lasers. *J Occup Environ Med* 2011;53:1302–9.
2. Barkana Y, Belkin M. Laser eye injuries. *Serv Opthamolol* 2000;44:459–78.
3. Kochevar IE, Taylor CR, Krutmann J. Fundamentals of cutaneous photobiology and photoimmunology. In: Goldsmith L, Katz S, Gilchrest B (Eds), *Fitzpatrick's Dermatology in General Medicine*. 8th ed. New York: McGraw-Hill; 2011.
4. Shulman S, Bichler I. Ocular complications of laser-assisted eyebrow epilation. *Eye (Lond)* 2009;23:982–3.
5. Parver DL et al. Ocular injury after laser hair reduction treatment to the eyebrow. *Arch Ophthalmol* 2012;130:1330–4.
6. Lin LT, Liang CM, Chiang SY, Yang HM, Chang CJ. Traumatic macular hole secondary to a Q-switch Alexandrite laser. *Retina* 2005;25:662–5.
7. Alam M, Chaudhry NA, Goldberg LH. Vitreous floaters following use of dermatologic lasers. *Dermatol Surg* 2002;28:1088–91.
8. Park DH, Kim IT. A case of accidental macular injury by Nd:YAG laser and subsequent 6 year follow-up. *Korean J Ophthalmol* 2009;23:207–9.
9. Smalley PJ. Laser safety: Risks, hazards, and control measures. *Laser Ther* 2011;20:95–106.
10. Brilakis HS, Holland EJ. Diode-laser-induced cataract and iris atrophy as a complication of eyelid hair removal. *Am J Ophthalmol* 2004;137:762–3.
11. Cao LY, Taylor JS, Vidimos A. Patient safety in dermatology: A review of the literature. *Dermatol Online J* 2010;16:3.

12. Minkis K, Whittington A, Alam M. Dermatologic surgery emergencies: Complications caused by systemic reactions, high-energy systems, and trauma. *J Am Acad Dermatol* 2016;75:265–84.

13. Ogle CA, Shim EK, Godwin JA. Use of eye shields and eye lubricants among oculoplastic and Mohs surgeons: A survey. *J Drugs Dermatol* 2009;8:855–60.

14. A clinician's guide to surgical fires: How they occur, how to prevent them, how to put them out. *Health Devices* 2003;38:314–32.

15. Waldorf HA, Kauvar ANB, Geronemus RG, Leffell DJ. Remote fire with the pulsed dye laser: Risk and prevention. *J Am Acad Dermatol* 1996;34: 503–6.

16. Batra S, Gupta R. Alcohol based surgical prep solution and the risk of fire in the operating room: A case report. *Patient Saf Surg* 2008;2:10.

17. Patel R, Chavda KD, Hukkeri S. Surgical field fire and skin burns caused by alcohol-based skin preparation. *J Emerg Trauma Shock* 2010;3:305.

Index

T - #0546 - 071024 - C640 - 280/210/28 - PB - 9780367778606 - Gloss Lamination